Manual of Natural Veterinary Medicine

SCIENCE *and* **TRADITION**

Manual of Natural Veterinary Medicine

Science and Tradition

SUSAN G. WYNN, DVM
Professional Member, American Herbalist Guild
IVAS Certified Veterinary Acupuncturist
Wynn Clinic for Therapeutic Alternatives
Marietta, Georgia

STEVE MARSDEN, DVM
Naturopathic Physician
Master of Science in Oriental Medicine
Licensed Acupuncturist
Diplomate of Chinese Herbology
Co-founder, Edmonton Holistic Veterinary Clinic,
The Natural Path Clinic, Edmonton, Alberta
Instructor, International Veterinary Acupuncture Society

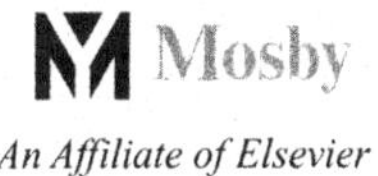

An Affiliate of Elsevier

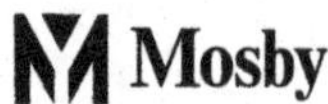

An Affiliate of Elsevier

11830 Westline Industrial Drive
St. Louis, Missouri 63146

MANUAL OF NATURAL VETERINARY MEDICINE
SCIENCE AND TRADITION

Notice

Veterinary medicine is an ever-changing field. Standard safety precautions must be followed, but as new research and clinical experience broaden our knowledge, changes in treatment and drug therapy may become necessary or appropriate. Readers are advised to check the most current product information provided by the manufacturer of each drug to be administered to verify the recommended dose, the method and duration of administration, and contraindications. It is the responsibility of the licensed prescriber, relying on experience and knowledge of the patient, to determine dosages and the best treatment for each individual patient. Neither the publisher nor the editor assumes any liability for any injury and/or damage to persons or property arising from this publication.

ISBN-13: 978–0–323–01354–3
ISBN-10: 0–323–01354–6

Acquisitions Editor: Elizabeth M. Fathman
Developmental Editor: Teri Merchant
Publishing Services Manager: Patricia Tannian
Project Manager: Sarah Wunderly
Book Design Manager: Gail Morey Hudson
Cover Designer: Teresa Breckwoldt

KI/QWF

Printed in the United States of America

Transferred to Digital Printing 2011

To my parents, teachers, and patients
for helping me explore what is best for the animals
SW

To my parents
Dave and **Shirley**
for always wanting the best for me

To my wife
Karen
for her selfless support and companionship
in every part of my life

To my "career cat"
Half Pint
for shepherding me this far

Most of all
to my patients
without whom I would have had nothing to offer

SM

Foreword

As a veterinary clinician and educator for the past 34 years, I have witnessed many changes in our profession. The practice of veterinary medicine has been altered by shifts toward a greater emphasis on companion animal medicine, wellness, and preventive medicine, by women in the profession, and by the increased influence of pharmaceutical companies, the pet food industry, and veterinary hospital corporations. I believe that the incorporation of complementary and alternative therapies into our current diagnostic and treatment strategies will have a profound effect on our profession. How we diagnose, treat, and view the pathophysiology of disease and the physiology of health will be greatly altered. I also believe that these new views will ultimately result in a more enlightened, effective, and personally rewarding approach to the practice of veterinary medicine.

Since we have become more globally connected, we have been exposed to medical paradigms of other cultures that challenge our traditional view of the body and health. The Internet has allowed veterinarians and clients rapid access to medical information and research. Armed with information from the Internet and other sources, clients often make demands on their veterinarians for alternative treatments, especially when the prognosis for their animal is poor by traditional standards. Client pressures force us to break out of our routines, explore other options, and grow in our practice of medicine. Interest in complementary and alternative medical approaches has also been generated by veterinarians with a strong desire to explore new ideas to enhance their practice of medicine and others who seek new markets for financial gain. Some people are more comfortable with change than others, and an often emotional dialogue occurs when new ideas are presented that may threaten the traditional paradigm. A lively interchange concerning complementary and alternative veterinary medicine has been observed in letters to the editor and opinions expressed in the *Journal of the American Veterinary Medical Association* in the past few years. Some veterinarians identify themselves as protectors of the tradition, and some see themselves as purveyors of change. Yet others are curious observers who find themselves somewhere in the middle. All types are essential to maintain some checks and balances on change yet allow us to continue to grow as a medical community. Our personal beliefs affect how we practice medicine, for example, the therapeutic tools we choose, the prognoses we give, and the analysis of our outcomes. Our goal is to practice evidence-based medicine as much as possible, yet at the same time our personal biases influence research funding, protocols and outcomes, and also the data we choose to publish or believe.

Interest in exploring complementary and alternative therapies continues to grow despite the controversy surrounding these new paradigms of medicine. Interest within the profession is evidenced by the formation of the American Holistic Veterinary Medical Association, other specialty groups, and an increasing number of continuing education and certification courses. Elective courses in complementary and alternative veterinary medicine are now offered in many veterinary colleges, and for the past 5 years I have coordinated such a course, which has received enthusiastic student support.

A positive change that has resulted from a more holistic view has been that veterinarians now consider the effect of nutrition, lifestyle, and environment on animal health and disease and explore new methods of disease prevention and treatment that enable the body's innate healing capabilities to function maximally. Both the increased interest in wellness and our frustrations with the limitations of current medical practices have led us to a desire to evaluate new paradigms in veterinary medicine.

The ancient Chinese physicians and veterinarians were well aware of the changes in the body's energy patterns that occurred before physical disease, and the initial focus of acupuncture was disease prevention. In veterinary medicine there has been particular interest in acupuncture, Chinese and other herbs, nutraceuticals, and homeopathy, which are all treatments that alter the energy system of the body to maximize its innate healing abilities.

As an easy-to-read, quick-reference handbook, the *Manual of Natural Veterinary Medicine: Science and Tradition* is ideal for busy veterinarians who are interested in applied acupuncture, homeopathy, and herbal medicine. Each chapter addresses common traditional diagnoses in a given organ system and makes specific, easy-to-follow suggestions for alternative therapeutic options. When possible, the research support for each option is noted so that veterinarians can refer quickly to the scientific basis of the therapy. This book represents a bridge between our traditional medicine and the traditional medicine of other cultures so that the best of both worlds can be fused to form an advanced system of integrative veterinary medicine.

Cheryl L. Chrisman, DVM, Ms, Eds

Diplomate of the American College of Veterinary Internal Medicine
Specialty of Neurology
Professor of Small Animal Clinical Sciences
Chief of the Neurology Service, Veterinary Teaching Hospital
College of Veterinary Medicine
University of Florida

This is the book that we have been waiting for, the next generation of the evolution of complementary and alternative veterinary medicine to truly *integrative*, combining the best of all therapies. Drs. Wynn and Marsden are the perfect writers to bring our ability to help animals to the next level.

Allen M. Schoen, DVM, MS

Affiliate Faculty, College of Veterinary Medicine
Colorado State University
Adjunct Professor, School of Veterinary Medicine
Tufts University

Preface

The major problems of medical practice are not greatly altered or diminished by the tremendous increase in our knowledge of the causes of specific diseases and our vast store of well tested remedies. What sort of art medicine is; to what extent the physician should let nature run its course; with what restraint or prudence the physician should apply general rules to particular cases; whether health is better served by the general practitioner treating the whole man or by a specialist treating a special organ; how the relation of the physician to his patient is itself a therapeutic factor and underlies the effectiveness of his skill in all other respects; to what extent mind and body interact both in the origin and in the cure of disease—these are the problems of medicine concerning which Hippocrates and Galen can converse with William Osler and Freud almost as contemporaries (Adler, M, 1992. Great Books: A Lexicon of Western Thought. McMillan Publishing Company, New York, p. 517).

In this book, we present natural medicine as a way to treat difficult problems in veterinary medicine.

The late acclaimed pharmacognosist Varro Tyler hypothesized that plant constituents were better candidates for drug research than novel molecules. His reasoning that nature had developed a limited number of molecules shared from the beginning by plants and animals suggests that natural molecules are a better "fit" and more worthy of investigation than novel molecules.

Natural medicine—herbs, nutrition, and nutraceuticals, and physical manipulation, including acupuncture and chiropractic—is not simply a consumer movement in revolt against the medical profession. Natural medicine, inasmuch as it explores the role of body responses and biologic response modifiers, represents the vanguard in medical care. As both a new development and a biologic necessity, natural medicine requires the attention of the veterinary profession now more than ever before.

We have tried in this book to present natural—or alternative, or complementary, or integrative—medicine in a way it has never been examined before. We agree with the many colleagues who call for evidence-based veterinary medicine, and we have striven to find supporting data—at least a foundation—for many alternatives now in use.

But let us face facts. There is *much* natural medicine in use in the United States and worldwide that has no scientific support. A great deal of this traditional medicine has years, decades, centuries, even millennia of use to tutor us on the appropriateness of these remedies for further study and controlled trial. We want to bring as much of this experience to light as possible for clinicians and researchers to scrutinize further. In fact, we may find that use of traditional medicines in traditional ways can be tested more efficiently than looking for single extracts that work in controlled trials, which might take much, much longer.

Knowledge is power. Herbs and food heal with great natural efficiency. Healing is a fundamental process, not some supernatural or mystical process. We can encourage the body to heal itself. What is so controversial about these truths?

This book is one we would gladly have bought ourselves, if it had been available. Since it was not available, we created it. It addresses the need of a growing number of practitioners for effective alternatives to conventional treatments that either do not work (despite research to the contrary), or have undesirable side effects. It is written for those who feel the debate about the ethical use of alternative medicine in veterinary practice cannot be settled by rationalization and dogma, but only by the acid test of clinical veterinary practice in the real world.

Why do we need to examine these remedies? Because in the twenty-first century, we can now diagnose a host of ills that we cannot treat. The real question is—why can they not be treated?

Susan G. Wynn
Steve Marsden

Acknowledgments

Previous texts on complementary and alternative veterinary medicine concentrated on describing the modalities themselves, but veterinarians have responded with the same question over and over: How do I treat this case? This book is a logical next step.

In my search for a coauthor, I knew I had to find someone with extensive education and practical experience in the traditions of alternative medicine. I found that author in Dr. Steve Marsden and, when asked to help, he unwittingly committed himself to a year of new lessons and continuing crises. I am grateful to him for his grace under pressure, and hope he will remain my friend after this collaboration!

I am also grateful to my patients and their people for their part in my practical research. My patients are, in the main, animals that have exhausted what conventional medicine has to offer, and their owners are special people who are willing to go the extra mile with their dogs and cats and give them more work, patience, and love than most owners will. I appreciate the owners' extra efforts in helping us to learn what works and what does not work.

I am especially grateful to our reviewers who applied their enormous knowledge and nearly nonexistent free time to improving this text. To Drs. Cheryl Chrisman, Greg Ogilvie, Tracey King, Frank Smith, William Thomas, Jane Armstrong, Rob Schick, Joni Freshman, and Rebecca Remillard—thank you! And to all my teachers who are experts in their areas and remain open to new ideas—Tony Buffington, Duncan Ferguson, Brenda Bonnett, Paul Pion, Julie Churchill, Robert Poppenga, Huisheng Xie, Janet Steiss, and Patricia Kyritsi Howell—thanks for your patience in answering my calls and e-mails! To all of you, and to our readers, be aware that any mistakes in this text are mine alone.

Teri Merchant, Sarah Wunderly, Linda Duncan, and Liz Fathman were constant in their gentle corrections and persuasive encouragement, and I thank them for helping us bring this project to fruition.

And finally, to my family and the animals with which they live: I am extremely grateful for the encouragement and experience you provided. If this book is considered any contribution to the practice of veterinary medicine, the credit is yours!

Susan G. Wynn

I would like to acknowledge the help of my wife, Karen Engel, in contributing some of the cases of this textbook, which show so clearly both the benefits of natural medicine and Karen's natural talent for it. I also want to thank Dr. Heiner Fruehauf, one of the great minds of twentieth-century Classical Chinese medicine, for showing me a world full of possibilities.

Steve Marsden

Introduction

This is a book about a new field: integrative medicine. It is an approach defined as "practising medicine in a way that selectively incorporates elements of complementary and alternative medicine into comprehensive treatment plans alongside solidly orthodox methods of diagnosis and treatment" (Rees, 2001).

There are veterinarians who believe that this approach dilutes and belittles the traditions embodied in such systems as traditional Chinese medicine or homeopathy and that the resulting "mongrel" cannot possibly be as holistic as the traditional systems. We disagree. We propose to bring potentially effective treatments to the larger part of the veterinary profession for further study, in order to help animals who suffer. Although truly competent use of Chinese herbs or homeopathy does require comprehensive knowledge of the system, we think you can use some of the tools presented here more easily than that.

This textbook is written to address a specific need of veterinarians for a clinical reference describing how to practice alternative medicine. It is designed so that a practitioner can look up the condition of concern and find descriptions of the alternative treatments that seem to hold the best chances for a favorable outcome. We hope that it will serve as a foundation from which to proceed, a life raft to help navigate a sea of alternatives to conventional therapies.

In no way can this book be considered the final word on alternative therapies. The reader should remember that we are presenting some of the best choices (in our view), but not the only choices. Rather, this text is best considered the initial word in a long discussion, which ideally will culminate in alternative treatments that can be recommended with confidence and certainty by veterinarians.

Although many of the therapies listed in this book were derived from a thorough review of the available literature on veterinary alternative medicine, we developed some of the therapies in our own practices. The goal of this text is to pass along to the reader not only those potential discoveries, but also the methods by which these effective therapies were identified. In this way, all practitioners can assist in the discovery and development of therapeutic alternatives to identify those that show the most promise for future investigation by clinical research.

Role of Evidence-Based Medicine in Alternative Therapy

Evidence-based medicine is the "gold standard" to which all of medicine should aspire. A large portion of this textbook is dedicated to reviewing currently available research supporting the use of alternative medicine in veterinary practice. Even so, by comparison to the amount of research supporting conventional veterinary practice, few such studies had been completed at the time this book was written.

"Alternatives" are by definition not well supported, so this collection represents dozens, hundreds, or even millions of opinions. Our choices were based on the clinical experiences of veterinarians and doctors using these therapies—both in modern times and from historical traditions. Not everyone agrees on the treatment choices for a given condition, but we felt that it was important to list the most popular in order to present those with the greatest potential for clinical use or further research.

It is possible that many alternative therapies, including those discussed in this book, do not work. The authors do not use the same therapies and do not always agree on the best treatment for a condition. This raises a red flag for many observers, suggesting that none of the recommendations work at all. We would suggest alternative explanations:

1. Alternative therapies represent such a huge number of new therapies that the choices are indeed wide ranging. Until the research is done, clinical practitioners offer the first line of investigation to identify effective therapies. There are those who point to the track record of alternative medicine research—in 7 years, the National Center for Complementary Medicine has funded millions of dollars of research and still has not clearly identified effective

therapies. We would counter that difficult problems require more effort—20 years of AIDS research has not yielded a cure or a vaccine, either.

2. Alternative therapies are usually applied "holistically," involving individualized attention to the patient's unique needs, as opposed to the practitioner's applying evidence-based recommendations for what works most of the time in a population of patients. Different patient populations may easily have variant characteristics, explaining why individual alternative practitioners obtain different results and have different treatment preferences. Fortunately, the paradigmatic recommendations for each condition in this book help the veterinarian individualize treatments above and beyond simply adding more drugs for more diseases. Perhaps this is one of alternative medicine's greatest future contributions to medicine in general.

This book is meant to serve as a jumping-off point for clinicians and researchers. We wonder how complementary and alternative veterinary medicine practitioners and skeptics alike can act as experts in every specialty. We cannot offer comprehensive expert advice on the treatment of every condition in every system—that is the purview of clinical and research specialists. The aim in providing systems-based information on treatment alternatives is to give clinicians ideas to apply in the difficult cases seen by us all, and researchers some ideas about promising areas for new discovery in their particular fields.

Infrastructure of This Book

Each condition or disease in this book is addressed in two main ways. The first is discussed under "Alternative Options with Conventional Bases." This section is roughly evidence-based, reflecting my (SW) interests and practice style. In other words, the most popular treatments are briefly analyzed with the extent and type of evidence that exists for their use. This section may also contain treatments that neither of us has used but that should be addressed because the treatments are in the popular literature or because they are being investigated by researchers.

The second heading, "Paradigmatic Options," addresses treatments that have centuries of use and that we may employ whether or not supporting data exist. Dr. Marsden summarizes these traditional practices clearly and comprehensively. Traditional systems of diagnosis and treatment lend themselves well to a problem-oriented approach, since traditional medicine did not make use of modern Western diagnostic methods. Some readers will notice that herbs or nutraceuticals are mentioned in both sections, which further underlines the fact that they can be analyzed in different ways.

In the "Authors' Choices" section, we note which treatments we find most useful and are first choices in our practices. In many cases we recommend Chinese herbs without specifying a particular formula. This should lead the reader to investigate the "Paradigmatic Section" to determine which formula is appropriate for a given patient.

Ultrastructure of This Book

Astute readers will note that the referencing in this book is occasionally inconsistent. We have tried to present the most useful supporting studies while avoiding those that would be difficult for readers to access. We have usually avoided foreign language journals, for instance, since most of our readers cannot obtain these papers or their translations. However, we may mention them without giving a reference, simply to alert the reader that a body of knowledge already exists on those treatments.

We relied heavily on a few sources that should be mentioned here. For single herb pharmacology and toxicity, the Natural Medicines Database and the Review of Natural Products were helpful. Our main source for pharmacology of Chinese herbs is Kee Chang Huang's book of the same name, but Kerry Bone's book *Clinical Applications of Ayurvedic and Chinese Herbs* was also helpful. For traditional Chinese (paradigmatic) options, class notes from the Chi Institute's herbal medicine course, as well as Dr. Huisheng Xie's text, were invaluable. Lectures and comments given by Drs. Heiner Fruehauf, Ri Hui Long, and Meng Ke Kou in the Department of Classical Chinese Medicine at the National College of Naturopathic Medicine embody lineages of Chinese medical thought that this book has inherited and now passes on to the reader. Yan Wu's book *Practical Therapeutics of Traditional Chinese Medicine* is the direct source of several Chinese herbal formulas that are now used across North America in veterinary practice. This text draws inspiration and recommendations for some of its Western herbal formulas from the major 19th- and early 20th-century works on Western herbalism, including *King's American Dispensatory, Cook's Physiomedical Dispensatory, Culpeper's Complete Herbal and English Physician, Boericke's Pocket Manual of Homeopathic Materia Medica,* and *John Christopher's School of Natural Healing.* Ironically, Chinese medicine aids in applying information in these texts to modern problems.

Conclusions

We are not neo-Luddites, espousing a return to nature for nature's sake. We are clinicians who strive to offer effective therapies to our patients. We eagerly await proof of the efficacy of any of these natural remedies; however, it could take centuries to fully investigate all of the nutraceutical and herbal therapies presented here. In the meantime, we believe that some offer relief for animals that are ill *now* and that find no relief with currently "proven" therapies.

As a social, political, and medical movement, alternative medicine has served two important purposes. First, it has brought, en masse, a number of potential new therapies to the testing fields, giving more hope to those with chronic diseases. More important, however, is that alternative medicine has served to refocus medical research (and, by extension, research funding) on clinical answers instead of molecular ones. We offer this as our contribution to clinical research: to hone the number of possibilities to a manageable number and to encourage clinical practitioners to be part of the research process.

Contents

Appendixes

PART ONE

Fundamentals of Chinese Medicine

1

The Cooking Pot Analogy

The Meat and Potatoes of Chinese Medicine

The *Nei Jing Su Wen,* the 2000-year-old seminal classic that gave rise to all of Chinese medicine, states that to be a master physician, one must master the use of metaphors as they apply to both medicine and the body. Perhaps the best metaphor for the inner workings of the body as understood by Chinese medicine is that of a cooking pot suspended over a fire (Fig. 1-1). Mastering the simple implications of this analogy eliminates much of the confusion surrounding Chinese medical physiology and pathophysiology and provides a solid foundation for understanding the Chinese medical treatments discussed in this textbook.

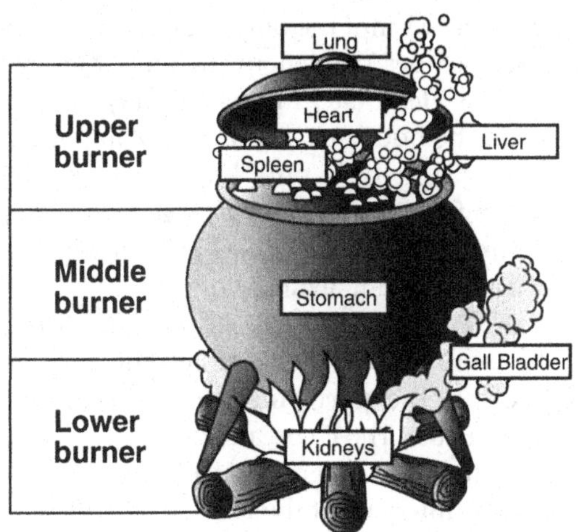

Fig. 1-1 The cooking pot analogy.

KIDNEYS AND BLADDER (LOWER JIAO)

The best place to begin a discussion of the cooking pot analogy is with the fire underneath the pot. In Chinese medicine this fire and the fuel that supplies it are the main contribution of the Kidneys. Just as the fire is located underneath the pot, the Kidneys are located in the lower third, or jiao, of the body. In animals this is equivalent to the caudal abdomen.

The "fuel" component of the Kidneys is Essence. Essence is Yin and Yang in a primordial, undifferentiated form. Although visualized as a sticky glutinous fluid, Essence contains the potential to become either Yin (Substance) or Yang (Energy).

Essence is made up of Prenatal and Postnatal types. Prenatal Essence is that part of Essence allotted to the organism before birth. It includes Heavenly Water, or what Western medicine recognizes as gonadal and developmental hormones. As in Western medicine, these can never be replaced by normal body function. Postnatal Essence is replenished throughout life, and is derived from the digestive and assimilative actions of the Spleen on food.

When necessary, the Yin and Yang stored in the Kidneys as Essence are mobilized and ignited to provide the fire under the pot, known as Source Qi or Yuan Qi. Yang acts upon Yin the way a spark ignites a puddle of fuel to create a virtual flame of life. Essence is not the only source of this Yang spark. The Heart also provides Yang energy to ignite Kidney Yin (see the section on the Heart later in this chapter).

All organs in the body are classified as Zang or Fu organs. The Zang organs store only pure life-giving substances and can never be too full. The Fu organs are generally hollow and interact directly with the environment, moving materials through the body and out again.

The Zang and Fu organs unite as a team to fulfill a vital body function. The more active, and therefore Yang, member of the duo is the Fu organ. The quiet, pure, and protected Zang organs are more Yin in nature. The Fu organ does the dirty work of fulfilling the body function assigned to each organ pair.

As the Yang counterpart of the Kidneys, the Bladder stores. It does the dirty work of storage by accumulating "turbid" liquid waste for elimination. However, the Bladder also is perceived to make a final attempt at absorbing useful body fluids from its lumen before the urine is voided. The Bladder's function in storage and absorption is powered directly by Kidney energy, and when Kidney Yang is deficient, incontinence and profuse urination of clear urine result. Kidney deficiency is thus an important aspect of many cases of urinary incontinence in dogs.

SPLEEN AND STOMACH (MIDDLE JIAO)

The major action of the Spleen and Stomach is to nourish the body by transforming food into usable energy. Not surprisingly, these organs that feed the rest of the body occupy the central region of the body, known as the middle jiao. The Spleen and Stomach equate to the cooking pot hung over the fire of the Kidneys.

The Stomach is the Yang counterpart of the Spleen. It is the organ in which the dirty work of digestion is initiated, the vessel in which cooking occurs. In the *Nei Jing* it is called the Sea of Grains. It equates with the mechanical process of digestion, including intestinal peristalsis and the secretion of digestive juices.

The Spleen is the part of digestion relating to assimilation. If Spleen function is inadequate, the products of the Stomach's efforts show up as watery, painless diarrhea with weight loss. The Spleen is thus akin to the wafting of vapors from the pot up to the underside of the cooking pot lid. It "raises the Clear," or pure, so that only the "Turbid," or impure, descends to form stool. The Clear substance that is raised is also termed Qi.

As well as extracting Qi from food, the Spleen extracts fluids. We can visualize this as fluid being drawn off from a stopcock at the bottom of the pot. All body fluids, including blood, synovial fluid, and cerebrospinal fluid, are manufactured by the Spleen. In addition, as mentioned in the section on the Kidneys and Bladder, some of these fluids drawn off by the Spleen are stored in the Kidneys as Postnatal Essence.

The Spleen is the source of not only healthful fluids, but also of pathologic fluids such as Dampness or Phlegm. Pathologic fluids are unusable by the body but accumulate as pollutants. They are considered a cause of many diseases from the Chinese veterinary medical perspective.

LUNGS AND LARGE INTESTINE

The major action of the Lungs and Large Intestine is to gather and descend. The Lungs are the lid of the cooking pot, gathering the Qi raised by the Spleen. In addition, they gather the Qi that is inhaled during respiration.

The Qi gathered by the Lungs is neither matter nor energy, but a mixture of both. Like a cloud of steam rising from a pot on the stove, it possesses the ability to both warm and moisten.

Qi is visualized to gather in the Lungs in the center of the chest, underneath the acupuncture point known appropriately as Dan Zhong (Chest Center; Conception Vessel 17). From here it descends to the Kidneys, where it is stored and used to augment the Source Qi. The deposit of Qi in the Kidneys is not passive, however. The Kidneys must have enough strength to reach up and actively grasp the descending Qi.

Not all of the Qi gathered in the chest descends to the Kidneys. Some also enters the pathways and meridians of the body, where it circulates in intimate association with the Blood. Qi and Blood both contain fluid (Yin) and energy (Yang). Of the two, however, Qi is relatively more Yang, and Blood relatively more Yin. The Yang energy of Qi drives the Blood, and together they circulate through the meridians and collaterals, restoring and balancing Yin and Yang in the farthest reaches of the body.

The farthest reach of Qi in the body is an insulating layer between the tissues and the external environment. This "shield" is made of Qi and is known as Wei Qi. It resists the invasion of pathogenic Xie Qi from the environment into the body and is partly akin to the lymphoid tissues that exist as a first line of defense along body surfaces and linings, especially in the upper airways. Wei Qi is also heavily concentrated along the dorsum. Aches and pains arising during inclement weather are considered to represent an attack upon the Wei Qi by invading pathogenic Qi, such as Dampness and Cold. Herbs considered to strengthen the Wei Qi layer frequently turn out to have immune-enhancing properties.

The Large Intestine is the Yang counterpart of the Lungs. It does the dirty work of gathering and descending, by moving ingesta from the Small Intestine back to the outside world. During this process an additional amount of pure fluid is absorbed from the Turbid contents of the lumen of the Large Intestine.

HEART AND SMALL INTESTINE

The Heart houses consciousness or Shen. The immediate survival of an organism hinges, above all else, on its ability to engage in an appropriate manner with its environment. The responsibility of the Heart for this power of discernment has earned it the title of Emperor of the body.

The Heart is nestled within the Lungs, which are filled with Clear pure Qi. Its location here gives it the clarity it needs to wisely rule the rest of the body. Consciousness is disturbed, and even lost, when this clarity is lost. In such a case the "orifices" of the Heart are said to be "obstructed." A common condition in which this occurs is grand mal seizures.

The Heart is a Yang organ, located in the clear and pristine upper reaches of the body. As such it is an important source of Yang energy for use by the Kidneys in the ignition of Yin to create Source Qi, which is also known as Ministerial Fire. However, as a source of Yang energy, the Heart has a tendency to become too hot (a condition known as Heart Fire). In this case the Kidneys reciprocate and help cool the Heart by using their fire to steam some of the Kidney Yin to the upper jiao, where it controls the Imperial Fire. A failure of the Heart and Kidneys to maintain this mutually controlling relationship causes the lower body to become too cold and the upper body to become too hot. A common clinical syndrome arising from this dynamic is chronic renal failure, in which the heat in the upper jiao creates uncontrollable thirst and the coldness of the lower jiao creates profuse watery urine.

Additional defense against pathologic Heart Fire is provided by the Pericardium. The Pericardium wraps around the Heart to nourish and cool it with Blood and Yin. It is the anteroom to the Imperial chamber and is the sole route of access to the Emperor. For this reason Pericardium channel points have historically been the main points to calm an agitated Heart, and are possibly more important in clinical practice than Heart channel points.

The Small Intestine is the Yang counterpart of the Heart. It does the dirty work of "prudent engagement with the environment" by discriminating the Clear from the Turbid in the chyme received from the Stomach. The pure water it extracts from the lumen is sent directly to the Bladder for final processing.

LIVER AND GALL BLADDER (MIDDLE JIAO)

The major action of the Liver is to initiate and facilitate movement through the regulation of circulation. The Liver guides or instructs Qi to maintain the smooth flow of Blood around the body. To do this, the Liver itself requires an adequate Blood supply. The Spleen is the source of all fluids, including Blood, and adequate Blood production by the Spleen ensures that the Liver has sufficient Blood to nourish the extremities.

The Yang counterpart of the Liver is the Gall Bladder. The Gall Bladder has an important influence on the smooth movement of the limbs just as the Liver has an important influence on the smooth movement of Qi and Blood. This role of the Gall Bladder is discussed more thoroughly in the following section on the Triple Burner.

TRIPLE BURNER (TRAVERSES ALL THREE JIAO)

The major action of the Triple Burner is to facilitate the activity of all other organs. The Triple Burner has no Western organ equivalent but is perceived to be a sort of internal axis or corridor that provides a conduit for the movement of Qi and fluids up and down the body. Within the Triple Burner, Lung Qi descends to the Kidneys, taking with it water and fluids obtained from the Spleen and digestive tract. Meanwhile, the Source Qi moves up from the Kidneys to supply the various organs of the body. The Triple Burner is therefore the intermediary between the rest of the body and the Source Qi of the Kidneys. Without the "stovepipe" properties of the Triple Burner, no organs could access the Ministerial Fire. The Triple Burner is thus somewhat equivalent to the stove that houses the fire and on which the cooking pot rests.

The Yin counterpart of the Triple Burner is the Pericardium. By wrapping itself around the Heart, the Pericardium is the intermediary between the power of the Emperor and the outside world.

The Pericardium channel traverses all three jiao, just like the Triple Burner. This results in the therapeutic usefulness of Nei Guan (Pericardium 6) in disorders in which Qi is not descending properly from the upper to the middle and lower burners. Common clinical examples are asthma and vomiting.

Like the Pericardium, the Gall Bladder is closely related to the Triple Burner. Both are classified as having a Shao Yang energetic and thus have similar functions. In particular, the Gall Bladder facilitates use of Source Qi for external body movement just as the Triple Burner allows the use of Source Qi by internal organs. It is said that if the Gall Bladder is not in harmony, the limbs cannot move.

Whereas the Triple Burner provides an internal axis or corridor for movement of Qi and fluids, the Gall Bladder provides an external axis for movement of the fore and hind limbs. This is the reason the Gall Bladder channel runs up the middle of the leg, trunk, head, and neck—to provide a framework on which the rest of the body is hung.

The Gall Bladder teams with the Triple Burner to govern the Dai Mai, or Girdling Vessel. This vessel provides a structural basis for movement by resisting lordosis and gathering the belly to the spine. It provides a basis for erect stature, whether in animals or in humans. Obstruction of the Dai Mai seems to be a leading cause of degenerative myelopathy in dogs because it squeezes off the flow of Qi that passes beneath it to the legs.

INTRODUCTION TO PATHOPHYSIOLOGY: WHAT CAN GO WRONG WITH THE COOKING POT

Kidneys

A deficiency of Kidney Essence or Yin is akin to an inadequate wood supply. As fuel dwindles slowly over the life span of an organism, the flame of the Source Qi flickers but cannot be strengthened because of a lack of Kidney Yang. Unless the situation is rectified, life will soon be extinguished. The dying fire means that the Spleen, or cooking pot, cannot properly do its job of generating fuel for the Kidneys. This leads to an acceleration of the decline, manifested as increasing weakness of the low back, knees, and pulse. The Spleen also cannot generate Blood, leading to tongue pallor and anemia. The accumulation of Dampness with the decline in Spleen function leads to visible tongue swelling.

The coldness of the dying flame is also felt directly. The Bladder does not receive the Yang needed to fulfill its role of absorbing Clear fluids back in the body and eliminating only Turbid waste fluids. In addition, a decline in Kidney Qi and Yang prevents Kidney Yin from becoming "steamed up" to the point at which it can condense, moisten, and cool the upper jiao. Increased thirst and profuse urination result and, together with chilliness, are the hallmarks of kidney failure in both Chinese and Western medicine.

Even before the flame dies, fuel is being consumed, resulting in a steadily increasing ratio of flame to fuel if the fuel is not replaced by the Spleen's generation of Postnatal Essence. Relatively deficient fuel, or Yin, produces relative signs of Heat. This is known as Empty Heat and is associated with a number of symptoms including heat intolerance, eye redness, a red tongue, a rapid pulse, and even a flaring of Yang energy upward as counterbalancing Yin is lost. Disorders in small animals characteristically associated with Empty Heat include some cases of idiopathic vestibular syndrome, renal failure, epilepsy, and cognitive deficiency. Other signs of dwindling Yin include a thin pulse, dry tongue, loss of weight, and thirst. Any excessive or pathological Heat in the body may dry up Yin reserves, making all such disorders appear Yin deficient in their late stages. Yin deficiency is commonly seen in advanced hyperthyroidism and diabetes mellitus.

Yin deficiency leads to deficiencies of particular fluids, not just fluid in general. Hormones are considered a form of Yin, but are a component of Prenatal Essence and cannot be replaced when lost. Hormone-responsive urinary incontinence is thus a form of Yin deficiency. Similarly, the Blood supply depends on adequate reserves of Kidney Yin. This is because the production of Blood is sacrificed in favor of more valuable Kidney Yin and Essence during Yin deficiency. Liver Blood deficiency can thus arise from Kidney Yin deficiency and is often a concern in older animals.

Spleen and Stomach

The function of the Stomach depends largely on the relative amount of Heat to which its contents are exposed. If it is too hot, its contents dry out and congeal, leading to an obstructive mass that blocks the descent of Stomach Qi and results in vomiting. Signs of Heat include an effort by the body to "restock the pot," thus lowering the relative amount of Heat to which its contents are exposed. Appetite and thirst increase. The direct access of the cooking pot contents to the upper jiao produces an excess Heat in the upper body, which agitates the Heart to produce mania and excitability. The Lung similarly dries out, leading to a dry cough and hemoptysis. The lack of moisture available in the Stomach to be passed on to the Large Intestine produces constipation.

Problems exist when the fire is too low under the Stomach. The fire may be relatively too low, because of too much food in the vessel, or truly low, because of a Spleen and Kidney Yang deficiency. The consequences are a generation of Dampness or Phlegm somewhat akin to surface scum forming on the contents of a cooking pot. These fluids are unusable by the body and represent a pathogen accumulation. They vary in tenacity from relatively fluid Dampness to relatively tenacious Phlegm.

Some of the pathogenic fluids may stay in the Stomach, resulting in the vomiting of a tenacious, slimy, clear mucus. The rebelling of Stomach Qi upward often carries some Phlegm with it into the normally clear and pristine upper jiao. Here it obscures the "vision" of the Heart, leading to disorders of consciousness, epilepsy, and idiopathic vestibular disease. If the Phlegm accumulates in the Lungs instead of around the Heart, pneumonia and asthma result.

Other pathogenic fluids enter the general circulation along the paths of normal fluid movement and accumulate anywhere normal moisture goes. They particularly follow the downward flow of gravity and descending Lung Qi to accumulate in the lower body. If they accumulate in the Large Intestine, colitis results. If they accumulate in the Bladder, cystitis results. If they accumulate in the legs, degenerative myelopathy results. The pathway to the lower body is the Triple Burner, and if pathogenic fluids accumulate in the Triple Burner, feline hyperthyroidism results.

Symptoms of Dampness and Phlegm accumulation are usually obvious. Mucus, catarrh, and phlegm may be present in discharges from virtually any mucous membrane. The patient may have a greasy coat and accumulations of earwax or debris. Anal glands become distended and uncomfortable. The tongue becomes wet and swollen, and the pulses are slippery. The saliva may be copious or tenacious.

Once Dampness and Phlegm accumulate anywhere in the body, they eventually turn to Phlegm Heat or Damp Heat. Exact pathologic mechanisms are seldom discussed in resources concerning traditional Chinese medicine (TCM), but we may envision that large accumulations "gum up the works." In other words, they interfere with normal Qi and Blood flow, generating Heat as a result of a sort of friction. This is the chief means by which pathogenic Heat is created in animal bodies.

Pathogenic Heat agitates the hot Yang organs of the body, particularly the Liver and Heart, to produce excitability, irritability, and aggression. Heat agitates the Blood to produce intense itch and hemorrhagic tendencies. The patient exhibits heat intolerance. The connection between accumulation of moisture and Heat generation is reflected in appetite and thirst patterns, in that one of the two is usually elevated and one depressed. Encounters with Damp Heat are exceedingly common in veterinary practice, since Damp Heat produces such disorders as allergic dermatitis, diabetes mellitus, and feline hyperthyroidism.

The Spleen stores fluids and so falls prey to Dampness accumulation just as many other organs do. In addition, the Spleen exhibits pathologic signs distinct from those of the Stomach.

One such disorder is a failure by the Spleen and Stomach to generate Qi to be raised up to the Lung. Because the Lung is the immediate "end user" of this Qi, signs of Spleen Qi deficiency are essentially signs of Lung Qi deficiency, namely, shortness of breath, pallor, weakness, a weak voice, and a weak pulse.

Sometimes Qi is generated but not raised, leading to Qi collapse. Indications of sinking Spleen Qi include not only the usual signs of Spleen Qi deficiency, but also urinary incontinence, pelvic organ prolapse, and lower abdominal bloating. Similarly, a failure to raise the Pure results in watery, painless diarrhea, usually equated with small bowel diarrhea in conventional medicine. An example of the loss of the "containing" power of the Spleen on the Blood is a chronic tendency to pale, watery hemorrhage.

When the Spleen fails in its function to generate fluids, Liver Blood deficiency commonly results. Symptoms include fear aggression, dry coat, powdery dander, tendency to muscle spasms, irritability, depression, failure of hair to grow back after surgery, alopecia without apparent cause, and corneal dryness. Examples of Liver Blood deficiency are keratoconjunctivitis sicca (KCS) and numerous skin conditions. A failure by the Spleen to generate fluids may also lead to Kidney Essence deficiency, eventually resulting in chronic renal failure, as discussed previously.

Chinese medicine also considers fluid generated by the Spleen to be what gives muscles their form. Emaciation and wasting thus arise from Spleen deficiency but can also be caused by a pathogenic Heat that consumes fluids or Yin in general. Thus Yin deficiency and Spleen Qi deficiency are the two main differential diagnoses for chronic weight loss in humans or animals.

Lung and Large Intestine

The Lung is where Qi, a fine mist, is gathered. For mist to persist, a fine balance in temperature is required. Too cold, and the mist congeals into water and Phlegm that obstruct the Lungs and interfere with the downward descent of Lung Qi. The warmth of the Kidney fire has a major impact on the warmth of the Lungs, and Kidney Yang deficiency is thus a major cause of asthmatic breathing in cats. Symptoms of water accumulation in the upper jiao include a moist rattling cough, regurgitation of food and water, vomiting of water after drinking, and cataracts. When Phlegm obstructs the orifices of the Heart, epilepsy and Shen disturbances occur. Excess Heat also damages the Lung Qi. When the Lungs are too hot the Qi evaporates and the Lungs dry out, leading to a dry cough with tenacious, stringy mucus and thirst.

Problems arise when too much or too little Lung Qi is gathered in the chest. Lung Qi deficiency arises from a failure of the Spleen to generate and raise adequate Qi, producing shortness of breath reminiscent of asthma. Asthma can also arise from a lack of Kidney Qi reserves. When the Lungs descend Qi to the Kidneys for storage, the Kidneys are supposed to reach up and grasp it. If Kidney Qi is deficient, this grasping action does not occur, causing Qi to accumulate in the Lungs and asthma to result.

If Lung Qi is either deficient or fails to disperse, the Wei Qi weakens. Deficient Wei Qi leaves the organism vulnerable to upper respiratory infections and to pathogenic Qi invasion of both the channels and the defensive Tai Yang area of the body, which is the dorsum. The result is stiffness, back pain, and hind-limb weakness in older animals and a tendency to facial edema and edema of the superficial layers of the body in patients exposed to pathogenic Wind-Damp. When Large Intestine Qi fails to descend, constipation can result.

Heart

Although it is the Emperor of the body, the Heart is at the mercy of the other organs in the body it oversees. This is why the Heart is the only organ that has another organ, the Pericardium, dedicated to serving as its buffer with the rest of the world. The Heart requires clarity to carry out its function as a judicious interface with the environment. Accumulations of Phlegm in the upper jiao from pathologic conditions in the Lung or Stomach lead to clouded mentation, epilepsy, fear, anxiety, aggression, and other behavioral disturbances. As mentioned previously, because the Heart is a Yang organ, it is agitated by any accumulation of Heat in the body. Symptoms of this include cognitive disorders, aggression, anxiety, and fear. The Heart also depends on an adequate Blood supply from the Spleen to provide the Yin force that will balance and hold its content of Yang energy, which in the Heart is Shen, or consciousness. Blood deficiency leads to Heart agitation and cognitive disorders.

The only other major function of the Heart is to provide the initial propelling force for Blood and Qi to leave the place where they have gathered in the chest and enter the general circulation via the channels and meridians. When the Heart fails in this duty, Heart Qi and Blood stasis result, producing congestive heart failure and a rapid, erratic pulse.

Liver and Gall Bladder

The Liver and Gall Bladder together regulate movement. True to its Shao Yang nature, the Gall Bladder uses the Source Qi of the

Kidneys to activate movement. A deficiency in Gall Bladder function is most commonly manifest in small animals as paralysis. The Liver governs the smooth movement of Qi within the channels. When this function is disturbed, Qi stagnation occurs, manifested as distending and shooting pains that develop suddenly anywhere in the body or as pain that is lessened by motion. Qi stagnation is a major cause of lameness without apparent structural cause; it also produces anxiety disorders, irritability, depression, dysphagia, and a tense or wiry pulse.

When Liver Qi stagnates, it also invades adjacent organs in the middle jiao, the Stomach and Spleen. Invasion of the Stomach leads to vomiting, poor appetite, and what is generally recognized as gastritis caused by inflammatory bowel disease. When Liver Qi invades the Spleen, diarrhea, poor appetite, and irritable bowel syndromes ensue.

Tendency to Liver Qi stagnation is aggravated by Blood deficiency, which in turn often arises from Spleen dysfunction. To a lesser extent, Kidney Yin and Essence deficiency may also cause Blood deficiency. Other signs of Blood deficiency that have not already been mentioned include muscle spasm and pain. The tendons depend on an adequate Blood supply to remain limber and relaxed; a deficiency in Blood and Yin causes tendons to dry out, producing spasms.

The smooth movement of Qi produces the smooth movement of Blood, and Qi stagnation leads to Blood stasis. Symptoms of Blood stasis include organomegaly, manifested as liver and spleen tumors; stabbing localized persistent pain, manifested as lameness; and focal blood accumulations, manifested as many tumors. Adequate circulation also ensures that adequate Blood is delivered to the extremities. Blood deficiency hampers this, producing lesions of peripheral dryness and malnourishment, including dry skin, powdery dander, corneal dryness, and a loss of hair or its failure to regrow. Common diseases arising from this Blood deficiency are KCS and allergic dermatitis.

Conclusions

The simple cooking pot model enables the practitioner to grasp much of TCM physiology and pathophysiology. Some trends become obvious as the model is contemplated, such as that multiple pathophysiologic mechanisms may be responsible for a given disease. To eliminate confusion in deciding which pathogenic mechanism is operative, we address the different diseases in detail throughout the text. The chief signs and symptoms that suggest the presence of one pathologic dynamic over another are included.

A particular organ failure in Chinese medicine may have multiple effects. A tendency to a weakness in one organ provides the basis for a variety of diseases over the lifetime of the patient. This has led some practitioners to claim that there are really no acute diseases, just multiple manifestations of one core imbalance. The common relationship between different disorders appears strong enough to have predictive value; for example, a feline prone to other Damp Heat syndromes arising from Spleen and Stomach Qi deficiency may be expected to eventually manifest feline hyperthyroidism. These associations may provide fodder for research toward better understanding and prevention of the conditions.

The sharing of a common root provides a basis for prevention of diseases on a wide scale for a given patient. Diet and lifestyle measures can be used early to counter the patient's single core tendency to imbalance. Even when causes of individual diseases are not known from a Western perspective, knowledge of the patient's tendencies to imbalance allows the veterinarian to practice at the highest possible level, that of preventing illness by providing causes of health.

2

Chinese Medicine as a Basis for an Alternative Medical Approach

Most medical systems in history were holistic and made heavy use of the metaphoric approach, until tools were developed that allowed medical science to understand the physical world in direct terms. Greek, Ayurvedic, Chinese, and early Western herbal traditions all offered a similar metaphoric perspective on medicine, disease, and health. However, Chinese medicine may hold an advantage over the use of other systems, since it is currently accessible through an abundance of high-quality educational resources. Although most works on Chinese medicine remain to be translated, enough key works exist in English to allow Western practitioners to effectively use the tools and techniques of Chinese medicine.

Traditional systems of medicine help transcend existing limits of scientific knowledge for difficult diseases, increasing therapeutic options when conventional medicine fails. This is especially true for Chinese medicine, given the multiple modalities this single field encompasses. Regardless of which modality is used, the practitioner begins by viewing the problem in the metaphoric terms offered by Chinese medical models of physiology and pathology. The practitioner uses these models to define the patient's condition and the metaphoric requirements of a feasible solution. A Chinese medical assessment of a patient may provide a blueprint for successful treatment. The use of an appropriate model to solve seemingly unanswerable problems is also known as the principle of approximate knowledge. Once the general features of a feasible solution have been determined using metaphoric thinking, available treatment options are assessed to see which are appropriate in terms of these metaphoric requirements.

An advantage of Chinese medicine is that clues to appropriate preventive measures may be obtained by analysis of the herbs and acupuncture points that were successfully used in the patient. In both Chinese and modern Western medicine, these preventive measures generally revolve around appropriate diets, relationships, and lifestyles. Thus, although the causes of certain diseases from the conventional perspective may not be known, the causes of health for a given patient according to his or her response to Chinese medicine may be abundantly clear.

The belief that an inappropriate lifestyle underlies all chronic illness seems to be the one tenet on which all medical systems, historical and present, can agree. Naturopathic medicine has defined itself according to this core belief and maintains that ideal living conditions not only prevent disorders, but also resolve them. Zoo medicine practitioners test and confirm these principles daily, having to rely on an ideal diet and physical environment as the main method of maintaining health in animal collections. Both Chinese and Western medicine agree that optimum factors such as diet, occupation, approach to interpersonal relationships, and level of physical activity are the foremost priorities in promoting health and preventing disease. In Western medicine, optimum lifestyle choices are determined by genetic and social factors. In Chinese medicine, appropriate lifestyle and diet are also dictated by the patient's environmental surroundings.

Throughout this chapter and the rest of the book, liberal use is made of the term "energetic." This term refers to the metaphoric impact of a treatment or influence, as determined by its effect in Chinese medical terms. Thus a thyroidectomy in a hyperthyroid cat would have a cooling energetic, since from a Chinese medical perspective it results in elimination of Heat signs (rapid pulse, aversion to heat, increased appetite, thirst). Not only herbs and acupuncture points, but any phenomena can be viewed in Chinese medical terms and thus can be assigned a particular energetic.

Throughout the Chinese medical sections of the text, readers will note that some terms are capitalized while seemingly related terms are not. For example, a patient may be described as appearing "hot," whereas at other times they will be suffering from Heat. The former is a descriptive term while the latter is a particular concept in Chinese medicine with specific signs and causes. As a general rule, this principle is followed throughout this text. Wherever terms are merely used descriptively they appear in lower case and the term is capitalized when it has specific implications and is being used to describe a Chinese medical diagnosis, organ, substance, or type of pathogenic Qi.

MEDICAL HISTORY

Understanding which strategies to employ in the treatment and prevention of a disorder using Chinese medical principles begins, as it does in conventional medicine, with obtaining a medical history. The history is usually much more detailed than that typically obtained in practice of conventional medicine, however. Following are some areas of inquiry that I (SM) find useful, together with some possible interpretations of some common answers in Chinese medical terms.

History of Present Illness

- Characterize the chief complaint as clearly as possible in terms of apparent causes.
  - Trauma: Examples are the absolute ruling out of trauma as a cause of a central nervous system (CNS) disturbance, or the linking of a cat's inappropriate urination to seeming acts of anxiety related to another animal.
  - Food sensitivities: Obvious relationships of particular foods and ingredients to the appearance of certain signs should be noted. The energetic of these foods might then be evaluated in metaphoric Chinese medical terms to shed light on the energetic that is probably at work in the patient. For example, if rich, oily foods or supplements aggravate the appearance of skin lesions, it suggests the lesions are Damp in nature and possibly due to a failure of the digestion or Spleen Qi to adequately "transform" these foods or supplements into a usable substance. Some perspectives of the energetic nature of various foods are listed in Appendix B.

- Drug effects: Drugs and pharmaceuticals also have an energetic that allows them to be combined with various herbal formulas to further the energetic goals of that formula. This energetic also gives drugs and vaccines the ability to cause disease. In homeopathy, the disease induced by the administration of a vaccine is termed "vaccinosis." In Chinese medicine, however, the apparent linking of signs to the administration of a particular drug or vaccine usually implies that the drug or vaccine merely aggravated latent tendencies toward illness in the organism. This tendency is usually of the same energetic nature as the drug itself. Cooling drugs such as antibiotics may thus aggravate latent tendencies to coldness in an organism. Similarly, infectious organisms are considered environmental toxins in Chinese medicine, and the injection of a vaccine into a latently toxic patient seems to elicit the sudden development of Toxic Heat.

- Critical details: The practitioner should be able to visualize clearly the clinical behavior of the animal based on the description of symptoms in the history. For example, if the complaint is of diarrhea, the practitioner should obtain a detailed description of the appearance of the stool along with an accurate idea of the times bowel movements are passed and the level of ease or discomfort.
- Modalities: A special emphasis is based on "modalities" of the complaint, such as what makes the problem better or worse, and the impact of weather, activities of daily living, and even time of day of the complaint.
  - Response to weather is a direct indicator of the nature of the patient's physiology, with Damp, Dry, and Hot conditions becoming worse on damp, hot, and dry days, respectively.
  - Conditions improved by motion reflect the likelihood that stasis exists in the circulation of Qi and Blood.
  - Certain phases of the day are dominated by a particular energetic. As the sun rises, for example, the activity of most animals increases. The energetic of dawn is thus that of rising energy, or Yang. In Chinese medicine the living organism is not considered to be a closed system, invulnerable to these exterior conditions or energetics.

Rather, it is an open system and is influenced by its environment. If its symptoms are born of the same energetic as the environment, they will become amplified as the environment cycles through that energetic over the course of each day. Thus conditions of rising Yang energy may be aggravated as the Yang energy of the environment increases during the early morning hours. Another impact of time of day is elicited when the organism is out of phase with its environment. Rather than resonating too strongly with the energy of that phase of the day, the body is completely out of step with it. Thus patients deficient in Yang energy will not rise as the day around them rises but will sleep late. Patients with too much Heat will not cool off as the day around them withdraws into night but will remain agitated and restless.

- Current therapy and doses of all drugs, herbs, and supplements
  - Avoid prescribing products that may have energetic or pharmacologic interactions or redundancy with current medications.
  - Previous therapies: Special attention should be given to previous treatments that have been very effective.
  - Supplements: Therapies should be chosen that have the same benefit in terms of Chinese medicine but go even further. For example, if an animal responds well to essential fatty acid supplementation for skin problems, it is more likely to be Blood deficient and to benefit from Blood tonic herbs. If the benefit of Blood tonic herbs is only partial, the real problem may be a Qi deficiency that is causing a secondary Blood deficiency.
  - Acupuncture points: If possible, obtain a list of acupuncture points that have been helpful.
    - ◊ Acupuncture points, like herbs and drugs, have a particular effect that, when correctly interpreted, can shed light on the underlying problem. Appendix E of this text gives the energetic of some of the major acupuncture points.
  - Drugs: Conventional medicines have their own energetics, and response to a particular therapy may

suggest the presence in the body of a particular dynamic. Examples of this are:

◊ Intravenous fluids are commonly indicated in cases of Yin deficiency and can help in their rapid correction.
◊ Nonsteroidal antiinflammatory drugs appear to clear excess Yang pathogens, most notably Damp Heat. Some, such as aspirin, also have moving properties.
◊ Antibiotics also frequently clear Damp Heat.
◊ Analgesic and antispasmodic drugs often help move stagnant Qi and Blood.
◊ Diuretics drain Damp and have a mild Heat-clearing effect. They can facilitate the movement of Qi and Blood by removing obstructing Dampness.

Past Medical History

- Obtain descriptions of all conditions that have occurred in the past along with their effective treatments and antecedent events. In other words, the same information gathered for the present illness should be gathered for previous illnesses.
- The nature of previous illnesses often sheds light on the current illness. The current illness may represent the progression of a previously untreated energetic dynamic reflected in earlier diseases, or may reflect the same dynamic as was present in earlier diseases.

Review of Systems

- Gastrointestinal
  - Obtain a thorough description of any significant or recurring episodes of vomiting, nausea, diarrhea, constipation, or gas.
    ◊ Malodorous flatus is often indicative of a Damp-Heat condition.
    ◊ Constipation is a result of several different possible dynamics, including Blood deficiency and Qi stagnation.
    ◊ Slimy vomitus suggests the obstruction of the Stomach by Phlegm, causing Stomach Qi to rebel upward.
    ◊ Diarrhea may be a form of colitis, which usually arises from Damp Heat, or small bowel diarrhea, which is more characteristic of Spleen Qi deficiency.
    ◊ Mucus in the stool suggests Dampness.

- Respiratory
  - Ascertain the details of any coughing, abnormal breathing, poor stamina, and the nature of any limitations on physical activity.
    - ◊ Apparent poor stamina may be caused by Qi deficiency, but also by a painful lesion, a marked degree of stiffness, or a high residual level of Heat in the body that makes further heat generated by exercise intolerable.
    - ◊ Wet or productive coughs imply Phlegm.
    - ◊ Difficult expectoration implies the presence of Phlegm congealed by dryness.
    - ◊ Shortness of breath may suggest Qi deficiency.
- Musculoskeletal
  - Obtain detailed information on any episodes of stiffness, soreness, and places that the animal resents being touched.
    - ◊ Symptoms that improve with movement imply that Qi or Blood stasis plays a role.
    - ◊ Pain, turgor, flaccidity, warmth, or coolness at sites associated with known acupuncture points suggests those points may be useful in treating the current ailment and that the energetics of the point can be helpful in obtaining a Chinese medical diagnosis. For example, if BL 17, the Blood association point, feels unusually swollen or warm relative to the surrounding area, a role of Blood in symptom development should be considered, such as Blood deficiency or Blood stasis.
    - ◊ Well-localized painful areas suggest Blood stasis. Deformities imply Blood stasis, possibly mingled with a Phlegm accumulation.
    - ◊ Lower lumbar stiffness that does not substantially resolve upon chiropractic adjustment suggests an underlying causative pattern perpetuating the lack of resilience. This pattern requires appropriate treatment with herbs and acupuncture.
- Integument
  - Obtain a detailed description of rashes, dryness, itching, and discharges of the skin. Take note of the meridians on which these lesions occur.

- ◊ Fine powdery dander suggests Blood deficiency.
- ◊ Large discolored flakes, even if dry, are associated with Dampness.
- ◊ Inguinal lesions are associated with the Liver, axillary lesions with the Pericardium, and ear lesions with the Gall Bladder.
- ◊ Extreme itch suggests extreme Heat.
- ◊ Purulent destructive skin lesions suggest Damp Heat that has "composted" to Toxic Heat.
- ◊ Even mild skin lesions in cats suggest an underlying Toxic Heat.
- ◊ Watery, moist, greasy, or malodorous skin discharges suggest Dampness.

- ■ Urologic
  - ○ Obtain a detailed description of any episodes of cystitis or urinary incontinence. Also note the color, volume, and odor of the urine, and the necessity for elimination during the night.
    - ◊ Tenesmus during urination or defecation implies the presence of Dampness in the Bladder and Large Intestine, respectively.
    - ◊ Incontinence after exertion implies a Qi or Yin deficiency.
    - ◊ Heat conditions often produce dark urine. Kidney Yang deficiency and Damp Heat both can produce polydipsia, which in turn leads to profuse clear urination.
    - ◊ Increased need for urination during the night implies a possible Kidney deficiency.
- ■ HEENT (head, ears, eyes, nose, throat)
  - ○ Inquire about loss of hearing or vision, the nature of infections or discharges from the eyes, nose, and ears, tendencies toward sneezing or snoring, and the presence of gum or dental disease and halitosis.
    - ◊ Hearing loss may stem from Kidney deficiency and from "catarrhal" deafness, in which closure of the Eustachian tubes inhibits equalization of the middle ear, thus restricting movement of the tympanum.
    - ◊ External eye disorders are often associated with the Liver and the Gall Bladder. Dryness implies Liver or Kidney Yin deficiency. Blepharitis implies

accumulation of Dampness in the Gall Bladder channel. Heat produces yellow discharges. Mucoid discharges imply Dampness.
        - ◊ Dampness can produce an excessive tendency to snore or to reverse sneezing.
        - ◊ Halitosis, when not clearly referable to accumulations of tartar, may suggest a pathologic condition in the Stomach or the accumulation of Damp Heat.
        - ◊ Stomatitis may reflect a Damp-Heat accumulation. While Stomach Yin deficiency is very commonly a cause for stomatitis in people, I (SM) have not found it to be so for animals.
- ▪ General physical signs
    - ○ Obtain owner ratings of the patient's appetite and thirst levels and apparent preferences for certain temperatures. Temperature sensations of various parts of the body reported by the owner should also be recorded. Confirm the basis for the owner's assessment of appetite, thirst, and temperature preferences. Regarding appetite and thirst:
        - ◊ Increases in one and decreases in the other suggest Damp Heat.
        - ◊ Increases in both suggest a true Heat condition leading to Dryness.
        - ◊ Poor appetite in the absence of Dampness suggests Qi deficiency.
        - ◊ Cool-seeking animals prefer to lie on tile floors or table-tops or in basements, bathtubs, shade, or holes dug in the yard. They usually have to leave beds after lying on them for a short while at night.
        - ◊ Heat-seeking animals seek out sunshine, computer or TV surfaces, and heat registers.
        - ◊ Coldness of paws in relation to the rest of the animal suggests Qi stagnation.
        - ◊ Damp Heat and Yin deficiency can produce Heat signs that are worse at night.
        - ◊ Qi and Yang deficiencies are associated with heat-seeking behavior.
- ▪ Sleep
    - ○ Inquire whether sleep is particularly deep or fitful, and about the frequency of dreaming.

        - ◊ Deep sleep suggests Dampness accumulations that contribute to decreased alertness.
        - ◊ Fitful sleep is associated with Heat conditions, especially Yin deficiency.
        - ◊ Blood deficiency produces dream-filled sleep.
        - ◊ Animals that are slow to rise in the morning are often Qi or Yang deficient.
- ▪ Mental and emotional signs
    - ○ Ask the owner to describe the animal's personality and its behavior in different situations. These situations include encounters with strange animals or people, as well as interactions with other people and animals in the household. Do not accept an interpretation of the animal's behavior by the owner, but rather seek to visualize and interpret the behavior for yourself.
        - ◊ When the Liver is affected, the patient's mood may be abruptly changeable, stuck in one emotion, or excessively subdued. The most common mannerisms exhibited by the animal that are associated with pathologic conditions in the Liver are anxiety and aggression. Stress-related changes in digestive function may be another indication of such conditions.
        - ◊ Heat signs are fully developed when the Fire element or Heart is in disarray. These include restlessness, insomnia, delirium, mental agitation, anger, and excessive joy.
        - ◊ Blood-deficient animals often exhibit fear aggression.

Although these symptomatic associations seem clear and perhaps intuitive, the skill of the practitioner is challenged when the animal has only a few presenting symptoms or a mix of seemingly conflicting symptoms (e.g., Heat and Cold, Dampness and Dryness). Such instances are frequently encountered, and it is at this point that the practitioner should rely heavily on the pulse and tongue features to decide which energetics predominate. Often the signs, pulse, and tongue will each offer a slightly different perspective on the patient, and when woven together, provide a complete assessment.

PHYSICAL EXAMINATION

The first priority in the practice of alternative veterinary medicine remains the establishment of a conventional medical diagnosis, or at least a list of differentials. Conventional medical interventions that are both safe and effective should not be overlooked in the eagerness to provide alternative treatment.

Establishment of a conventional medical diagnosis also provides a foundation for retrospective studies to determine which alternative treatments are helpful in which disorders. Successful treatments, when investigated, can improve our conventional medical understanding of alternative treatments and the pathophysiology of the conditions they resolve.

In the area of scientific research the two spheres of medicine are not competing, but complementing each other. Each of them serves as a lens through which the other system may examine and find ways to improve itself. While alternative medicine provides "approximate knowledge" that can eventually inspire conventional medical research, conventional medicine helps ground alternative medicine approaches by suggesting the general pathophysiologic qualities an effective alternative therapy will most likely possess.

Once a conventional medical examination has been conducted, the practitioner is ready to assess the case from a metaphoric Chinese medical perspective. Arguably, the two most important sources of information for this evaluation are the descriptions of the pulse and tongue. The tongue and pulse illuminate the general dynamic pervading the case, which can then be used to confirm the interpretation of the symptoms and signs of the patient. Tongue and pulse diagnosis also exposes hidden influences in the case that, although not symptomatically apparent, should be considered in the choice of therapy.

Tongue Diagnosis

The tongue is an indicator of the cumulative effects of Qi, Blood, Yin, and Yang on the tissues of the body, and the various parameters noted when the tongue is examined are given high priority in the interpretation of physical and behavioral signs.

- Color: a normal tongue is pink and vital. Redness indicates Heat caused by excess or deficiency and pallor indicates Blood, Qi, or Yang deficiency. A mauve or lavender tint implies stagnation, and the deeper the mauve, the more severe the stagnation. Purple hues indicate that stagnation has progressed from the Qi to the Blood level. Tension in the muscles of the tongue causes the appearance of a mauve hue in almost all animals; however, the rate at which the hue appears is variable. Animals that are tenser and therefore more prone to stagnation develop the deeper mauve and purple colors more rapidly.
- Shape: a normal tongue fills the floor of the mouth and the edge of the healthy tongue has a sharp edge, like a healthy liver or spleen. When the tongue shows indentations or scallops from the teeth, or is swollen with round edges, large, or flabby, Dampness accumulation is implied. When the tongue is unduly small it generally coincides with other signs of tissue wasting and signifies deficiencies of Yang or Yin.
- Coating: tongue coatings are not as common in dogs or cats as they are in people. Coatings in animals generally appear as a tenacious foam or froth. Sometimes the only evidence of a coating is an obvious difference in color between the top of the tongue, which appears quite pale, and the bottom of the tongue, which is pink or red. Tongue coatings imply the accumulation of Phlegm (a tenacious or congealed form of Dampness) somewhere in the body.
- Moisture: a normal tongue does not appear dry, but it is free of copious moisture. A wet tongue implies Dampness, particularly if it has strings of saliva. A tongue that looks coarse and dry implies Yin deficiency.
- Features: some disorders are accompanied by the appearance of pathologic features on the tongue. Focal ulcers imply Heart Heat since the Tongue is said to express the Heart and Shen in Chinese medicine. Dark purple spots or the appearance of veins in the tongue indicates Blood stasis. Lesions that appear along the sides of the tongue denote Liver involvement and lesions at the tip of the tongue imply Heart involvement.

Observation and collation of the various parameters of the tongue allow the practitioner to assess Qi, Blood, Yin, and Yang, and their influence on the tissues. Certain features of the tongue that are commonly observed together automatically imply certain diagnoses:

- Excess Heat: manifests as a red, dry tongue. If the Heat is caused by Yin deficiency the tongue is sometimes small.
- Yang Deficiency: both Spleen deficiency and Kidney Yang deficiency can be accompanied by a pale, swollen, scalloped, or wet tongue. The tongue may be small in severe cases.
- Damp Heat: a bright red, swollen, scalloped, and moist tongue signifies the accumulation of Damp Heat or Toxic Heat. This tongue is commonly observed in cystitis.
- Qi Stagnation arising from Phlegm accumulation: a lavender tongue with a thick coating signifies this condition. This type of tongue is commonly observed in chronic lung disorders and also in epilepsy when Phlegm clouds consciousness.

Pulse Diagnosis

If we embrace the Chinese View that all parts are an expression of an underlying Yin/Yang dynamic that permeates the whole, any pulse on the body will theoretically serve to illuminate this dynamic. The radial artery is thus palpated in human pulse diagnosis, whereas the femoral artery is palpated in dogs and cats. Pulse location is not nearly as important as finding a pulse that can be readily evaluated. The parameters of interest include the following:

- Tension: how easily both the pulse and the vessel wall can be extinguished with digital pressure.
- Force: the force with which the pulse hits the fingers; roughly equivalent to pulse pressure; note whether this force is dedicated more to lifting the finger or to pushing its way underneath.
- Diameter: the surface area the pulse occupies across the fingertips.
- Depth: how hard the fingers must be pressed before the maximum intensity of the pulse beat is felt.

- Rate: a subjective assessment of pulse rate, as well as an actual count.
- Rhythm: how readily one pulse beat follows the others.

The interpretation of each of these parameters is logical:

- Tension: the ease of flow of Qi in the body; increased vessel wall tension with a forceful beat (a Wiry pulse) implies increased stasis.
- Force: the amount of Qi in the body; a forceless pulse is indicative of Qi deficiency. A component of force is its vector; strong pulse beats that "whip past" the fingertips rather than force them upward (i.e., a Slippery pulse) indicate systemic repletion promoting ease of flow; the Slippery pulse can also indicate internal accumulations such as Dampness, Phlegm, tumors, or pregnancy.
- Diameter: the amount of Blood or Yin in the body; a Thin pulse implies Yin or Blood deficiency, but it also can indicate Damp accumulations in the tissues that squeeze the Blood out of the vessels.
- Depth: the location of the Yang energy and Righteous Qi of the body; Deep or Sinking pulses imply Qi and Yang are being conserved or cannot be mobilized from where they are stored in the lower jiao; Floating pulses imply that the Qi or Yang is at the surface of the body and are most often seen in animals in with conditions of Yin deficiency, in which the relatively stronger Yang begins to escape upward and outward. They are also associated with Spleen Qi deficiency, which is essentially a type of Yin deficiency, since the Spleen is the source of all postnatal Yin.
- Rate: a Rapid pulse implies excess or deficient Heat; a Slow pulse implies Coldness caused by Yang deficiency.
- Rhythm: occasional subtle hesitancy between beats (i.e., a Choppy pulse) or variations in both pulse amplitude and rate (i.e., a Knotted pulse) implies Blood stasis; rapid rhythms with occasional dropped beats (i.e., a Skipping pulse) imply a severe excess of Heat or exuberance of Yang; regular pauses (i.e., an Intermittent pulse) imply critically low levels of Source Qi, to the point that the heart must periodically pause to gather itself.

By observing the characteristics and collating their diagnostic implications, the practitioner can create a coherent picture of the current status of Yin and Yang and their Qi and Blood derivatives within the body. Further understanding of pulse diagnosis is not technically necessary for making sound interpretations of many pulses in animal patients. It can, however, make pulse diagnosis a little easier.

Early Chinese medical practitioners noted that certain variations of the five pulse characteristics are frequently observed together, to produce 27 classically recognized pulse types. Recognition of a pulse type served as a shortcut to interpretation, automatically implying the presence of a specific dynamic of Qi, Blood, Yin, and Yang.

About half of these pulse types are commonly observed in veterinary medicine, including the aforementioned Wiry, Floating, Sinking, Slippery, Thin, Choppy, Skipping, Intermittent, Rapid, and Slow pulses. Other pulse types include the following:

- Soft: a Thin, Floating, forceless pulse that indicates depletion of Qi and Blood, commonly associated with Spleen Qi deficiency. An even more forceless version (the Minute pulse) is seen after a prolonged illness and signifies the exhaustion of Qi and Yin.
- Weak: a Thin, Deep, forceless pulse that indicates depletion of Qi and Blood, with Qi unable to rise.
- Flooding: a Floating, broad, often Rapid pulse that rises forcefully but falls without strength, like waves crashing on a beach; it indicates abundant Heat, often with accompanying Yin deficiency.
- Moderate: a pulse that is moderate in all respects, signifying a normal pulse.
- Firm: a Sinking, Wiry and forceful pulse that indicates internal accumulations of either pathogenic or normal Qi.

Positional Pulse Diagnosis

While the general pulse characteristics illuminate the general pathologic dynamic affecting the patient from a Chinese medical perspective, palpation of the pulse at specific positions along the artery helps the practitioner determine the channel in which the most useful acupuncture points in managing the condition are located. Identification of these points provides further diagnostic information since each is associated with a particular pathologic dynamic (Fig. 2-1).

The practitioner should be aware that opinions differ as to the associations between different positions on an artery and the acupuncture channels of the body. In small animals the prevailing opinion is that the upper jiao organs correspond to the most proximal position of the femoral pulse where it exits the abdomen and enters the leg. The next most proximal position is said to correspond to the middle jiao, and the distalmost position corresponds to the lower jiao. (Table 2-1)

I (SM) wish to advance an alternative interpretation, however, in which the femoral artery is best palpated as close to the knee as possible (Fig. 2-2). In this schema the distal pulse corresponds to the upper jiao; slightly (1 cun) proximally is the pulse corresponding to the middle jiao; a little further (another cun) proximally gives the pulse corresponding to the lower jiao (Table 2-2). (Box 2-1 gives the definition of a cun.)

Although at odds with prevailing expert opinion, the technique yields good results in practice. It is also logical from a hemodynamic perspective. When an animal is active, with its Yang energy mobilized and dispersed, the pulse is felt more distally. The distalmost pulse thus should correspond to the upper jiao, which represents the maximum reach to which mobilized Yang energy can be dispersed from its usual storage position in the lower jiao. In keeping with this logic, the distal radial pulse of humans corresponds to the upper body.

The most proximal of the three positions is the pulse that is most likely to be felt in even a weak animal, when Yang energy cannot be raised from its position of storage in the lower jiao. The proximal pulses in both the wrist and the hind limb are thus the pulses of the lower jiao. The intervening space between the proximal and distal positions on the femoral and radial arteries corresponds to the middle jiao.

Upper, lower, and middle jiao pulses are further subdivided into Yin organs on the left side of the body and Yang organs on the right side of the body. The Yin organs are the Lungs of the upper jiao, the Liver of the middle jiao, and the Kidney of the lower jiao. They thus correspond to the distal, middle, and proximal positions, respectively, of the left femoral artery. The

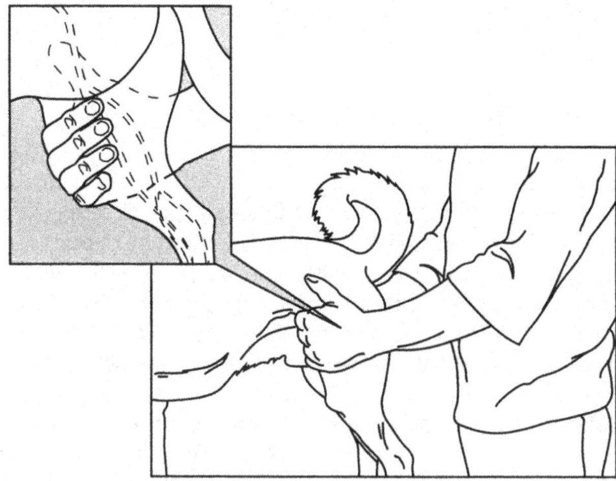

Fig. 2-1 Canine pulse diagnosis—common technique.

Table 2-1 Canine Pulse Diagnosis—Common Technique*

		Proximalmost Pulse Position Is Associated with the Upper Jiao	
Area of the Body	**Type of Pulse**	**Organ Indicated on the Left Femur**	**Organ Indicated on the Right Femur**
Upper Jiao	Superficial	Small Intestine	Large Intestine
	Deep	Heart	Lungs
Middle Jiao	Superficial	Gallbladder	Stomach
	Deep	Liver	Spleen
Lower Jiao	Superficial	Bladder	Triple Burner
	Deep	Kidneys	Pericardium†
		Distalmost Pulse Position Is Associated with the Lower Jiao	

*Frequently, only the deeper Yin organs are evaluated.

†In one classical system the lower jiao pulses are associated with Kidney Yin on the left and Kidney Yang on the right.

BOX 2-1 Definition of a Cun

"Cun" means "little measurement." In Chinese medical dictionaries it is defined as slightly more than 3 cm. Cun measurements are commonly used in acupuncture to help define the precise location of a point. For example, Stomach 36 is three cun distal to Stomach 35, and one cun lateral to the tibial crest. In acupuncture the precise length of a cun varies fom patient to patient and is defined as approximately the width of the patient's thumb.

Because dogs, cats, and horses do not reliably have thumbs, some other definition of cun has to be used in animals. Fortunately, certain body dimensions are considered to be a standard number of cun in length. For example, there are:

- 12 cun from the transverse cubital crease to the transverse carpal crease
- 19 cun from the prominence of the greater trochanter to the midpatella
- 16 cun from the center of the patella to the tip of the lateral malleolus
- 5 cun from the center of the umbilicus to the upper border of the pubic symphysis

These measurements are used in people and have been adapted for use in animals, particularly dogs and cats.

To define a cun in a dog or cat, a veterinary acupuncturist typically divides the distance from the elbow to the carpus into 12 equal units, then selects one of these units as equivalent to a cun. To accomplish this, the practitioner places an elastic tape that will be divided into small equal segments numbered from 0 to 19 over the region of interest. For the wrist, the tape is stretched so that the distance between the wrist and the elbow spans the distance on the tape from 0 to 12. One of the segments on the tape is then considered to equal a cun.

For horses, a measure of convenience has been identified that avoids the necessity of measuring distances using an elastic tape. The main definition of a cun in a horse is the width of the 16th rib taken level with the tuber coxae. Some authors also feel that it is approximately equal to the width of the dorsal spinous process of the first caudal vertebra, or about 3 cm.

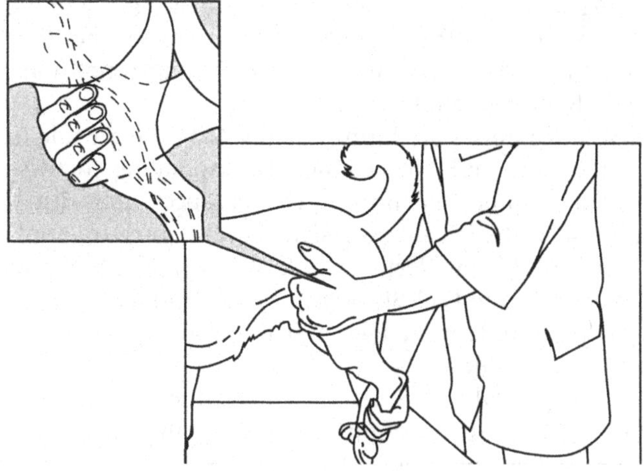

Fig. 2-2 Proposed new system of pulse diagnosis.

Table 2-2 Proposed New System of Pulse Diagnosis

		Proximalmost Pulse Position Is Associated with the Lower Jiao	
Area of Body	**Type of Pulse**	**Organ Associated with the Left Side of the Body**	**Organ Associated with the Right Side of the Body**
Lower Jiao	Superficial	Bladder	Triple Burner
	Deep	Kidney	Pericardium
Middle Jiao	Superficial	Gallbladder	Stomach
	Deep	Liver	Spleen
Upper Jiao	Superficial	Large Intestine	Small Intestine
	Deep	Lung	Heart
		Distalmost Pulse Position Is Associated with the Upper Jiao	

Yang organs are the Heart of the upper jiao, the Spleen of the middle jiao, and the Triple Burner of the lower jiao. They thus correspond to the distal, middle, and proximal positions, respectively, of the right femoral artery.

These three pulses are further subdivided on each side to reflect the Yang and Yin channels corresponding to these organs. For example, the most superficial aspect of the distalmost pulse on the left side is assigned to the Large Intestine. The Lung pulse is the deeper aspect of this same pulse position. Similarly, the Gall Bladder pulse is the outer aspect of the Liver pulse and the Bladder pulse is the outer aspect of the Kidney pulse position.

On the right side the Small Intestine is the outer or Yang aspect of the pulse position assigned to the Heart. The Stomach is the Yang aspect of the Spleen pulse. The Triple Burner is actually the outer aspect of the proximalmost pulse on the right side, with the Pericardium corresponding to the deeper aspect of this same pulse.

When superficially palpating these various pulse positions, the practitioner is looking for relative differences in beat force among the three positions. When palpating deep aspects of the pulse, the practitioner is comparing the different positions to see which position can be most easily extinguished. An especially strong superficial pulse and a deep pulse that particularly resists digital compression suggest that the associated channel is an especially important source of efficacious points for the treatment of that particular patient's condition.

The exact location of pulse positions changes according to body size, making interpretation of pulse position findings problematic. Some general anatomic landmarks are that the middle pulse overlies the insertion of the adductors on the distal femur; the upper body pulse spans the gap between the adductors and the popliteal fossa, where the artery disappears; the lower body pulse is the portion of the artery just proximal to the segment that lies atop the adductors. Some other general guidelines are that each position is approximately 0.75 cm in length in a large-breed dog, ranging down to perhaps only a few millimeters in a cat or small-breed dog.

Differences between positions cannot always be felt in animals or humans, even though "active" acupuncture points can be found to treat their condition. Furthermore, not all "active" points are represented in pulse position findings, and the practitioner will have to palpate other meridians not suggested by the pulse findings to be sure all the best points with which to treat the case have been found. The clinician is occasionally unable to find an "active" point to correspond to pulse findings, despite even the most thorough palpation.

Acupuncture Point Palpation

Once various pulse positions have been palpated with the view to finding out the most involved meridians, the practitioner can begin palpating the corresponding channels to find the "active" points. Japanese acupuncturists have developed point and channel palpation to a high art beyond simply assessing Shu and Mu points. Veterinary practitioners are encouraged to study with a Japanese-style acupuncturist, if possible, in order to further develop their skill.

In palpating points, the practitioner must consider the texture and resilience of the immediately surrounding tissue. Points that have become active to an extreme feel thicker and less resilient than adjacent areas, as though an extra layer of tough tissue has been deposited at the site underneath the skin. This thickening is transitory and does not correspond to the anatomy of clinically normal animals. It may involve a large area around the active point.

Points that are active to a lesser degree but are still of significant benefit feel rounded, raised, and slightly turgid. In humans, this swelling may consolidate into a hard nodularity, but in animals it remains as a rounded wheal, which may be 1 to 2 cm in diameter bulging up under the skin. At their subtlest level of development, in both humans and animals, active points offer merely a slight source of skin drag and a sensation of warmth to a fingertip lightly dragged across them.

The Conception Vessel is palpated by gentle ballottement along its length, from the xiphisternum to the pelvic brim, using only the fingertips. Active points along the Conception Vessel frequently feel tauter than surrounding regions.

As the practitioner gains experience in the subtleties of point palpation, cruder methods of looking for heightened point sensitivity in response to digital pressure will eventually be abandoned. The quest for active points can be done quickly, looking for areas of thickening and warmth merely by lightly sweeping, brushing, kneading, or tickling along the length of a channel. The practitioner will no longer have to inflict pain when examining Shu and Mu points, and pain referred from spinal nerve root compression at the site of vertebral fixations will no longer confuse physical findings.

Once active points are found, the area of greatest heat, thickening, or swelling within the point is identified and the needle is inserted at that point. On referral to human point guides, the practitioner will often find that the needle corresponds to the position of a known acupuncture point.

Use of palpation as a primary means of locating points removes some of the controversy over whether human points can be transposed onto animal bodies. Active points usually correspond well to known human acupuncture points, helping to confirm their existence on animal bodies. In addition, the identification of consistently active points will suggest their inclusion in future revisions of veterinary acupuncture point curricula.

Each acupuncture point embodies a certain type of energetic. For example, SP 6 is an important point for the relief both of Blood and Yin deficiency, and of Qi stagnation in the lower jiao. Finding this point to be active would suggest to the practitioner that Blood or Yin deficiency is involved in the development of the patient's symptoms. Location of active points is not therefore just a method of finding the points most likely to be of benefit. The energetics of the points identified as active often suggest the dynamic creating the symptoms and are therefore of diagnostic value.

Manual Thermal Diagnosis

Manual Thermal Diagnosis is a descriptive term for evaluating a patient for localized areas of warmth or coolness. In Manual Thermal Diagnosis the hand is held approximately 1 to 2 cm above the skin and moved down channels and over body regions. Sudden temperature gradations that can be consistently felt, and especially those that are asymmetric relative to the opposite side of the body, are considered significant in denoting areas of Qi stagnation manifesting as heat, and Qi deficiency manifesting as coolness. Needles are placed in the warm areas and downstream along the affected channel in an effort to draw the Qi from the area where it has welled up. Needles are placed in cool areas and just upstream to draw Qi into areas where it is deficient. Typical findings include coolness over GB 29 and GB 30 in animals suffering from hip pain, and sudden gradations in heat along the Bladder channel in animals suffering from back pain. Qi can be drawn to GB 30 from the distal reaches of the Bladder channel, with which it connects.

Homeopathy

The repertorization, selection, and potentization of a homeopathic remedy for a given patient also constitute an assessment, but without the benefit of the perspective of other medical systems, the repertorization of a remedy does not lead to a detailed metaphoric evaluation of a patient. If the patient responds well to the remedy, there are no implications for specific preventive measures that might be used to perpetuate the benefits of the remedy.

Chinese medicine offers a perspective that translates a response to a particular remedy into preventive measures that perpetuate the therapeutic benefits already realized. If a practitioner skilled in both homeopathy and Chinese medicine notices that a particular homeopathic remedy is repeatedly indicated for a given Chinese medical diagnosis, a response to that remedy confirms an associative link between that particular diagnosis and the remedy. Preventive lifestyle recommendations can now be made based on a response to the homeopathic remedy. In addition, homeopathic prescribing now becomes less time consuming and laborious. *Lachesis,* for example, can now be quickly prescribed with confidence in any Liver Blood deficiency case in dogs with throat conditions, bleeding tendencies, dominance, and pronounced aggression. *Lycopodium* can be used to reliably treat Blood-deficient, possessive, fear-aggressive animals. *Rhus toxicodendron* will regularly be effective in "rusty gate" lameness in Blood-deficient dogs. Thus, although the field of homeopathy is notable for its self-reliance, much can be gained if it uses the lens of other medical systems to analyze itself.

ASSESSMENT

A conventional medical diagnosis is the first priority in a holistic assessment. Based on this assessment, provisional plans are made for treatment using conventional medicine, either in tandem with alternative medicine or in its place should alternative therapies prove ineffective.

After the conventional assessment has been made, a "metaphoric" diagnosis is made. Chinese medicine, for reasons previously explained, is perhaps the best medical system currently available for making an "energetic" assessment of a patient, but this may change if sophisticated educational resources in the areas of Greek, early Western herbal, and Ayurvedic medicine become more available. All of these medical systems, including Chinese medicine, probably shared many fundamental perspectives that permit the skilled practitioner to fulfill Chinese medical goals, for example, with Western herbal medicines or even homeopathic remedies.

In Chinese medical assessments the tongue and pulse provide the context for the interpretation of the signs detailed in the history and physical examination. Active or "alive" acupuncture points further flesh out this assessment when consideration is given to their usual symptomatic and energetic indications. A thorough understanding of Chinese medical pathophysiology aids greatly in the assessment process, and a large portion of this text is directed toward providing that understanding.

The final assessment provides a basis for evaluating the improvement of the patient, if it is detailed in the chart together with the aspects of the case that support it. When the patient is reevaluated, the physical signs, and pulse and tongue findings that specifically support the assessment are reviewed to see whether they have improved. If pervasive improvements in all are noted, the patient is responding well.

Treatment goals can be formulated from the detailed assessments to ensure as complete an improvement in the patient as possible. Treatment goals should be formulated for both the conventional and alternative medical assessments, and the fewest therapies that satisfy all of the identified goals should be chosen. Ensuring that an alternative therapy addresses pharmacologic goals even as it addresses goals arising from the metaphoric assessment of the patient seems to help ensure positive outcomes. To increase the chances of a favorable outcome, however, it appears more important to satisfy alternative medical goals.

As long as they share a common purpose, multiple modalities can be employed synergistically in the treatment of a patient, helping to speed the rate and to improve the completeness of patient outcomes. At the same time, the practitioner can enjoy the satisfaction that comes with specifically diagnosing a patient's disorder, and not feel he or she has succumbed to a "shotgun" approach.

TREATMENT PLAN IMPLEMENTATION

Chinese herbal therapy is increasingly popular among integrative practitioners. This textbook makes reference to scores of Chinese herbal formulas that seem to show promise in treating particular conditions. As with pharmaceuticals, generous expiration dating allows the stocking of many formulas with the reasonable expectation that they will be completely used up before their shelf life has expired. Financially, however, carrying a large formula inventory may not be feasible. Most Chinese herbalists prefer to stock a favorite group of 20 or 30 formulas, and adapt them to the most commonly encountered clinical conditions by adding single herbs to them or adjusting the ratios of their constituents. Tables 2-3 and 2-4 show examples of the inventory I (SM) carry, together with the general conditions under which each herb or formula is considered for use.

Dosage strategies for granular concentrates of all of these herbs and formulas are similar, with a *recommended starting dose* of ¼ tsp per 10 to 15 lb of body weight per day, or 60 to 75 mg/kg of body weight, divided into two doses. When the formula seems to be particularly appropriate, with no observable adverse side effects, larger doses may be contemplated, up to double or triple the recommended starting dose. This is especially true if improvements seen thus far in the patient with use of the formula are pervasive but not complete.

Table 2-3 Inventory of Single Herbs and Their Uses

Single Herb	Use
Bo He *(Peppermint)*	Combine with Gou Qi Zi, Ju Hua, and Man Jing Zi for external eye redness and corneal disorders
Cang Zhu *(Red Atractylodes)*	Warms and tonifies the Spleen; stimulates the Spleen and improves appetite
Chai Hu *(Bupleurum)*	Moves Qi; useful in hepatitis and hyperlipidemia where Qi stagnation is present
Chuan Bei Mu *(Fritillaria)*	Strongly reduces Phlegm accumulations in the airways
Dan Shen *(Salvia)*	Moves Blood; calms; reduces blood cholesterol; consider for congestive heart failure
Dang Gui *(Angelica sinensis)*	Blood mover and tonic; combine with Si Miao San when a Blood mover is needed
Dang Shen *(Codonopsis)*	Tonifies Spleen Qi
Du Zhong *(Eucommia)*	Tonifies Kidney Yang; descends energy; good additive for geriatric animals receiving down-bearing formulas for neurological conditions such as Ban Xia Bai Zhu Tian Ma Tang
E Zhu *(Zedoaria)*	With San Leng, a good additive for Blood-moving formulas to increase their antineoplastic activity
Fu Ling *(Poria)*	Drains Dampness and supports the Spleen; add with Dang Shen or Ren Shen to Si Wu Xiao Feng Yin in Spleen-deficient patients
Gou Qi Zi *(Lycium)*	Nondampening Liver Yin tonic; use with Ju Hua as additive to Liu Wei Di Huang Wan for eye dryness; also see comments for Bo He above
Hua Shi *(Talc)*	Drains Damp Heat; combine with Shao Fu Zhu Ye Tang to address Blood stasis in the Bladder
Huai Niu Xi *(Achryanthes)*	Consolidates Yin; relaxes low back stiffness; moves Blood
Huang Bai *(Phellodendron)*	Use with Zhi Mu in Liu Wei Di Huang Wan to create Zhi Bai Di Huang Wan to address Yin deficiency with Empty Heat
Huang Lian *(Coptis)*	Clears Heat from Blood, Heart, Stomach, and upper jiao
Huang Qi *(Astragalus)*	Powerful Spleen and Wei Qi tonic; use with Dang Gui in a 5:1 ratio as a powerful Blood tonic
Jiang Can *(Silkworm casing)*	Transforms Phlegm; useful in neurologic conditions arising from Phlegm; add to Ban Xia Bai Zhu Tian Ma Tang

Table 2-3 Inventory of Single Herbs and Their Uses—cont'd

Single Herb	Use
Jue Ming Zi *(Cassia seed)*	Useful herb in ophthalmologic conditions arising from Liver Heat
Jin Yin Hua *(Lonicera)*	Use with Lian Qiao and Pu Gong Ying for the treatment of pustular skin lesions; additive to Si Wu Xiao Feng Yin
Ju Hua *(Chrysanthemum)*	See Gou Qi Zi and Bo He
Lian Qiao *(Forsythia)*	See Jin Yin Hua
Mai Men Dong *(Ophiopogon)*	Use to moisten the Yin of the upper body; with Wu Wei Zi for chronic dry cough and mild urinary incontinence in Yin-deficient patients; add to Liu Wei Di Huang Wan
Man Jing Zi *(Vitex fruit)*	See Bo He
Mu Dan Pi *(Moutan)*	Moves and cools Blood
Mu Gua *(Chaenomeles)*	Antispasmodic; add to Blood tonics
Mu Tong *(Akebia)*	Drains Dampness; opens the channels to relieve pain
Pu Gong Ying *(Taraxacum)*	See Jin Yin Hua
Ren Shen *(Panax ginseng)*	Powerful Qi tonic; use with Fu Ling as additive to Si Wu Xiao Feng Yin when Spleen Qi deficiency and Dampness accompany Blood deficiency
San Leng *(Sparganium)*	Use with E Zhu as antineoplastic Blood mover; see E Zhu above
San Qi *(Pseudoginseng)*	Moves Blood; stops acute bleeding
Shan Zha *(Crataegus)*	Lowers cholesterol and improves myocardial perfusion; use with Dan Shen or formulas such as Bu Gan Tang and Dang Gui Shao Yao San
Sheng Di Huang *(Rehmannia)*	Clears Empty Heat and nourishes Yin; moistens Dryness
Wu Wei Zi *(Schizandra)*	Astringes coughing and urine flow; see Mai Men Dong above
Yi Yi Ren *(Coix)*	Leaches out Dampness; tonifies Spleen; clears Heat
Zhi Mu *(Anemarrhena)*	See Huang Bai
Zi Cao Gen *(Lithospermum)*	Use with tapazole to lower required dose; cools the Blood

Table 2-4 Inventory of Common Formulas and Their Uses

Formula	General Use
Ba Wei Di Huang Wan	Kidney failure in chilly cats; Kidney Qi or Yang deficiency
Ban Xia Bai Zhu Tian Ma Tang	Idiopathic vestibular syndrome; epilepsy; conditions in which Qi rebels upward because of accumulations of Phlegm
Bu Gan Tang	Blood deficiency without Dampness in dogs; fear aggression; muscle tightness and spasm
Dang Gui Shao Yao San	Hyperlipidemia; persistent crystalluria in Blood-deficient animals; conditions in which both Blood deficiency or stasis and Dampness accumulation are evident
Du Huo Ji Sheng Tang	Low back stiffness and hind end weakness or pain in animals with Kidney, Yin, or Blood deficiency and cold intolerance; pulses are often wiry
Er Xian Tang	Combined conditions of extreme Heat, Yang deficiency and Yin deficiency; late-stage hyperthyroidism
Ge Xia Zhu Ye Tang	Liver or Spleen enlargement
Liu Wei Di Huang Wan	Any condition arising from Yin deficiency
Long Dan Xie Gan Tang	Excess Damp Heat in the Liver or its channels; conditions might include severe toxic skin lesions such as pemphigus and uncontrolled epilepsy; pulses are forceful
San Ren Tang	Any Damp-Heat condition arising from Spleen deficiency; feline hyperesthesia syndrome
Sang Piao Xiao San	Enuresis arising from Kidney and Heart deficiency; hormonally responsive urinary incontinence
Shao Fu Zhu Ye Tang	Any Blood stasis in the lower abdomen, including Bladder tumors
Si Miao San	Any condition in which Damp Heat arises from Spleen deficiency; a stronger formula than San Ren Tang; hind limb proprioceptive disorders; recurrent cystitis or colitis
Si Wu Xiao Feng Yin	Skin disorders arising from Blood deficiency in dogs

Table 2-4 Inventory of Common Formulas and Their Uses—cont'd

Formula	General Use
Su Zi Jiang Qi Tang	Chronic productive cough associated with Kidney deficiency; asthma in older cats; chronic coughs in old dogs
Xiao Feng San	Skin lesions in Blood-deficient animals that also exhibit Dampness
Xiao Yao San	Cases with Blood deficiency, Qi stagnation, Spleen Qi deficiency, and mild Dampness accumulation; loss of appetite; Liver disorders
Tian Ma Gou Teng Yin	Yin deficiency leading to cognitive disorders
Tao Hong Er Chen Tang	Phlegm accumulations that cause chronic vomiting; early hyperthyroidism; chronic vomiting in cats
Wei Ling Tang	Any case of Spleen Qi or Yang deficiency that leads to Dampness accumulation; diabetes mellitus; lymphangiectasia; hypoalbuminemia
Modified Wei Ling Tang	Damp-Heat skin lesions in which Dampness predominates and signs of Spleen deficiency are clear; Blood deficiency may also be present
Modified Wen Dan Tang	Feline hyperthyroidism
Xiao Huo Luo Dan	Localized pain in chilly animals with Blood stasis and Phlegm
Xue Fu Zhu Ye Tang	Any condition with Qi stagnation, Blood deficiency, and Blood stasis; chronic coughing; malignancies of the chest; recurrent mast cell tumors; thyroid tumors
Yi Guan Jian	Any condition with Liver or Kidney Yin deficiency, with Liver Blood deficiency, or in which stronger Yin tonifiers are being avoided because of risks of Spleen Dampness; chronic gastritis; halitosis; costal arch pain; upper abdominal pain

BOX 2-2 References for Chinese Herbal Formulas

Ehling D. *The Chinese Herbalist's Handbook*, revised ed. Santa Fe, NM, 1996, Inword Press.

Naeser MA. *Outline Guide to Chinese Herbal Patent Medicines in Pill Form.* Boston, Mass, 1990, Boston Chinese Medicine.

Yan W. *Practical Therapeutics of Traditional Chinese Medicine,* Brookline, Mass, 1997, Paradigm Publications.

Yeung H. *Handbook of Chinese Herbs.* Los Angeles, Calif, 1996, Self-published.

Yeung H. *Handbook of Chinese Herbal Formulas.* Los Angeles, Calif, 1995, Self-published.

Although self-published, the latter two books are commonly found in the bookstores of institutions where Chinese medicine is taught.

Strangely, the converse is also true: a well-chosen Chinese herbal formula may also be effective in lower than normal doses. Consider this strategy if poor patient compliance or formula palatability is proving to be a major issue.

A detailed list of ingredients of the Chinese herbal formulas mentioned in this text can be found in one of the five references in Box 2-2. If Chinese herbal formula companies do not stock the formula of interest, practitioners may find the formula in one of the references and either order the ingredients to make it up themselves or have an herbal company make it up specially for them.

ASSESSING OUTCOME

It is important that the practitioner reevaluate the patient when assessing outcomes. Although the placebo effect is commonly said to be inoperative in veterinary medicine, it is indeed a consideration. Animal owners or veterinarians heavily invested in the positive outcome of a case managed by alternative medicine may inadvertently attempt to convince themselves that an improvement has been seen. Similarly, some clients focus on the presence or absence of just one symptom in formulating their impression of whether the treatment has been successful.

In either case the same strategy is used to objectify the evaluation of patient outcomes. The patient is reexamined, and the entire checklist of findings that supported the practitioner's initial assessment is reviewed for changes. The pulse and tongue are reassessed to see whether they reflect a change in the patient's condition. Laboratory findings can be reassessed to determine whether the alternative therapy can be considered effective from a conventional medical perspective. Most of the features that formed the basis for the assessment of the patient should improve or resolve if the treatment was an unqualified success. If only one or two of these features improve, the case should be reevaluated. Treatment using alternative medicine is ideally continued until the tongue and pulse revert completely to normal.

PREVENTION OF DISEASE

Disease prevention remains the highest goal in medicine, even when alternative modalities are used. Preventive measures that help preserve health in improved patients can be recommended, even when the cause of the disease remains unknown from a conventional perspective. This is possible because acupuncture and herbs are forms of focused intervention that counter and correct aberrant "energy" patterns in the body. Diets are perceived to have this same metaphoric effect, but are less forceful in their action. They provide a background influence that supports and enhances the actions of herbs and acupuncture. Once aberrations are corrected, the gentle but pervasive influence of diet, and even other lifestyle factors such as daily activities and climate, maintains the balance of the organism and prevents it from remanifesting its pathologic energetic, which in turn can manifest as a number of different diseases. This text attempts to illuminate, in at least broad strokes, the dietary strategies that, thus far, seem indicated in an animal that has responded to a particular acupuncture and herbal strategy.

PART TWO

Clinical Strategies by Organ System

3

Therapies for Behavioral Disorders

ANXIETY

Therapeutic Rationale

- Reduce anxiety.
- Behavior modification.

Alternative Options with Conventional Bases

Nutrition

- **Phosphatidylserine, acetyl-L-carnitine, and antioxidants** may be useful in older dogs and are discussed in the section on cognitive dysfunction. Anxiety is sometimes a component of cognitive dysfunction, since older dogs may respond with anxiety to increasing debility of senses, increasing pain, and so on.

Herbs

- **Valerian** *(Valeriana officinalis)*: has been studied primarily for insomnia and appears to be effective, but the greatest effect is noted after a few weeks of treatment (Beaubrun, 2000). Valerian's mechanism of action is thought to be mediated through gamma-aminobutyric acid A (GABA-A) receptors and perhaps benzodiazepine receptors (Houghton, 1999; Mennini, 1993). The most active principles appear to be contained in the essential oils and terpenes so alcohol extracts and the whole herb may be more effective than water extracts.
- **Kava** *(Piper methysticum)*: has established anxiolytic activity (Cauffield, 1999). Kava contains multiple major active constituents which have complex activities, including analgesia. In a study measuring human

anxiety, 100 mg tid of an extract standardized to 70% kavalactones significantly reduced signs of anxiety compared with subjects receiving a placebo (Warnecke, 1991). Long-term use of Kava results in an ichthyosiform dermatitis and more recent reports of hepatotoxicity in Europe and the U.S. require that Kava be used with caution. In traditional societies in which the herb is masticated and drunk as a "tea" only the dermatitis has been reported, whereas recent hepatotoxicity reports may involve extracts as well as herb or drug interactions. I (SW) now use the dried herb only and avoid the use of extracts.

- **Hops** *(Humulus lupulus)*: an ingredient in beer, and has been used for insomnia. However, there is little support for this use. There is a single report of five dogs that had malignant hyperthermia after ingestion of spent hops used in beer making; four of these dogs were greyhounds (Duncan, 1997).
- **Passion Flower** *(Passiflora incarnata)*: a traditional mild anxiolytic. Experimental animal studies confirm this effect (Petry, 2001; Sopranzi, 1990; Soulimani, 1997), but it has not been studied in humans or companion animals.
- **Oats** *(Avena sativa)*: are a traditional remedy for insomnia and anxiety. There is little support for this use, but Oats are not associated with adverse effects.
- **Skullcap** *(Scutellaria lateriflora)*: a traditional anxiolytic, but its use is not supported by studies at this time.
- **St. John's Wort** *(Hypericum perforatum)*: often recommended for anxiety, but there is little support for this use. It is better recognized as an effective treatment for some types of depression in humans.

Paradigmatic Options

- Anxiety amounts to a disturbance of the consciousness, or Shen, of an animal. The Shen is housed in the Heart, and the Heart's location and vulnerabilities indicate the types of circumstances in which the Shen or consciousness becomes disturbed. In Shen disorders manifesting as anxiety, things are not perceived as they really are, but rather as they are feared to be.

Heart Fire

- The Heart is equated with the element Fire and is the source of pure Yang energy in the body. Because of this purity and clarity the Heart has been allocated the duty of serving as the consciousness of the body. The strength of every organ is also its weakness, however, and the Heart's Yang tendencies sometimes result in its becoming too hot. Often, in animals, this Heat is a Damp Heat, and a formula that may be considered in such a case is **Huang Lian Wen Dan Tang** (Warm the Gall Bladder Decoction with Coptis). Huang Lian Wen Dan Tang is made by adding 9 g of Huang Lian (Coptis) to 50 g of Wen Dan Tang (Warm the Gall Bladder Decoction). Animals that benefit from this formula have slippery, rapid pulses and red, wet tongues. Irritability, eye redness, aggressive or destructive tendencies, poor appetite, and sudden outbursts all may manifest from Phlegm Fire. To make the formula more powerful in calming the Shen, add 9 g of Yu Jin (Curcuma) per 60 g of base formula. A *recommended starting dose* is ¼ tsp per 10 to 15 lb of body weight, or 1 mg/kg of body weight. Administer in divided doses, twice daily.
- Another formula is commonly prescribed for excess Heart Fire leading to anxiety and is known as **Zhu Sha An Shen Wan** (Cinnabar Sedative Pills). While effective, this formula is toxic because of its content of Cinnabar, a mercury compound. As a result, it cannot be recommended for general use.
- Deficiency Heart Fire may also cause anxiety. In this case the Heart has an appropriate amount of Yang energy but is deficient in Yin. Severe Heart Yin deficiency is treated with **Huang Lian E Jiao Tang** (Coptis and Donkey-Hide Decoction). Coptis clears Heart Fire and gelatin made from Donkey Hide nourishes the Yin of the Heart, which is Blood. This is a very rich formula and should not be used for patients with wet tongues and slippery pulses. It should be used only when the tongue is a deep red or purple-red and the pulses are rapid and thready. For this formula to be of benefit, the patient should be thirsty, have an elevated appetite, and be agitated and restless. A *recommended starting dose* is ¼ tsp per 10 to 15 lb of body

weight, or 1 mg/kg of body weight. Administer in divided doses, twice daily.

- A less severe form of deficiency, or Empty Heat, calls for **Tian Wang Bu Xin Dan** (Heavenly Emperor's Nourish the Heart Pill). Patients that benefit from this formula have Empty Heat because of deficient Kidney Yin as well as deficient Heart Blood. In the normal body, Kidney Yin is steamed up from the lower jiao to keep the Heart cool and moist. When Yin deficiency is present, a Deficiency Heat arises that leads to signs of mild Heat and Dryness, including heat intolerance, thirst, eye redness, dry stools, and panting. In addition, there may be signs the Kidney is affected, such as possible nocturia and hind limb weakness or stiffness. The Heart appears more agitated, manifesting such signs as insomnia and restlessness. A *recommended starting dose* is ¼ tsp per 10 to 15 lb of body weight, or 1 mg/kg of body weight. Administer in divided doses, twice daily.
- Acupuncture points that may be beneficial include GV 14, GV 26, GV 16, ST 40, CV 12, LIV 3, ST 44, and PC 6. LIV 3, ST 44, and GV 14 drain excessive Heat from the body. ST 40, CV 12, and PC 6 stop the formation of Dampness and Phlegm. PC6 also clears Heart Fire, and GV 26 and GV 16 regulate the Governing Vessel to control Brain activity and pierce the turbidity that obscures rational thought.

Qi Stagnation

- In the natural world, when things do not flow smoothly past each other there is tension. When Qi does not flow smoothly, tension manifests on all levels. On the physical level it manifests as distending pain. On the mental level it manifests as anxiety or irritability. The smooth movement of Qi is governed by the Liver. It is injured by smoldering anger and constraint and the general presence of tension in the environment. When an animal's anxiety is suspected to be a reflection of its owner's anxiety, the formula **Chai Hu Shu Gan San** (Bupleurum Disperse the Liver Powder) should be considered. Animals that benefit will have wiry pulses and a normal- to lavender-appearing tongue. They may also have periods of depression and signs of poor appetite, excessive belching, nausea or vomiting, and constipation. Their blood pressure may be elevated. A *recommended starting dose* is ¼ tsp per 10 to 15 lb of body weight, or 1 mg/kg of body weight. It should be administered in divided doses, twice daily.

- Often, Liver Qi stagnation is not the primary complaint but is secondary to Liver Blood deficiency. An adequate Liver Blood supply strengthens and emboldens an animal, making it less prone to anxiety. In addition, an adequate amount of Blood soothes the Liver, enabling it to perform its function of smoothly moving Qi. As previously mentioned, when Qi does not flow smoothly there is tension, including mental emotional tension. In extreme states anxiety can manifest as fear aggression. *Liver Blood deficiency, in my practice (SM), is the most important cause of fear aggression, and can be treated successfully with the appropriate Blood-tonifying formula.* The role of Blood deficiency in other diseases of the dog is discussed in other chapters. When these other disorders are not present, and when Spleen Qi deficiency is not an underlying cause of Liver Blood deficiency, **Bu Gan Tang** (Nourish the Liver Decoction) should be considered. This is a rich formula, filled with Blood and Yin tonics, and it should not be used in Damp animals. Animals that may benefit from Bu Gan Tang have pale or lavender tongues, thin and/or wiry pulses, a tendency to soft tissue lameness that is not associated with radiographic lesions, overt muscle spasms and tightness, powdery, fine dander on the fur, a tendency to dream frequently, and a dull coat or poor hair regrowth. A *recommended starting dose* is ¼ tsp per 10 to 15 lb of body weight, or 1 mg/kg of body weight. Administer in divided doses, twice daily.

Western Herbs

- Once a Chinese medical diagnosis has been established, Western herbs may be used instead of Chinese herbal formulas to relieve anxiety in animals. They may be used alone or in combination. They are classified as follows according to their theoretical action in Chinese medical terms.

Herbs that move Qi

- Valerian Root: appears especially effective in relaxing muscle spasms and nervous tension (i.e., moving Qi) in animals with Blood deficiency. Some herbalists consider Valerian to be warming and claim that it is contraindicated in nervous animals with signs of Heat (such as a red tongue and rapid pulses). Passion Flower has a strong down-bearing action, serving not only to move Qi but also to descend it from the head. It may be more effective in relaxing animals with signs of Dampness and Phlegm.

Phlegm-transforming herbs

- In situations in which Dampness is obstructing the Heart orifices, making it difficult for the Shen to "see clearly," Hops can be considered. Hops may be even more effective in these cases when combined with Passion Flower.

Cooling herbs

- For deficiency Heart Fire, Skullcap can be considered. The combination of Skullcap and Oats provides a better foundation of Yin to aid in cooling the Heart.

Cautions

- Most of the herbal anxiolytics have ill-defined mechanisms of action. It is wise to avoid combining these herbs with pharmaceutical anxiolytics until more is known about the interactions.

AUTHORS' CHOICES:

SM: Appropriate Chinese herbal formulas for clinical presentation; Western herbs appropriate to their energetics.
SW: Kava; Valerian; behavior modification.

COGNITIVE DYSFUNCTION

C Therapeutic Rationale

- Inhibit dopaminergic degradation in the central nervous system (CNS).
- Little understood pathophysiology.

Alternative Options with Conventional Bases

Nutrition

- **Phosphatidylserine:** in a large controlled trial of elderly people with cognitive decline, 300 mg/day for 6 months led to significant improvement as compared with a placebo (Cenacchi, 1993). Clinical experience suggests treatment with 100 to 500 mg daily.
- **Acetyl-L-carnitine:** appears to reduce decline in Alzheimer's disease and other cognitive problems of elderly humans (Brooks, 1998; Salvioli, 1994; Thal, 2000). Doses in those studies ranged from 1500 mg daily to 1 g tid. Suggested dosage for dogs may range from 10 to 20 mg/lb of body weight bid.
- **Melatonin:** frequently useful for old dogs that pace at night. It has also been studied in people and, in addition to improving sleep, improved some cognition measures (Jean-Louis, 1998). The dose is variable at approximately 50 μg/lb of body weight, at least 1 hour before bedtime, and is best taken on an empty stomach. Use for 1 to 2 weeks may be enough to effect changes that last for a period of time without further treatment.
- **Antioxidants:** these, especially Vitamin E, have shown potential in clinical trials with humans who have Alzheimer's disease (Flynn, 1999; Grundman, 2000). Since antioxidants are increasingly recognized as beneficial for many conditions of aging pets, a broad-spectrum antioxidant supplement is a reasonable recommendation, although in the Grundman study Vitamin E was supplied at very high doses—2000 IU daily. Doses recommended in companion animals are closer to 10 to 20 IU/lb of body weight, topping out at 800 IU daily. Recent trials by Hills Pet Nutrition highlight alpha-lipoic acid, Vitamin E, Vitamin C and L-carnitine as possibly particularly effective in combination.
- **Red Yeast Rice,** a natural lipid-lowering agent that acts like a statin, may help prevent worsening cognitive decline. In human studies, statin use was associated with a lower incidence of Alzheimer's disease (Rockwood, 2002; Scott, 2001).

Herbs

- **Ginkgo** *(Ginkgo biloba)*: when supplied as the standard extract EGb Ginkgo has repeatedly been found effective in improving cognitive measures in people with certain mental disorders (Le Bars, 2000). While we understand little of how canine cognitive dysfunction relates to Alzheimer's and other cognitive disorders in humans, anecdotal reports suggest some success. Benefits of Ginkgo are thought to be due at least in part to its ability to increase perfusion and oxygen delivery to the cerebrum.
- **Qian Ceng Ta** *(Huperzia serrata)*: commonly used in China for the treatment of Alzheimer's disease. It has been shown to reduce reactive oxygen species formation and reduce beta-amyloid formation in neurons (Xiao, 2002).
- **Curcumin,** an extract of Turmeric *(Curcuma longa)*: has antiinflammatory and antioxidant properties. In a mouse trial Curcumin was shown to reduce beta-amyloid and plaque burden (Lim, 2001).
- **Other herbal preparations** being investigated for their ability to enhance cognitive dysfunction in people include Gotu Cola *(Centella asiatica)* and Brahmi *(Bacopa monniera)*.

Other Treatments

- **Treatment with an oxygen-enriched atmosphere** often provides temporary relief to dogs with cognitive dysfunction. In my experience (SW), 3 to 5 hours in an oxygen cage often helps dogs for 2 to 4 weeks.

Paradigmatic Options

- The Chinese medical perspective of cognitive dysfunction is similar to that of Western medicine, in which the main therapeutic thrust is at improving oxygen delivery and blood flow to the cerebrum. In Chinese medicine, because consciousness is a metaphoric function of the Heart, adequate Heart Yin and Blood are considered paramount in maintaining cognitive abilities.

Heart and Kidneys Disconnected

- One possible cause of the Heart's "drying out" is disconnection of the upper and lower jiaos, or halves, of the body. When this occurs, there is inadequate Kidney

Yin in the lower jiao to be "steamed up" to where it can "moisten" the Heart. Likewise, the Heart has too little Qi, or Yang, to warm the Kidney Yin to provide this steaming action. The chief formula to address this complaint is **Sang Piao Xiao San** (Mantis Egg–Casing Powder). The therapeutic efficacy of the formula may be enhanced by adding 9 g each of Wu Wei Zi (Schizandra) and Suan Zao Ren (Jujube seed) to about 60 g of base formula. Patients that benefit from Sang Piao Xiao San may appear distracted and become easily fatigued and confused. Nocturia may be present, and appetite may be finicky. The pulse may be thin, weak, and difficult to find. The tongue may be light red or pale. There is not usually much tongue coating, nor are there usually pronounced signs of Heat or Coldness. A *recommended starting dose* is ⅛ tsp per 5 to 10 lb of body weight, or about 1 mg/kg of body weight, divided into two daily doses.

- Useful acupuncture points include GV 20 to calm the Shen; ST 36, SP 6, and KI 3 to nourish Qi, Yin, and Blood; BL 15 and 23 to nourish the Heart and Kidneys; and PC 6 to calm the Heart.

Blood Deficiency

- When Heart Blood deficiency is considered to be causing cognitive dysfunction, **Gui Pi Tang** (Restore the Spleen Decoction) is indicated. This formula nourishes Heart Blood by strengthening the Spleen, since the Spleen is the source of Blood from the Chinese medical perspective. Guiding signs for use of this formula include poor appetite, loose stools, insomnia, frequent dreaming (often seen in Blood-deficient animals), and fatigue. Other signs of Blood deficiency may be present, including a lusterless coat with fine, powdery dander and timidity. Pulses are thin or soft, and the tongue is pale and perhaps slightly swollen. A *recommended starting dose* is ⅛ per 5 to 10 lb of body weight, or about 1 mg/kg of body weight, divided into two daily doses.
- Useful acupuncture points include PC 6 to calm the Heart; GV 20 to calm the mind; LIV 3, ST 36, and SP 6 to nourish Blood; BL 15, 20, and 23 to tonify the Heart, Spleen, and Kidney; and CV 6 or 12 to tonify Spleen Qi.

Qi and Blood Deficiency

- When both Qi and Blood deficiency are more pronounced, **Ren Shen Yang Ying Tang** (Ginseng Nutritive Decoction) is indicated. This formula bears many similarities to Gui Pi Tang described previously but has an even greater Blood- and Yin-tonifying action. In addition, it contains a small amount of Rou Gui to address Spleen Qi deficiency that has progressed to early Spleen and Kidney Yang deficiency. Guiding signs for this formula are otherwise similar to Gui Pi Tang, except the patient may have increased signs of Coldness and fatigue. A *recommended starting dose* is ⅛ tsp per 5 to 10 lb of body weight, or about 1 mg/kg of body weight, divided into two daily doses.
- Useful acupuncture points include PC 6 and GV 20 to calm the mind; LIV 3, ST 36, and SP 6 to nourish Blood; BL 15, 20, and 23 to tonify the Heart, Spleen, and Kidney; and CV 6 or 12 to tonify Spleen Qi.

Yin Deficiency

- A more fundamental and deep-seated fluid deficiency of the Heart is Yin deficiency. When Yin deficiency is present, a Deficiency Heat arises that leads to signs of mild Heat and Dryness, including heat intolerance, thirst, eye redness, dry stools, and panting. The Heart, as well as the Kidney, is affected, leading to possible nocturia and hind limb weakness or stiffness. The Heart appears more agitated, manifested as such signs as insomnia, restlessness, panting, and nocturnal vocalizations. Blood deficiency is often simultaneously present, since Yin is the foundation of Blood. Liver enzyme levels may be elevated, and the pulse is floating and somewhat forceful, or thin and rapid. The tongue is red and dry.
- The formula for Kidney and Heart Yin deficiency causing Empty Fire is **Tian Wang Bu Xin Dan** (Heavenly Ruler's Nourish the Heart Pellet). A *recommended starting dose* is ⅛ tsp per 5 to 10 lb of body weight, or about 1 mg/kg of body weight, divided into two daily doses.
- When Yin deficiency is primarily affecting the Kidney and Liver, **Zuo Gui Wan** (Replenish the Left Pill) should be considered. All of the signs calling for Tian Wang Bu

Xin Dan may be present, along with loss of hearing, increased heat intolerance and the seeking of cool places to rest, fatigue, thirst, insomnia, urinary incontinence, hind limb weakness, low back stiffness, and emaciation. The animal is usually elderly and may have some tendencies to develop idiopathic vestibular syndrome. The tongue is dry and red, and the pulse is rapid and thin.

- Useful acupuncture points include PC 6 and BL 15 to calm the mind; KI 2 or 6 to clear Empty Heat and nourish Kidney Yin; GV 20 to calm the mind; and BL 23, SP 6, and CV 4 to tonify the Kidneys.

Cautions

- Drugs with cholinergic or anticholinergic effects are known to interact with anti-Parkinsonian drugs and may have to be used with caution for patients with dementia that are taking Ginkgo.
- Ginkgo should also be used with caution for patients taking monoamine oxidase inhibitors, such as selegiline.
- Ginkgo has also been associated with clotting disorders and it should be withdrawn days to weeks before surgery.
- Melatonin has been associated with dysregulating effects in human diabetics; blood sugar levels should be monitored carefully in diabetic patients when melatonin is used. Melatonin may also suppress fertility.

AUTHORS' CHOICES:

SM: Appropriate Chinese herbal formulas and acupuncture points.
SW: Combinations of antioxidants, phosphatidylserine, acetyl-L-carnitine and Ginkgo.

COMPULSIVE DISORDERS (TAIL-CHASING, FLY-SNAPPING, LIGHT-CHASING, SOME AGGRESSION)

Therapeutic Rationale

- Psychomotor seizure, attention-seeking behavior, adult-onset hydrocephalus should be ruled out.

Alternative Options with Conventional Bases

- **Overvaccination should be avoided,** especially with rabies vaccine, which has been noted by some veterinarians to immediately worsen these disorders. It is theorized that some of these dogs have a subclinical form of immune-mediated meningitis that may be stimulated by vaccination and may be responsive to steroids.
- **Melatonin** may have a role in regulating brain function in compulsive disorders (Pacchierotto, 2001) and may be given a trial course.

Paradigmatic Options

- **Xiao Huo Luo Dan** (Minor Invigorate the Collateral Circulation Pill) has been recommended for use in compulsive disorders. This formula may relieve pain or discomfort that might cause tail-chasing or other signs of obsession with a body area. This formula is potentially toxic; it should be used only in appropriate cases and is not for extended use. Chapter 12 gives more information on this formula and recommendations regarding its use.
- Another formula that has been proposed for use in compulsive disorders is **Zhen Gan Xi Feng Tang** (Subdue the Endogenous Liver Wind Decoction). This is a strong formula for subduing Liver Wind and its various manifestations (dizziness, apoplexy, stroke, coma) when it arises secondary to Liver Yin deficiency. Listed among its indications for human use is an inability to control body movement. It may therefore prove useful for compulsive disorders in animals, provided the underlying cause is a Liver Yin deficiency. Guiding clinical signs include a red, dry tongue and a wiry, forceful pulse.
- When cases are predominated by clinical findings that suggest Blood stasis or Damp Heat, the practitioner should use **Xue Fu Zhu Yu Tang** (Dispel Stasis from the Mansion of Blood Decoction) or **Long Dan Xie Gan Tang** (Gentian Drain the Liver Decoction), respectively. For all formulas in this section, the dosage is about ¼ tsp per 15 to 20 lb of body weight, or 1 mg/kg of body weight, divided into two daily doses.

Cautions

- Melatonin has been suggested to alter blood glucose control in diabetic patients and may suppress fertility.

AUTHORS' CHOICES:

SM: Rule out and address physical causes of irritation.
SW: Avoid overvaccination; rule out physical disorders causing pain; attempt behavior modification.

FELINE INAPPROPRIATE URINATION

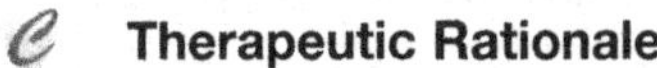

Therapeutic Rationale

- Rule out physical causes (e.g., infection, stone, inflammation, tumors).
- Reduce anxiety.

Alternative Options with Conventional Bases

- See section on Anxiety—any of the herbs recommended for anxiety may be considered for cats that urinate inappropriately because of stress or anxiety.

Paradigmatic Options

- Although an effort should be made to distinguish inappropriate urination resulting from inflammatory causes from inappropriate urination resulting from behavioral causes, many times they coexist. Thus resolution of cystitis reduces what seems to be a behavior problem. Treatment suggestions that focus on cystitis are given in Chapter 18.
- Formulas that primarily address behavioral problems are listed in the section on Chinese medicine that follows. Calming a distressed cat also reduces bladder inflammation and illustrates a tie that is recognized in the treatment of human interstitial cystitis. The close relationship between inflammation and behavioral problems in cats urinating outside of the litter box underscores the philosophy of Chinese medicine that there need not be a separate field of medicine for contending with psychological disorders. Rather, the mind and the body together are just arenas in which an

BOX 3-1 Environmental, Behavioral, and Other Approaches to Feline Inappropriate Urination

- Clean litter boxes daily.
- Keep litter boxes out of high-traffic or noisy areas.
- Increase the number of litter boxes (at least one per cat).
- Change litter types.
- Do not use litter box liners.
- Uncover covered boxes.
- Consider covering uncovered boxes if cat is seeking hidden areas in which to urinate.
- Offer a "smorgasbord" of litters—a variety of litter types (clumping, clay, pine/alfalfa pellets, etc.) in a line of litter boxes to determine substrate preference.
- Move food bowls to areas where the cat is eliminating.
- Move litter boxes to areas where the cat is eliminating; if the cat begins using the litter box, gradually move back to desired spot.
- If cat is eliminating in defined areas, cover them with aluminum foil or sheet plastic to give an undesirable substrate.
- Change dynamics of a multicat household—separate cats when not monitored or use gates or crates; cover outside windows, gradually reintroduce the cats after behavior is satisfactory.
- Treat soiled areas with odor removers and citrus-type sprays—cats are said to dislike citrus odor.
- Use Feliway to decrease territorial pressure.
- Confine the offender—use a small space and provide food and water; a small space will require the cat to use the litter box unless it wants urine and feces near its food.
- Give a favored treat as a reward when the cat uses the litter box.
- Punish the cat for going outside of the box *only by using a squirt gun if at all*—do not let the cat associate the owner with punishment.

underlying energetic dynamic is expressed by the body, and an appropriate treatment for the body is an appropriate treatment for the mind as well.

Chinese Medicine

- For the irritable cat that clearly urinates more when agitated or stressed, **Wu Yao Tang** (Lindera Decoction) can be considered. Cats that benefit may be chilly, experience forms of abdominal pain (e.g., colitis) when upset, have a wiry pulse, and a pale to lavender tongue.

This formula warms the abdomen and bladder and relieves abdominal pain when it is due to Liver Qi stagnation and perhaps Liver Blood deficiency. A *recommended starting dose* is ¼ tsp per 10 to 15 lb of body weight, or 1 mg/kg of body weight, administered in divided doses, twice daily.

- Acupuncture points to consider in tandem with Wu Yao Tang include BL 28 and CV 3 to influence the Bladder, and SP 6 and LIV 3 to nourish Liver Blood and move Qi in the lower abdomen.
- For anxious hot cats with hematuria and stranguria, **Dao Chi San** (Guide out the Red Powder) can be considered. A cat that will benefit will have a red, and perhaps even ulcerated, tongue. The cat may be thirsty and have a rapid and perhaps wiry pulse. Dao Chi San treats cystitis caused by Heart Fire, which manifests as a Shen disturbance. When the Heart Fire flares up, some of its Yang energy is transferred to the Small Intestine, which is the Yang organ paired with the Heart. The main function of the Small Intestine in the body is to transfer water from where it has been absorbed in the small intestinal tract to the Bladder. When Heart Fire blazes, its Heat is also conducted by the Small Intestine to the Bladder, where it manifests as cystitis. A *recommended starting dose* is ¼ tsp per 10 to 15 lb of body weight, or 1 mg/kg of body weight, administered in divided doses, twice daily.
- Acupuncture points to consider in tandem with Dao Chi San include PC 6 to calm the Shen and clear Heart Fire, and BL 28 and CV 3 as local points for the Bladder. SP 9 can be used to reduce the formation of Damp Heat in the Bladder.

Homeopathy

- **Staphysagria:** practitioners should consider this for the "sweet, downtrodden" cat that does not express irritation as aggression, but merely as vocalization. Often, this cat is very affectionate. There may be a history of chronic or recurrent cystitis. One pulse may be wiry and one slippery. The cat may show clear indications of resentment toward another animal or person, often manifesting as jealousy. A *recommended starting dose* is 30C once daily for 5 days, then as needed. When the case is obvious single doses of higher potencies may be considered.

Cautions

- See entry under Anxiety.

AUTHORS' CHOICES:

SM: Staphysagria 30C; treat cystitis as appropriate.
SW: Kava and Valerian for 4 to 8 weeks, combined with thorough investigation and correction of behavioral causes if physical cause is ruled out.

FELINE PSYCHOGENIC ALOPECIA, FUR-PULLING

Therapeutic Rationale

- Identify behavioral, neurologic, immunologic, parasitic, hormonal, or neoplastic causes.

Alternative Options with Conventional Bases

- **Rule out allergies** and other physical causes. These cats should undergo elimination diet trials.
- **St. John's Wort:** has been recommended by some practitioners. Interestingly, it has been historically used for skin lesions as well as peripheral neuropathy and may be worth trying for approximately 1 month.

Paradigmatic Options

- Feline hyperesthesia syndrome should be ruled out in cases of psychogenic alopecia in cats. This is especially true when the hair pulling is occurring on the flanks or back and not on the abdomen. See Chapter 14 for more information on treating feline hyperesthesia.

Homeopathy

- **Arsenicum album:** this should be considered for cats exhibiting psychogenic hair pulling. Signs suggesting that it may be of benefit include increased thirst, general tendencies to fearfulness and anxiety, restlessness and crying at night, increased appetite, relentless seeking of heat, a tendency to lose weight, and separation anxiety. A hallmark indication for its use in hair-pulling in particular is a tendency for the patient to experience profound skin irritation despite the absence of any lesions. A *suggested starting dose* is 30C once daily on an as-needed basis. Arsenicum should be discontinued if no improvement is shown after 1 week.

Cautions

- St. John's Wort causes photosensitivity. It also activates hepatocyte receptors that regulate expression of cytochrome P450 (CYP) enzymes and may increase the metabolism of some drugs, including indinavir, cyclosporin, and oral contraceptives.

AUTHORS' CHOICES:

SM: Anxiety herbs and approaches; address allergies; homeopathic Arsenicum.

SW: Investigate potential for allergies; acupuncture; anxiety approaches if physical causes are thoroughly investigated.

HYPERACTIVITY

Therapeutic Rationale

- Identify underlying hormonal or other disorder.
- Identify underlying anxiety.

Alternative Options with Conventional Bases

- **Increase** physical exercise and mental activity.

Paradigmatic Options

- Any Heat condition can manifest as hyperactivity. Heat in the body agitates the organs that are already Hot by nature, particularly the Heart. When Heat leads to the manifestation of other disorders such as colitis or skin disease, use of the appropriate formula for that condition often calms hyperactivity. When hyperactivity is the only concern, the formulas below can be considered.
- For Heat that is present in relative excess because of Yin deficiency, **Er Yin Jian** (Two Yin Brew) can be used. Guiding signs are a red, dry tongue or a tongue that

appears "delicate and clean" and varies from pink to red, a rapid and thin or thready pulse, insomnia, weight loss, tiredness aggravated by physical exertion, restlessness, nighttime vocalizations, and fearfulness. A *suggested starting dose* is about ⅛ tsp per 5 to 10 lb of body weight, or 1 mg/kg of body weight, divided into two daily doses. For Damp animals this formula should be used only with caution, if at all. They may be recognized by a tendency to weight gain, mucoid stools, weeping skin lesions, and otitis externa with yeast overgrowth.

- Acupuncture points that may be beneficial in cases of Heart Fire caused by Empty Heat include PC 6, SP 6, KI 2 or KI 6, BL 15, and BL 23. PC 6 and BL 15 cool the Heart, and BL 23 and SP 6 nourish Kidney Yin. KI 2 or 6 strongly nourishes Yin and clears Empty Heat.
- For Excess Heat that is due to Phlegm Fire Flaring Upward, **Wen Dan Tang** (Warm the Gall Bladder Decoction) can be considered. Animals that benefit have slippery, rapid pulses and red, wet tongues. Irritability, eye redness, aggressive or destructive tendencies, poor appetite, and sudden outbursts all may manifest from Phlegm Fire. To make the formula more powerful in clearing Heart Fire, the practitioner can add 6 to 9 g each of Huang Lian (Coptis) and Yu Jin (Curcuma) per 50 g of base formula.
- Acupuncture points that may be beneficial include GV 14, GV 26, GV 16, ST 40, CV 12, LIV 3, ST 44, and PC 6. LIV 3, ST 44, and GV 14 drain excessive Heat from the body. ST 40, CV 12, and PC 6 stop the formation of Phlegm. PC 6 also clears Heart Fire. GV 26 and GV 16 regulate the Governing Vessel to control Brain activity and pierce the turbidity that obscures rational thought.

Cautions

- None recognized.

AUTHORS' CHOICES:

SM: Appropriate Chinese herbal formula.
SW: Structured activity, such as agility, flyball, herding.

THUNDERPHOBIA

Therapeutic Rationale

- Reduce fear while instituting behavior modification.

Alternative Options with Conventional Bases

- **Melatonin:** a case report suggested that giving thunderphobic dogs melatonin 0.1 mg/kg of body weight bid (up to 3 mg tid), in combination with anxiolytics and behavior modification, was helpful in managing these dogs (Aronson, 1999). Melatonin can be given for a few days during times that thunderstorms are expected.

Paradigmatic Options

Homeopathy

- Several remedies are famous for treating fear of thunderstorms. A "true" fear of thunderstorms is suggested when the dog does not respond in a similar manner to comparable loud noises. If thunderstorms are just one of many noises to which an animal is sensitive, remedies for "noise sensitivity" in general should also be considered.
- **Phosphorus:** the classic remedy for animals fearing thunderstorms. Animals that benefit may appear Yin or Blood deficient from a Chinese medical perspective. It is common for animals that need Phosphorus to be abruptly affectionate to humans and a nuisance to other animals in the house. The nuisance behavior is best described as "excessive teasing" of other pets. Both extreme affection and teasing seem to arise from a tendency to have little concept of boundaries, which also characterizes some human patients benefiting from Phosphorus. Animals that benefit from Phosphorus are often thirsty. They are classically considered to desire cool places, although some animals may be chilly and desire warmth. They may vomit food or water shortly after eating. Colitis may be part of the past medical history, with a peculiar orange or yellow color to the stool. These animals commonly show a tendency toward weight loss, coughing, bleeding disorders, and

throat affectations, including dysphagia and loss of voice. A *suggested starting dose* is 30C given once daily as needed to address accompanying signs, with prophylactic doses given up to a few times before and during the actual storm.

- **Rhododendron:** a less well known remedy for thunderstorms. Its use should be considered when a fear of thunderstorms accompanies a significant history of rheumatic pains. Pains are typically worse on rising and with overexertion and better with gentle motion. When pain is directly aggravated by thunderstorms, Rhododendron may be especially appropriate. A *suggested starting dose* is 30C given once daily as needed to address accompanying signs, with prophylactic doses given up to a few times before and during the storm.
- **Aconitum napellus:** the general all-purpose remedy for fear and anxiety used by veterinary homeopaths. Patients that benefit may be alarmed even by gusts of wind. The animal may be extremely fearful, with forceful, rapid pulses, red eyes, and intense thirst. A *suggested dose* is 30C every 15 minutes. Discontinue if no benefit is seen after 45 minutes to an hour. Prophylactic doses may be needed before the storm. Give two doses separated by 1 to 2 hours before the storm.
- **Belladonna:** this has been used successfully to calm animals with a violent fear of thunderstorms. Even between storms, animals that benefit from Belladonna have dilated pupils and may seek to hide in dark places. Gums and eyes may be very red. A *suggested starting dose* is 30C given once daily as needed to address accompanying signs, with prophylactic doses given up to a few times before and during the storm.
- **Gelsemium:** the practitioner should consider this for fear of thunderstorms that manifests in dogs as urinary incontinence and cowering in a stationary position. Prophylactic doses (30C potency) may need to be given several times before and during the storm. Doses should be separated by at least 15 minutes, and treatment should be discontinued if no benefit is seen after 45 minutes to an hour.

- **Nat Mur:** patients that benefit from this are perhaps the most noise sensitive of all patients. Any loud noise may irritate or antagonize these patients, which are otherwise refined, quiet, and dignified. They frequently seek out quiet solitude and are loner animals. Other health complaints may include back pains or stiffness, allergic rhinitis, or urinary incontinence. From a Chinese perspective, this patient may appear to be Qi deficient. A *suggested starting dose* is 30C given once daily as needed to address accompanying signs, with prophylactic doses given up to a few times before and during the storm.

Chinese Medicine

- Fear of thunderstorms in animals in Chinese medicine is often considered merely an expression of a general tendency toward anxiety. In particular, many dogs exhibiting intractable noise sensitivity are also Blood deficient from a Chinese medical perspective, and treatment of this underlying disorder together with its symptomatic manifestations should also reduce attending tendencies to anxiety and noise sensitivity. The relevant chapters should be consulted for blood-tonifying formulas for problems in other organ systems. When no other problem is present, use of **Bu Gan Tang** as previously discussed in the section on Anxiety can be considered.

Cautions

- Melatonin may affect blood glucose regulation in diabetics and may suppress fertility.
- Some owners use the sedative herbs (Kava, Valerian, etc.), which may interact with or enhance the effects of anxiolytic drugs.

AUTHORS' CHOICES:

SM: Address underlying blood deficiencies; homeopathic remedies as appropriate.
SW: Melatonin; counterconditioning.

3 CASE REPORT
Inappropriate Urination by a Cat

HISTORY

Beauty, a 13-year-old, spayed female, black Domestic Shorthair cat, was brought for treatment with a chief complaint of inappropriate urination for the past year. Beauty especially preferred urinating on objects on the floor, including plastic bags, but she also urinated in other places, including the bed. Initial evaluation at a conventional veterinary medical facility included a urinalysis, complete blood count, and serum chemistry profile, all of which were within normal limits. Amitriptyline was prescribed and formulated for topical application in the pinna to relieve anxiety. The drug was effective in stopping inappropriate urination but seemed to have the side effect of depressing Beauty. A reduction of the dose minimized inappropriate urination to once every 3 to 4 weeks, but failed to lift Beauty's spirits. Further reductions in the dose resulted in a complete relapse of the condition. Unable to take Beauty off the medication but concerned about her depression, the owner sought alternatives.

At the time of presentation to the holistic veterinary medical clinic, Beauty was urinating only in the bedroom. The urine appeared to be dilute and clear, but Beauty's thirst was normal. A recent repeat of the complete blood count and serum chemistry profile showed results that were still within normal limits. The owner thought Beauty considered the bedroom a haven of sorts.

Beauty shared the house with two other cats, one of which was a male neutered Domestic Shorthair cat named Timmy. Timmy had been found to have lymphosarcoma a year earlier when he was hospitalized during the acute phase of the illness. He was currently asymptomatic under holistic care. Careful questioning established that Beauty's behavior problems started when Timmy was brought home from the veterinary clinic and he was commanding a lot of the owner's attention.

Despite the history, the owner did not feel that Beauty was inordinately jealous. Indeed, Beauty was observed by the owner to act submissively toward the other cats. Occasionally she would hiss if Timmy approached while she was in the owner's lap or if she entered the room to find Timmy in the owner's lap. Otherwise, Beauty was best described as timid and nervous but very affectionate to the owner.

Beauty's behavior toward Timmy marked a departure from their previous relationship. Beauty had been introduced to the household long after the other two cats. Although she was never "browbeaten" by either cat, only Timmy appeared to accept her. At this time, Timmy and Beauty were regularly observed to sleep together.

Additional questioning revealed no signs of abnormalities in other organ systems, except for a dull hair coat. Appetite and thirst were normal, and Beauty's body weight was stable. The only other visits to a veterinary clinic had been to receive annual vaccinations and routine dental hygiene. The last vaccination had been 18 months earlier

PHYSICAL EXAMINATION

During her examination Beauty was timid but affectionate. She had a slightly red tongue with strands of viscid saliva visible in the mouth. Her pulses were wiry and thin. The linea alba, or Conception Vessel, seemed especially taut in the lower abdomen over CV 3. BL 27 and 28 also seemed turgid and bulging relative to the surrounding area.

ASSESSMENT

Although no evidence of cystitis was found and Beauty's inappropriate urination seemed to be purely "behavioral" in origin, physical examination findings suggested the possibility of bladder inflammation. CV 3 and BL 28 are the "alarm" and "association" points of the bladder, respectively. Also, in Chinese medicine cystitis arises most commonly in dogs and cats from the accumulation of Damp Heat in the Bladder, which is usually accompanied by a red, wet tongue with wiry pulses.

TREATMENT

The Western herbal bladder formula containing Hydrangea *(Hydrangea arborescens)*, Corn Silk *(Zea mays)*, Gravel Root *(Eupatorium purpureum)*, and Stone Root *(Collinsonia canadensis)* was prescribed to address possible cystitis. Other considerations were the administration of homeopathic Cantharis for cystitis, homeopathic Staphysagria for inappropriate urination triggered by resentment in passive cats, and **Wu Yao Tang** (Lindera Decoction) for inappropriate urination associated with irritability and stress. Only the herbal formula was prescribed at the time of the first visit, however, at a dose of 0.2 ml per 5 lb of body weight, divided into three daily doses. If no episodes of inappropriate urination were seen after 1 month, the owner was to attempt to wean Beauty off amitriptyline.

OUTCOME

Follow-up after 3 weeks revealed a persistence of inappropriate urination, even though Beauty was still taking amitriptyline. The herbs had been given consistently for the entire 3 weeks. Physical examination revealed some improvement in the wetness of the tongue and the wiriness of the pulses. Nevertheless, Beauty was assessed as unchanged. Staphysagria 30C was then prescribed, at a dose of three pellets once daily for 1 week, tapering gradually to a dose of once weekly or as needed.

Two weeks later the owner reported that Beauty had been an "angel," and had been more even tempered than usual. She had once again started to sleep with Timmy. Her tongue had returned to normal, and her pulses were soft and pliable. After another 6 weeks of weekly doses of the homeopathic prescription, inappropriate urination had still not been observed, and the amitriptyline was discontinued. Two months later, while still being given Staphysagria weekly, Beauty remained affectionate to Timmy and had not urinated outside of the litter box.

DISCUSSION

The consistency of Beauty's inappropriate urination before the administration of the Staphysagria, as well as its sudden and complete cessation even off amitriptyline after use of the remedy, suggests the remedy had a genuine effect. Beauty also illustrated how all other signs of illness tend to normalize when a homeopathic medicine has been used effectively, including pulse and tongue findings and any other signs that were cited as a basis for the original assessment. In Beauty's case this included, most notably, an abrupt cessation of her long-standing animosity toward Timmy.

SM

REFERENCES

Aronson L. Animal behavior case of the month. *J Am Vet Med Assoc* 215(1):22-24, 1999.

Beaubrun G, Gray GE. A review of herbal medicines for psychiatric disorders. *Psychiatr Serv* 51(9):1130-1134, 2000.

Brooks JO III, Yesavage JA, Carta A, Bravi D. Acetyl L-carnitine slows decline in younger patients with Alzheimer's disease: a reanalysis of a double-blind, placebo-controlled study using the trilinear approach. *Int Psychogeriatr* 10(2):193-203, 1998.

Cauffield JS, Forbes HJ. Dietary supplements used in the treatment of depression, anxiety, and sleep disorders. *Lippincotts Prim Care Pract* 3(3):290-304, 1999.

Cenacchi T, Bertoldin T, Farina C, Fiori MG, Crepaldi G. Cognitive decline in the elderly: a double-blind, placebo-controlled multicenter study on efficacy of phosphatidylserine administration. *Aging* (Milano) 5(2):123-133, 1993.

Day C. *The Homeopathic Treatment of Small Animals: Principles and Practice.* Saffron Walden, England, 1990, C.W. Daniel.

Duncan KL, Hare WR, Buck WB. Malignant hyperthermia–like reaction secondary to ingestion of hops in five dogs. *J Am Vet Med Assoc* 210(1):51-54, 1997.

Ehling D. *The Chinese Herbalist's Handbook,* revised ed. Santa Fe, NM, 1996, Inword Press.

Flynn BL, Ranno AE. Pharmacologic management of Alzheimer disease. II. Antioxidants, antihypertensives, and ergoloid derivatives. *Ann Pharmacother* 33(2):188-197, 1999.

Grundman M. Vitamin E and Alzheimer disease: the basis for additional clinical trials. *Am J Clin Nutr* 71(2):630S-636S, 2000.

Houghton PJ. The scientific basis for the reputed activity of Valerian. *J Pharm Pharmacol* 51(5):505-512, 1999.

Jean-Louis G, von Gizycki H, Zizi F. Melatonin effects on sleep, mood, and cognition in elderly with mild cognitive impairment. *J Pineal Res* 25(3):177-183, 1998.

Mennini T, Bernasconi P, Bombardelli E, Morazzoni P. In vitro study on the interaction of extracts and pure compounds from *Valeriana officinalis* roots with GABA, benzodiazepine and barbiturate receptors. *Fitoterapia* 64:291-300, 1993.

Le Bars PL, Kastelan J. Efficacy and safety of a *Ginkgo biloba* extract. *Public Health Nutr* 3(4A):495-499, 2000.

Lim GP, Chu T, Yang F, Beech W, Frautschy SA, Cole GM. The curry spice curcumin reduces oxidative damage and amyloid pathology in an Alzheimer transgenic mouse. *J Neurosci* 21(21):8370-8377, 2001.

Pacchierotti C, Iapichino S, Bossini L, Pieraccini F, Castrogiovanni P. Melatonin in psychiatric disorders: a review on the melatonin involvement in psychiatry. *Front Neuroendocrinol* 22(1):18-32, 2001.

Petry RD, Reginatto F, de-Paris F, Gosmann G, Salgueiro JB, Quevedo J, Kapczinski F, Ortega GG, Schenkel EP. Comparative pharmacological study of hydroethanol extracts of *Passiflora alata* and *Passiflora edulis* leaves. *Phytother Res* 15(2):162-164, 2001.

Rockwood K, Kirkland S, Hogan DB, MacKnight C, Merry H, Verreault R, Wolfson C, McDowell I. Use of lipid-lowering agents, indication bias, and the risk of dementia in community-dwelling elderly people. *Arch Neurol* 59(2):223-227, 2002.

Salvioli G, Neri M. L-Acetylcarnitine treatment of mental decline in the elderly. *Drugs Exp Clin Res* 20(4):169-176, 1994.

Scott HD, Laake K. Statins for the prevention of Alzheimer's disease (Cochrane Review). *Cochrane Database Syst Rev* 4:CD003160, 2001.

Sopranzi N, De Feo G, Mazzanti G, Tolu L. Biological and electroencephalographic parameters in rats in relation to *Passiflora incarnata* L. *Clin Ter* 132(5):329-333, 1990.

Soulimani R, Younos C, Jarmouni S, Bousta D, Misslin R, Mortier F. Behavioural effects of *Passiflora incarnata* L. and its indole alkaloid and flavonoid derivatives and maltol in the mouse. *J Ethnopharmacol* 57(1):11-20, 1997.

Thal LJ, Calvani M, Amato A, Carta A. A 1-year controlled trial of acetyl-L-carnitine in early-onset AD. *Neurology* 55(6):805-810, 2000.

Warnecke G. Psychosomatic dysfunctions in the female climacteric: clinical effectiveness and tolerance of Kava extract WS 1490. *Fortschr Med* 109:119-122, 1991.

Xiao XQ, Zhang HY, Tang XC. Huperzine A attenuates amyloid beta-peptide fragment 25-35-induced apoptosis in rat cortical neurons via inhibiting reactive oxygen species formation and caspase-3 activation. *J Neurosci Res* 67(1):30-36, 2001.

Yan W. *Practical Therapeutics of Traditional Chinese Medicine.* Brookline, Mass, 1997, Paradigm Publications.

Yeung H. *Handbook of Chinese Herbal Formulas.* Los Angeles, 1995, Self-published.

Yeung H. *Handbook of Chinese Herbs.* Los Angeles, 1996, Self-published.

4

Therapies for Cardiovascular Disorders

CONGESTIVE HEART FAILURE

Therapeutic Rationale

- Correct treatable inciting causes.
- Improve cardiac output (optimize heart rate, control arrhythmias, vasodilate, improve myocardial function).
- Reduce workload.
- Block excessive activation of neuroendocrine systems.
- Control the consequences of failure, such as congestive signs (pulmonary edema, ascites, and arrhythmias) and low output signs (like weakness, syncope, arrhythmias, increased sympathetic tone, and azotemia) (Nelson and Couto, 1998).

Alternative Options with Conventional Bases

- This is an introduction to complementary, integrative and unconventional therapies for heart disease in general. Since the specific cardiovascular conditions that follow may all lead to signs of congestive failure, herbal and nutritional supplements and the traditional Chinese medicine (TCM) pathologic principles may be identical to those listed for heart failure and therefore will not be repeated.

Herbs

- **Hawthorn** *(Crataegus oxyacantha):* may increase myocardial contractility, and reduce peripheral vascular resistance. Most trials indicate greatest effect after 6 to 8 weeks of use. May increase effect of cardiac glycosides (Jellin, 1999).

BOX 4-1 Herbs for the Cardiovascular System: Potential Activities

Decrease Peripheral Resistance
Hawthorn
Garlic
Ginkgo
Evodia
Coleus
Salvia

Antiarrhythmics
Berberine-containing herbs
Stephania

Negative Chronotropes
Garlic
Evodia

Positive Inotropes
Hawthorn
Evodia
Coleus

Antiatherosclerotics
Garlic
Terminalia

Anticoagulants
Garlic
Salvia

- **Garlic** *(Allium sativum):* popular in management of human cardiovascular disease; evidence suggests that the primary focus of action is on modulating blood lipids and controlling atherosclerotic disease, although one study in dogs indicated capacity to reduce diastolic blood pressure and heart rate (Martin, 1992; Nagourney, 1998).
- **Ginkgo** *(Ginkgo biloba):* traditional treatment that appears to have vasodilatory effects in peripheral circulation and has antioxidant capacity by virtue of the flavonoids it contains.
- **Coptis** *(Coptis chinensis),* Barberry *(Berberis vulgaris),* Oregon Grape *(Mahonia aquifolium):* a primary constituent that determines the actions of these three herbs is berberine, which decreases heart rate and may act like a class III antiarrhythmic (Huang, 1992; Riccioppo, 1993).
- **Evodia** *(Evodia rutaecarpa):* used in Chinese herbal combinations and known as Wu Zhu Yu, this herb is not used as a single herb. Various extracts have negative chronotropic, vasorelaxant, and vasodilatory actions in vitro; one study showed that an extract had positive inotropic action; the only published study in cats showed

no cardiorespiratory effects, but the extract did enhance cerebral blood flow (Haji, 1994).

- **Coleus** *(Coleus forskolii)* (Baumann, 1990): the forskolin extract increases myocardial contractile strength and peripheral vasodilation and may also reduce cardiac preload and afterload, possibly by activating adenylate cyclase.
- ***Terminalia arjuna*** (Bharani, 1995): used for a variety of cardiovascular diseases; most appropriate for humans, rather than animals as evidence to date points to beneficial effects on cholesterol levels and coronary artery disease.
- ***Salvia miltiorrhiza:*** traditionally used in Chinese herbal combinations (the pinyin name is Dan Shen or Tan Seng), this herb may increase coronary circulation, decreases resistance, and has anticoagulant activity (Huang, 2000). A study in perfused rat hearts suggested greater recovery after ischemic insult when Dan Shen was used (Takeo, 1990). Studies measuring relaxation in peripheral vasculature taken from dogs showed that Dan Shen induces a dose-related hypotension (Lei, 1986).
- **Korean Ginseng** *(Panax ginseng):* known in Chinese as Ren Shen, this herb is used singly and in combinations of Chinese herbs. It increases heart rate, prolongs contraction time (may act like a calcium channel blocker), and acts as a vasoconstrictor in small doses and a vasodilator in large doses (Huang, 1998).
- **Stephania** *(Stephania tetranda):* known as Fang Ji and seen in Chinese herbal combinations. This herb is a calcium channel blocker (Bone, 1997). Avoid products in which the Stephania is labeled Mu Tong—it may be substituted with Aristolochia, a toxic herb that has been shown to cause renal failure and cancer. At this time Chinese herbal products are routinely screened in Canada and the United States prior to sale to ensure they do not contain Aristolochia but it is recommended that practitioners be thoroughly familiar with their supplier's policies.
- **Other herbs** with less well documented cardiovascular effects:

Bugleweed *(Lycopus virginicus):* see section on hyperthyroidism.

Motherwort *(Leonurus cardiaca).*

Cayenne *(Capsicum nanum):* capsaicin, a single extract of Capsicum, caused hypertension in dogs and cats when given intravenously. Peripheral vasoconstriction in anesthetized dogs (followed by hypotension) and isolated arterial strips appeared mediated through cholinergic mechanisms (Toda, 1972). How this demonstrated effect is related to oral ingestion of the whole herb is unknown.

- Herbs with cardioactive glycosides—indicated in traditional texts; may be useful but toxic and potentially fatal!

  Lily of the Valley *(Convallaria majalis).*

  Foxglove *(Digitalis purpurea).*

  Scilla *(Scilla maritima).*

Nutrition

- **Marine lipid/ω-3 fatty acids**: modulates cytokines (insulin-like growth factor 1, interleukin-1 beta, tumor necrosis factor), which affect survival in canine chronic heart failure (Freeman, 1998). Reduces electrical excitability, increases refractory period, and reduces calcium availability and release, reduces potential for arrhythmia (Billman 1999; Negretti, 2000; Leaf, 1998). *Recommended dose:* 150 mg EPA and DHA/kg of body weight, but best researched dose (Freeman, 1998) is EPA 40 mg/kg of body weight and DHA 25 mg/kg of body weight.
- **Coenzyme Q_{10}**: catalyses ATP production and supports energy metabolism; also an antioxidant. Indicated in ischemic disease (Rush, 1996; Jellin, 1999). May take months for evidence of effects. More indicated in human cardiovascular conditions as a primary indication is ischemic heart disease. *Dose:* Dogs—2.2 to 22 mg/kg of body weight daily.
- **Vitamin E:** rising levels of free radicals resulting from oxidative stress are thought to promote myocardial decompensation. Vitamin E levels may be decreased in dogs with naturally occurring idiopathic dilated cardiomyopathy (Freeman, 1999). Cats with dilated cardiomyopathy and hyperthyroid heart disease also

had low Vitamin E levels (Fox, 1993). Vitamin E may be supplemented at approximately 5 to 10 IU/lb of body weight sid.

- **Selenium:** an antioxidant mineral that enhances the effects of Vitamin E and a cofactor for glutathione peroxidase, both properties that help reduce oxidative stress. In addition, selenium is involved in arachidonic acid metabolism, which may also affect prostanoid levels. Supplement as part of combination antioxidant products, at approximately 2 to 50 μg daily.
- **Magnesium:** prevents arrhythmias in human ischemic heart disease, regulates vascular smooth muscle tone, and may have inotropic effects. *Dose:* 10 mg and up qd (1 to 2 mEq/kg of body weight per day, roughly equivalent to 5 mg/lb of body weight per day); contraindicated in renal disease.
- **Carnitine:** improves myocardial metabolism and has been shown to be protective in one human myocardial disease model. Carnitine was shown to be effective in American Cocker Spaniels with dilated cardiomyopathy at a dose of 1 g tid (Kittleson, 1997), and a family of boxers with dilated cardiomyopathy at 2 g tid (Keene, 1991). The response in other breeds with dilated cardiomyopathies is less consistent. *Dose:* approximately 50 to 150 mg/kg of body weight tid.
- **Taurine:** improves clinical parameters in human patients with congestive heart failure. *Dose:* 50 to 100 mg/kg of body weight sid to tid. (American cocker spaniels with their unique cardiomyopathy should be treated at 500 mg tid.)
- **Glandular (heart),** or dietary raw heart: dietary administration of heart to patients with heart disease is an ancient practice with little supporting data. Theoretically, healthy slaughterhouse heart would contain higher concentrations of nutritional factors important to the function of that tissue.

Paradigmatic Options

- A number of Chinese herbal formulas have been suggested for use in different types of heart failure, as assessed from the Chinese medical perspective. A small number of them are listed below, with dozens more Heart formulas available in texts on Chinese herbal medicine.

- For Qi and Blood stagnation (purple tongue, irregular pulse, obvious pain), consider **Fu Fang Dan Shen Pian** (Compound Dan Shen Pill). This pill contains only Dan Shen *(S. miltiorrhiza)* and is used for coronary artery disease in humans. Dan Shen is to some extent an all-in-one heart drug, since it has been credited with the following functions:
  - Improved capillary microcirculation
  - Coronary artery dilation
  - Tissue regeneration and repair
  - Blood clotting reduction and fibrinolysis enhancement
  - Lowering of blood cholesterol

  A *suggested starting dose* is 1 tablet per 7 lbs of body weight per day, in divided doses. Larger doses may be used with appropriate supervision, since the herb is quite safe.
- For Kidney, Liver, and Heart Yin deficiency (red, dry tongue, thready, fast pulse, hyperactivity or restlessness, thoracic pain, insomnia, hind limb weakness, dizziness, declining body weight), consider **Zuo Gui Yin** (Restore the Left Drink). This formula is very rich and should not be used in animals with a history of Dampness symptoms (e.g., cystitis, colitis, seborrhea oleosa, weight gain). For painful animals, to 75 g of base formula, add:
  - 9 g Dang Gui
  - 12 g Dan Shen
  - 6 g Chuan Xiong
  - 9 g Yu Jin
- Alternatively, some authors have recommended combining **Zuo Gui Wan** and **Xue Fu Zhu Yu Tang** for patients with marked chest pain, which is difficult to document, if it occurs, in animals. For hypertensive animals, to 75 g base formula, add:
  - 12 g He Shou Wu
  - 12 g Nu Zhen Zi
  - 9 g Gou Teng
  - 15 g Shi Jue Ming
  - 15 g Mu Li
  - 15 g Bie Jia

Recommended starting dose of granular concentrate is 60 mg per lb of body weight, or approximately ¼ tsp per 15 to 20 lb of body weight, divided into two daily doses.

- For cases in which it is suspected that Phlegm is Obstructing the Heart Blood a formula based on **Wen Dan Tang** (Warm the Gall Bladder Decoction) has been suggested. Patients that benefit have a deep, slow pulse, unusual behaviors such as hyperactivity or depression, and low appetite. Traditional indications of Wen Dan Tang also suggest it should be considered for hot patients with red, moist, coated tongues, heat intolerance, irritability, and rapid, slippery, and wiry pulses. The ingredients are as follows:

Ban Xia	13%
Chen Pi	6%
Zhu Ru	17%
Zhe Ke	6%
Fu Ling	15%
Dang Shen	20%
Gan Cao	6%

All of the ingredients are found in Wen Dan Tang except for Dang Shen, which is added as a Spleen Qi tonifier. For cases in which Phlegm obstructs the Heart orifices (lethargy, fearfulness, mania, full abdomen, slippery pulse, foam in mouth, chest stuffiness), consider Wen Dan Tang itself.

- **Xue Fu Zhu Yu Tang** (Drive Out Stasis in the Mansion of Blood Decoction) is used to treat obstruction of the Heart by Blood stasis. This is quite a commonly indicated formula for the dog, a species that is especially prone to Blood stasis. The formula addresses Blood stasis arising from Blood deficiency and subsequent Qi stagnation. It may be useful in early heart failure and especially when there is evidence of pulmonary congestion. Other guiding signs to its use include a dry alopecic coat with fine dander, fear aggression, a history of recurrent mast cell tumor or allergic dermatitis, a thin and wiry pulse, a pale to lavender tongue, and sensitivity over the thoracic vertebrae and chest regions. *Recommended starting dose* of granular concentrate is 60 mg per lb of body weight, or approximately ¼ tsp per 15 to 20 lb of body weight, divided into two daily doses.

- When an Accumulation of Yin Cold (dyspnea, palpitation, cold extremities, pale tongue, weak pulse) is present, **Qiang Xin Yin** (Strengthen Heart Decoction) or **Zhen Wu Tang** should be considered. Qiang Xin Yin tonifies Yang and Qi in addition to nourishing Yin and activating Blood. Signs in patients that benefit include a pale or purple, wet tongue, weakness, and weak pulses. The formula contains the following:

Yin Yang Huo	12%
Fu Zi	5%
Huang Qi	12%
Dang Shen	12%
Huang Jing	9%
Mai Men Dong	12%
Dan Shen	12%
Yi Mu Cao	21%
Gan Cao	5%

- **Zhen Wu Tang** (Water Controlling God Decoction) is especially indicated in cold, weak patients with substantial edema accumulation. The diuretic action of this formula can be further enhanced with the addition of 12 g each of Ze Xie, Yi Yi Ren, and Che Qian Zi to 40 g of the base formula. *Recommended starting dose* of granular concentrate is 60 mg per lb of body weight, or approximately ¼ tsp per 15 to 20 lb of body weight, divided into two daily doses.
- For Oppression of the Heart by Water and Phlegm, manifested as arrhythmias, dyspnea, edema of extremities, cold extremities, a gray-purple tongue, and a rapid, irregular pulse, a modification of **Zhen Wu Tang** can be considered. This formula is actually closer in content and design to **Wu Ling San** (Five Ingredients with Poria Powder), which is a strong diuretic formula. Its ingredients are as follows:

Gui Zhi	20%
Gan Jiang	16%
Bai Zhu	16%
Fu Ling	16%
Zhu Ling	16%
Bai Shao Yao	16%

- For Deficiency of Qi and Yin (signs worse after moving, "dizziness," red tongue, weak irregular pulse, shortness of breath), a combination of 30 g of **Sheng Mai San** (Restore the Pulse Beverage) with 100 g of **Ren Shen Yang Rong Tang** (Ginseng Construction Nourishing Decoction) should be considered. When the pulse has become erratic or intermittent in Qi- and Yang-deficient patients, **Zhi Gan Cao Tang** (Honey-Fried Licorice Decoction) should be considered. *Recommended starting dose* of granular concentrate for both formulas is 60 mg per lb of body weight, or approximately ¼ tsp per 15 to 20 lb of body weight, divided into two daily doses.
- For complete collapse or shock with pallor, faint pulse, and coldness, **Shen Fu Tang** (Ginseng and Aconite Decoction) can be used to rescue the patient's Qi and Yang. This formula is for emergency use only and should not be used long term. *Recommended starting dose* of granular concentrate is 60 mg per lb of body weight, or approximately ¼ tsp per 15 to 20 lb of body weight, given every half hour until the shock is improved.

Western Herbs

- In my practice (SM), cases of congestive heart failure in animals refractory to conventional therapy seem frequently to not match the indications of the various Chinese herbal formulas listed previously. Western herbal medicine seems to hold more promise for stabilizing the condition in these patients. Although experimentation with different herbal formulas is still ongoing, some principles of general herbal formula design for congestive heart failure now seem apparent. A successful herbal formula generally fulfills the following three key functions.

Slowing of the heart rate

- A rapid heart rate is usually interpreted in alternative medicine as a sign of Heat. In the case of congestive heart failure, however, a rapid heart rate is best considered a form of spasm. Relaxant herbs are needed to relieve this "spasm." Some relaxants are sweet tasting, including Honey-Fried Licorice in Chinese herbal medicine and

Lime Blossoms *(Tilia vulgaris)* and Mistletoe *(Viscum album)* in Western herbal medicine. Antispasmodic herbs also are often Qi and Blood movers by nature, including Motherwort, Bugleweed, Passion Flower, Valerian, and Lily of the Valley. Even Lily of the Valley, known in herbal folklore as the "poor man's digitalis," seems to lack adequate moving power in severe cases of refractory heart failure. Dan Shen *(Salvia miltiorrhiza)* in Chinese medicine may be one possible treatment, but early Western herbalism had another solution, namely, the accentuation of the blood-moving action of these cardiac herbs with the addition of a small amount of Lobelia *(Lobelia inflata)*. Lobelia seems to interact synergistically with virtually any other Qi mover, as well as contribute symptomatic benefits of its own, such as a reduction of pulmonary edema through the promotion of expectoration (Brinker, 1995).

- Other herbs that are potentially useful in slowing a rapid heart rate include Hawthorn, Barberry, and Skullcap *(Scutellaria laterifolia)*. These herbs rein in "excess energy" in the Heart by clearing Heat (Skullcap, Barberry) or astringing Heart Qi and nourishing Heart Blood (Hawthorn). Green Oat Seeds *(Avena sativa)* combine with either of these two herbs to help nourish the Yin and Blood of the Heart.

Reduction of afterload

- Herbs that help open the vascular beds of the body to reduce afterload include the "diffusives" of 19th-century Western herbalism. These herbs include Pleurisy Root *(Asclepias tuberosa)*, Cayenne, and Prickly Ash Bark *(Xanthoxylum americanum)*. Garlic may also be considered here, and has the added benefit of reducing platelet aggregation and the tendency toward thrombus formation in cases prone to "sludging." These warming herbs also enhance the action of the Qi and Blood movers used to slow heart rate, creating a valuable synergy. Cayenne is also used to strengthen the pulse of chilly, weak patients and to cryptically slow the pulse of patients who feel hot in the upper body and cold in the lower body. Juniper *(Juniperus communis)* is another plant that can be considered as a diffusive. Juniper is contraindicated in patients with chronic renal failure and patients with glomerulonephritis. All the herbs in this section are very powerful and should make up a relatively small amount of formulas in which they are used.

Reduction of preload

- A means of reducing preload is through the use of diuretics. Dandelion *(Taraxacum officinalis)* has been categorized as a potassium-sparing diuretic, but the diuretic most commonly used in herbal management of heart disease in 19th-century Western herbalism is probably Parsley *(Petroselinum crispum)*. Long-term use of parsley in large doses may, however, lead to nerve damage.

Western Herbal Formulas

- Knowledge of the energetics of Western cardiac herbs gives us a foundation for understanding some formulas for heart disease that have been suggested for the management of human cardiac disease.
- A formula directed at improving cardiac output advocated by David Winston of the company Herbalist and Alchemist is Hawthorn Compound. It contains Hawthorn Flower and Berry, Ginkgo Leaf, Lemon Balm *(Melissa officinalis)*, Lime/Linden Flowers *(Tilia* spp.*)*, Prickly Ash Bark, Bugleweed, and Cactus *(Selenicereus grandiflorus)*. Cactus is a potentially toxic plant. In this formula, Hawthorn and Gingko serve as Blood tonics, Lemon Balm moves Qi, Lime Flowers relax the heart, and the rest of the herbs move Blood. A *recommended starting dose* is 0.1 ml of tincture per 5 lb of body weight, divided into two or three doses per day.
- Hoffman has suggested a formula for "heart weakness" that may also have antiarrhythmic properties. It consists of 2 parts Hawthorn, 2 parts Motherwort, and 1 part Lily of the Valley (potentially toxic). This formula primarily nourishes and moves Blood and would be expected to help slow tachyarrhythmias from Blood deficiency or "heart muscle spasm." The pulse of the patient benefiting from this formula will be thin, fast, and wiry. A *recommended starting dose* is 0.1 ml of tincture per 5 lb of body weight, divided into two or three doses per day.

- Hoffman also advocates a formula more specific for cardiac arrhythmias, consisting of 2 parts Motherwort, 1 part Mistletoe (toxic), and 1 part Valerian. This formula moves Qi, moves Blood, and "softens" the heart muscle. A *recommended starting dose* is 0.1 ml of tincture per 5 lb of body weight, divided into two or three doses per day.
- A formula for severe congestive heart failure might consist of 10 ml Lobelia (potentially toxic), 20 ml Parsley, 15 ml Pleurisy Root, 10 ml Skullcap, 15 ml Prickly Ash Bark, and 15 ml Lily of the Valley. In this formula, Lobelia and Lily of the Valley move Qi and Blood, potentiated by the diffusive action of Pleurisy Root and Prickly Ash Bark. Skullcap cools the upper body to slow the heart, and Parsley and Lobelia remove accumulated edema. A *recommended starting dose* is 0.1 ml of tincture per 5 lb of body weight, divided into two or three doses per day. Continued use in high doses will result in Lobelia toxicity, manifested as retching and vomiting. This side effect wears off over several days when the formula is discontinued.
- Much work remains to be done in identifying consistently effective herbal formulas for congestive heart failure in animals. Practitioners are encouraged to use these formulas as a starting point from which to mount their own exploration of the role of herbs in the management of heart disease.

Cautions

- Hawthorn may enhance the effects of digitalis and cardiotonic herbs such as Lily of the Valley.
- Garlic may potentiate the effect of anticoagulants, may potentiate the hypoglycemic effect of insulin, and may aggravate bleeding tendencies.
- Ginkgo potentiates the effect of anticoagulants and may potentiate the effect of monoamine oxidase inhibitors.
- Ginseng may potentiate the hypoglycemic effect of insulin.
- Evodia is to be used with caution in the presence of hypotensives and vasodilators, although Chinese medical literature and clinical experience with the herb in humans suggests Evodia can also have a mild hypertensive effect.

- Coleus theoretically may potentiate the positive inotropic action of digoxin, Foxglove, Hawthorn, and Lily of the Valley.
- Carnitine is a competitive inhibitor of thyroxine at peripheral receptors.
- Magnesium is contraindicated for patients with renal disease because of risk of hypermagnesemia.

AUTHORS' CHOICES:

SM: Magnesium; CoQ_{10}; appropriate Western herbal formula; Chinese herbal formulas may be less useful.
SW: Fish Oil; Magnesium; Western herbs; Carnitine; Taurine.

DILATED CARDIOMYOPATHY (SEE CONGESTIVE HEART FAILURE)

Therapeutic Rationale

- Optimize cardiac output (increase contractility and decrease peripheral resistance).
- Prevent arrhythmias.
- Decrease oxidative stress caused by circulatory insufficiency.
- Rule out metabolic and nutritional abnormalities such as hypothyroidism, use of lamb- and rice-based diets, and taurine deficiency.

Alternative Options with Conventional Bases

- **See introductory section** for possible applicability of Carnitine, Taurine, Fish Oil, antioxidants, and Coenzyme Q_{10}.
- **Herbs** that are theoretically useful include Ginseng, Coleus, Hawthorn, Lily of the Valley, and Scilla (the last two are too toxic to be considered routinely and should be used only by prescription of an herbalist experienced in formula design).
- **Magnesium** deficiency is associated with cardiomyopathy in several species, and magnesium may help suppress ventricular arrhythmias. The myocardium depends on large amounts of magnesium for proper

function, with magnesium concentrations in the heart muscle typically exceeding plasma concentrations by 23 times. Magnesium supplementation may be attempted orally; however, absorption of magnesium from the gastrointestinal (GI) tract is self-limiting because of its tendency to produce osmotic diarrhea, thereby accelerating gut motility and decreasing transit times. Accordingly, magnesium may be given by injection to affected patients. A *suggested starting dose* of magnesium sulfate is 10 mg/kg of body weight given twice weekly by subcutaneous injection. Frequency can be reduced as clinical improvement is noted. Renal failure is a contraindication for magnesium administration.

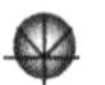

Paradigmatic Options

- For cats with aortic thrombus, **Qi Bu San** (Seven Tonification Powder) has been advocated. This formula warms Yang, moves Blood, and eliminates stasis. On analysis, it does not seem specific for the cat with aortic thrombosis, but contains the following:

Codonopsis	Dang Shen	10%
Atractylodes	Bai Zhu	10%
Poria	Fu Ling	10%
Dioscorea	Shan Yao	8%
Astragalus	Huang Qi	10%
Angelica	Dang Gui	10%
Zizyphus	Suan Zao Ren	10%
Gentiana	Qin Jiao	7%
Hordeum	Mai Ya	5%
Melia	Chuan Lian Zi	5%
Cyperus	Xiang Fu	5%
Citrus	Chen Pi	5%
Licorice	Gan Cao	5%

Cautions

- Hawthorn may enhance the effects of digitalis and cardiotonic herbs such as Lily of the Valley.
- Garlic may potentiate the effect of anticoagulants, may potentiate the hypoglycemic effect of insulin, and may aggravate bleeding tendencies.
- Ginkgo potentiates the effect of anticoagulants and may potentiate the effect of monoamine oxidase inhibitor.

- Ginseng may potentiate the hypoglycemic effect of insulin.
- Evodia is to be used with caution in the presence of hypotensives and vasodilators, although Chinese medical literature and clinical experience with the herb in humans suggests Evodia can also have a mild hypertensive effect.
- Coleus theoretically may potentiate the positive inotropic action of digoxin, Foxglove, Hawthorn, and Lily of the Valley.
- Carnitine is a competitive inhibitor of thyroxine at peripheral receptors.
- Magnesium is contraindicated for patients with renal disease because of risk of hypermagnesemia.

AUTHORS' CHOICES:

SM: Appropriate Chinese herbal formula from general section.
SW: Taurine; Carnitine; Fish Oil; Western herbal formulas.

HEARTWORM DISEASE (SEE CONGESTIVE HEART FAILURE)

Therapeutic Rationale

- Kill parasites.
- Reduce intimal damage.
- Control secondary heart failure.
- Prevent thromboembolism.

Alternative Options with Conventional Bases

- **Black Walnut** *(Juglans nigra)*: a popular treatment for gastrointestinal (GI) parasites as well as heartworm disease, for which there are no data. Black Walnut Hull has also been recommended for heartworm prevention at a dosage of approximately 1 capsule of ground herb per day, but long-term safety is unknown. Therapy should be discontinued if diarrhea arises.
- **Homeopathic heartworm nosodes:** popular for the prevention and treatment of canine heartworm disease. Efficacy is unknown, but prophylactic use of nosodes is not generally endorsed in human homeopathic medicine, and anecdotal reports of heartworm infection

while using heartworm nosodes make this alternative inadvisable.

- **Ginger** *(Zingiber officinalis):* 100 mg/kg of body weight of alcoholic extract of Ginger, given subcutaneously by 12 injections to dogs infected with heartworms, caused 98% reduction in microfilarial counts and appeared to have some adulticide activity (Datta, 1987). How this study relates to oral dosing is uncertain.
- **Andrographis** *(Andrographis paniculata):* Three subcutaneous injections of water extract at 0.06 ml/kg of body weight reduced *Dipetalonema reconditum* numbers by 85% (Dutta, 1982).

Paradigmatic Options

- The reported efficacy of Ginger, an aromatic herb, in the management of heartworm disease in dogs is consistent with a general clinical approach to internal parasitism that has existed in China for well over 1000 years.
- Internal parasitism was known then as Gu syndrome and herbal formulas to address this problem contained heavy amounts of aromatic herbs. Modern pharmacology credits the aromatic constituents of many of these herbs with significant antimicrobial properties, including action against internal nematodes. Chinese medicine selected aromatic herbs for Gu syndrome because of their apparent ability to be readily absorbed by virtually every tissue. The lipid solubility of aromatic herbal constituents accounts for their high absorption, lending them a strong theoretical clinical advantage over less readily absorbed astringent herbs such as Black Walnut. Aromatic herbs also have the advantage of helping improve circulation, an important consideration in canine heartworm disease.
- Several aromatic herbs have been identified to contain antinematodal aromatic compounds, including Garlic, Wormwood *(Artemisia absinthum)*, Thyme *(Thymus vulgaris)*, Cinnamon *(Cinnamonum* spp.*)*, Peppermint *(Mentha piperita)*, and Ginger. Wormwood, Thyme, and Peppermint are classed as cooling herbs, and Ginger, Garlic, and Cinnamon are classed as warming herbs. They can therefore be combined into a "thermally"

balanced formula for the treatment of canine heartworm disease. Garlic has the added advantage of reducing platelet aggregation, thus helping to reduce thrombus formation in severely compromised cardiac patients.

- A suggested formula including some of the above herbs is 14 ml Ginger, 9 ml Wormwood, 4 ml Garlic, 14 ml Thyme, and 9 ml Cinnamon. A *recommended starting dose* is 0.1 ml of tincture per 5 lb of body weight, divided into two or three doses per day. Additional amounts may be given at the practitioner's discretion.
- Use of similar formulas in tandem with Bromelain (see following paragraph) has been effective in converting heartworm-positive dogs to heartworm-negative status in my practice (SM). The formula should be discontinued if no reduction in heartworm antigen is observed within 2 months. The formula should also be discontinued in the event of any evidence of abnormal behavior or neurotoxicity, which is a potential side effect of Wormwood in high doses or over long periods of administration. Owners may wish to give the tincture in gelatin capsules with food to reduce side effects of GI irritation and to compensate for the low palatability of the formula.
- The potent vermifugal effects of aromatic herbs have led some practitioners using these herbs to be concerned about the risks of pulmonary thrombosis from sudden heartworm die-offs. Accordingly, Bromelain has been advocated as a supplement to break down dead worms through systemic proteolysis or by disrupting antigen-antibody complexes. Bromelain has also been observed to have antinematodal effects within the digestive tract. Bromelain is given 2 hours before or after meals. A *recommended starting dose* is approximately 30 mg per lb of body weight, divided into two or three daily doses.

Cautions

- Ginger, in high doses, may interfere with calcium channel blocker therapy.

AUTHORS' CHOICES:

SM: Western herbal formula with Bromelain.
SW: Conventional treatment; possibly Ginger, Black Walnut, or Western herbal formulas.

HYPERTENSION (SEE CONGESTIVE HEART FAILURE)

Therapeutic Rationale

- Reduce blood pressure (decrease cardiac output or vasodilate).

Alternative Options with Conventional Bases

- **Garlic:** has mild antihypertensive properties in humans.
- **Stephania** *(Stephania tetrandra):* known in Chinese medicine as Fang Ji, may act as a calcium channel blocker but should be used only in traditional formulas until it is better investigated as a single agent.
- **Uncaria** *(Uncaria rhynchophylla):* Gou Teng in Chinese formulas. This herb mediates endothelium-dependent relaxation in spontaneously hypertensive rats in in vitro studies. One extract resulted in peripheral vasodilation in anesthetized dogs (Ozaki, 1990).
- ***Clerodendron trichotomum:*** extract given intravenously to anesthetized dogs resulted in increased renal blood flow and led to reduced blood pressure in spontaneously hypertensive rats (Lu, 1994).
- **Berberine-containing herbs:** Coptis, Barberry, and Oregon Grape are negative chronotropes.
- **Acupuncture** may assist in modulating blood pressure (Williams, 1991; Yao, 1993).

Paradigmatic Options

- Hypertension is usually considered a form of rising energy, in the form of either Heat or Qi. Heat can be truly excessive, such as when there is an excess of a Yang pathogen, or present in relative excess, resulting from a Yin deficiency. In addition, hypertension may be caused by a rise of Qi resulting from obstruction of its normal downward path. From a Chinese medical perspective, hot pungent herbs like Garlic are contraindicated much of the time for the management of hypertension. The exception might be cases in which the normal descent of Qi is obstructed by Dampness accumulations.

For excess Yang pathogens

- Excess Yang pathogens usually affect the hot organs of the body, namely the Liver and the Heart. **Long Dan Xie Gan Tang** (Gentian Purge the Liver Decoction) is a formula useful for hypertension arising from excess Liver Fire and resultant excess Heart Fire. The pulse of affected patients is fast, wiry, and forceful, and the tongue is red and wet or frothy. Patients often have a history of Dampness-related complaints such as moist eczema, cystitis, colitis, and seborrhea oleosa. They may also be aggressive or hyperactive and are frequently heat intolerant. Thirst and appetite may be elevated, and patients may have a tendency to gain weight. Cool places are sought. Possible additives to 75 g of base formula include:
  12 g Gou Teng to further reduce blood pressure in mild cases; for severe cases, add:
  30 g Zhen Zhu Mu
  30 g Shi Jue Ming

  A *recommended starting dose* of granular concentrate is 60 mg per lb of body weight, or approximately ¼ tsp per 15 to 20 lb of body weight, divided into two daily doses. Use should be discontinued if the patient's appetite becomes depressed or diarrhea ensues.
- Acupuncture may be used to augment the effects of Long Dan Xie Gan Tang. LIV 2 clears Heat from the Liver, and GB 43 clears Heat from the Gall Bladder channel, with which the Liver is connected. Points to descend rising energy include GB 20 and ST 8 (located in the temporal area just rostral to the ear). LI 11 clears Damp Heat in general from the body and SP 6 nourishes Yin when it has been dried out by Excessive Heat.
- For patients that have little or no history of Dampness or Dryness, **Tian Ma Gou Teng Yin** (Gastrodia and Uncaria Decoction) can be considered. This formula addresses Liver Yang Rising, which is suspected when the pulse is wiry or taut and rapid and the tongue is red or pale. A

recommended starting dose of granular concentrate is 60 mg per lb of body weight, or approximately ¼ tsp per 15 to 20 lb of body weight, divided into two daily doses.

- **Er Xian Tang** (Curculigo and Epimedium Decoction) can be considered when an Extreme Fire has consumed Yin and Yang. This condition is especially common in hypertension in cats with advanced hyperthyroidism and chronic renal failure. Patients that may benefit usually have a small red or pale tongue, and a rapid, floating, weak pulse. To nourish Yin, add the following to 50 g of base formula:
  12 g Shu Di Huang
  30 g Gui Ban
  To warm Yang, add the following to 35 g of base formula:
  15 g Du Zhong
  12 g Lu Jiao Jiao
  Recommended starting dose of granular concentrate is 60 mg per lb of body weight, or approximately ¼ tsp per 15 to 20 lb of body weight, divided into twice daily doses.
- Acupuncture points that support the main action of the formula are those that support the Qi and Yang of the body, including BL 23, ST 36, CV 4, GV 20, CV 6, BL 20, KI 3, SP 6, and GV 4.

For Yin deficiency

- **Qi Ju Di Huang Wan** (Lycium, Chrysanthemum, and Rehmannia Pill) is used for Liver and Kidney Yin deficiency. From a Western perspective, it is perhaps especially appropriate for hypertension caused by renal failure. Guiding symptoms include a red, dry tongue, a floating, rapid pulse, thirst, heat intolerance, weight loss, oliguria, and increased appetite. To 100 g of base formula, add the following:
  30 g Gui Ban to nourish Yin
  30 g Mu Li to descend Yang
  12 g Dan Shen to move Qi and Blood
  Recommended starting dose of granular concentrate is 60 mg per lb of body weight, or approximately ¼ tsp per 15 to 20 lb of body weight, divided into two daily doses.
- Acupuncture can be used to augment the effects of Chinese herbal medicine. KI 2 is an important point to

relieve the effects of Empty Fire. Although this technique is not commonly taught in veterinary acupuncture courses, the point can be accessed by passing a needle horizontally from just ventral to the navicular bone posterior to SP 4 caudally toward KI 3. KI 3 may also be used to nourish Kidney Yin, as may be BL 23. LIV 3 and BL 18 are used to nourish Liver Yin, and SP 6 is used to nourish the Yin of the Liver and Kidney simultaneously. GB 20 and GV 20 are needled to suppress rising energy.

- For hypertension from kidney failure when the pulse is weak and deep and the tongue is pale, **Shen Qi Wan** (Kidney Qi Pill) should be considered. Both Shen Qi Wan and Qi Ju Di Huang Wan contain herbs that may enhance renal blood flow (see chronic renal failure in Chapter 18). Patients benefiting from Shen Qi Wan are chilly, thirsty, and may be weak in the hind limbs. *Recommended starting dose* of granular concentrate is 60 mg per lb of body weight, or approximately ¼ tsp per 15 to 20 lb of body weight, divided into two daily doses.
- A Western herbal tincture that may be considered for Yin-deficient types of hypertension contains 20 ml Skullcap, 20 ml Oats, 5 ml Lobelia, and 5 ml Mistletoe. In this formula, Skullcap clears Empty Heat and Oats nourishes Yin. Lobelia increases the forcefulness of the downbearing action of Skullcap and Mistletoe softens and relaxes tension. A *recommended starting dose* is 0.1 ml of tincture per 5 lb of body weight, divided into two or three doses per day. Lobelia and Mistletoe are potentially toxic, but ill effects are not anticipated when used in appropriate cases and at these ratios. Tincture use should be discontinued if vomiting is observed.
- A Western herbal high blood pressure formula suggested by David Hoffman consists of 2 parts Hawthorn, 2 parts Lime Blossom, 2 parts Yarrow *(Achillea millefolium)*, and 1 part Mistletoe. Analyzed from a Chinese medical perspective, this formula might be especially appropriate in weakened, debilitated, overwrought, hypertensive patients. Hawthorn astringes and gathers escaping Qi and nourishes Heart Yin. Lime Blossom and Mistletoe share an ability to soften and relax patients without depleting them. Yarrow gently moves the circulation to relieve stasis and tension. A

recommended starting dose is 0.1 ml of tincture per 5 lb of body weight, divided into two or three doses per day.

For rebellious uprising of Qi

- Qi rebellion is usually caused by an accumulation of obstructing Dampness in the middle burner. Signs of this disorder include vomiting of slimy, clear fluid, vomiting after eating, lethargy and sluggishness, weight gain, and mental dullness. The pulse is soft or slippery, and the tongue coated or wet. A history of food sensitivities may be noted. The formula for this disorder is **Ban Xia Bai Zhu Tian Ma Tang** (Pinellia, Atractylodes and Gastrodia Decoction). To 50 g of base formula, add the following:

  12 g of Gou Teng
  6 g of Shi Chang Pu
  9 g of Jiang Can

  Recommended starting dose of granular concentrate is 60 mg per lb of body weight, or approximately ¼ tsp per 15 to 20 lb of body weight, divided into twice daily doses.
- Acupuncture may be used to augment the effects of the formula. CV 12, ST 40, and PC 6 act to stop the formation of Phlegm and harmonize the Stomach. ST 8 and GB 20 descend rebellious Qi. ST 36 and SP 9 regulate the middle jiao to stop the formation of obstructing Dampness.

Cautions

- Garlic may potentiate the effect of anticoagulants, may potentiate the hypoglycemic effect of insulin, and may aggravate bleeding tendencies.

AUTHORS' CHOICES:

SM: Appropriate herbal formula; exercise in overweight animals.
SW: Conventional medications; appropriate herbal formula.

HYPERTROPHIC CARDIOMYOPATHY (SEE ALSO CONGESTIVE HEART FAILURE, HYPERTENSION)

Therapeutic Rationale

- Relax the myocardium.
- Enhance ventricular filling.
- Control signs of failure such as pulmonary edema.
- Manage arrhythmias.
- Rule out hyperthyroidism, systemic hypertension, and acromegaly (rare).

Alternative Options with Conventional Bases

- **See the following herbs** and their formulas under Congestive Heart Failure: *S. miltiorrhiza, S. tetranda, G. biloba, C. chinensis, B. vulgaris, M. aquifolium.*
- **Echocardiographic monitoring** of the progress of patients receiving alternative treatment for hypertrophic cardiomyopathy suggests that hypertrophic changes are occasionally reversible. Hawthorn was a component of therapy in my patients (SM) that showed apparent improvements in myocardial thickening function. Hawthorn scavenges free radicals, improves blood flow through the coronary arteries, and improves cardiac contractility. A *suggested starting dose* of the liquid extract is 0.1 ml of tincture per 5 lb of body weight, divided into two or three doses per day. Hawthorn is a safe herb and can be given liberally if the patient is under veterinary supervision.
- **Dan Shen** *(Salvia)* has effects similar to and compatible with Hawthorn. In China this herb is often taken by itself for coronary artery disease and is widely considered the single most important herb for cardiac disease in Chinese hospitals. According to Chinese studies, its application to hypertrophic cardiomyopathy is suggested by several of its effects, including an ability to improve capillary microcirculation, dilate coronary arteries, mediate tissue regeneration and repair, and reduce blood clotting by enhancing fibrinolysis, according to Chinese studies. Dan Shen is available as a pill, known as **Fu Fang Dan Shen Pian.**

- **Magnesium** deficiency is associated with cardiomyopathy in several species, and magnesium supplementation may also be considered for feline hypertrophic cardiomyopathy. The myocardium depends on large amounts of magnesium for proper function, with magnesium concentrations in the heart muscle typically exceeding plasma concentrations by 23 times. The wide use of magnesium-restricted diets in cats prone to feline lower urinary tract disease (FLUTD) raises the question of whether this practice may increase susceptibility of cats to cardiomyopathy (Freeman, 1997). Magnesium supplementation may be attempted orally (in the Freeman study, it was administered as 210 mg MgCl orally for 12 weeks), but absorption of magnesium from the GI is self-limiting because of its tendency to produce osmotic diarrhea, thereby accelerating gut motility and decreasing transit times. Accordingly, magnesium may be given to affected patients by injection. A *suggested starting dose* of magnesium sulfate is 10 mg/kg of body weight subcutaneously, given twice weekly. Frequency can be reduced as clinical improvement is noted.

Paradigmatic Options

- Hypertrophic cardiomyopathy is sometimes associated with hypertensive tendencies. When hypertension cannot be documented in cats with feline hypertrophic cardiomyopathy, patients should still be evaluated for the various Chinese medical diagnoses associated with hypertension in the preceding section. If Kidney, Liver, and Heart Yin deficiency is identified, one formula that may be considered is **Zuo Gui Yin** (Left Restoring Beverage). Suggestive signs include a red, dry tongue, a thready, fast pulse, hyperactivity or restlessness, thoracic pain, insomnia, hind limb weakness, dizziness, and declining body weight. This formula is very rich and should not be used for animals with a history of Dampness symptoms (e.g., cystitis, colitis, seborrhea oleosa, and weight gain). For painful animals, to 75 g base formula, add the following:

9 g Dang Gui
12 g Dan Shen
6 g Chuan Xiong
9 g Yu Jin

Recommended starting dose of granular concentrate for either formula is 60 mg per lb of body weight, or approximately ¼ tsp per 15 to 20 lb of body weight, divided into twice daily doses.

- A Western herbal formula that may be considered for use in hypertrophic cardiomyopathy is Hawthorn Compound (Herbalist and Alchemist). It contains Hawthorn Flower and Berry, Ginkgo Leaf, Lemon Balm, Lime/Linden Flowers, Prickly Ash Bark, Bugleweed, and Cactus. Cactus is a potentially toxic plant. In this formula, Hawthorn and Gingko serve as Blood tonics, Lemon Balm moves Qi, Lime Flowers relax the Heart, and the rest of the herbs move Blood. A *recommended starting dose* is 0.1 ml of tincture per 5 lb of body weight, divided into two or three doses per day.

AUTHORS' CHOICES:

SM: Appropriate Chinese or Western herbal formula.
SW: Dan Shen; Fish Oil; antioxidants; appropriate Western or Chinese formula.

VALVULAR DISEASE (SEE CONGESTIVE HEART FAILURE)

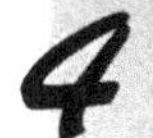

CASE REPORT
Reverse Patent Ductus Arteriosus in a Dog

HISTORY

Crystal, a 10-year-old American cocker spaniel, presented with a chief complaint of severe coughing and dyspnea secondary to a reverse patent ductus arteriosus (PDA).

The condition was diagnosed when Crystal was approximately 5 years old. At that time, she had exhibited periodic hind end collapse that improved with rest. Physical examination by the veterinarian revealed a tendency to patellar luxation, which was assumed to be the cause of Crystal's reluctance or inability to walk. No treatment was advised.

Three years later, Crystal was boarded at the same clinic, and the veterinary staff observed Crystal's inability to walk more than a few steps at a time without collapsing. They also noticed that Crystal's tongue and rectum exhibited a blue discoloration at the time she collapsed, and a cough had also recently developed. A cardiac condition was suspected based on these observations and survey radiographs of the thorax were obtained. Right-sided heart enlargement and hilar edema were evident on the radiographs. Furosemide (10 to 20 mg twice daily) and a hypotensive medication (type and dose unknown) were prescribed. Crystal's condition worsened on these medications and Crystal was referred for cardiac evaluation by the Western College of Veterinary Medicine at the University of Saskatchewan 6 months later.

Further evaluation at the veterinary college using echocardiography and electrocardiography revealed that Crystal had an axis of deviation consistent with right ventricular enlargement, proximal pulmonary artery dilation, distal pulmonary artery attenuation, and marked right ventricular hypertrophy. A contrast echocardiogram was performed and contrast media injected intravenously immediately became visible in the abdominal aorta. Based on these findings, Crystal was suspected to have a right-to-left shunt secondary to a reverse patent ductus arteriosus.

Crystal's medications were discontinued and phlebotomy was prescribed to relieve hyperviscosity that resulted in a hematocrit of 76%. This increase in packed cell volume was considered secondary to chronic renal hypoxia that resulted in increased synthesis of erythropoietin. The phlebotomy produced a dramatic improvement in Crystal's exercise intolerance and was repeated 6 months later when Crystal's condition had declined. When she declined again after only 3 months, the owners elected to consult me (SM) to determine if there were any alternative treatment options for Crystal.

At the time of examination, Crystal was unable to walk more than a few steps without sitting down. She had been unable to walk around the block without stopping repeatedly for many years. She was also now exhibiting a chronic "barking" cough that was aggravated by cold air and that improved with occasional administration of diphenhydramine (Benadryl). The cough seemed dry and nonproductive.

Crystal had numerous chronic eye problems, including distichiasis, skin tags along the lid margins, and keratoconjunctivitis sicca (KCS). Her eyes had a chronic tendency to redness and mucoid eye discharge that was relieved through the use of dexamethasone eyedrops twice daily as needed. Between bouts of dexamethasone usage, sterile saline drops were administered several times daily to relieve eye dryness.

Crystal also had a history of periodontal disease and dental tartar accumulation. Her history of cardiac problems had precluded any prospects of general anesthesia for the purpose of dental scaling and polishing. At times, Crystal seemed to exhibit pain while eating, possibly because of the periodontal disease.

Other problems included nasal hyperkeratosis and occasional development of a variety of benign cysts and nodules.

Crystal's past medical history included ongoing tendencies to psychogenic polydipsia and urinary incontinence that were partially responsive to water restriction. She had a history of periodic superficial pyoderma, managed with periodic administration of 250 mg twice daily of Cephalexin and weekly use of a benzoyl peroxide–based shampoo. She also had a history of recurrent but mild yeast otitis externa that was managed with topical medications.

Regarding her general physical tendencies, Crystal was easily chilled and shivered after any exposure to cold. She sought warm places to rest. She exhibited occasional tendencies to dream when sleeping, and woke quickly at the slightest disturbance. Crystal exhibited good energy in the mornings after sleeping and also after periods of rest. She had a poor appetite, however, unless offered a homemade meat-based diet.

Mentally, Crystal appeared to be well adjusted and cheerful. She was not afraid to assert herself with the other dogs in the household when necessary, but declined from engaging in any play activity with them.

PHYSICAL EXAMINATION

On physical examination, Crystal's tongue was lavender. After moving just a few steps in the exam room, she would sit down and her tongue would have turned a deep purple. Her pulse was choppy on the left side and slightly wiry on the right side. No abnormal heart or lung sounds could be auscultated, but her spleen was palpably enlarged. She had a pronounced apical beat palpable bilaterally over her chest wall.

Acupuncture points that felt swollen, turgid, thickened, or warm included BL 17, SP 6, CV 10, and CV 17. In addition,

Crystal had mild surface pyoderma over the dorsum of the nose with yellow-green crusty exudate.

ASSESSMENT

Crystal's conventional medical diagnosis is reverse patent ductus arteriosus.

A choppy or irregular pulse in tandem with a purple tongue is pathognomonic for Blood stasis in Chinese medicine and is the cause of Crystal's symptoms from a Chinese perspective. Crystal's wiry pulse suggests Qi stagnation may be contributing to Blood stasis since Qi is the motive force for Blood. Spleen enlargement is viewed quite literally as stagnant Blood in Chinese medicine, and Blood stasis is also a chief cause of a chronic deep cough. The active points in this case, especially CV 17, BL 17, and SP 6, are instrumental in relieving Blood stasis in the chest.

Several factors may have contributed to Crystal's Blood stasis from a Chinese medical perspective. Blood deficiency is a latent problem in many canines and contributes to Blood stasis in the same way a river is more likely to break into stagnant pools when its volume is low. Signs of Blood deficiency include a history of KCS and a tendency to sleep lightly.

Cold is also known to contribute to Blood stasis and is known in Chinese medicine as Cold Coagulation. The worsening of Crystal's cough in cold air suggested this, as did her intolerance for cold in general.

TREATMENT

There are several Chinese herbal formulas to relieve Blood stasis in the chest and Heart. **Xue Fu Zhu Yu Tang** was prescribed for Crystal. The granular concentrate form of the herbal formula was prescribed at a dose of ½ teaspoon twice daily. In addition, from a Chinese medical perspective, vitamin A is a Blood or Yin tonic. An injection of 100,000 IU of vitamin A was administered subcutaneously.

OUTCOME

After 1 month, Crystal's response to therapy markedly exceeded that observed after phlebotomy. Her cough had decreased dramatically, and her exercise tolerance was significantly increased. She was now participating in play activity with the other dogs in the household, which she had not done in many years. Rather than collapsing, Crystal now exhibited only occasional stumbling. Only the eye redness and poor appetite had not improved. After 2 months, her cough was resolved and her exercise tolerance had further increased.

The case was still in progress at the time of writing and a 3- or 4-month follow-up was not yet available to contrast with the declines seen 3 months after the second phlebotomy. The steady improvements seen in Crystal under Chinese herbal treatment exceeded those seen with phlebotomy, which were typically at their maximum within the first few days after the procedure.

COMMENTS

Reverse PDA is an uncommon congenital heart defect in dogs. It is thought to arise secondary to pulmonary hypertension at birth, which is sufficient to force blood from the pulmonary artery through the still patent ductus arteriosus. Although it is a congenital defect, reverse PDA is not usually manifested clinically in dogs until they are 2 or 3 years old.

Reverse PDA creates a right-to-left shunt, with poorly oxygenated blood being delivered to the abdomen and lower limbs. Signs and symptoms related to this hypoxia include a compensatory increase in erythropoiesis by the kidneys, seizures, cyanosis of the anus, and, in some animals, hind limb weakness. Crystal exhibited all of these symptoms except seizure activity. Murmurs are not typically auscultated in reverse PDA.

There is no effective treatment for reverse PDA. Duct ligation results in immediate right-sided heart failure, since the pulmonary hypertension is irreversible. Hyperviscosity is relieved by periodically withdrawing 10% of the blood volume and replacing it with intravenous fluids. Life expectancy of affected animals is 4 to 6 years and the cause of death usually is embolic disease.

Given these conventional perspectives of reverse PDA, Crystal's longevity is already atypical and impressive. Her further response to Xue Fu Zhu Yu Tang is understandable given the tendency to hyperviscosity and embolism in dogs with reverse PDA. The ingredients of this formula have demonstrated significant "blood thinning" activity that helps increase perfusion and reduce coagulation. Dang Gui *(Angelica sinensis)* has shown clinical benefit in the treatment of thromboangiitis obliterans and in improving coronary artery blood flow. Bai Shao Yao *(Paeonia lactiflora)* reduces platelet aggregation. Chuan Xiong *(Ligusticum* spp.*)* induces peripheral vasodilation, lowers blood pressure, reduces platelet aggregation, and increases perfusion of the abdomen and lower limbs.

SM

REFERENCES

Baumann G, Felix S, Sattelberger U, Klein G. Cardiovascular effects of forskolin (HL 362) in patients with idiopathic congestive cardiomyopathy—a comparative study with dobutamine and sodium nitroprusside. *J Cardiovasc Pharmacol* 16(1):93-100, 1990.

Billman GE, Kang JX, Leaf A. Prevention of sudden cardiac death by dietary pure omega-3 polyunsaturated fatty acids in dogs. *Circulation* 99(18):2452-2457, 1999.

Bone K. *Clinical Applications of Ayurvedic and Chinese Herbs: Monographs for the Western Herbal Practitioner.* Warwick, Queensland, Australia, 1997, Phytotherapy Press.

Brinker F. *Formulas for Healthful Living.* Sandy, Ore, 1995, Eclectic Medical Publications.

Chen CF, Chen SM, Lin MT, Chow SY. In vivo and in vitro studies on the mechanism of cardiovascular effects of Wu-Chu-Yu *(Evodiae fructus). Am J Chin Med* 9(1):39-47, 1981.

Dutta A, Sukul NC. Antifilarial effect of *Zingiber officinale* on *Dirofilaria immitis. J Helminthol* 61(3):268-270, 1987.

Dutta A, Sukul NC. Filaricidal properties of a wild herb, *Andrographis paniculata. J Helminthol* 56(2):81-84, 1982.

Fox PR, Trautwein EA, Hayes KC, Bond BR, Sisson DD, Moise NS. Comparison of taurine, alpha-tocopherol, retinol, selenium, and total triglycerides and cholesterol concentrations in cats with cardiac disease and in healthy cats. *Am J Vet Res* 54(4):563-569, 1993.

Freeman LM, Rush JE, Kehayias JJ, Ross JN Jr, Meydani SN, Brown DJ, Dolnikowski GG, Marmor BN, White ME, Dinarello CA, Roubenoff R. Nutritional alterations and the effect of fish oil supplementation in dogs with heart failure. *J Vet Intern Med* 12(6):440-448, 1998.

Freeman LM, Brown DJ, Smith FW, Rush JE. Magnesium status and the effect of magnesium supplementation in feline hypertrophic cardiomyopathy. *Can J Vet Res* 61(3):227-231, 1997.

Freeman LM, Brown DJ, Rush JE. Assessment of degree of oxidative stress and antioxidant concentrations in dogs with idiopathic dilated cardiomyopathy. *J Am Vet Med Assoc* 215(5):644-646, 1999.

Haji A, Momose Y, Takeda R, Nakanishi S, Horiuchi T, Arisawa M. Increased feline cerebral blood flow induced by dehydroevodiamine hydrochloride from *Evodia rutaecarpa. J Nat Prod* 57(3):387-389, 1994.

Huang KC. *The Pharmacology of Chinese Herbs.* Boca Raton, Fla, 1998, CRC Press.

Huang WM, Yan H, Jin JM, Yu C, Zhang H. Beneficial effects of berberine on hemodynamics during acute ischemic left ventricular failure in dogs. *Chin Med J* 105(12):1014-1019, 1992.

Jellin JM, Batz F, Hitchens K. *Pharmacists Letter/Prescribers Letter Natural Medicines Comprehensive Database.* Therapeutic Research Faculty, Stockton, Calif, 1999.

Keene BW, Panciera DP, Atkins CE, Regitz V, Schmidt MJ, Shug AL. Myocardial L-carnitine deficiency in a family of dogs with dilated cardiomyopathy. *J Am Vet Med Assoc* 198(4):647-650, 1991.

Kittleson MD, Keene B, Pion PD, Loyer CG. Results of the multicenter spaniel trial (MUST): taurine- and carnitine-responsive dilated cardiomyopathy in American cocker spaniels with decreased plasma taurine concentration. *J Vet Intern Med* 11:204-211, 1997.

Leaf A, Kang JX, Xiao YF, Billman GE. Dietary n-3 fatty acids in the prevention of cardiac arrhythmias. *Curr Opin Clin Nutr Metab Care* 1(2):225-228, 1998.

Lei XL, Chiou GC. Studies on cardiovascular actions of *Salvia miltiorrhiza*. *Am J Chin Med* 14(1-2):26-32, 1986.

Lu GW, Miura K, Yukimura T, Yamamoto K. Effects of extract from *Clerodendron trichotomum* on blood pressure and renal function in rats and dogs. *J Ethnopharmacol* 42(2):77-82, 1994.

Martin N, Bardisa L, Pantoja C, Roman R, Vargas M. Experimental cardiovascular depressant effects of garlic *(Allium sativum)* dialysate. *J Ethnopharmacol* 37(2):145-149, 1992.

Marz RB. *Medical Nutrition from Marz,* ed 2. Portland, Ore, 1997, Omni-Press.

Murray MT. *The Healing Power of Herbs,* ed 2. Roseville, Calif, 1995, Prima Publishing.

Nagourney RA. Garlic: medicinal food or nutritional medicine? *J Medicinal Foods* 1(1):13-28, 1998.

Negretti N, Perez MR, Walker D, O'Neill SC. Inhibition of sarcoplasmic reticulum function by polyunsaturated fatty acids in intact, isolated myocytes from rat ventricular muscle. *J Physiol (Lond)* 523 (pt 2):367-375, 2000.

Ozaki Y. Vasodilative effects of indole alkaloids obtained from domestic plants, *Uncaria rhynchophylla* Miq. and *Amsonia elliptica* Roem. et Schult. *Nippon Yakurigaku Zasshi* 95(2):47-54, 1990.

Riccioppo Neto F. Electropharmacological effects of berberine on canine cardiac Purkinje fibres and ventricular muscle and atrial muscle of the rabbit. *Br J Pharmacol* 108(2):534-537, 1993.

Rush JE. Alternative Therapies in Heart Failure Patients. In Proceedings of the 14th Annual Conference of the American College of Veterinary Internal Medicine, May 23-26, San Antonio, Tex, Lakewood, Colo, 1996, ACVIM.

Takeo S, Tanonaka K, Hirai K, Kawaguchi K, Ogawa M, Yagi A, Fujimoto K. Beneficial effect of tan-shen, an extract from the root of Salvia, on post-hypoxic recovery of cardiac contractile force. *Biochem Pharmacol* 40(5):1137-1143, 1990.

Toda N, Usui H, Nishino N, Fujiwara M. Cardiovascular effects of capsaicin in dogs and rabbits. *J Pharm Exp Ther* 181(3):512-521, 1972.

Weiss RF, Volker F. *Herbal Medicine,* ed 2. Stuttgart, Germany, Thieme.

Williams T, Mueller K, Cornwall MW. Effect of AP-point stimulation on diastolic blood pressure in hypertensive subjects: a preliminary study. *Physical Therapy* 71(7):523-529, 1991.

Wu Y, Fischer W. *Practical Therapeutics of Traditional Chinese Medicine.* Brookline, Mass, 1997, Paradigm Publications.

Yao T. AP and somatic nerve stimulation: mechanism underlying effects on cardiovascular and renal activities. *Scand J Rehab Med Suppl* 29:7-18, 1993.

Yeung HC. *Handbook of Chinese Herbs.* Los Angeles, 1996, Self-published.

5

Therapies for Dermatologic Disorders

GENERAL PARADIGMATIC PERSPECTIVES OF SKIN DISEASE (SEE SPECIFIC DISORDERS TO FOLLOW)

One of the more satisfying applications of Chinese medicine is in the treatment of skin disease. Most patients can experience significant and enduring relief through the application of the appropriate herbal formula. Response to a particular Chinese herbal formula also suggests that certain dietary strategies may be effective in preventing further skin problems and promoting long-term resolution or stability of skin problems without the need for continued use of drugs or herbs.

Chinese herbal therapy seems to be more consistently successful in the treatment of skin disorders than the standard homeopathic and dietary treatment strategies of lay publications. A relatively simplistic view in some of these books suggests that most skin disorders are due to only one or two causes—induced either by a vaccine, vaccinosis, or by feeding an animal commercially prepared diets with preservatives. The standard recommendations of treating with homeopathic Thuja to reverse the vaccinosis and of feeding a home-cooked or raw food diet are often unrewarding. Although these approaches can be successful, skin disease remains a complex syndrome that defies rote methods of treatment. Home-cooked diets that contain antigens to which the animal is sensitive may be more irritating to the skin than commercially prepared diets. Homeopathic Thuja fails in the majority of cases to which it is applied unless the patient resembles the homeopathic picture of the remedy, with a greasy and sweet-smelling coat, warty excrescences, and general evidence of Spleen deficiency from a Chinese medical perspective. Preservatives are probably not nearly as important a source of toxins in animals with skin disorders as those toxins that are autogenously generated from the action of ordinary digestive or metabolic processes. The challenge to the serious alternative practitioner dealing with skin problems remains the same as the challenge to the conventional practitioner coping with skin disorders—differentiate the condition from one of several possibilities, and render a treatment specific to the diagnosis.

In Chinese medicine the system of diagnosis used by an alternative practitioner to select an appropriate therapy is considerably different from that used by conventional veterinarians. As a result, the same Chinese herbal formula will apply to a host of different skin disorders, yet one conventional diagnosis may be treatable by up to half a dozen different herbal approaches. This is the observation behind the Chinese medical dictum, "Same disease, different treatments; same treatment, different diseases." *For all skin conditions the basic approach in Chinese medicine is to identify the pattern affecting the patient and select the appropriate formula to address that pattern.* The first step in this process is to identify whether the patient has an "excessive" or "deficient" type of skin disorder.

Excess Skin Disorders

The Excess inflammatory skin disorder corresponds fairly well to the prevailing naturopathic perspective of skin disorders, which is that the patient is "toxic" from the inside out. Specifically, the naturopathic "toxemia" model of disease holds that all chronic inflammation of epithelial surfaces represents a vicarious method of "burning" off or shedding toxic material that has formed as a result of some deficiency of the internal detoxification methods, most notably liver function. "Leaky Gut Syndrome" is another postulated method by which toxemia occurs (see Chapter 6 for more information on Leaky Gut Syndrome).

Chinese medicine considers that perhaps half of all small animal skin disorders arise from an overwhelming accumulation of toxins, which are referred to as Dampness in Chinese medicine. As Dampness lingers in the body, it becomes hot (Damp Heat) and perhaps toxic (a severe form of Damp Heat).

Prevailing Signs of Excess, Toxic, or Damp Heat

- Inflamed suppurative yellow lesions (yellow is the color of Heat in Chinese medicine).
- Either elevated appetite or thirst, but often not both.
- Preference for cool surfaces (tile, shade, holes in the dirt, the floor rather than the bed, hard surfaces, bathtubs, or basements).
- Skin that is hot to the touch.
- Lesions that bleed bright red blood.
- Extremely agonizing itch (according to Chinese medicine Heat in the Blood causes an itch).

Other Signs of Dampness

- Greasy or "clumped" coat.
- Lichenification and thickening of the skin.
- Large flakes of dander, often tinted; note that they are often dry even though the underlying cause is Dampness.
- Slimy vomitus.
- Tendency to sleep very deeply.
- Reverse sneezing, snoring during sleep.
- Strong skin or ear odor.
- Strong breath odor or yeast otitis externa.
- Copious exudates.
- Aggravation during humid weather.
- Loose or mucoid stools.
- Past medical history of cystitis or colitis.
- Anal gland inflammation, infection, and impaction.

Role of Diet in the Management of Excess Skin Disorders

According to Chinese medicine, the sources of all Damp Heat are the Spleen and Stomach. Spleen and Stomach functions equate approximately with the activity of the small intestine, stomach, and pancreas. Response to therapy for a Damp condition therefore suggests that long-term prevention and control of a skin disorder will hinge, at the very least, on enhancing the completeness of digestion and reducing or eliminating food allergens.

Diets to eliminate food allergies should include changing previous protein and carbohydrate sources. For many cases of food intolerance the underlying pathophysiologic or biochemical mechanisms are unknown. From a Chinese medical perspective the Spleen is injured by an excess of the "sweet" taste, which is assigned to carbohydrate-laden plants and foods.

Given that cats and, to a lesser extent, dogs are not biologically designed to use carbohydrates as a main energy source, carbohydrates may be significant contributing factors in disorders referable to the diet and digestive tract. Practitioners should exercise prudence in the selection of protein sources for elimination diets in Damp Heat animals, however, since many of the "novel" protein sources on the market are rich, "hot," heavy meats, such as lamb and duck. In my practice (SM), it is becoming more common for food sensitivity cases initially not to respond to hypoallergenic diets, perhaps because these fundamental aspects of chinese dietetics are being ignored. The reader is referred to Appendix B, Chinese Food Therapy, for further information on the characteristics of individual foods.

Raw food diets (ground raw meat, vegetables, and bone) may be important in the management of Damp Heat animals. In my opinion (SM), raw diets take longer to digest, and this longer digestion time means there is no deluge of absorbed calories that may dampen the Spleen. Spleen-deficient animals with Damp Heat and strong pulses may fare well on a raw food diet. The longer digestion time may present a burden for the Spleen-deficient animal with a weak pulse, however, and should not as a rule be given to such animals. The main concerns surrounding raw food diets include perforation or irritation of the gastrointestinal tract by bone fragments and the growth of pathogens such as *Salmonella*, and care must be taken in the handling and processing of raw food diets to minimize these concerns. Ground raw food diets specifically prepared for small animals that are deep frozen immediately after manufacture may pose less risk in this regard.

Mention should be made of some supplements frequently used by veterinarians in the management of Excess or Damp Heat skin disorders. Essential fatty acids and diets that have been enriched with them theoretically have a dampening influence in Spleen-deficient animals. These fatty acids should initially be used at low doses and should be discontinued if a greasy coat or digestive upset develops. Digestive enzymes, however, may be especially useful as a supplement for Spleen-deficient Damp Heat animals.

Chinese Herbal Approaches to Excess Skin Disorders

A large number of formulas are potentially useful in the management of Damp Heat skin disorders. The formulas are described below, in approximately descending order of the intensity of their cooling actions. The most important formulas are marked with an asterisk.

- **Huang Lian Jie Du Tang** (Coptis Decoction to Relieve Toxicity) is mentioned in the chapter on Ear Disorders as a very strong formula to treat severe acute bacterial infections. Animals that have purulent bleeding lesions, forceful, rapid pulses, and wet red or purple-red tongues may respond to this formula. A *suggested starting dose* of granular concentrate is ¼ tsp per 15 to 20 lb of body weight, or 60 to 75 mg/kg of body weight, divided into two daily doses.
- ***Modified Long Dan Xie Gan Tang** (Modified Gentian Drain the Liver Decoction) consists of **Long Dan Xie Gan Tang** combined with **Er Miao San** (Two Marvels Powder), which improves Heat-clearing ability and provides Spleen support. Other herbs may be added to 100 g of this combined formula, including 12 g of Bai Xian Pi, 16 g of Di Fu Zi, 21 g of Sheng Di Huang, and 12 g each of Chi Shao Yao and Mu Dan Pi. The additional herbs help the formula relieve intense itch and cool the skin. Signs that an animal may benefit from this formula are intense itch, heat intolerance, agitation, suppurative lesions and moist pyoderma, a preponderance of lesions over the rump and in the inguinal area, elevated thirst or appetite, dominance aggression, and suppurative otitis externa. A good rule of thumb is to use this formula for Damp Heat animals in which Heat dominates the clinical picture. The pulse may be rapid, wiry, or slippery, but is forceful. The tongue is deep red or purple-red and wet. A *suggested starting dose* of granular concentrate is ¼ tsp per 15 to 20 lb of body weight, or 60 to 75 mg/kg of body weight, divided into two daily doses. Use should be discontinued in the event of appetite suppression or the advent of painless, watery diarrhea.
- **Wu Wei Xiao Du Yin** (Five Ingredient Decoction to Eliminate Toxin) is a superficially acting formula that is used to treat suppurative boils or sores. The pulse may be

rapid and the tongue red or dry. A *suggested starting dose* of granular concentrate is ¼ tsp per 15 to 20 lb of body weight, or 60 to 75 mg/kg of body weight, divided into two daily doses.

- **Long Dan Xie Gan Tang** and **Wu Wei Xiao Du Yin** are sometimes used together to achieve a more systemic effect than Wu Wei Xiao Du Yin alone. In this combination the efficacy of Long Dan Xie Gan Tang in treating superficial bacterial infections is enhanced. The patient that benefits from this combination may have less itch and more infection than the patient described for **Modified Long Dan Xie Gan Tang,** but otherwise the indications are similar. A *suggested starting dose* of granular concentrate is ¼ tsp per 15 to 20 lb of body weight, or 60 to 75 mg/kg of body weight, divided into two daily doses.
- **Fang Feng Tong Shen San** (Pills of Ledebouriella with Magical Therapeutic Effects) is a complex formula usually reserved for febrile animals with associated acute skin eruptions. It is especially indicated in cases of acute hives with accompanying abdominal pain, nausea, vomiting, constipation, or diarrhea. The pulse is forceful and rapid, and the tongue red and perhaps wet. A *suggested starting dose* of granular concentrate is ¼ tsp per 15 to 20 lb of body weight, or 60 to 75 mg/kg of body weight, divided into two daily doses.
- ***Si Miao San** (Four Marvels Powder) should be one of the top considerations for an animal with pronounced Heat signs and obvious Spleen Qi deficiency signs, particularly a soft or weak pulse or a pale, swollen tongue. Other signs suggesting this formula may be especially effective are low back stiffness; a predilection of lesions for the lower half of the body, including the hind limbs, lower abdomen and rump; an obvious line of demarcation between normal skin and the affected regions encircling the trunk just caudal to the rib cage; and a history of recurrent cystitis or colitis. A *suggested starting dose* of granular concentrate is ¼ tsp per 15 to 20 lb of body weight, or 60 to 75 mg/kg of body weight, divided into two daily doses.
- **Jia Wei Er Miao San** (Modified Two Marvels Powder) contains the same ingredients as Si Miao San except that Yi Yi Ren has been removed and Fang Ji, Bi Xie, Dang Gui Wei,

and Gui Ban have been added. (Gui Ban is tortoise shell, a Yin tonic, and should probably be omitted for the maximum benefit in Damp Heat eczema cases, and Yi Yi Ren should perhaps be added back in.) Fang Ji and Bi Xie both hasten the drainage of Dampness through the Bladder. Dang Gui Wei is the portion of Dang Gui root that has exceptional Blood-moving properties. It moves Blood that has stagnated because of Dampness accumulation. If whole Dang Gui is added in small amounts, the formula may be helpful in addressing Damp Heat Spleen deficient animals when a component of Blood deficiency is present (see the section on Blood deficiency). Jia Wei Er Miao San is classically indicated for more "liquid" forms of Dampness in which Toxic Heat signs are less pronounced and the main concerns are cellulitis, edema, a greasy coat or loose stools, and excessive anal gland secretions. It should also be considered for use in treating perianal fistulae. The pulse of patients that may benefit is soft and rapid, and the tongue is wet, swollen, and red. Signs similar to those indicating *Si Miao San* may also be present. A *suggested starting dose* of granular concentrate is ¼ tsp per 15 to 20 lb of body weight, or 60 to 75 mg/kg of body weight, divided into two daily doses.

- **Bi Xie Shen Shi Tang** (Fish Poison Yam Dampness Percolating Decoction) is a mild Heat-clearing, strong Damp-draining formula. It may be combined with **Wu Shen Tang** (Five Spirits Decoction) to enhance its effectiveness in treating Damp Heat conditions. The formula is most commonly used in humans for acute, rapidly spreading skin infections such as erysipelas. The patient may have lesions that appear as blisters or vesicles with mild purulent tendencies, irritability, thirst, low appetite, vomiting, and joint swelling. The pulse is soft and rapid, and the tongue is wet or heavily coated and red. A *suggested starting dose* of granular concentrate is ¼ tsp per 15 to 20 lb of body weight, or 60 to 75 mg/kg of body weight, divided into two daily doses.
- ***San Ren Tang** (Three Seeds Decoction) is the penultimate formula for tonifying the Spleen while draining accumulated Dampness from all three burners. It may be extremely important in a modified form in the management of

hyperesthetic syndromes in felines (see Feline Hyperesthesia Syndrome in Chapter 14). Even without modification it can be very useful in Damp Heat syndromes of dogs and cats when Heat signs are not pronounced relative to Dampness signs. Indications that an animal may respond to this formula are greasy ears, joint stiffness, recurrent cystitis, a greasy coat, elevated thirst or appetite but not usually both, malodorous flatulence, weight loss or gain, and lethargy. The pulse is soft, and the tongue is wet and either pale or red. A *suggested starting dose* of granular concentrate is ¼ tsp per 15 to 20 lb of body weight, or 60 to 75 mg/kg of body weight, divided into two daily doses. This formula is quite palatable.

- ***Chu Shi Wei Ling Tang** (Modified Wei Ling Tang; Modified Decoction to Dispel Dampness in the Spleen and Stomach) is reserved for Spleen-deficient cases in which Dampness definitely dominates the clinical picture and Heat is slightly evident. In some cases the patient benefiting from this formula may demonstrate some heat-seeking tendencies even as other signs cryptically point to the presence of excessive Heat. Chu Shi Wei Ling Tang is made by the modification of 75 g of the base formula of **Wei Ling Tang** with the addition of 12 g Hua Shi, 9 g Fang Feng, 6 g Shan Zhi Zi, 12 g Mu Tong, and 9 g Deng Xin Cao. These added herbs help to reduce pruritus and promote the drainage of Dampness. Patients benefiting from this formula may have fairly obvious signs of Spleen Qi deficiency, including poor appetite, loose mucoid painless diarrhea, tendencies to weight gain and bloat, lethargy and sluggishness, bland watery discharges and exudates, and perhaps even signs of Blood deficiency (see section on Blood Deficiency in this chapter). Their pulses are slippery or soft, and the tongue may be swollen and pale or mildly red with abundant moisture. A *suggested starting dose* of granular concentrate is ¼ tsp per 15 to 20 lb of body weight, or 60 to 75 mg/kg of body weight, divided into two daily doses. This formula is also quite palatable.
- **Wu Ling San** (Powder of Five Drugs with Poria) is a subformula of **Wei Ling Tang** that has primarily diuretic properties. Some authors have advocated its use in Damp Heat skin conditions with an underlying Spleen Qi or Yang

deficiency. A *suggested starting dose* of granular concentrate is ¼ tsp per 15 to 20 lb of body weight, or 60 to 75 mg/kg of body weight, divided into two daily doses.

- **Xiao Feng San I** (Dissipate Wind Powder I) may be helpful when there are fewer signs of internal Dampness, but the skin has wet "hot" lesions. See the section on Chinese herbal treatment of Deficient disorders of the skin for more information on this formula.

Western Herbal Approaches to Excess Skin Disorders

Western herbs such as Yellow Dock *(Rumex crispus)*, Nettle *(Urtica dioica)*, and Burdock *(Arctium lappa)* most often advocated for skin problems will be most applicable to Excess or Damp Heat disorders in animals. Many of these herbs were classed as "alteratives" by early Western herbalists. They were believed to "alter" or "purify" the Blood by removing "toxins" through the bolstering of flagging internal detoxification mechanisms. Although their effectiveness in the treatment of small animal skin disorders pales in comparison to Chinese herbs, there is one notable exception commonly known as the **Hoxsey Formula.**

Harry Hoxsey, an early 20th-century herbalist, popularized the use of the Hoxsey Formula. Hoxsey claimed that his grandfather developed the formula in Kentucky in 1840 by assembling the herbs his horse had allegedly naturally sought out to cure itself of cancer. However, this claim has been called into question given that the bulk of the formula was published in the 1926 edition of the National Formulary shortly after Hoxsey went into practice.

The Hoxsey Formula is a proprietary formula. Hoxsey was somewhat evasive about the contents of the formula during several legal "inquisitions" as to his methods. Some of the inconsistencies in formula ingredients reported by Hoxsey at different inquiries may reflect changes he made over time. The herbs in the 1956 version of the Hoxsey Formula included Licorice Root *(Glycyrrhiza glabra)*, Red Clover Blossoms *(Trifolium pratense)*, Burdock Root, Stillingia Root *(Stillingia sylvatica)*, Oregon Grape *(Mahonia aquifolium)*, Poke Root *(Phytolacca americana)*, Cascara Sagrada *(Rhamnus purshiana)*, Prickly Ash Bark *(Xanthoxylum americanum)*, and Buckthorn Bark *(Rhamnus frangula)*. Alfalfa *(Medicago sativa)* had been included in earlier milder versions of the formula. Ratios of ingredients were never disclosed and remain a trade secret of Hoxsey's descendants and followers. However, knowledge of the dynamics between herbal ingredients afforded by Chinese medicine allows us to devise a therapeutically useful formula using these ingredients. A suggested ratio of whole herb tincture extracts of the above herbs, based on my (SM) work and experience with the formula, is 25 ml Oregon Grape, 20 ml Burdock, 5 ml Poke Root, 5 ml Stillingia, 20 ml Red Clover, 5 ml Cascara, 5 ml Buckthorn, 5 ml Licorice, and 10 ml Prickly Ash Bark. Alfalfa (10 to 15 ml) may be added for Blood-deficient animals (see section on Blood-Deficient Disorders), and Ginger *(Zingiber officinale)* (10 to 15 ml) may be added for animals with evidence of Spleen Qi or Yang deficiency.

Although this formula does show promise in the treatment of cancer as the Hoxsey family suggested (see Chapter 13), it is also highly efficacious in the treatment of severe destructive Damp Heat lesions that have progressed to a Toxic Heat state. This formula thus finds application in severe skin disorders, including pemphigus foliaceus. Guiding signs to its use are wiry, forceful, or rapid pulses; a red or purple-red wet tongue; evidence of liver hypofunction in serum chemistry screens (including abnormal cholesterol levels, low blood urea nitrogen level, and low albumin level); and crusting, purulent, or bleeding lesions on the most Yang surfaces of the body, including the pinnae, top of the head, and nasal dorsum.

True to the theories of early naturopaths, the Hoxsey Formula appears to work in pemphigus foliaceus by increasing liver function and decreasing toxemia. Deficient liver metabolism may be related to both the production of autoantibodies and the accumulation of abnormally high levels of tissue plasminogen activators. Deposition of plasminogen activators in the skin may lead to increased plasmin-mediated lysis of desmosomes, resulting in acantholysis and pemphigus foliaceus. Improved liver function may lead to enhanced clearance of tissue plasminogen activators and reduce the production of autoantibodies against desmosomes.

Most feline inflammatory skin disorders, even when the lesions appear mild, seem to be underpinned by significant amounts of Toxic Heat. The Hoxsey Formula thus finds potential use in cats with miliary dermatitis, severe pruritus, and even eosinophilic granulomas. Forceful, rapid pulses and red, wet, or yellow-coated tongues in cats with these signs are indications sufficient to warrant its use. Whether in feline or in canine pemphigus foliaceus, complete lesion resolution can require several months. However, initial signs of improvement should be seen after 2 to 3 weeks of formula use. The action of the formula may be potentiated by administration of Vitamin A. A *suggested starting dose* of the formula is 0.2 ml per 5 lb of body weight, administered at least once daily. Administration should be stopped if vomiting, inappetence, or diarrhea develop. The addition of Ginger to the formula should be considered for more intolerant patients. The formula is poorly palatable and may have to be encapsulated to be administered consistently.

Another Western herbal tincture formula I (SM) have used that shows promise in the treatment of Damp Heat skin disorders with excruciating itch comprises equal parts of Linden Flowers *(Tilia vulgaris)*, Nettles, and Passion Flower *(Passiflora incarnata)*. These are mild herbs and should be used in quantity. The formula is as much a nervine or calming formula as it is a skin formula, although Nettles exerts a slow detoxifying effect on the skin and is reputed to have significant antihistamine properties. The formula should be *considered whenever amitriptyline is being used effectively as a deterrent to scratching and when the dog's pruritus appears to have a psychoemotional component.* It may also be beneficial for similar conditions in cats. If the animal has only a partial response, the dose can be increased, or the animal simultaneously treated with another herbal formula that seems appropriate. A *suggested starting dose* is 0.2 ml per 5 lb of body weight, given two or three times daily.

Acupuncture Point Prescriptions for Excess Skin Disorders

Acupuncture can play a strong supportive role to the use of the herbal formulas described in the previous section in the treatment of Excess skin disorders. Points that feel especially turgid, painful, or warm should be selected from the following:

- For Spleen tonification to eliminate Dampness generation: BL 20, CV 12, BL 21, and SP 9.

- For Spleen Yang deficiency: needle SP 4 and KI 3.
- To drain Dampness: needle BL 22, BL 39, and SP 9.
- To clear Damp Heat: needle BL 25, LI 11, SP 9, GB 41, LIV 3, and CV 3.
- To cool the Blood to relieve itch: needle LI 11, LI 4, BL 40, SP 10, and GV 14.

Deficient Skin Disorders

Blood deficiency is the main deficiency in dogs with skin disorders. Feline skin disorders are almost never of the deficient type, except in the sense that a Spleen deficiency has led to them. The chief mechanism of skin disease in felines appears to be the generation of damp and toxic heat through Spleen Qi deficiency.

Dogs, on the other hand, seem unusually susceptible to Blood deficiency, which seems to be associated with a host of canine disorders besides skin disease. These disorders include recurrent mast cell tumors, fear aggression, thyroid adenocarcinoma, hypothyroidism, superficial hemangiomas, hyperlipidemia, chronic active hepatitis, and inflammatory bowel disease of the gastric mucosa. Blood deficiency skin disorders respond poorly to typical Western herbal approaches, since these are often considered detoxifying and Dampness draining according to the principles of Chinese medicine. Indeed, detoxifying approaches, whether through the use of Chinese or Western herbs, may actually be deleterious in the management of Blood-deficient skin disorders because of their drying effects in an already dry patient.

In Chinese medicine Blood deficiency is metaphorically understood to leave the skin vulnerable to invasion by external Wind, usually Wind-Heat or Wind-Damp, or both. Blood nourishes the skin and the hair coat. When Blood is deficient, the skin lacks integrity and a sort of vacuum is present that an external Wind can invade. In treatment of Blood deficiency rashes the rash is "expelled" and Blood is added to the skin to fill the resulting void. The dynamics of this strategy stand in contrast to those of Damp Heat approaches, in which the Damp Heat pathogen is effectively drawn into the body and voided through the urine. From this perspective, therefore, drawing a pathogen inward in a Blood-deficient dog makes the dog much worse, since the previously protected inner layers of the body become polluted and exposed. In order to obey the first credo of medicine and "do no harm," the practitioner must generally expel Blood deficiency rashes.

Hallmark Signs of Blood Deficiency in the Dog

- Pale or pale-lavender tongue.
- Thin and possibly tense or taut pulses.
- Very fine, powdery dander.
- Coat dryness or dullness.
- Alopecia; fine hair coat.
- Failure of hair to grow back after surgery.
- Restless dream-filled sleep.
- Low-grade, very pruritic lesions.
- Preponderance of lesions along the sides of the body, in the axillae, and in the inguinal region.
- Fear aggression, timidity, and anxieties of all types.
- Keratoconjunctivitis sicca.
- Chronic lameness of soft tissue origin; tendency to muscle spasm.
- The practitioner may have the diagnostic impression that there is reduced immunity in the skin, resulting in recurrent pyoderma, generalized demodectic mange, and similar disorders.

Typical Signs That Blood Deficiency Is Secondary to Spleen Deficiency

- Soft or slippery pulses.
- Swollen or scalloped tongue; coated tongue.
- Greasy coat and waxy ears.
- Undigested food in the stool.
- Coprophagy, a predilection for consuming rotting (i.e., predigested) debris.
- Episodic diarrhea with pale mucus in the stool.
- Depressed appetite.
- Lethargy.
- Weight gains.

Role of Diet in the Management of Blood-Deficient Skin Disorders

Essential fatty acids (EFAs) are much more useful in the treatment of Blood deficiency skin diseases than of Damp Heat excessive skin disorders. If Blood deficiency is secondary to a

Spleen deficiency, long-term use of these fatty acids may cause the coat to become greasy or oily because the richness of the EFA supplement overwhelms the digestive power of the Spleen, inducing the formation of pathologic Dampness. Although Blood tonic herbs (see following section) may initially appear useful in these cases, they have a similarly Dampening effect.

Chinese herbal medicines evolved out of dietary approaches to the treatment of disease and were added to foods and dishes that were believed to address the patient's problem. Dietary strategies for the treatment of disease thus often predate herbal strategies. Organ meats, most notably liver, have been considered Blood tonics for two millennia, and Blood-deficient dogs seem often to respond to the use of organ meats as Blood tonics. Efforts by the manufacturers of commercial pet diets to provide a higher grade of meat may have resulted in a backlash of avoidance of the inclusion of viscera, since liver, lungs, glands, and other potentially useful meats may fall under the Association of American Feed Control Officials (AAFCO) "by-product" label. Viscera may contain large numbers of different "nutraceuticals," the value of which is only beginning to be appreciated by scientists in nutrition and medicine. Accordingly, the degree to which they are required by an optimally healthy body as components of the diet is unknown and they are not part of current nutritional guidelines for humans or animals.

Liver contains high quantities of Vitamin A, which is proving to be a useful adjunct in the treatment of cancer (see Chapter 13) in both Blood-deficient animals and those receiving the **Hoxsey Formula**. Existing recommendations for vitamin A levels in food may need to be revised, given its apparent therapeutic usefulness in a variety of conditions.

Raw meat diets include organ meats and may be suitable for Blood-deficient animals if they show no evidence of Spleen Qi deficiency underlying the Blood deficiency. In such a case the animal's pulses may be thin but are forceful. However, if pulses are frail and feeble, Spleen deficiency may be an underlying cause of the Blood deficiency and raw meat diets should be introduced very gradually, to animal tolerance, if they are used at all. In Spleen-deficient animals it may be as important to exclude carbohydrates for a period and assess the animal's response to the diet change as it is to supply viscera in raw or cooked form.

Chinese Herbal Approaches to Deficient Skin Disorders

Formulas used to treat skin disorders arising from Blood deficiency are described in the following sections. They include formulas to address simple Blood deficiency, Blood deficiency secondary to Spleen Qi deficiency, and Blood deficiency in which a significant amount of Dampness and a disharmony between the Liver and the Spleen are present. Formulas to address related disorders of Blood Heat, Heat in the Ying layer, and Yin deficiency are also included. Formulas and herbs for topical use are briefly discussed. Major formulas are indicated with an asterisk.

Simple Blood deficiency

- ***Si Wu Xiao Feng Yin** (Four Materials Dissipate Wind Beverage) is the main formula used in my practice (SM) to address skin disease arising from Blood deficiency. The **Si Wu Tang** (Four Materials Decoction) component of the formula nourishes Blood, and the **Xiao Feng San** (Wind Dissipating Powder) component disperses the invading pathogenic Wind. In dogs responding well to the formula, visible lesions, if present, are typically mild maculopapular rashes, sometimes in areas of thin papery skin. Pruritus is usually evident. The tongue is usually lavender or pale pink, and the pulse is thin or wiry. Some of the signs of Blood deficiency mentioned previously may be present. A *recommended starting dose* of granular concentrate is ¼ tsp per 10 to 15 lb of body weight, divided into two daily doses.
- When dryness and itch are more pronounced than skin lesions, **Dang Gui Yin Zi** (Dang Gui Beverage) should be considered. A *recommended starting dose* of granular concentrate is ¼ tsp per 10 to 15 lb of body weight, divided into two daily doses.
- ***Yi Guan Jian** (One Linking Decoction) is a major formula to consider when simple Blood deficiency is associated with chronic vomiting, as in inflammatory bowel disease. Dampness should not be in evidence. A *recommended starting dose* of granular concentrate is ¼ tsp per 10 to 15 lb of body weight, divided into two daily doses.

Blood deficiency secondary to Spleen deficiency

- **Chu Shi Wei Ling Tang** (Modified Decoction to Dispel Dampness in the Spleen and Stomach) is commonly the final formula used in cases that start as Blood deficiency but turn into Dampness cases. In such cases the Spleen deficiency is the original problem but has led to a secondary Blood deficiency. Replacement of Blood losses brings signs of the Spleen deficiency to the fore. A *recommended starting dose* of granular concentrate is ¼ tsp per 10 to 15 lb of body weight, divided into two daily doses.
- **Si Wu Xiao Feng Yin** is composed of two formulas, **Si Wu Tang** (Four Materials Decoction), a Blood tonic, and **Xiao Feng San** (Dissipate Wind Powder), a formula to disperse pathogenic Wind. The latter formula has three versions labeled appropriately I, II, and III. **Xiao Feng San II** may be helpful in its own right in Blood-deficient skin disorders secondary to Spleen Qi deficiency, since it contains Fu Ling, Ren Shen, and Chen Pi to support the Spleen and regulate its Qi. An even better strategy would be simply to add 12 g of Fu Ling, 12 g of Ren Shen, and 6 g of Chen Pi to 100 g of Si Wu Xiao Feng Yin. If Spleen Qi tonification is the main goal, Dang Shen is a less expensive substitute for Ren Shen, used in the same proportion.
- ***Xiao Yao San** (Rambling Ease Powder) is an extremely important formula in human Chinese herbal medicine and is possibly the most commonly prescribed formula for women. Women, too, are prone to Blood deficiency, and Xiao Yao San tonifies the Spleen Qi to nourish Blood and "ease" the tension of the Liver. In my practice (SM) generalized demodectic mange is often characterized by a Blood deficiency arising from a Spleen deficiency. Patients that respond well have signs of both Blood and Spleen deficiency (previously mentioned). It is not known exactly how the formula works to benefit these patients, although cases refractory to ivermectin alone seem to resolve with the combined use of ivermectin and Xiao Yao San. A *recommended starting dose* of granular formula is ¼ tsp per 10 to 15 lb of body weight, divided into two daily doses.
- **Dang Gui Yin Zi** (Dang Gui Beverage) was previously mentioned for simple Blood deficiency. When Spleen Qi deficiency accompanies Blood deficiency, but itch and

dryness are more prominent than visible lesions, 40 g of **Yu Ping Feng San** (Jade Screen Powder) can be added to 100 g of Dang Gui Yin Zi. A *recommended starting dose* of granular formula is ¼ tsp per 10 to 15 lb of body weight, divided into two daily doses. This formula might be especially important as an intercurrent formula between bouts of lesion development in animals with recurrent skin infections caused by a seeming immune deficiency. This is because Yu Ping Feng San helps tonify not only Spleen Qi, but also the "shield" of Wei Qi that surrounds the body and resists the invasion of pathogenic Wind. The combination of Dang Gui, He Shou Wu, and Huang Qi contained within this formula also seems effective in resolving chronic low-grade human acne and is worth considering for the same condition in dogs. This formula may prove to be important in the near future, given its numerous applications.

Blood deficiency with prominent Dampness

- ***Dang Gui Shao Yao San** (Dang Gui and Peony Powder) is used when Blood-deficient skin problems accompany signs of internal Dampness. Chief among them might be recurrent crystalluria or recurrent cystitis. Another condition that calls for this formula is Blood deficiency lesions in dogs with hyperlipidemia. A *recommended starting dose* of granular concentrate is ¼ tsp per 10 to 15 lb of body weight, divided into two daily doses.
- ***Xiao Feng San I** (Dissipate Wind Powder, version I) is the classic version of the formula **Xiao Feng San.** It may be helpful to disperse Wind Heat related to Blood deficiency. When Heat signs are not exaggerated, Shi Gao and Zhi Mu can probably be eliminated from the formula. Lesions in patients responding to this formula may be quite Damp and oozing. The patient probably exhibits a solid mix of Dampness signs and Blood deficiency signs.

Blood Heat

- Hot patients may have rashes that resist efforts to disperse them with Blood tonic formulas and efforts to draw them inward for internal drainage with Dampness-draining formulas. In these unusual cases the Heat pathogen is considered to have successfully invaded through the Wei, Qi, and Ying levels to finally lodge in the Xue, or Blood, level. The classic formula to expel Heat pathogens from the Blood is **Xi Jiao Di Huang Tang** (Decoction of Rhinoceros Horn and Rehmannia). Rhinoceros horn is no longer used in the formula but is substituted with Shui Niu Jiao (Water Buffalo Horn), as water buffalo is a domesticated species in China. In animals likely to benefit from this formula, the tongue will be dark-red or purple and perhaps covered with a dry yellow coat. The pulse will be rapid and thin. A *recommended starting dose* of granular concentrate is ¼ tsp per 10 to 15 lb of body weight, divided into two daily doses. This formula may be hard to obtain in North America.

- When the pathogen has not quite penetrated the Blood level but is stuck in the Ying (Constructive or Nutritive Qi) layer of the body, **Qing Ying Tang** (Clear the Ying Layer) should be considered. The patient exhibits symptoms similar to those calling for Xi Jiao Di Huang Tang. Skin lesions are macular, the tongue is dark, dry, and red, and the pulse is rapid and thin. The patient also may demonstrate some signs of Yin deficiency and Empty Fire such as heat intolerance, nighttime restlessness, skin dryness, and thirst. A *recommended starting dose* of granular concentrate is ¼ tsp per 10 to 15 lb of body weight, divided into two daily doses.
- A more common manifestation of Blood Heat is extreme itch. Qing Ying Tang seems routinely effective in significantly alleviating extreme puritus.

Yin deficiency

- Adequate Blood levels require adequate Kidney Yin and Essence. If valuable Kidney Yin is compromised, other body fluids must be compromised for its sake and Blood becomes deficient. In some cases this is manifested as alopecia, coat dryness, and perhaps hyperpigmentation in elderly animals. There may also be a mild itch and nighttime restlessness. Pulses are weak and thready, and the tongue is often pale (because of the accompanying Blood deficiency) with a thin coating. The formula indicated for this type of alopecia is **Shen Ying Yang**

Zhen Dan (Wondrous Response True-Nourishing Elixir). A *recommended starting dose* of granular concentrate is ¼ tsp per 10 to 15 lb of body weight, divided into two daily doses.

- For elderly dogs with red, hot, itchy feet, powdery dander, heat intolerance, thirst, thin floating pulses, and a pale or red, dry tongue, **Zhi Bai Di Huang Wan** (Amenarrhena, Phellodendron, and Rehmannia Pill) should be considered. A *recommended starting dose* of granular concentrate is ¼ tsp per 10 to 15 lb of body weight, divided into two daily doses.

Acupuncture Point Prescriptions for Deficient Skin Disorders

- To cool the Blood to relieve itch: LI 11, LI 4, BL 40, SP 10, and GV 14.
- To nourish Blood through the Spleen: ST 36, LI 4, CV 12, and BL 20.
- To nourish Blood directly: LIV 3, BL 18, BL 17, and SP 6.

Acupuncture Points for Skin Inflammation in Particular Areas

- For eruptions in the lower part of body: SP 10, ST 44, SP 6, GV 3, Bai Hui, and SP 6.
- For eruptions of the front feet: HT 5, HT 6, HT 7, PC 4, LI 4, LI 11; LU 5, LU 10, GV 14, PC 6, TH 5, and Bai Hui.
- For eruptions of the rear feet: KI 7, SP 6, BL 23, Bai Hui, SP 6, SP 9, and KI 6.
- For eruptions of the lips: ST 2, ST 44, ST 45, SP 6, SP 9, BL 20, and BL 21.
- For eruptions around the ears: LIV 3, GB 1, GB 2, GB 8, and GB 20.

Topical Treatments with Chinese Herbs

- Huang Bai plus Pu Gong Ying plus Ju Hua to resolve exudates; dust on three times daily (antibacterial effect).
- Qing Dai San in sesame oil for aftercare or for chronic dry lesions; apply three times daily (antibacterial effect).

Topical Treatments with Western Herbs

- Calendula *(Calendula officinalis)* for hot spots; this herb rapidly soothes, promotes reepithelialization, and is mildly antimicrobial; apply liberally as needed.

- Thuja Oil *(Thuja occidentalis* as an oil extract*)*: seems helpful in reducing or eliminating proliferative lesions. Apply liberally two to three times daily as needed.

Vitamin A

- Vitamin A may be given by injection to help reduce hyperkeratotic lesions although type I hypersensitivity reactions may be observed with some injectable preparations, manifested chiefly as acute hives. A *suggested dose* is 5000 IU per lb of body weight in animals with no evidence of liver disease, up to a maximum dose of 500,000 IU. Repeat monthly or as needed, unless ineffective.

ACNE

Therapeutic Rationale

- Identify and address cause (parasitic, allergic, abnormalities of sebum production).
- Remove sources for contact sensitivity such as plastic food and water bowls.

Alternative Options with Conventional Bases

Nutrition

- **Elimination diet** to determine whether food allergy plays a part.

Herbs

- **Topical herbs:** Calendula tincture is recommended by some practitioners. Calendula has shown antiinflammatory activity in experimental animal trials (Akihisa, 1996; Lievre, 1992). Tea Tree Oil *(Melaleuca alternifolia)* is commonly recommended for human acne; however, Tea Tree Oil is very toxic to cats and potentially so to dogs. Tea Tree Oil is not generally recommended for use in animal acne, since it can be easily ingested by the animal.

Paradigmatic Options

Traditional Chinese Medicine

- Acne is usually a Damp-Heat–related condition, although some mild forms may be a manifestation of

Blood deficiency. Review the previous section for assistance in selecting an appropriate Chinese herbal formula and acupuncture protocol to best address the patient.

- In addition to these formulas, others have been recommended specifically for use in acne in dogs. **Pi Pa Ye Yin** (Eriobotyra Beverage) contains Pi Pa Ye 12 g, Sang Bai Pi 9 g, Huang Qin 6 g, Ju Hua 6 g, Lian Qiao 9 g, Jin Yin Hua 6 g, Pu Gong Yin 6 g, Zi Hua Di Ding 9 g, Chi Shao 9 g, Mu Dan Pi 9 g, Zhi Zi 6 g, and Rhubarb 6 g. These ingredients clear Heat from the upper body through their various antimicrobial and antibacterial properties. The formula also has a Blood-moving and Blood-cooling effect that aids in decongesting lesions and relieving itch. Animals that may benefit have a rolling, rapid pulse and a red tongue. A *suggested starting dose* of granular concentrate is ¼ tsp per 15 lb of body weight, or 60 to 75 mg/kg of body weight, given in divided doses, usually twice daily.
- **Pu Ji Xiao Du Yin** (Universal Antiphlogistic Beverage) was originally developed to address acute viral infections such as mumps in humans. It has been suggested as being helpful in acne as well. Like Pi Pa Ye Yin the formula dispels pathogenic Heat and toxins from the upper body, but it does not move or cool the Blood. Patients that benefit may have a red tongue and a rapid or wiry pulse. A *suggested starting dose* of granular concentrate is ¼ tsp per 15 lb of body weight, or 60 to 75 mg/kg of body weight, given in divided doses, usually twice daily.
- Consideration should probably also be given to the use of **Siler and Coix Decoction**, mentioned in Chapter 7. This formula contains 3 g each of Chuan Xiong, Bai Zhi, Yi Yi Ren, Huang Qin, Jie Geng, Zhi Zi, and Fang Feng. It also contains 1.5 g each of Jing Jie, Zhi Shi, Huang Lian, Gan Cao, and Bo He. The formula is designed to treat inflammation of the head in almost any form (stomatitis, acne, furuncles) when it is secondary to an internal accumulation of Damp Heat. This formula is especially appropriate for cases

that probably also have a Wind-Heat component (i.e., sudden onset) of the rash. The pulse in these patients is wiry and rapid and the tongue is red or purple-red and wet. A *suggested starting dose* of granular concentrate is ¼ tsp per 15 lb of body weight, or 60 to 75 mg/kg of body weight, divided into two equal portions.

- For severe infections when the patient has pronounced inflammation and cellulitis, a red or purple tongue, and a rapid, wiry pulse, consider **Huang Lian Jie Du Tang** (Antiphlogistic Decoction of Coptis). This formula should never be used in mild or deficient cases. A *suggested starting dose* of granular concentrate is ¼ tsp per 15 lb of body weight, or 60 to 75 mg/kg of body weight, given in divided doses, usually twice daily.

AUTHORS' CHOICES:

SM: Use appropriate Chinese herbal formulas and diets to address the animal's general presentation.
SW: Remove plastic bowls; use elimination or homemade diet; Calendula tincture topically; possibly Chinese herbal formulas.

ALOPECIA, IDIOPATHIC

Therapeutic Rationale

- Identify endocrine, allergic, parasitic, or other underlying conditions.

Alternative Options with Conventional Bases

Nutrition

- **Diet changes:** anecdotally, elimination or homemade diets have resolved some cases of chronic, noninflammatory alopecia in dogs.
- **Melatonin:** for seasonal alopecia of boxers and possibly other alopecia of unknown origin in other breeds. The *recommended dose* is 3 to 6 mg tid.

Paradigmatic Options

Traditional Chinese Medicine

- The two main causes of hair loss are Toxic Heat, which is usually attended by evidence of pronounced inflammation, and Yin or Blood deficiency, which is usually indicated by few or no lesions. See the section on Deficient Skin Disorders for assistance in selecting an appropriate Blood- or Yin-tonifying formula. **Shen Ying Yang Zhen Dan** (Wondrous Response True-Nourishing Elixir) is a formula developed specifically for idiopathic alopecia in people and it may be useful in animals, especially dogs. Guiding signs for the use of this formula are mild itch and nighttime restlessness, weak and thready pulses, and an often pale (because of the accompanying Blood deficiency) and thinly coated tongue. Other authors also advocate this formula for dogs with irritability, an oily coat, and hair loss when stressed. These authors describe the pulse indicating appropriateness of the formula as stringy and rapid, and the tongue as red on the edges. Use of a plum blossom hammer on the denuded areas to help restore circulation is also recommended by some TCM practitioners. A *suggested starting dose* of granular concentrate is ¼ tsp per 15 lb of body weight, or 60 to 75 mg/kg of body weight, given in divided doses, usually twice daily.
- For cases in which the animal has dry hair that is easily broken or epilated, thready pulses, and a pale tongue, some authors also advise using **Gu Ben Tang,** an aggressive Yin and Blood tonic. The formula's ingredients are Sheng Di Huang 9 g, Shu Di Huang 9 g, Tian Men Dong 9 g, Mai Men Dong 9 g, Fu Shen 9 g, Ren Shen 6 g, Dang Gui 9 g, and Ce Bai Ye 5 g. Ce Bai Ye is a specific herb used to address alopecia areata in humans. A *suggested starting dose* of granular concentrate is ¼ tsp per 15 lb of body weight, or 60 to 75 mg/kg of body weight, given in divided doses, usually twice daily. Plum blossom hammers applied to the alopecic areas are also advocated to help draw circulation to the area to support the action of the formula.

Cautions

- Melatonin has been associated with inhibited fertility and diabetic dysregulation, although these effects are not commonly recognized.

AUTHORS' CHOICES:

SM: Blood tonic herbs and diets.
SW: Diet changes; Chinese herbs.

ALLERGIC DERMATITIS (ATOPIC, FLEA)

Therapeutic Rationale

- Suppress pruritus.
- Manage secondary infection.
- Remove offending allergens.
- Consider hyposensitization.
- Control fleas.

Alternative Options with Conventional Bases

Nutrition

- **Diet improvement:** virtually every veterinarian who is interested in alternative or emerging treatments has learned, through trial and error, that dogs and cats with allergies improve when the quality of their diets is improved. There are a number of possible explanations, including the following:
  - A reduction in the number of food allergens. Higher quality diets are often composed of limited ingredients, such as only one to two meat, dairy, or grain ingredients, as opposed to lower quality commercial diets that may contain various animal products under the AAFCO labels "meat by-products" or "poultry by-products," or multiple grains.
  - Higher quality diets are of fixed formulation, whereas lower quality diets may contain ever-changing ingredients under AAFCO labeling rules, making identification of the offending ingredient difficult.

- Higher quality diets may contain more digestible products or higher levels of ingredients particularly needed by the animal for its skin condition (conditional essentiality).
- Homemade diets may contain phytonutrients or other constituents that are beneficial to sick animals but not available in any processed diet.
- If the owner is not willing to prepare homemade food for the animal, many high-quality, limited-ingredient diets are on the market. Educating the owner that a trial of more than one diet may be necessary is important. If the owner can prepare food at home for their pet, a number of different systems and philosophies can be tried (Berschneider, 2002). Homemade diets have the advantage of offering flexibility to cover all of the animal's individual requirements. Improving the diet of any pet with allergic dermatitis is vital, regardless of other treatments that are considered.

- **Fatty acids:** a great many fatty acid supplements are on the market for treatment of atopic dermatitis, but many veterinarians consider them ineffective. Much greater clinical success can be obtained with these supplements if they are given as DHA/EPA only (from fish body oil). The *recommended dose* is approximately 100 to 200 mg of fatty acids (not fish oil) per kg of body weight, divided into 2 to 3 doses daily (Remillard, 1998). This translates realistically to at least 1 capsule of Fish Oil (containing 300 mg of EPA and DHA) for 10 lb of body weight.
- **Bioflavonoids:** given alone or in combination with Vitamin C, have been recommended for treatment of atopic dermatitis. This is probably based on preliminary studies suggesting that quercetin may be effective in the treatment of allergic rhinitis in humans, but there are no studies on bioflavonoids and allergic dermatitis. Presumably, the antiinflammatory and antioxidant properties of some flavonoids may be useful for inflammatory skin disorders.
- **Vitamin C:** administration may suppress blood histamine levels (Johnston, 1992), and the occasional

animal appears to benefit from supplementation. The *recommended dose* is 5 to 10 mg/lb of body weight, tid.

- **Bee pollen:** has been recommended for treatment of allergies, probably on the idea that ingestion of the pollens may induce immunologic tolerance and reduce signs over time. Use of locally produced bee pollen is important, and it should be remembered that the administration of antigens may worsen allergies. Oral tolerance should be accomplished by a gradual increase in an initial low dose of pollen.
- **Enzymes:** frequently recommended as an adjunct treatment for allergic dermatitis. Whether digestive enzymes enhance digestibility and increase absorption of dietary nutrients, leading to an effect similar to improving the diet, or whether another mechanism is at work is unknown. Some veterinarians claim that enzymes are absorbed systemically and actually destroy circulating immune complexes, although no direct evidence has been found for this theory.

Herbs

Systemically administered herbs

- **Burdock Root:** a traditional Western alterative that is often a part of herbal allergy treatments. There are no studies to support and no reason to believe that Burdock Root is effective if used alone. On the other hand, Burdock Seed is used in Chinese medicine and is often part of prescriptions for skin disorders.
- **Oregon Grape Root:** a traditional antiinflammatory that has shown unique antibiotic activity against *Staphylococcus aureus* (Stermitz, 2000).
- **Nettles and Cleavers** *(Galium aparine):* traditional herbs that are often included in both systemic and topical formulas, but no support can be found for this use.
- **Licorice:** often recommended as a substitute for corticosteroids. A constituent, glycyrrhizin, does in fact have mineralocorticoid activity (see Appendix C for a summary table that includes undesirable side effects of Licorice).

- **Zemaphyte:** a number of controlled studies have shown that a specific combination of Chinese herbs is helpful in managing atopic eczema in human patients (Xu, 1992, 1995, 1997). Long-term use has not been fully evaluated but may be associated with hepatic enzyme changes in children. Zemaphyte is a combination of 10 herbs: *Clematis armandii* (Chuan Mu Tong), *Dictamnus dasycarpus* (Bai Xian), Licorice (Gan Cao), *Ledebouriella saseloides* (Fang Feng), *Lophatherum gracile* (Zhu Ye), White Peony *(Paeonia lactiflora)* (Bai Shao), *Potentilla chinensis* (Fan Bai Cao), Rehmannia (*Rehmannia glutinosa*) (Di Huang), *Schizonepeta tenuifolia* (Jing Jie), and *Tribulus terrestris* (Ji Li).
- **Zemaphyte derivative:** a recent study from the University of Minnesota College of Veterinary Medicine investigated three herbs contained in Zemaphyte for control of pruritus in atopic dogs. Fifty dogs with atopic dermatitis were assessed by both owners and veterinarians and given either a placebo or a combination of Licorice, White Peony, and Rehmannia. These herbs were chosen on the basis of company (Phytopharm, LLC, United Kingdom) bioassay and palatability. Of the dogs receiving herbs, 37.5% improved compared with 13% of the placebo group, and the deterioration scores were worse in the placebo group at the final visit. Although neither result reached statistical significance, the researchers were encouraged at the results and suggested further study (Nagle, 2001).
- **Byakko-ka-ninjin-to:** a Kampo formula composed of Gypsum, Anemarrhena Root *(Anemarrhenae asphodeloides)*, Licorice, Ginseng *(Panax ginseng)*, and Rice inhibited pruritus in a mouse allergy model (Tohda, 2000).

Topically administered herbs

- Although little supporting data are available, the following herbs are frequently used for focal pruritus, acute moist dermatitis, and other focal inflammatory skin disorders: Chickweed *(Stellaria media)*, Jewelweed *(Impatiens capensis, I. biflora,* other

Impatiens spp.), Plantain *(Plantago major)*, Calendula, Chamomile *(Matricaria recutita)*, and Tea *(Camellia sinensis)*.

Paradigmatic Options

- Atopic dermatitis may be manifested as either an Excess or a deficient skin syndrome. The initial section of this chapter can be consulted for help in selecting the appropriate herbal formula to deal with this condition. The most useful formulas are usually **Si Wu Xiao Feng Yin** (Four Materials Dissipate Wind Beverage), **Xiao Feng San** (Dissipate Wind Powder), **Zhi Bai Di Huang Wan** (Anemarrhena, Phellodendron, and Rehmannia Pill), **Chu Shi Wei Ling Tang** (Modified Decoction to Dispel Dampness in the Spleen and Stomach), **Si Miao San** (Four Marvels Powder), and **Modified Long Dan Xie Gan Tang** (Modified Gentian Drain the Liver Decoction).
- **Wu Ling San** (Powder of Five Herbs with Poria), **Bi Xie Shen Shi Tang** (Fish Poison Yam Dampness Percolating Decoction), and **Long Dan Xie Gan Tang** (Gentian Drain the Liver Decoction) were also mentioned previously and are especially advocated by other authors. For Blood-deficient cases, other authors advocate **Si Wu Tang** (Four Materials Decoction), **Yi Guan Jian** (One Linking Decoction), and **Dang Gui Yin Zi** (Dang Gui Beverage). The initial section of this chapter should be consulted for specific indications of these formulas.
- For cases of Toxic Heat with papules, pustules, and furuncles, **Wu Wei Xiao Du Yin** (Five-Ingredient Antiphlogistic Decoction) and **Pu Ji Xiao Du Yin** (Universal Antiphlogistic Decoction) have been advocated. The former is a dispersing formula for cases with fairly superficial involvement. The latter is for more internally or severely affected patients, especially those with possible attending lymphadenopathy associated with the sores. The tongue of these patients is red, and the pulse is wiry and rapid. A *suggested starting dose* of granular concentrate for either formula is ¼ tsp per 15 lb of body weight, or 60 to 75 mg/kg of

body weight, given in divided doses, usually twice daily.

Cautions

- Diuretic herbs may enhance diuresis if corticosteroids are being used.
- Licorice may enhance adverse effects of corticosteroids unless the deglycyrrhizinated (DGL) form is used.

AUTHORS' CHOICES:

SM: Diet changes; appropriate Chinese herbal formula; Fish Oil.
SW: Diet changes; Fish Oil; appropriately chosen Chinese herbs; tea bags for hot spots.

ANAL GLAND PROBLEMS

Therapeutic Rationale

- Unknown causes—keep emptied and evaluate for infection.
- Increase stool bulk using fiber supplements.

Alternative Options with Conventional Bases

- **Control weight and encourage exercise**—sedentary animals appear to be at increased risk.
- **Evaluate for concurrent signs of allergy** because controlling allergies appears to help in some dogs.

Paradigmatic Options

- Anal gland impaction and inflammation usually attend the accumulation of Damp Heat. Chinese herbal and dietary strategies to address Damp Heat should be considered, including **Si Miao San** (Four Marvels Powder), and herbal formulas specifically designed to address lower body disorders. Other useful formulas and strategies, including **Jia Wei Er Miao San** (Augmented Two Marvels Powder), are listed in the section at the beginning of this chapter dealing with Excess skin disorders.

AUTHORS' CHOICES:

SM: Formulas and diets to address Damp Heat.
SW: Increase dietary fiber; increase exercise; address allergies.

DEMODICOSIS

Therapeutic Rationale

- Eliminate parasites.
- Manage immunodeficiency, where possible.

Alternative Options with Conventional Bases

Nutrition

- **Diet** plays a critical role in combating this condition. When the diet of dogs eating medium- or poor-quality commercial diets is improved, they appear to develop better defenses and clear generalized demodectic mange. This diet improvement involves either very high-quality commercial diets or, preferably, homemade diets.
- **Carotenoids:** in one study the supplementation of up to 20 mg crystalline lutein in beagles led to increases in serum lutein within 2 weeks and was associated with augmentation of both cellular and humoral immune responses (Kim, 2000). Since most other carotenoids have not been tested in dogs but have been shown to have beneficial effects on immune function in other species, a mixed carotenoid supplement (containing beta-carotene, lycopene, Vitamin A, or others) may be most useful. Carotenoids are relatively safe, so dosage determination according to the animal's weight as a proportion to the human dose is recommended.
- **Minerals:** Zinc and Selenium have been shown to enhance immune function and prevent infections in humans (Girodon, 1999; Sazawal, 1998).
- **Antioxidant vitamins:** Vitamins C and E appear to enhance immune function in various species, including humans, mostly in elderly humans (Grimble, 1997). Treatment of demodectic mange using Vitamin E alone

has been found ineffective. Whether similarities exist between the depressed immune function seen in dogs with generalized demodectic mange and normal immune senescence is unknown, but a reevaluation, using a combination of Vitamins C and E, Zinc, Selenium, and Carotenoids, might be warranted.

Herbs

Systemic herbs

- Systemic herbs center primarily on immune stimulants. An herbal immunostimulant that has traditional Chinese indications for skin disease is Astragalus *(Astragalus membranaceus)*, which enhances immune function according to results of in vitro and laboratory animal trials. Medicinal mushrooms may also be considered.
- **Plant sterols**, and in particular one sterol product (Moducare), have been shown to beneficially alter the TH1/TH2 balance in conditions when an immunopathologic condition causes disease signs (Bouic, 1999). Some studies have suggested that adult demodectic mange may be accompanied by TH1 defects and abnormalities in CD4/CD8 ratios (Birkett, 1996; Lemarie, 1996). Anecdotal reports suggest that giving Moducare supplements to dogs with chronic demodectic mange is helpful.

Topical herbs

- **Neem** *(Azadirachta indica):* extracts have been shown to have variable efficacy (usually dose dependent) on a variety of parasitic arthropods (Guerrini, 1998; Mulla, 1999; O'Brien, 1999). It has not been tested against demodex mite species, but clinical experience suggests that topical application of Neem can suppress mite numbers.
- **Tea Tree Oil:** has antimicrobial, fungicidal, and insecticidal properties. Unfortunately, it can be toxic to dogs, notably small breeds, and should be used only in combination with other herbs or in extremely low concentrations.
- **Essential oils:** Lavender, Eucalyptus, and other plant oils have been recommended for control of external

parasites. Many of these oils are toxic if used undiluted and this limits their usefulness in animals that will certainly groom themselves and ingest the oils.

Paradigmatic Options

- One herbal formula that consistently has been shown to be of benefit in my practice (SM) is **Xiao Yao San** (Rambling Ease Powder). It is prescribed in Blood-deficient cases, as described in the initial section of this chapter. It seems to exceed the benefits seen with other Blood tonic formulas, but the reason is unknown at present. It can safely be used with other miticidal treatments. A *suggested starting dose* of granular concentrate is ¼ tsp per 15 lb of body weight, or 60 to 75 mg/kg of body weight, given in divided doses, usually twice daily.

Cautions

- Essential oils are potentially very toxic, with a few exceptions (such as lavender).

AUTHORS' CHOICES:

SM: Xiao Yao San.
SW: Immunomodulatory nutritional supplements, especially plant sterols (Moducare); Neem on focal areas or as a bath and dip treatment.

DERMATOPHYTOSIS

Therapeutic Rationale

- Eradicate fungal organisms on animal and in environment.
- Identify predisposing factors such as immunologic defects.
- Clip hair to reduce parasite numbers and substrate.

Alternative Options with Conventional Bases

Nutrition

- **Immunostimulant vitamins and minerals** (see section on Demodex). A combination supplement containing Vitamins A, C, and E, Selenium, Zinc, Lutein, and perhaps plant sterols may be ideal.

Herbs

- **Immunostimulant herbs** that may be useful for stimulating immune function include Astragalus (see Demodex section) and Reishi mushroom *(Ganoderma lucidum)*.
- **Eucalyptus Oil** *(Eucalyptus paucifolia)*: exhibited antifungal activity against *Trichophyton mentagrophytes, Microsporum canis,* and *M. gypseum*. There were no adverse effects when this oil was applied to mammalian skin at 0.5% concentration (Shahi, 2000). Unforunately, Eucalyptus Oil is potentially quite toxic or fatal if ingested and this limits its use in animals, especially in cats.
- **Garlic** *(Allium sativum)*: showed antifungal activity in vitro against *T. mentagrophytes* and *M. canis* (Venugopal, 1995). However, it is unclear whether oral treatment with Garlic would affect clinical cases of dermatophytosis and topical treatment is probably too unpleasant to contemplate.

Paradigmatic Options

- Dermatophytosis should be treated according to its presenting signs if Chinese medicine is to be used by the veterinarian. The initial section of this chapter describes specific indications for the use of a large variety of Chinese herbal formulas. Low-grade lesions may respond to Blood-tonifying formulas, which can be viewed as enhancing the local immunity of the skin. Excessive purulent lesions often respond to Damp Heat formulas.
- Tea Tree Oil is reported to be effective against dermatophytes. It is potentially toxic unless used in minute doses.

Cautions

- Essential oils are potentially very toxic.

AUTHORS' CHOICES:

SM: Use the appropriate herbal formula.

SW: Immunostimulant herbs; Chinese herbal formulas as appropriate; Neem topically; clipping when appropriate; itraconazole in resistant cases.

DISCOID LUPUS

Therapeutic Rationale

- Suppress immune-mediated inflammation.
- Prevent scarring.
- Reduce ultraviolet exposure.
- Manage secondary pyoderma.

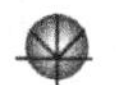

Alternative Options with Conventional Bases

- **Oral and topical applications of Vitamin E** have anecdotal support for resolving milder lesions.

Paradigmatic Options

- Consult the initial section of this chapter for signs that call for the use of different herbal formulas. Select the most appropriate formula for the patient's overall condition. Siler and Croix Decoction, especially when used in tandem with Vitamin E, is of particular benefit. Long-term remissions are possible, even after herbal treatment is discontinued.

Cautions

- None recognized.

AUTHORS' CHOICES:

SM: Vitamin E.

SW: Vitamin E and niacinamide; tetracycline if necessary; Chinese herbal formulas.

EOSINOPHILIC GRANULOMAS, INDOLENT ULCERS, EOSINOPHILIC PLAQUES

Therapeutic Rationale

- Control hypersensitivity reactions.
- Identify and treat allergies.
- Control fleas and exposure to other biting insects.

Alternative Options with Conventional Bases

- **Interferon:** many cats with these lesions are thought to have some form of allergy, although some dermatologists consider viruses may contribute and many cases are truly idiopathic. A trial with interferon is probably safe and may yield benefit in a few cases.

Paradigmatic Options

- Current experience with the treatment of eosinophilic granulomas in cats reveals them to be, like other skin lesions in cats, a manifestation of Damp or Toxic Heat. For patients that have red tongues and relatively forceful and rapid pulses, the **Hoxsey Formula** should be considered. Some practitioners have reported at least temporary success with the use of other Western herbs, including a combination of Yellow Dock, Agrimony *(Agrimonia eupatoria)*, Sarsaparilla *(Smilax officinalis)*, and Burdock. A *suggested starting dose* for either formula is 0.2 ml per 5 lb of body weight, given at least once daily.

AUTHORS' CHOICES:

SM: Western herbs.
SW: Diet changes; herbs if cat will tolerate them.

FLEA INFESTATION

Therapeutic Rationale

- Control all stages of flea life cycle.

Alternative Options with Conventional Bases

Nutrition

- **Diet:** most practitioners interested in alternative therapies have noted that fleas cause serious irritation in dogs eating poor-quality diets and that these same dogs do not experience such irritation when the diet is improved. Flea numbers may or may not change from year to year despite the change in skin response. Attention to diet is crucial for dogs with chronic serious flea bite dermatitis.
- **Yeast:** the use of yeast is popular among pet owners and we suspect that brewer's yeast simply acts as a nutritional supplement, providing the same benefit

noted with diet improvements. In a study in which dogs were administered brewer's yeast at 14 g per day no effect against fleas was seen (Baker, 1983).

Herbs

- **Neem**: in a study using topical Neem extract on both dogs and cats, 1000 to 2400 ppm azadirachtin reduced fleas on greyhounds and cats by 53% to 93% in a dose-dependent manner for 19 days (Guerrini, 1998). Clinical experience suggests that Neem spray should be applied every few days.
- **Garlic**: although orally administered Garlic has a reputation for repelling fleas, the literature is filled with warnings that Garlic will cause Heinz body anemia when administered to dogs and cats. However, a thorough search of the literature fails to locate any reports of Garlic's causing Heinz body anemia in dogs. Toxicologists suggest that this may be a dose-related phenomenon, since anemia after onion administration has been reported, and onions are usually used at higher "doses" in cooking. In practice, there appear to be differences in the susceptibility of individual animals. Considering the many pet owners who feed Garlic to dogs and cats, it may be safer than is usually assumed. The efficacy of Garlic against fleas, however, is still questionable; in studies so far, it has not been effective.
- **Fleabane** *(Erigeron canadense)*: has been used for many centuries (Aristotle mentions it). The traditional recommendation is to repel fleas by burning the herb, but some sources also recommend rubbing the herb on the clothes (or fur for animals) or applying extracts topically. There are no data supporting use of fleabane for fleas.
- **Essential oils:** Lavender, Eucalyptus, Citronella *(Cymbopogon nardus)*, Pennyroyal *(Mentha pulegium)*, Tea Tree, and other plant oils have been recommended for control of external parasites. Many of these oils are toxic if used undiluted, which limits their usefulness in animals that will certainly groom themselves and ingest the oils. Pennyroyal Oil ingestion in particular has been

associated with the death of at least one dog (Sudekum, 1992).

- **Pyrethrum** *(Tanacetum cinerarifolium* or *Chrysanthemum cinerarifolium):* the source of pyrethrins, and the powdered flowers have been used topically on dogs and cats.

Environmental control

- **Diatomaceous earth:** has been recommended as a desiccant to kill flea larvae. It may be irritating to the respiratory tract.
- **Sodium polyborate powders:** are offered by various companies and seem to work well.

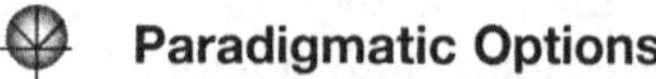

Paradigmatic Options

- Control of skin inflammation probably represents an important means of flea control. Active inflammation is usually attended by an increased blood supply to the skin, thus providing an increased food supply for fleas. Reduction of skin inflammation through the use of herbal formulas seems to result in gradual attenuation of flea numbers in most cases. To use Chinese medicine to reduce dermatitis, consult the initial section of this chapter.

Cautions

- Essential oils are potentially toxic.

AUTHORS' CHOICES:

SM: Address the skin disorder with the appropriate herbal formula; sodium polyborate environmental control as needed.

SW: High-quality or homemade diets; sodium polyborate environmental control; flea combs.

LICK GRANULOMA

Therapeutic Rationale

- Identify predisposing conditions such as allergy, local fungal, parasitic, or bacterial infection, endocrinopathy, foreign body, neoplasia, or psychogenic causes.

Alternative Options with Conventional Bases

- See section on Allergic Dermatitis, especially regarding diet.

Herbs

Topical herbs

- **Aloe** *(Aloe vera, A. barbadensis)* has been shown to enhance healing in surgically induced wounds (Swaim, 1992). Aloe also may have antiinflammatory properties (Vazquez, 1996), although the relative strength of these properties in relation to the sometimes-effective steroids is weak. Anecdotally, Aloe is rarely effective in treating lick granulomas.

Other

- **Chiropractic:** one theory about the origin of lick granulomas suggests that spinal subluxation or malalignment leads to peripheral nerve irritation. Chiropractic examination and adjustment may be helpful.
- **Acupuncture** is often helpful. See the information on technique later in this section.

Paradigmatic Options

- Lick granuloma may involve a mental-emotional component, a general skin inflammatory component, and a local inflammatory component. Treatment directed simultaneously at all three components may be beneficial in reducing these lesions.
- As described in the initial section of this chapter, for the mental-emotional component the practitioner should consider using an herbal tincture that comprises equal parts of Linden Flowers, Nettles, and Passion Flower (see discussion under Western herbal approaches to Excess skin disorders).
- Consideration might also be given to use of the calming herbs mentioned in Chapter 3. The approach most appropriate to the animal's overall condition should be chosen.
- For any coinciding general skin disorder, the most appropriate herbal formula from those described at the beginning of this chapter should be chosen.

- For control of local irritation and inflammation a number of options may be considered. Infection of the wound should be controlled, with antibiotics if appropriate. Homeopathic *Silicea* 12C or 30C given once or twice daily for a couple of weeks may assist discharge of infectious material from the lesion and possibly reorganization of the granuloma itself. However, sustained use of low-potency *Silicea* will result in a perpetual discharge and should be stopped at least temporarily after 2 to 3 weeks of use. Administration may be restarted for another couple of weeks at a time if it appears the *Silicea* is having a beneficial, not an aggravating, effect.
- Another means of relieving local inflammation and irritation is through the topical application of oils or ointments containing St. John's Wort *(Hypericum perforatum)*, since one of the traditional uses of St. John's Wort is for soothing irritated nerve endings.
- "Ring the dragon" is an acupuncture technique commonly used to address the lesion at a local level. The lesion is encircled by needles and one needle is placed at the center of the lesion. Needle stimulation may be by moxibustion, hand manipulation, or injection. Treatments should initially be repeated once or twice weekly.

Cautions

- None recognized.

AUTHORS' CHOICES:

SM: Silicea; nervine or calming herbal formulas; address underlying skin problems; local application of St. John's Wort.

SW: Address underlying problems such as allergy; acupuncture; antibiotics for deep infections.

PERIANAL FISTULAE

Therapeutic Rationale

- Surgically debride or remove.
- Keep area very clean.
- Control bacterial infection.
- Control inflammation.
- Control pain.

Alternative Options with Conventional Bases

- **Taro Root:** anecdotally, slices of this root vegetable applied as a compress have been successful.

Paradigmatic Options

- Success has been achieved in the treatment of perianal fistulae using formulas to address Damp Heat in the lower jiao. Herbs can be added to address the Blood stasis that creates the pain associated with these lesions. The initial section of this chapter should be reviewed for further guidance on formula selection. **Si Miao San** (Four Marvels Powder) and **Jia Wei Er Miao San** (Augmented Two Marvels Powder) can be especially considered. If the treatment is effective, use of the formulas can be continued until all lesions have completely resolved.

Cautions

- None recognized.

AUTHORS' CHOICES:

SM: Si Miao San or Jia Wei Er Miao San.
SW: Elimination diet and probiotics; Taro Root compresses; Chinese herbs; low-dose (homeopathic in low potency) Silica.

PYODERMA, RECURRENT

Therapeutic Rationale

- Identify underlying factors including allergy, fungal or parasitic infections, immunologic defects, and endocrine disorders.

Paradigmatic Options

- The initial section of this chapter should be consulted for recommended Chinese herbal formulas for recurrent pyoderma. Low-grade lesions often respond to Blood-tonifying formulas. Excessive purulent lesions often respond to Damp Heat formulas.

AUTHORS' CHOICES:

SM: Appropriate Chinese herbal formula; diet changes.
SW: Diet; Chinese herbs; possibly plant sterols (see explanation under Demodectic Mange) for prevention; antibiotics for active infection.

SEBACEOUS ADENITIS

Therapeutic Rationale
- Prevent buildup of sebum and scales with topical therapy.
- Prevent secondary pyoderma.
- Control hyperkeratosis.

Alternative Options with Conventional Bases
- For a big dog, Vitamin A 8000 to 20,000 IU daily bid for 4 to 8 weeks.

Paradigmatic Options
- Sebaceous adenitis is usually a Dampness problem. Formulas and dietary strategies to address the accumulation of Dampness and Damp Heat in the skin are given earlier in the chapter.
- Homeopathic Thuja 30C should be considered for dogs with a watery, sweet-smelling sebum. It should be given once daily for 10 days, then as needed.

Cautions
- Vitamin A is toxic when used at high doses for a long time.

AUTHORS' CHOICES:

SM: Appropriate diet and Chinese herbal formula; Vitamin A; Thuja.
SW: Diet changes; Chinese herbs; Vitamin A.

WARTS (VIRAL PAPILLOMAS)

Therapeutic Rationale
- Differentiate from less benign masses.
- Remove if lesions are frequently traumatized or for cosmetic reasons.

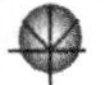

Paradigmatic Options

- Ointments or oil extracts containing Thuja have been effective when applied topically 3 times daily to affected patients. These products are sold for human use and can be adapted to animals.

AUTHORS' CHOICES:

SM: Thuja applied topically.
SW: Crushing under anesthesia or autogenous vaccines; Thuja topically or systemically as low-potency homeopathic (essentially a very low-dose herbal); laser removal.

WOUNDS/TRAUMA

Therapeutic Rationale

- Promote wound healing.
- Prevent infection.
- Reduce pain.

Alternative Options with Conventional Bases

- **Honey:** when it is applied topically honey enhances wound healing and has been shown to have antimicrobial properties (Moore, 2001).
- **Aloe:** may accelerate wound healing when applied topically (Swaim, 1992).
- **Fresh juice** (i.e., "succus") from Calendula: believed to have mild antimicrobial properties and to promote wound healing. It can be used diluted as part of wound lavage.

Other

- **Laser:** low-level laser therapy has efficacy in promoting wound healing; some lasers even work through wound dressings (Lilge, 2000).

Paradigmatic Options

Homeopathy

- ***Arnica montana*** 30C: to control passive hemorrhage and relieve aching and bruised sensations. Give up to three times daily.

- *Hypericum perforatum* 30C: to relieve stinging pain associated with superficial erosions and ulceration (i.e., "road rash"). Give up to three times daily.
- *Silicea* 30C: for chronic indurations and to expel foreign bodies. Give once daily for 2 to 3 weeks.
- *Calcarea sulphuricum* 30C: for yellow discharges from chronic fistulae. Give once daily. Use of this remedy should be followed by *Silicea* 30C once daily to "complete the case."

Cautions

- None recognized.

AUTHORS' CHOICES:

SM: Conventional wound management techniques, augmented by appropriate homeopathics; Calendula washes.
SW: Honey; aloe; Silica low-potency homeopathic (low dose); Silvadene and insulin for chronic wounds.

5 CASE REPORT
Dermatitis in a Dog

HISTORY

Cody, a 5-year-old, male, neutered Lhasa Apso, presented with a chief complaint of dermatitis and anxiety. The anxiety manifested as quivering, cowering, shaking, barking, and fearfulness in response to loud noises. Valium on an as-needed basis seemed to significantly reduce Cody's anxiety level. Exact dose levels used were not discussed. Cody was also fearful when he encountered large-breed dogs, and he was quite territorial.

Cody's dermatitis manifested as a constant licking of the paws and an obsessive scratching of the flanks and belly despite his having only minimal lesions. The few lesions that were present were located in the inguinal, perineal, and axillary regions. In the past, the lesions had tended to improve during the winter and worsen during the summer but they had not shown a seasonal improvement over the last year. The lesions were chiefly epidermal collarettes, which suggested a pyoderma. Cody's poor response to a number of antibiotics suggested the pyoderma was not primary, but secondary to an underlying disorder such as allergic dermatitis. A medicated shampoo (Pyoben) seemed to relieve his skin discomfort temporarily.

Cody's ears were chronically inflamed. Although discharge was usually minimal, the inside surfaces of the pinnae were perpetually covered by a brown dry scale. A topical combination antibiotic, antiinflammatory, and antifungal medication (Otomax), massaged into the pinnae and ear canals on an as-needed basis, seemed to relieve much of Cody's ear discomfort. A lotion containing Tea Tree Oil applied to his ears had also provided relief, but the owner did not know the name or exact composition of this product.

Cody suffered from chronic conjunctivitis that was relieved by topical administration of a combination antibiotic and anti-inflammatory ophthalmic drop (Gentocin Durafilm).

Cody had been given numerous diets in the past in case he had a food sensitivity underlying his various complaints. Although no one food tended to aggravate his condition, Cody seemed to itch less on the commercial diet he was currently being given (Arcana). Cody exhibited a strong preference for table scraps over commercial diets. His appetite was otherwise poor; he routinely refused to eat for 2 to 3 days at a time.

Cody had been immunized in the past, but vaccines had recently been avoided in case they further irritated his skin. Various alternative treatments had been tried for his skin irritation, including essential fatty acid supplements, various vitamins and mineral supplements, and digestive enzymes. None of these seemed particularly beneficial.

Cody demonstrated few other complaints. He had had sporadic episodes of vomiting yellow bile and occasional bouts of "reverse sneezing"; at one point both of Cody's eyes had swollen shut.

Regarding his general tendencies, Cody sought shade if outdoors, or drafts if indoors, suggesting that he felt warm as a rule. His body weight was stable.

Because of financial constraints, intradermal skin testing and histopathologic tests had not been performed to confirm allergic dermatitis as the primary skin lesion. Neither had any laboratory studies been performed to assess for underlying systemic disorders, such as hypothyroidism.

PHYSICAL EXAMINATION

Cody constantly either paced or scratched his abdomen while his history was being taken. He had a pale tongue, and thin, wiry pulses. The acupuncture point BL 17 felt slightly domed and turgid relative to the surrounding area.

Collarettes were noted on Cody's posterior hind limb over the semimembranosus and semitendinosus muscles. He had one healing lesion on the lower left abdomen.

Cody's ears appeared generally clean but roughened over the inside surface of the left pinna, and they had a slightly sour odor.

A general physical examination was otherwise unremarkable. Given that a relatively clear diagnosis was suggested from a Chinese medical perspective, the owner chose not to pursue laboratory studies before treatment.

ASSESSMENT

Physical examination strongly suggested Liver Blood deficiency as the source of Cody's skin and anxiety complaints. Activity at BL 17, the "Blood association point," suggested an underlying problem with Blood. Cody's thin pulses and pale tongue suggested a Blood deficiency, as did his itch in the absence of overt skin lesions and his skin and ear lesions of a generally dry nature. Blood deficiency lesions tend to occur in the axillary, inguinal, and even perineal regions, since these are the zones associated with the Liver and Pericardium, which are organs dependent on an adequate Blood supply for proper function. Cody's general anxiety and restlessness, and even his covetous or territorial nature, were also strongly suggestive of Blood deficiency.

Blood deficiency can be either primary or secondary. Primary Blood deficiency exists of itself and has no apparent cause other than an inappropriate diet. Spleen deficiency is the main cause of secondary Blood deficiency. Cody's signs that suggested a possible underlying Spleen deficiency were symptoms of Dampness. These included sporadic vomiting, skin lesions with thick scales and collarettes, eyelid swelling, and a presumed swelling of the palate and throat that led to reverse sneezing. In addition, mild Damp Heat tendencies can result in a preference for cool places, and Spleen deficiency can lead to a very low appetite. The possible role of Spleen deficiency as an underlying cause of Cody's Blood deficiency was acknowledged, but the Blood deficiency seemed much more prominent.

TREATMENT

Cody was initially prescribed a formula to tonify Blood and disperse Wind-Heat invasion, with the knowledge that a Spleen-tonifying formula might eventually be needed to effect complete resolution of the skin problems. A granular concentrate of **Si Wu Xiao Feng Yin** was supplied at a dosage of approximately ¼ teaspoon twice daily.

OUTCOME

After 3 weeks of therapy the owners reported that Cody was less itchy and anxious and the collarettes were replaced by a few small scabs. Cody's appetite remained poor. Si Wu Xiao Feng Yin was continued.

Cody's improvement continued over the next month, with declining itch and reduced anxiety. Focal collarettes were still found on his lower abdomen, along with mild redness and hyperpigmentation. His pulses were still thin, and his tongue was still pale. Si Wu Xiao Feng Yin was continued.

After an additional 40 days further improvements were seen. The itch persisted but was very mild, as was the ear inflammation. Eye discharges were reduced or absent. Collarettes were absent. Cody was also uncharacteristically hungry and starting to gain weight. On this visit, active points included BL 22, BL 17, ST 36, and CV 8, suggesting as a group that although Blood deficiency was still the cause of most of Cody's symptoms, an underlying Spleen deficiency was becoming more apparent. In addition, his weight gain and elevated appetite were considered to possibly reflect a tendency to Damp Heat accumulation, given his past history of symptoms related to Dampness and Damp Heat. Accordingly, ½ tsp twice daily of Xiao Feng San I, the original version of Xiao Feng San, was prescribed to address both his Blood deficiency and the possible presence of Dampness and Damp Heat. More information on the various forms of Xiao Feng San can be found in this chapter.

More than 2 months later, Cody's clinical presentation had changed. He was slow to rise in the mornings and was seeking more warmth. He was also continuing to gain weight but still could not be considered obese. His coat was mildly greasy, his tongue was pale, and his pulses were slippery. CV 6 and BL 24 were especially taut and swollen, and he was again having reverse sneezing. Cody was assessed as fully manifesting Spleen Qi deficiency with a secondary Dampness accumulation. His prescription was switched to **Chu Shi Wei Ling Tang.**

Seven weeks later, and 7 months after his initial presentation, Cody's skin had improved significantly and all of his skin and ear lesions had resolved. As of his last examination 3 months later, these improvements had been sustained.

COMMENTS

Cody's case illustrates how, as Blood-deficiency symptoms are successfully addressed, signs of Dampness related to an underlying Spleen deficiency can emerge. Practitioners sometimes begin treatment of skin disease in dogs with Blood-tonifying and Wind-dispersing formulas, but eventually switch to Spleen-tonifying and Dampness-draining formulas to complete resolution of symptoms.

Not all Spleen-deficient animals need herbal formulas for the long term, and diet may maintain skin health once lesions have been resolved. Cody showed no interest in raw foods when the owner provided them, which is typical of very Spleen-deficient animals. Usually these dogs are attracted to commercial diets, presumably because of the predigested state of their components as a result of cooking during their manufacture. Interestingly, however, Cody did not like commercial pet food as a rule and given his interest in table scraps a home-cooked diet probably should be considered for him.

SM

REFERENCES

Akihisa T, Yasukawa K, Oinuma H, Kasahara Y, Yamanouchi S, Takido M, Kumaki K, Tamura T. Triterpene alcohols from the flowers of compositae and their anti-inflammatory effects. *Phytochemistry* 43(6):1255-1260, 1996.

Baker NF, Farver TB. Failure of brewer's yeast as a repellent to fleas on dogs. *J Am Vet Med Assoc* 183(2):212-214, 1983.

Bensky D, Gamble A. *Chinese Herbal Medicine Materia Medica,* revised ed. Seattle, 1993, Eastland Press.

Bensky D, Barolet R. *Chinese Herbal Medicine Formulas and Strategies.* Seattle, 1990, Eastland Press.

Berschneider H. Alternative diets. *Clin Tech Small Anim Pract* 17(1):1-5, 2002.

Birkett G, Frank L. Immunology of dogs with juvenile onset demodecosis as determined by lymphocyte blastogenesis and Cd4:CD8 ratio. *Veterinary Allergy and Immunology* 4(2):46-52, 1996.

Bouic PJ, Lamprecht JH. Plant sterols and sterolins: a review of their immune-modulating properties. *Altern Med Rev* 4(3):170-177, 1999.

Ehling D. *The Chinese Herbalist's Handbook,* revised ed. Santa Fe, NM, 1996, Inword Press.

Girodon F, Galan P, Monget AL, Boutron-Ruault MC, Brunet-Lecomte P, Preziosi P, Arnaud J, Manuguerra JC, Herchberg S. Impact of trace elements and vitamin supplementation on immunity and infections in institutionalized elderly patients: a randomized controlled trial. MIN. VIT. AOX. geriatric network. *Arch Intern Med* 159(7):748-754, 1999.

Grimble RF. Effect of antioxidative vitamins on immune function with clinical applications. *Int J Vitam Nutr Res* 67(5):312-320, 1997.

Guerrini VH, Kriticos CM. Effects of azadirachtin on *Ctenocephalides felis* in the dog and the cat. *Vet Parasitol* 74(2-4):289-297, 1998.

Johnston CS, Martin LJ, Cai X. Antihistamine effect of supplemental ascorbic acid and neutrophil chemotaxis. *J Am Coll Nutr* 11(2):172-176, 1992.

Kim HW, Chew BP, Wong TS, Park JS, Weng BB, Byrne KM, Hayek MG, Reinhart GA. Dietary lutein stimulates immune response in the canine. *Vet Immunol,* 74(3-4):315-327, 2000.

Lemarie S. Evaluation of IL-2 production and receptor expression in dogs with generalized demodecosis. *Vet Derm* 7 (4): 213-219, 1996.

Lievre M et al. Controlled study of three ointments for the local management of second and third degree burns. *Clin Trials Metaanal* 28:9-12, 1992.

Lilge L, Tierney K, Nussbaum E. Low-level laser therapy for wound healing: feasibility of wound dressing transillumination. *J Clin Laser Med Surg* 18(5):235-240, 2000.

Moore OA, Smith LA, Campbell F, Seers K, McQuay HJ, Moore RA. Systematic review of the use of honey as a wound dressing. *BMC Complement Altern Med* 1(1):2, 2001.

Mulla MS, Su T. Activity and biological effects of neem products against arthropods of medical and veterinary importance. *J Am Mosq Control Assoc* 15(2):133-152, 1999.

Nagle TM, Torres SM, Horne KL, Brover R, Stevens MT. A randomized, double-blind, placebo-controlled trial to investigate the efficacy and safety of a Chinese herbal product (P07P) for the treatment of canine atopic dermatitis. *Vet Dermatol* 12(5):265-274, 2001.

O'Brien DJ. Treatment of psoroptic mange with reference to epidemiology and history. *Vet Parasitol* 83(3-4):177-185, 1999.

Remillard RL. Omega 3 fatty acids in canine and feline diets: a clinical success or failure? *Vet Clin Nutr* 5(2):6-11, 1998.

Sazawal S, Black RE, Jalla S, Mazumdar S, Sinha A, Bhan MK. Zinc supplementation reduces the incidence of acute lower respiratory infections in infants and preschool children: a double-blind, controlled trial. *Pediatrics* 102(1 Pt 1):1-5, 1998.

Shahi SK, Shukla AC, Bajaj AK, Banerjee U, Rimek D, Midgely G, Dikshit A. Broad spectrum herbal therapy against superficial fungal infections. *Skin Pharmacol Appl Skin Physiol* 13(1):60-64, 2000.

Sheehan MP, Stevens H, Ostlere LS, Atherton DJ, Brostoff J, Rustin MH. Follow-up of adult patients with atopic eczema treated with Chinese herbal therapy for 1 year. *Clin Exp Dermatol* 20(2):136-140, 1995.

Sheehan MP, Rustin MH, Atherton DJ, Buckley C, Harris DW, Brostoff J, Ostlere L, Dawson A, Harris DJ. Efficacy of traditional Chinese herbal therapy in adult atopic dermatitis. *Lancet* 340(8810):13-17, 1992.

Stermitz FR, Lorenz P, Tawara JN, Zenewicz LA, Lewis K. Synergy in a medicinal plant: antimicrobial action of berberine potentiated by 5′-methoxyhydnocarpin, a multidrug pump inhibitor. *Proc Natl Acad Sci USA* 97(4):1433-1437, 2000.

Sudekum M, Poppenga RH, Raju N, Braselton WE Jr. Pennyroyal oil toxicosis in a dog. *J Am Vet Med Assoc* 200(6):817-818, 1992.

Swaim SF, Riddell KP, McGuire JA. Effects of topical medications on the healing of open pad wounds in dogs. *J Am Anim Hosp Assoc* 28(6):499-502, 1992.

Tohda C, Sugahara H, Kuraishi Y, Komatsu K. Inhibitory effect of Byakko-ka-ninjin-to on itch in a mouse model of atopic dermatitis. *Phytother Res* 14(3):192-194, 2000.

Vazquez B, Avila G, Segura D, Escalante B. Antiinflammatory activity of extracts from *Aloe vera* gel. *J Ethnopharmacol* 55(1):69-75, 1996.

Venugopal PV, Venugopal TV. Antidermatophytic activity of garlic *(Allium sativum)* in vitro. *Int J Dermatol* 34(4):278-279, 1995.

Xu XJ, Banerjee P, Rustin MH, Poulter LW. Modulation by Chinese herbal therapy of immune mechanisms in the skin of patients with atopic eczema. *Br J Dermatol* 136(1):54-59, 1997.

Yan W. *Practical Therapeutics of Traditional Chinese Medicine.* Brookline, Mass, 1997, Paradigm Publications.

Yeung H. *Handbook of Chinese Herbal Formulas*. Los Angeles, 1995, Self-published.

Yeung H. *Handbook of Chinese Herbs*. Los Angeles, 1996, Self-published.

6

Therapies for Digestive Disorders

GENERAL SIGNS OF GASTROINTESTINAL DISEASE—SYMPTOMATIC TREATMENTS

CONSTIPATION

Therapeutic Rationale

- Increase water content of colonic contents.
- Retain water with fiber bulking agents.
- Initiate colonic mucosal water and mucus secretion.
- Rule out obstructive or painful lesions such as strictures, masses, or perianal disease.
- Increase exercise.
- Rule out underlying disorders such as hypothyroidism.

Alternative Options with Conventional Bases

- **Supply fiber** in the diet with herbs or with a homemade diet that includes whole grains (barley, oats, whole wheat), vegetables, and fruit.
- **Magnesium** and **Vitamin C**: given in sufficient doses, these create an osmotic diarrhea that limits their own absorption. This can be used to support the action of any herbal formula that seems well suited to the patient but is not quite sufficient to make bowel movements regular and reliable. Doses of both or either can be increased until a softening effect is detected in the stool. A *recommended starting dose* is 500 mg of Vitamin C or 100 mg of Magnesium as a single oral dose. Adjust dose as needed until desired stool consistency is obtained.

Herbs

Herbs that supply fiber

- **Fiber** accelerates the transit of colonic contents by increasing weight and water content of feces. Fiber also optimizes intestinal bacterial populations and may have a trophic effect on intestinal mucosal epithelium. Herbs that supply soluble fiber include Psyllium *(Plantago ovata)*, Flaxseed *(Linum usitatissimum)*, and Guar Gum *(Cyamopsis tetragonolbas)*. All herbs supply insoluble fiber in the form of cellulose, but only those that can be given in relatively large doses should be used this way. Vegetables, whole grains, and fruits are a better way to supply insoluble fiber.

Herbs that act as osmotic or stimulant laxatives

- **Anthranoid-containing herbs:** contain precursors that are broken down to anthrones and anthraquinones, which themselves pass unchanged through the colon. These compounds cause water and electrolyte secretion in the colon, possibly through prostaglandin$_2$ (PGE_2)- or nitric oxide–mediated mechanisms (Beubler, 1985; Izzo, 1997). Chronic use of anthranoid laxatives has been suggested to predispose to colorectal cancer (Siegers, 1993). Different anthraquinone precursors lead to different absorbed versus retained moieties. This suggests that Cascara *(Rhamnus purshiana)* or Buckthorn *(Rhamnus frangula)* may be preferred choices, especially in cats because some require glucuronidation for elimination from the body (de Witte, 1990).
- **Aloe** *(Aloe vera, A. barbadensis)*: contains barbaloin and other anthraquinone precursors that increase colonic water and mucus secretion (Ishii, 1994).
- **Senna** *(Cassia acutifolia, C. angustifolia)*: Sennosides are converted to anthraquinones. Human dose is 1 to 4 g, which will produce loose stool within 5 to 7 hours.
- **Cascara:** anthraglycosides are generally retained unchanged in the colon. Not as powerful clinically as Senna or Aloe.
- **Buckthorn:** A species related to Cascara.
- **Rhubarb** *(Rheum palmatum, R. tanguticum)*: clinically rhubarb is said to have a biphasic effect; lower doses

are used for treating diarrhea, but at higher doses the effects of the anthranoids (rhein, chrysophanol, and others) are used to loosen stool to treat constipation. The rhizome is used in herbal medicine; however, it should be noted that the stalk and leaf (a common human food) are oxalate rich and its administration to individuals prone to oxalate urolithiasis is considered risky.

Paradigmatic Options

Homeopathy

- *Nux vomica:* a remedy of major importance for constipation in cats. Cats that respond are typically irritable or aggressive, have low back pain or lameness, and often vomit hairballs in the morning. The practitioner should try a dose of 30C once daily for 1 week and then as needed.

Western Herbs

- **Cascara Sagrada, Ginger** *(Zingiber officinalis),* and **Licorice** *(Glycyrrhiza glabra)* have traditionally been combined in Western herbal formulas to address constipation and promote vigorous intestinal contractions. The Licorice and Ginger are included in the formula partly to modulate the sometimes strong contractions elicited by Cascara. This formula is especially useful for cats with megacolon, in which any ability of the colon smooth muscle to contract seems lost. The herbs should be used in a 4:1:2, respectively ratio. A *suggested starting dose* of the combined tincture is 0.2 ml per 5 lb of body weight, divided into two daily doses. Higher volumes can be given if needed, and if the formula is well tolerated by the animal.

Chinese Medicine

- In Chinese medicine constipation has a number of potential causes. Movement of the stool requires, as do all fluids in the body, the motive force of Qi. Qi stagnation or Qi deficiency can thus lead to constipation. Sometimes the stool cannot slide easily through the colon because of excessive dryness caused by Blood or Yin deficiency. Such dryness is aggravated by the presence of excessive amounts of Heat in the Large Intestine. Excessive Cold in the abdomen can also lead to constipation by coagulating and binding the Qi.

- For all of the following formulas, a *recommended starting dose* of granular formula is ¼ tsp per 10 to 15 lb of body weight, or 60 to 75 mg/kg of body weight, administered daily in divided doses.
- Qi stagnation as a cause of constipation may be signaled in the patient by irritability, belching, flatulence, abdominal distention and pain, variable stool, a lack of mucus in the stool, lack of thirst, lateral abdominal pain, a purple tongue, and a wiry pulse. Acupuncture points to move Liver Qi and relieve constipation caused by Qi stagnation are GB 34, TH 6, LIV 3, and GV 1. **Liu Mo Tang** (Six Milled Herb Decoction) is considered for cases in which constipation is aggravated by tension or stress, and the patient exhibits belching, abdominal pain, and a preference for warmth. If the patient is heat intolerant, adding any or all of Huang Qin, Zhi Zi, Huang Lian, and Long Dan Cao to the base formula to clear Heat should be considered. Once constipation has been relieved, more constitutional formulas to address general tendencies to Liver Qi stagnation can be considered.
- Qi deficiency is suspected when the patient has chronic constipation with a constant urge to defecate but a lack of completeness to the bowel movement. The stools are normal in moisture but small with no mucus. The patient may also be tired after efforts to pass stool and may have low energy, low thirst, a tendency to seek warmth, polyuria, a lack of abdominal pain, a pale wet tongue, and a weak pulse. Acupuncture points that may assist in the management of the condition are ST 36, SP 6, CV 6, BL 21, and BL 25. A formula to address the problem is **Huang Qi Tang** (Astragalus Decoction). This formula contains Huang Qi, Chen Pi, Ma Zi Ren, and Honey. The first ingredient tonifies Spleen Qi, the second descends the Qi, and the last two moisten the colon. Dang Shen and Bai Zhu can be added when

Spleen Qi deficiency is even more pronounced. **Bu Zhong Yi Qi Tang** (Tonify the Center and Boost the Qi Decoction) is another formula that may be added to Huang Qi Tang to address constipation caused by Spleen Qi deficiency.

- Colon dryness is an important cause of constipation. A purely emollient formula to address nonspecific colon dryness is **Wu Ren Wan** (Five Seeds Pill). Blood and Yin deficiency as a cause of constipation can be manifested in general as chronically dry stools, mucus on the stools, thirst, little urine, mouth odor, a preference for cool areas, a pale or red and dry tongue with no coating, and a thin pulse. For these patients, **Run Chang Wan** (Moisten the Intestines Pill) should be considered. This is a small formula to address colon dryness and combined Yin and Blood deficiency. It also helps move Blood and Large Intestinal Qi downward in a gentle fashion. **Dang Gui Cong Rong Tang** (Angelica and Cistanche Decoction) contains 35 g Dang Gui, 16 g Rou Cong Rong, 10 g Fan Xie Ye, 6 g Hou Po, 3 g Mu Xiang, 3 g Xiang Fu, 6 g Zhi Qiao, 10 g Shen Qu, 6 g Qu Mai, and 2 g Tong Cao. This formula is much more forceful in its propulsive action than Run Chang Wan, which is more suited for frail patients. Acupuncture points to assist the actions of these formulas are BL 17, BL 23, BL 25, ST 37, CV 4, SP 6, SP 9, SP 10, and GV 1.
- When Yin deficiency seems to be the more prevalent cause of constipation, various herbs can be combined with **Run Chang Wan** to nourish Yin and clear Empty Heat in the aged. Any or all of Mai Men Dong, Xuan Shen, Rou Cong Rong, He Shou Wu, and Zhi Mu can be included.
- When intestinal dryness has arisen from excessive Heat in the Large Intestine, the patient may exhibit acute constipation, dry stool, mucus on the stool, strong thirst, a lack of abdominal pain, abdominal distention, foul mouth odor, an intolerance of heat, a red and dry tongue with a yellow coating, and a fast, wiry pulse. Acupuncture points used to address this can include LI 4, LI 11, BL 25, BL 21, ST 44, and ST 37. The classically indicated formula for this syndrome, which is known

as Large Intestine Yang Ming Syndrome, is **Da Cheng Qi Tang** (Major Rectify the Qi Decoction). It is a very strong purgative and should not be used on weak or deficient animals. **Tong Shun Wan** is a milder formula for use after major Heat episodes. It contains Huo Ma Ren, Tao Ren, Dang Gui Wei, Da Huang, Qiang Huo, and Fan Xie Ye, all of which still provide a strong moving effect on the bowels. **Ma Zi Ren Wan** (Hemp Seed Pill) is used when a moderately strong moving action is required but the patient is elderly or perhaps debilitated by previous episodes of Heat.

- **Wen Pi Tang** (Warm the Spleen Decoction) is the classically indicated formula for excess Cold coagulation of the abdomen. It should be used when the patient has constipation, abdominal pain relieved by warmth, coldness of the extremities, a deep, taut pulse, and a pale tongue. **Ji Chuan Jian** (Benefit the River Decoction) with added Rou Gui is the formula to be used when there is a deficiency Cold that has accumulated as a result of Kidney Qi or Yang deficiency. In this patient the pulse is deficient, deep, minute, and weak.

Cautions

- Aloe has been shown to improve the hypoglycemic action of glibenclamide.
- All herbs that reduce intestinal transit time may decrease absorption of drugs and vice versa.
- Purgative herbs may augment loss of potassium and other electrolytes, which may be a consideration with concomitant use of diuretics or in cases of heart or renal disease.
- Iron and other supplements and drugs can potentially worsen constipation.

AUTHORS' CHOICES:

SM: Appropriate homeopathic remedy; Western herbal formula; Chinese herbal formula.

SW: Dietary fiber; short-term anthranoid-containing herbs; Chinese herbal formulas for more chronic cases.

DIARRHEA, SMALL BOWEL

Therapeutic Rationale

- Remove or add bulk to stool.
- Maintain hydration.
- Normalize intestinal motility.
- Reduce inflammation or heal mucosal defects.
- Eliminate parasites.
- Identify and manage food intolerances.

Alternative Options with Conventional Bases

Nutritional Supplements

- **Probiotics:** indigenous bacterial populations appear to maintain normal immune responses in the gut and systemically (Erickson, 2000), help animals resist colonization with enteropathogens (Phuapradit, 1999; Shu, 2000), and assist in metabolizing certain drugs. Probiotic supplementation has a great deal of support in the treatment of intestinal inflammatory diseases and acute diarrhea (Rolfe, 2000). Different strains may have different effects, and in any event indigenous bacterial populations in the dog and cat are not well characterized. *Lactobacillus rhamnosus* strain GG is the most promising according to studies in people (Weese, 2002).
- **Glutamine:** decreases mucosal atrophy and supports enterocyte metabolism. This makes it useful in some cases of intestinal injury (Hickman, 1998).

Herbs

- **Tormentil** *(Potentilla tormentilla):* a traditional remedy for diarrhea. It is principally an astringent and has antioxidant capacity. In traditional thought, astringent herbs such as Tormentil and Blackberry *(Rubus fructicosis)* shrink swollen tissues, "coagulate" the inflamed mucosa, and may provide a kind of collyrium until the disorder is resolved.
- **Uzara** *(Xysmalobium undulatum):* a traditional African herb that is said to slow peristalsis.
- **Hange-Shashin-To:** a Kampo formula that inhibited castor oil–induced diarrhea at a dose of 1000 mg dried

herb/kg of body weight. The most active herbal constituents appear to be Skullcap *(Scutellaria baicalensis)*, Licorice, Ginseng *(Panax ginseng)*, and Coptis *(Coptis chinensis)* (Kase, 1999).

- **Gui Zhi Jia Shao Yao Tang:** appears to inhibit artificially accelerated small intestinal movement, and suppressed diarrhea caused by pilocarpine, barium chloride, or castor oil in rats (Saitoh, 1999).

Paradigmatic Options

- The pathologic cause of small intestinal diarrhea is broadly classified in Chinese medicine in the same way as colitis. Acute infectious causes (bacterial, protozoal) are deemed to rise from the invasion of an external Pathogen. Diarrhea can also result from some failure of the Spleen and Stomach. Examples include diarrhea from Food stasis, the Liver overacting on the Spleen, and Spleen Qi deficiency. Diarrhea over a long period can weaken the Kidney reserves and may require Kidney tonification. For all of the following formulas, a *recommended starting dose* of granular concentrate is ¼ tsp per 10 to 15 lb of body weight, or 60 to 75 mg/kg of body weight, administered daily in divided doses.
- For general exterior invasion, perhaps the most popular treatment in human Chinese medicine is **Pill Curing**, or **Kang Ning Wan.** Patients that benefit may have abdominal pain, nausea, vomiting, diarrhea, regurgitation and hyperacidity in the stomach, abdominal distension, poor appetite, low-grade fever, slight chills, and headache. If symptoms agree, it may be used to treat motion sickness and bacterial or viral diarrhea. A *suggested dose* is one vial of pills per 20 lb of body weight, divided into three daily doses.
- For exterior invasion by Wind and Cold, **Huo Xiang Zheng Qi San** (Agastache Powder to Rectify the Qi) is commonly used. Patients that benefit have diarrhea, nausea, vomiting, headache, fever, chills, a white frothy coated pale tongue, and a slippery pulse. **Wei Ling Tang** (Decoction to Dispel Dampness in the Spleen and Stomach) is considered when Dampness accumulations are obvious in the form of edema or

watery discharges. There may also be cramping pain, poor appetite, regurgitation of water, a weak and slippery pulse, and a wet or frothy pale tongue.

- Patients that suffer exterior invasion by Heat and Dampness or by Damp-Heat Toxin have an acute onset of diarrhea that is voluminous, brown or yellow color, possibly blood tinged, and malodorous. They may also be thirsty and have abdominal pain, a fast, forceful pulse, and a red and wet tongue with a yellow coating. Acupuncture points to assist in the management of the patient include LI 11, LI 4, ST 39, and GV 14. Formulas to address the problem include **Shao Yao Tang** (Peony Decoction) and **Ge Gen Huang Qin Huang Lian Tang** (Pueraria, Scutellaria, and Coptis Decoction). Both of these are powerful formulas and should be used only for excess patients. Shao Yao Tang moves Qi to relieve pain, clears Heat, and eliminates toxins, nourishes and moves Blood to stop bleeding and relax spasms, and warms the lower jiao to prevent damage to the Spleen from cooling herbs and to enhance action of moving herbs. The addition of Jin Yin Hua, Mu Tong, Fu Ling, and Che Qian Zi to Shao Yao Tang allows the formula to more aggressively drain watery accumulations of Dampness and Damp Heat. Ge Gen Huang Qin Huang Lian Tang is adapted to patients with a high fever and perhaps associated gastritis.
- When diarrhea arises secondary to indigestion and Food stasis, the patient has a history of dietary indiscretion, anorexia, abdominal distention and pain, bloating, smelly breath, a thick tongue coating, a slippery or forceful pulse, belching, and perhaps vomiting. The main formula to address this problem is **Bao He Wan** (Preserve Harmony Pill). It has mild Heat-clearing properties but is primarily geared toward strongly increasing the power of digestion.
- When the Liver overacts on the Spleen to produce diarrhea, the patient has subacute to chronic diarrhea, soft or watery stool, aggravation from stress, irritability, possible flank pain, a history of food allergies, a lavender tongue, and a wiry pulse. **Tong Xie Yao Fang** (Important Formula for Painful Diarrhea) is used

specifically in these patients, which may also exhibit loud borborygmi and marked abdominal pain that is alleviated by a bowel movement. If this condition has persisted for a long time, some practitioners resort to a more tonifying formula known as **Xiao Yao Wan** (Rambling Ease Pill) that harmonizes the Liver and Spleen.

- Chronic watery or soft stool that has no particular distinguishing color or no particularly offensive odor indicates Spleen and Stomach deficiency. The patient may also exhibit weight loss, low thirst, and abdominal discomfort after eating. The tongue may be pale and wet and the pulses weak, deep, and soft. Acupuncture points to address this problem include ST 36, BL 20, BL 21, and GV1. Various formulas are applicable, including **Xiang Sha Liu Jun Zi Tang** (Six Gentlemen Decoction with Saussurea and Cardamon) and **Bu Zhong Yi Qi Tang** (Tonify the Center and Boost the Qi Decoction). Xiang Sha Liu Jun Zi Tang is more of a consideration when the patient has abdominal pain and cramping and perhaps nausea in the morning. Bu Zhong Yi Qi Tang may be more useful when the Spleen-deficient patient has incontinence or rectal prolapse. **Shen Ling Bai Zhu San** (Ginseng, Poria, and Atractylodes Powder) is used to astringe diarrhea when no further evidence of a pathogen exists (e.g., tenemus, blood, fever, yellow stools) and the diarrhea is beginning to take a greater toll on the patient's energy reserves. **Fu Zi Li Zhong Wan** (Cultivate the Center Pill with Added Aconite) is a generic Spleen Qi tonic to be considered when the patient strongly seeks warmth.
- Special mention must be made of cats with pancreatic insufficiency that leads to a ravenous appetite, progressive weight loss, and fetid, soft stools. These cats generally have both a deficient Spleen and an accumulation of Damp Heat. Formulas such as **Si Miao San** (Four Marvels Powder) and **Xiang Lian Wan** (Aucklandia and Coptis Pill) should be considered as treatment options. Si Miao San is one of the more important herbal formulas in veterinary medicine. It

acts to tonify and warm the Spleen as it leaches Damp and Toxic Heat out of the lower burner. Patients with low back pain or stiffness may respond well to this formula. These patients often have obvious Spleen Qi with perhaps a soft pulse and the tongue is usually vivid pink to red. Xiang Lian Wan should be considered when an even more warming action on the Spleen is desired. Although it is not often used, this is a potentially very useful formula, since it warms the Spleen, cools the intestines, relieves pain, and addresses Damp Heat diarrhea. Signs calling for its use include obvious presence of Spleen and Stomach deficiency in the past medical history of the patient, a slippery, rapid pulse, sticky saliva, and a coated tongue.

- Kidney Yang deficiency is marked by "daybreak diarrhea," diarrhea of long duration, perhaps kidney failure, a pale, wet tongue, and a deep, weak pulse. Acupuncture points to address this disorder include BL 23, KI 3, GV 4, BL 20, and CV 4. Formulas to address it include the following:
  - **Zhen Ren Yang Zang Tang** (Upright Man's Nourish the Internal Organs Decoction) in cases with prolapse of the rectum, bowel incontinence, chronic diarrhea, and pain. Because the formula is an astringent formula, it should never be used in acute cases, since this will only aggravate the symptoms.
  - **Si Shen Wan** (Four Miraculous Drugs Pill) is used when the patient has painless diarrhea in the early morning and low back weakness.
  - **Gui Fu Li Zhong Tang,** which is **Fu Zi Li Zhong Tang** (discussed in the section on Colitis) with Cinnamon added for extra Yang tonification.
  - **Tao Hua Tang** (Peach Blossom Decoction) is a small formula specifically designed to treat chronic diarrhea containing dark blood or pus.

Cautions

- Uzara may increase cardiac contractile strength while slowing the heart rate; may potentiate the effects of digoxin and digitoxin.

AUTHORS' CHOICES:

SM: Appropriate Chinese herbal formulas; conservative dietary management in simple acute noninfectious cases.
SW: Diet management; probiotics; Chinese herbs.

VOMITING, NAUSEA

Therapeutic Rationale

- Dietary indiscretion: reduce exposure to offending food or nonfood items
- Rule out foreign body obstruction and any anatomic bases for vomiting.
- Rule out internal disorders arising from endocrine, pancreas, liver, and kidney disorders; apply specific treatment when these are found.
- Stop medications that may be causative, especially nonsteroidal antiinflammatory drugs (NSAIDs).
- Rest the gastrointestinal (GI) tract for 12 to 24 hours in acute cases.

Alternative Options with Conventional Bases

Herbs

- **Ginger:** some trials have shown Ginger to be helpful for seasickness, morning sickness, and chemotherapy-induced nausea in humans (Ernst, 2000).
- **Licorice:** See entry under Gastritis, Gastric Ulceration.

Other Therapies

- **Acupuncture:** effective for nausea and vomiting, especially at the point known as PC 6 or Nei Guan (NIH, 1997; Roscoe, 2002).

Paradigmatic Options

Homeopathy

- **Cocculus indicus 30C:** may be helpful in alleviating nausea caused by motion sickness. One or two doses should be given in the hour before travel, and then repeat doses as necessary en route.
- **Ferrum metallicum 30C:** especially in cats for vomiting of food immediately after eating or for vomiting of

undigested food hours after ingestion. Pulses in affected animals are soft. The *recommended dose* is up to three times daily as needed.

- ***Nux vomica* 30C:** effective for morning nausea in irritable cats with low back pain and stiffness. The *recommended dose* is once daily as needed.
- **Ipecacuanha 30C:** effective for intractable nausea and vomiting, especially when the emesis contains traces of blood. The *recommended dose* is up to three times daily as needed.

Chinese Medicine

- Vomiting is tantamount to Stomach Qi rebellion, in which Stomach Qi does not flow downward but rebels upward. Various reasons can underlie this problem, including physical obstruction to the descent of Stomach Qi, such as Phlegm accumulations, Food stasis, and Stomach contents congealed by Excess Heat. Liver Qi stagnation can also disrupt Stomach Qi descent. Vomiting also may arise because of Spleen Stomach deficiency, secondary Kidney deficiency, and external Pathogen invasion. For all the formulas in the following list, the *recommended starting dose* of granular concentrate is ¼ tsp per 10 to 15 lb of body weight, or 60 to 75 mg/kg of body weight, given daily in divided doses.
- Phlegm obstruction is characterized by vomiting of clear, slimy fluid or mucus, a poor appetite, occasional balance problems, a frothy coated tongue with tenacious saliva, and a wiry or slippery pulse. **Er Chen Tang** (Two Cured Herbs Decoction) is a long-standing formula for this problem. It seems especially effective for reducing vomiting of food by cats immediately after eating. It is an important formula in the first stages of feline hyperthyroidism, which is often characterized by vomiting.
- **Ling Gui Zhu Gan Tang** (Decoction of Poria, Cinnamon Twig, Atractylodes, and Licorice) with added **Xiao Ban Xia Tang** (Minor Pinellia Decoction, consisting of Sheng Jiang and Ban Xia) may also be considered for Phlegm obstruction of the Stomach. This formula may be particularly appropriate if the patient vomits water soon after drinking as well as eating.
- When vomiting arises secondary to obstruction by Food stasis, the patient may have anorexia, abdominal

distention and pain, bloating, smelly breath, a thick tongue coating, a slippery or forceful pulse, belching, and vomiting of undigested food. The main formula to address this problem is **Bao He Wan** (Preserve Harmony Pill). It has mild Heat-clearing properties but is geared primarily toward strongly increasing the power of digestion. If pronounced Heat signs are present, Huang Lian and Zhu Ru may be added to the formula.

- When the patient has obstructions caused by congealed stomach contents from Stomach Heat and Yin deficiency, signs include chronic gastritis, occasional fever, weight loss, frequent vomiting of small amounts, a dry mouth, dry stool, a red tongue with little coating, and a rapid, thready pulse. Acupuncture points advocated to treat this disorder are SP 6, ST 36, PC 6, BL 21, and GB 34. A typical formula for this condition is **Mai Men Dong Tang** (Ophiopogon Root Decoction). For severe Yin damage, Shi Hu, Tian Hua Fen, Zhi Mu, and Zhu Ru may be added to the formula. Alternatively, **Yu Nu Jian** (Fair Maiden Decoction) may be used when Stomach Heat seems exceptionally intense, manifested as gingivitis, great thirst, frontal head pain, epistaxis, and a floating, gigantic pulse.
- When the patient has Liver Qi stagnation, signs include frequent vomiting of small amounts, irritability, costal arch pain, eye redness and dryness, thirst, eructations, a tender pink to lavender tongue, and a thin and perhaps wiry pulse. An acupuncture protocol advocated for this condition is BL 21, LIV 3, CV 12, LIV 13, LIV 14, GB 34, ST 36, and PC 6. The main formula for this condition is **Yi Guan Jian** (One Linking Decoction), a Liver Blood and Yin tonic. Chronic cases with more evidence of Spleen involvement such as undigested food in the stool, soft pulses, anemia, hypoalbuminemia, and inappetence may benefit from **Xiao Yao Wan** (Rambling Ease Powder).
- Stomach and Spleen Yang deficiency manifests with chronic occasional vomiting of large amounts of ingesta, fatigue, loose stool, low thirst, cold limbs, a pale and wet tongue, and a weak, slow, thready pulse. Acupuncture points that may be used to address this

condition include ST 36, BL 20, BL 21, BL 23, BL 24, CV 6, and KI 3. Moxa may be helpful in stimulating these points. A useful formula is **Li Zhong Tang** (Cultivate the Center Decoction), with Sha Ren and Ban Xia added. For severe Cold, add Wu Zhu Yu to more vigorously warm the Spleen and Stomach. Rou Gui and Fu Zi may also be added; this creates **Gui Fu Zi Li Zhong Wan** to be used for Kidney Yang–deficient cases.

- For external Pathogen invasion, **Pill Curing** and **Huo Xiang Zheng Qi San** can be considered. External Pathogen invasion is characterized by acuteness of onset, chills and fever, abdominal pain, a pale tongue, and a floating pulse. Acupuncture points recommended for this condition include GB 34, ST 36, L I4, GB 20, and PC 6. Pill Curing may be especially helpful in motion sickness. A suggested dose for Pill Curing is one vial of pills per 20 lb of body weight, divided into three daily doses.

Dietary Considerations

- Chronic vomiting should prompt the practitioner to rule out food allergens. When none exist, the practitioner may wish to experiment with avoidance of carbohydrate ingestion in cats and a reduction of processed foods for dogs.

AUTHORS' CHOICES:

SM: Dietary changes; appropriate Chinese herbal formula; homeopathics are often very effective.
SW: Elimination diet; Ginger; Chinese herbal formulas.

SPECIFIC GASTROINTESTINAL DISORDERS

ANAL SAC DISEASE

Therapeutic Rationale

- Manage firmness of feces (increasing bulk and firmness may express glands on every defecation).
- Manage excessive glandular secretions from sacculitis.
- Be aware of poor muscle tone.
- Manage allergies.

Alternative Options with Conventional Bases

- **Feed a homemade diet.** Be conscious of fiber content, and add whole grains or vegetables if increased stool bulking is necessary. Be aware that food allergy may have to be ruled out.

Paradigmatic Options

- Increased accumulation of anal gland contents is interpreted in Chinese medicine quite literally as an excessive accumulation of Dampness. The belief that the anal glands are located on the Gall Bladder meridian is consistent with this interpretation, since the Gall Bladder has a tendency to accumulate Dampness and, in particular, Damp Heat. In dealing with anal gland problems, general approaches to reduce Dampness accumulation are recommended, including both herbal formulas and dietary measures. Dampening foods include processed and high-carbohydrate foods, and food allergens are also considered a Dampening influence. Elimination of these three dampening factors can be achieved by providing a balanced raw meat and vegetable diet with an appropriate protein source. These diets also help create firm stool consistency, and vegetable fiber may increase bowel movement frequency. These two features may help increase passive pressure on the anal glands, promoting emptying. Raw diets can be introduced slowly to test tolerance of patients with weak pulses.
- Chinese herbal formulas to address Dampness should be chosen based on the signs the animal exhibits. See other chapters for formulas recommended for various clinical presentations of Dampness and Damp Heat. When distended anal glands are the only feature exhibited, support using more "constitutional" formulas for Dampness should be considered. **San Ren Tang** (Three Seeds Decoction) is a mild-tasting but effective formula to tonify the Spleen and leach out Damp Heat accumulations from any of the three burners or jiao. **Wei Ling Tang** (Decoction to Dispel Dampness in the Spleen and Stomach) can be used

when evidence of Dampness is more fluid, such as watery gland secretions and "perspiration." **Si Miao San** (Four Marvels Powder) to which 25 g of Dang Gui has been added to 100 g of the base formula can be used for more "heated" dogs and cats with pruritus ani and previous anal gland abscesses. Appropriate diets should be recommended.

- For active anal sac infection, inflammation, and abscesses, more aggressive Damp Heat–clearing formulas are needed, such as **Long Dan Xie Gan Tang** (Gentian Drain the Liver Decoction). **Zhu Dan Tablets**, available from the Institute for Traditional Medicine in Portland, Oregon, have been advocated by some practitioners to address anal gland problems. The tablets contain equal portions of Zhu Dan (Pig Bile), Jin Qian Cao, Huang Qin, Zhe Bei Mu, Zhen Zhu Mu, Dan Shen, Yin Chen Hao, Tu Fu Ling, Ban Xia, and Yu Jin. The formula is designed to increase biliary clearance in humans but is believed by some to be an effective treatment for anal sac disease because of its content of Damp Heat–clearing herbs that enter the Gall Bladder meridian. Doses for animals can be prorated down from the recommended human dose on the bottle. For all of the listed formulas, a *recommended starting dose* of granular concentrate is ¼ tsp per 10 to 15 lb of body weight, or 60 to 75 mg/kg of body weight, administered daily in divided doses.
- Acupuncture points to drain Dampness and Damp Heat from the lower jiao and tonify the Spleen include SP 9, CV 3, and BL 25. Local points to regulate the perineal region include BL 34, BL 35, and GV 1. Distant points include BL 40, LV 5, and BL 58.

AUTHORS' CHOICES:

SM: Appropriate Chinese herbal formulas; dietary measures.
SW: Evaluate for allergies; manage diet; Chinese herbal formulas.

COLITIS

Therapeutic Rationale

- Eliminate parasites (*Trichuris, Ancylostoma, Giardia,* and others).
- Correct bacterial imbalances by supplying probiotic species or their substrates.
- Rule out foreign material being ingested.
- Identify and manage food allergy or intolerance.
- Reduce inflammation of any origin.
- Enhance energy substrates for colonocytes by supplying soluble fiber.

Alternative Options with Conventional Bases

- **Probiotics:** have been shown to have immunomodulatory activity; in one trial, they suppressed relapses in human patients with Crohn's disease who were in clinical remission (Shanahan, 2000).

Diet

- **Elimination diets** should be considered, as some colitis cases appear to be a manifestation of food allergy. A homemade diet may supply a limited array of antigens or may supply potential food allergens in a different form than previously supplied in commercial processed foods. See Appendix A for diet formulation guidelines.
- **Pumpkin,** as a source of insoluble fiber, may be effective in alleviating colitis. The added bulk acts to keep the colon mildly distended which may prevent development of spasms, and absorbs excess water and bacterial toxins. Other fiber sources include Citrus Pectin, Psyllium Seed (both sources of soluble fiber), and many others.

Herbs

Demulcent herbs

- Demulcent herbs are traditionally defined as soothing to mucous membranes; this is usually via mucilage contained in the herb. Demulcent herbs are popular traditional remedies for intestinal inflammation, though they haven't been examined experimentally. Most of them probably contain different soluble fibers.

Soluble fiber may have a trophic effect on intestinal villi as well as forming metabolites (butyrate), which are antiinflammatory (Andoh, 1999). Choices include Slippery Elm *(Ulmus fulva)*, Marshmallow *(Althea officinalis)*, Psyllium (Fernandez-Banares, 1999), Comfrey Root (*Symphytum officinalis*—potentially toxic), and Irish Moss or Carageenan *(Chondrus crispus)*.

Herbs that stimulate mucosal reepithelialization

- **Licorice:** one study indicated amelioration of NSAID-induced intestinal damage (Russell, 1984), but the mechanism by which the herb works remains unclear, and NSAID damage usually occurs in the upper GI tract. Although Licorice has mineralocorticoid effects and may cause hyperaldosteronism, it is used in almost every Chinese herbal combination as a "harmonizer" or flavoring agent. Long-term use of the herb by itself therefore is not well supported and not as safe as use in herbal combinations. Deglycyrrhizinated forms of licorice (DGL) are safe for long-term use, but their efficacy is questionable.
- **Chamomile** *(Matricaria recutita):* a traditional spasmolytic for GI distress. This herb may accelerate epithelial repair in dermal wounds (Glowania, 1987) and may support healing of GI ulcers if it acts on mucosal surfaces as it does on skin.

Smooth muscle relaxant (spasmolytic) herbs

- **Peppermint** *(Mentha piperita)*: relaxes ileal smooth muscle, possibly through calcium channel blocking activity (Hawthorn, 1988). In spastic colitis, controlling spasm is probably more important than correcting epithelial defects, so Peppermint is among the most important herbs for consideration in painful, spastic colitis.

Antiinflammatory herbs

- **Oren-gedoku-to** (Huang Lian Jie Du Tang): reduced inflammatory mediators and inflammation in a rat model of colitis (Zhou, 1999).

Other herbal approaches

- A modern Chinese herbal formula significantly improved symptoms of irritable bowel syndrome in a randomized controlled trial in human patients (Bensoussan, 1998). This trial compared patients given placebo, individualized Chinese herbal prescriptions, and the standard formula that is described in Table 6-1. Initially, both treatment groups improved significantly compared with the placebo group; at follow-up 14 weeks later, only those receiving individualized prescriptions maintained improvement.

Treatment Note: **The value of herbal teas given as enemas should not be overlooked.**

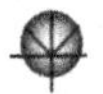

Paradigmatic Options

Homeopathy

- **Mercurius solubilis 30C:** is a very commonly indicated remedy in colitis of any cause. Dogs that benefit may have bloody mucoid stools, pronounced straining during bowel movements, and aggravation of these symptoms after midnight and through to 5 AM.

Table 6-1 Chinese herbal formula in Bensoussan trial

Chinese Name	Latin Name	Amount in Formula (g)
Dang Shen	*Codonopsis pilosulae*	7.0
Huo Xiang	*Agastaches seu pogostemi*	4.5
Fang Feng	*Ledebouriella sesiloidis*	3.0
Yi Yi Ren	*Coicis lacryma-jobi*	7.0
Chai Hu	*Bupleurum chinense*	4.5
Yin Chen	*Artemisia capillaris*	13.0
Bai zhu	*Atractylodes macrocephalae*	9.0
Hou Po	*Magnolia officinalis*	4.5
Chen Pi	*Citrus reticulata*	3.0
Pao Jiang	*Zingiber officinalis*	4.5
Qin Pi	*Fraxinus rhynchophylla*	4.5
Fu Ling	*Poria cocos*	4.5
Bai Zhi	*Angelica daihurica*	2.0
Che Qian Zi	*Plantago asiatica*	4.5
Huang Bai	*Phellodendron amurense*	4.5
Zhi Gan Cao	*Glycyrrhiza uralensis*	4.5
Bai Shao	*Paeonia lactiflora*	3.0
Mu Xiang	*Aucklandia lappa*	3.0
Huang Lian	*Coptis sinensis*	3.0
Wu Wei Zi	*Schisandra chinensis*	7.0

Associated symptoms in human homeopathic provings also include ptyalism, a swollen tongue, pronounced halitosis, muscle fasciculations after heavy exercise, and a marked tendency to appear suspicious or paranoid. Thirst and appetite may be increased, and the patient may avoid heat. The *recommended dose* is once daily for 1 week and then as needed.

- **Arsenicum album 30C:** should be considered for colitis in animals that have symptoms to support a diagnosis of Blood or Yin deficiency associated with long-term Damp Heat. Specific guiding signs include both vomiting and diarrhea often occurring together, bloody stool, marked abdominal cramping and pain, worsening of colitis symptoms after midnight and particularly around 2 AM, increased thirst, chilliness (tendency to seek warm spots), increased appetite, weight loss, and fearfulness, irritability, separation anxiety, or restlessness. The *recommended dose* is once daily for 1 week and then as needed.
- **Podophyllum 30C:** is a consideration when malodorous, "spluttering," painless diarrhea occurs around 5 AM. The *recommended dose* is once daily for 1 week and then as needed.
- **Colocynthis 30C:** should be considered for agonizing abdominal pain that causes the animal to sit hunched. Colitis may contain abundant gelatinous mucus and may be immediately stimulated by food consumption. The practitioner may recognize in the patient an association between colitis and what appears to be anger or resentment. The *recommended dose* is once daily for 1 week and then as needed.
- **Veratrum album 30C:** should be considered for violent painful lower abdominal contractions with scanty diarrhea in Kidney Yang–deficient patients. The recommended dose is once or twice daily as needed.

Chinese Medicine

- In Chinese medicine colitis develops because the distal large intestine has a tendency to accumulate Damp Heat. Dampness can obstruct Blood circulation, which leads to bleeding and severe abdominal pain. Heat can further increase bleeding by agitating the Blood. Tenesmus is viewed much as it is in conventional medicine, as a byproduct of tissue engorgement by edema. Edema and mucus in the stool are taken quite literally by Chinese medicine to represent an accumulation of Dampness.

- Damp Heat can enter the Large Intestine from a number of sources. Invasion of pathogenic Damp Heat from the immediate environment or food corresponds roughly to acute infection of the colon by bacteria or parasites. More commonly, the Dampness is internally generated by improper function of the Spleen and Stomach. These organs may be genuinely weak or may be relatively dysfunctional because of an inappropriate diet or overburdening by too much food.
- Treatment goals in colitis are to drain Dampness, clear Heat, move Blood, and stop bleeding. These objectives are often fulfilled by the use of bitter-tasting herbs, which unfortunately tend to weaken the Spleen and promote further Dampness formation. Thus bitter, strong formulas are used more for simple acute infectious causes, and more gentle and balanced formulas that warm and tonify the Spleen are sought when colitis is seen to be a chronic and remittent problem.
- Probably the main formula for colitis is **Shao Yao Tang** (Peony Decoction). Some practitioners add Jin Yin Hua to the formula to make it more effective at clearing Heat. The formula moves Qi to relieve tenesmus, clears Heat, and eliminates toxins. It nourishes and moves Blood to stop bleeding and relax spasms, yet warms the lower jiao to prevent damage to the Spleen from cooling herbs and to enhance the action of moving herbs. Despite this slight warming nature, this formula is still best suited to the patient in the throes of Damp Heat, with a red and wet or yellow-coated tongue and soft, slippery, and rapid pulses.
- Other formulas are arrayed above and below Shao Yao Tang in terms of Heat-clearing properties, with some being more Spleen supportive and others more adapted

to treating severe acute infection. They are listed below, with more bitter formulas listed first. A formula that best matches the symptomatic presentation of the patient should be chosen. For all of the formulas below, a *recommended starting dose* of granular formula is ¼ tsp per 10 to 15 lb of body weight, or 60 to 75 mg/kg of body weight, administered daily in divided doses.

- **Bai Tou Weng Tang** (Pulsatilla Decoction) and **Ge Gen Huang Qin Huang Lian Tang** (Pueraria, Scutellaria, and Coptis Decoction) can be used somewhat interchangeably in acute cases. Bai Tou Weng Tang is more focused on colitis, and Ge Gen Huang Qin Huang Lian Tang is more adapted to patients with a high fever and perhaps associated gastritis. Patients that receive these formulas should have red and wet or yellow-coated tongues and rapid, wiry, or slippery pulses.
- **Huang Lian Jie Du Tang** (Antiphlogistic Decoction of Coptis) can also be considered for these same acutely infected patients. The action of this formula is not restricted to the Large Intestine or Stomach but can be applied to acute infections anywhere in the body when the patient has a rapid and forceful pulse and a red or purple-red tongue.
- **Zhi Shi Dao Zhi Wan** (Immature Bitter Orange Pill to Guide Out Stagnation) is a formula to consider when some Spleen support is desired, perhaps based on the past medical history, but symptoms are still quite excessive and include abdominal distention and pain, malodorous diarrhea, mucus in the stool, and perhaps alternating diarrhea and constipation. The patient has a red tongue with a sticky yellow coat, as well as a slippery, rapid, forceful pulse.
- **Xiang Lian Wan** (Aucklandia and Coptis Pill) can be considered when an even more warming action on the Spleen is desired. Although it is not often used, this is a potentially very useful formula because it cools, relieves pain, and addresses colitis signaled by mucoid stools but with less blood in the stool. Signs calling for its use include obvious presence of Spleen and Stomach

deficiency in the past medical history and perhaps in the current presentation, but it is still best adapted for patients with a slippery, rapid pulse, sticky saliva, and a coated tongue.

- **Si Miao San** (Four Marvels Powder) is one of the more important herbal formulas in veterinary herbal medicine, in my opinion (SM). It acts to tonify and warm the Spleen as it leaches Damp and Toxic Heat out of the lower burner. Mild to moderate colitis with low back pain or stiffness may respond well to this formula. Spleen Qi deficiency signs are often obvious, with the patient perhaps having a soft pulse. The tongue is usually still vivid pink to red.
- **Wei Ling Tang** (Decoction to Dispel Dampness in the Spleen and Stomach) is considered in obvious Spleen Qi– or Yang-deficient patients with soft pulses and pale tongues. Dampness accumulations should be obvious but may seem less viscous with, for example, the saliva appearing wet rather than tenacious. Some practitioners add Shao Yao, Dang Gui, Mu Xiang, and Pao Jiang or Gan Jiang to the formula to enhance its ability to relieve pain, stop bleeding, relax spasms, and warm the lower abdomen.
- **Tong Xie Yao Fang** (Important Formula for Painful Diarrhea) is used specifically in cases in which the Spleen is perceived to be deficient from being overcontrolled by the Liver. Borborygmi may be loud and the colitis may specifically be known to be allergic in origin. Marked abdominal pain that is alleviated by a bowel movement is often present. Colitis may worsen when Liver Qi stagnation is accentuated, as when the patient is irritable or anxious.
- **Zhen Ren Yang Zang Tang** (Upright Man's Nourish the Internal Organs Decoction) is a formula to consider when colitis has affected the patient long enough to deplete Spleen and Kidney Yang. Signs that this formula may be effective include cases in which prolapse of the rectum, bowel incontinence, chronic diarrhea, and pain are present. Because the formula is an astringing formula, it should not be used in acute cases since it will aggravate the signs.

- When Spleen deficiency seems relatively uncomplicated by Dampness and the patient exhibits more classic signs of Spleen Qi deficiency, **Xiang Sha Liu Jun Zi Tang** (Six Gentlemen Decoction with Saussurea and Cardamon) or **Bu Zhong Yi Qi Tang** (Tonify the Center and Boost the Qi Decoction) should be considered. Both are candidates for consideration when the patient exhibits loose stools or diarrhea, reduced appetite, weakness of the extremities, weight loss, a pale tongue, and deep weak and possibly slippery pulses. Xiang Sha Liu Jun Zi Tang is more of a consideration when abdominal pain and cramping and perhaps morning nausea are present. Bu Zhong Yi Qi Tang is more of a consideration when a Spleen-deficient patient has incontinence or rectal prolapse.
- As the Kidneys become increasingly affected by a failure in their supply of Qi and Essence, other, more Kidney-oriented formulas become important. These should be considered when the patient has chronic or unremitting diarrhea that may contain blood, limb edema, anorexia, no thirst, cold extremities, abdominal pain made worse by cold, weakness, a long-term history of colitis managed by corticosteroids, a pale, puffy, lavender tongue, and a deep, weak pulse. **Si Shen Wan** (Four Miraculous Drugs Pill) is used when the patient has painless diarrhea in the early morning and low back weakness. **Shi Pi Yin** (Spleen Pill for Edema) is used when the patient has azotemia, abdominal pain or tenesmus, edema accumulation anywhere, and scanty urination. **Fu Zi Li Zhong Tang** (Cultivate the Spleen Decoction with Added Aconite) is a more generic formula to support Spleen and Kidney Yang, and **Zhen Wu Tang** (Water Controlling Decoction) is used when edema is pronounced along with abdominal pain and marked intolerance to cold.
- For colitis manifested as frank hemorrhage, short-term use of **Yunnan Bai Yao** (San Qi) may stop bleeding. A more specific formula to stop intestinal hemorrhage is **Huang Tu Tang** (Yellow Earth Decoction). It is

indicated when the Spleen is not controlling Blood, causing melena, hematemesis, a pale tongue, and deep, thin, weak pulses.

Western Herbs

- **Fennel** *(Foeniculum vulgare)*: seems to be a safe but powerful antispasmodic for violent colon spasms in chilly animals. The dosage is one capsule of dried herb as needed per 10 to 20 lb of body weight.
- **Cranesbill** *(Geranium maculatum)* and Agrimony *(Agrimonia eupatoria)*: have historically been combined to stop intestinal hemorrhage caused by the presence of Damp or Toxic Heat. They can be combined with Prickly Ash Bark *(Xanthoxylum americanum)* to help warm the Spleen and move Blood to stop bleeding. A recommended ratio is 3 parts each of Cranesbill and Agrimony to 2 parts Prickly Ash Bark. The *recommended dose* of combined tincture is 0.2 ml per 5 lb of body weight, divided into two daily doses. Higher volumes can be given if needed and the formula is tolerated well by the animal.
- **Black Walnut** *(Juglans nigra)* and Goldenseal *(Hydrastis canadensis)*: can be administered to kill protozoa in acute infectious cases. They can be given either alone or as part of a larger formula.

Dietary Strategies

- **Feeding low-carbohydrate and unprocessed diets** can keep an otherwise normal Spleen from being overwhelmed. The Spleen is more often truly deficient in animals with feeble or weak pulses.

Cautions

- Licorice may potentiate the action of glucocorticoids.

AUTHORS' CHOICES:

SM: Appropriate Chinese herbal formula or homeopathic remedy; dietary management for chronic cases.
SW: Elimination diets, fiber; Chinese herbs.

FLATULENCE

Therapeutic Rationale

- Identify food intolerances (especially lactose and poorly digestible foods such as soybean).
- Increase diet digestibility and reduce fermentable foods.
- Avoid rapid food changes.
- Manage aerophagia.
- Identify any intrinsic causes of malassimilation such as pancreatic insufficiency, small intestinal bacterial overgrowth, or *Giardia*.

Alternative Options with Conventional Bases

Nutritional Supplements

- **Enzyme products** such as Beano may be effective in some animals. The drops or tablets can be used in doses proportional to those recommended for humans on a per-weight basis.

Herbs

- **Traditional carminative herbs** include Anise *(Illicium verum)*, Fennel *(Foeniculum vulgare)*, and Caraway *(Carum carvi)*. Fennel is recognized as a carminative by the Commission E monographs.

Paradigmatic Options

- Flatulence is generally a Damp Heat condition and will respond to whatever formulas are addressing other manifestations of Damp Heat. Diets that are low in carbohydrates and less processed often improve flatulence dramatically. Any diet changes should be made slowly in affected animals, and treats should be avoided. Acupuncture can be employed to provide general Spleen support by needling BL 25, BL 20, and BL 26.

AUTHORS' CHOICES:

SM: Dietary management; appropriate herbal formula for other problems that may be present.

SW: Dietary management; investigate for food intolerances; combinations of Fennel, Peppermint, and Ginger.

FOOD ALLERGY

Therapeutic Rationale

- Eliminate food allergens.

Alternative Options with Conventional Bases

- **Probiotics,** or lactic acid–producing bacteria: believed to have a role in the development and expression of allergy, particularly atopy (Cross, 2001). Whether this is true for food allergy is unknown; however, probiotic bacteria are probably beneficial for inflamed gut mucosa and would be recommended in any case.
- **Nambudripad's Allergy Elimination Technique (NAET):** a new technique that combines mechanical stimulation of acupressure or acupuncture points and applied kinesiology. However, point selection and use are not dependent on Chinese medical theory but on a completely different rationale. We do not use the technique and are skeptical of its efficacy. Because NAET practitioners frequently use diet changes and other alternative modalities simultaneously, the efficacy of NAET is difficult to isolate. Anecdotal reports suggest, however, that NAET has been helpful in certain cases and may be worth considering. For more information, see http://www.vetnaet.com and http://www.naet.com.

Paradigmatic Options

- Select one of the formulas and strategies listed in the sections on Diarrhea, Colitis, and Vomiting that seem to best fit the patient's symptoms. **Tong Xie Yao Fang** (Important Formula for Painful Diarrhea) is traditionally recommended for food allergies manifesting with GI signs. Patients may exhibit signs of the Liver overacting on the Spleen, such as diarrhea, aggravation from stress, irritability, possible flank pain, borborygmi, abdominal pain that is relieved by bowel movements, a lavender tongue, and a wiry pulse. A *recommended starting dose* of granular concentrate is

¼ tsp per 10 to 15 lb of body weight, or 60 to 75 mg/kg of body weight, administered daily in divided doses.

AUTHORS' CHOICES:

SM: Appropriate Chinese herbal formula; avoid allergens.
SW: Elimination diet, then rotate through various hypoallergenic diets on a schedule determined by when patient develops new allergic responses; probiotics.

GASTRIC DILATATION, BLOAT (RECURRENT TENDENCIES)

Therapeutic Rationale

- Definitive emergency treatment for gastric dilatation is necessary, although long-term prevention of recurrence or temporary management for postsurgical ileus may include complementary therapies.

Alternative Options with Conventional Bases

Herbs

- **Carminative herbs** (such as those listed under Flatulence) include Fennel, Cardamom *(Elettaria repens)*, and Peppermint, which should be safe as daily additions to the diet in either fresh or dried form.

Paradigmatic Options

- Predispositions to gastric dilatation and volvulus appear to exist in animals with a Liver Stomach disharmony. This has a variety of symptoms, including costal arch tightness and pain, belching, nausea and eructations, anxiety, elevated or depressed appetite, thin and wiry pulses, and cranial abdominal distention. A formula that can address this presentation is **Xiang Lian Wang** (Aucklandia and Coptis Pill), which clears Stomach Fire, warms the Liver, and moves the Qi of the middle jiao. Acupuncture points that may help in the treatment of this syndrome include LIV 13 and 14, ST 36, CV 12, PC 6, GB 34, and TH 6.

AUTHORS' CHOICES:

SM: Yi Guan Jian; acupuncture.
SW: Carminative herbs in food; small meals often during the day.

GASTRITIS, GASTRIC ULCERATION

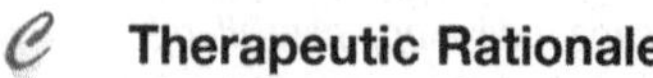

Therapeutic Rationale

- Identify cause (e.g., NSAID use, hepatic or renal failure, cancer, mast cell tumor).
- Protect ulcerated tissue.
- Reduce gastric acid secretion.
- Control vomiting.
- Control bacterial infection, such as spirochetes, as necessary.

Alternative Options with Conventional Bases

Herbs

- **Licorice:** contains glycyrrhizin, which is the source of the synthetic derivative carbenoxolone. Carbenoxolone is effective in accelerating gastric ulcer resolution. Like Licorice itself carbenoxolone is associated with high blood pressure, sodium and water retention, and hypokalemia. DGL was shown in one study to reduce aspirin-induced ulceration in rats, but at a high dose (350 mg per rat) (Rees, 1979). Most human clinical studies do not support its efficacy.
- **Gotu Cola** *(Centella asiatica):* inhibited ethanol-induced gastric ulcers in an experimental rat model (Cheng, 2000).
- **Turmeric** *(Cucurma longa):* the extract significantly inhibited formation of gastric ulcers in rats given 500 mg/kg of body weight. Turmeric extract inhibited ulcers caused through a number of different mechanisms in rats and humans (Prucksunand, 2002; Rafatullah, 1990).
- **Dang Shen** *(Codonopsis pilosula):* a component of many Chinese herbal combinations for digestive disorders. Codonopsis alone appears to inhibit gastric acid and pepsin secretion and prevented ulcer development in three of five different animal models (Wang, 1997).

However, in a Chinese study of five dogs, Dang Shen increased serum gastrin levels, making the advisability of its use in dogs suspect.

- ***Evodia rutaecarpa***, a Chinese herb called Wu Zhu Yu (the Kampo name is Gosuyu): has demonstrated activity against *Helicobactor pylori* (Hamasaki, 2000).
- **Huanglian Jie Du Tang** (Kampo: Oren-gedoku-to): was shown to reduce development of stress-induced gastric ulceration in rats (Ohta, 1999).

Paradigmatic Options

Western Herbs

- A formula that has been traditionally used for gastric ulcers in humans is Marshmallow Root, Indigo Root *(Baptisia tinctoria)*, Cranesbill, and Agrimony. These herbs are some of the ingredients in several commercially available formulas, such as GI Caps (Wise Woman Herbals) and Robert's Formula (various distributors). The formula acts to coat the lining of the stomach with a polysaccharide layer found in the Marshmallow. Early versions of the formula also included Comfrey, which has now been made unavailable because of concerns about its potential hepatotoxicity. Slippery Elm can be used in place of Comfrey, and is effective on its own as a demulcent in dogs with mild stomach ulcers. Without the benefit of endoscopy or imaging studies mild gastric ulceration can be hard to diagnose. It should be suspected in dogs with an obstinately poor appetite despite an interest in food, and in abdominal pain without apparent cause, although esophagitis should also be ruled out. Because of viscerosomatic reflexes gastric pain may manifest as severe back pain at the thoracolumbar junction, prompting a search for evidence of intervertebral disk (IVD) and a resultant delay in diagnosis.

Chinese Herbs

- The underlying cause of chronic gastritis and mild ulceration in dogs is a Blood and Yin deficiency that affects the Liver and Stomach. **Yi Guan Jian** (One Linking Decoction) is probably the single most important herbal formula for treatment of this condition. Guiding signs and symptoms to its use are pain in the epigastrium and across the costal arch; belching and acid regurgitation; mouth dryness; red, dry eyes; powdery dander and a dry coat; a tender tongue with no coating; and a thin and perhaps wiry pulse. The addition of 9 g of Huang Lian to 60 g of the base formula may be necessary to clear Stomach Heat. Diets that are rich in organ meat may reduce tendency to Liver Blood deficiency. A *recommended starting dose* of granular concentrate is ¼ tsp per 10 to 15 lb of body weight, or 60 to 75 mg/kg of body weight, administered daily in divided doses.

AUTHORS' CHOICES:

SM: Slippery Elm; Yi Guan Jian; Robert's Formula.
SW: Combinations of herbs including Slippery Elm; Chinese herbal formulas.

GINGIVITIS, STOMATITIS, DENTAL AND PERIODONTAL DISEASE

Therapeutic Rationale

- Identify anatomic, metabolic, immune-mediated, infectious, traumatic, or toxic causes.
- Treat accompanying dental or periodontal disease; inhibit plaque formation.
- Treat inflammation when appropriate.
- Suppress bacterial growth.

Alternative Options with Conventional Bases

- **Raw meaty bones:** bones such as femur ends, shanks, large intact poultry necks, and ox tails may physically prevent and destroy plaque, depending on the size of the animal (Brown, 1968). Raw (uncooked) bones are said to be harder and less likely to splinter than cooked bones and they contain marrow that assists in tartar control, although evidence for these claims is lacking. Dangers of feeding bones are the potential for dental fractures, swallowing and obstruction, perforation and infection with enteropathogens. Despite the risks, feeding bones is an old practice that has recently grown in popularity. Enteropathogens can be destroyed by immersion of the bone in boiling water for 30 to 60 seconds. It is recommended that owners carefully monitor animals given bones.

- **Lactoferrin:** has been reported useful in managing some cats with stomatitis, used topically (Sato, 1996). The dose is 40 mg/kg of body weight per day in syrup, milk, or liquefied baby food.
- **Coenzyme Q_{10}:** has been advocated for treatment of gingivitis and periodontal disease in humans and animals. The evidence is slight; one study showed that topical application improved human periodontal disease (Hanioka, 1994). Although older case series in human patients were intriguing, clinical experience in dogs and cats has not been promising. Anecdotal reports suggest that CoQ_{10} may be helpful for some animals when no conventional therapy has been effective making it worth trying in chronic cases. The dose range is 2 mg/kg of body weight to 20 mg/kg of body weight orally daily, or it can be used as a mouthwash.
- **Ascorbate:** Vitamin C is often recommended on the basis of its role in collagen synthesis and prevention of scurvy. Supplementation of Vitamin C for periodontal disease in pets has not been investigated but would appear to be safe.
- **Propolis:** a product of the honeybee, Propolis has well-recognized antimicrobial properties and may be an effective oral antiseptic (Koo, 2000). Topical application of Propolis also significantly improved healing of lesions in human genital herpes (Vynograd, 2000) indicating potential in the treatment of feline viral stomatitis. Allergic contact dermatitis has been recognized after use of Propolis in sensitive humans, probably related to which plants bees had pollinated.

- **Glutamine:** has been reported to relieve radiation- and chemotherapy-induced stomatitis and mucositis in numerous studies.
- **Cinnamon Oil** and **Clove Oil:** inhibit many oral bacteria (Saeki, 1989). Irritation to the oral mucous membranes may limit use in animals unless the oils are very diluted.
- **Coptis:** contains berberine. Has been shown to inhibit growth of many oral bacteria (Hu, 2000). Coptis or other berberine-containing herbs may be used systemically or as a mouthwash, but these herbs are extremely bitter.

Herbs

Topical herbs

- **Bloodroot** *(Sanguinaria canadensis):* extract of Bloodroot has been shown to have antimicrobial and antiinflammatory activity. Sanguinarine is approved by the Food and Drug Administration (FDA) as a topical agent for use in rinses and pastes for the prevention of plaque in people.
- **Bistort** *(Polygonum bistorta):* a traditional mouthwash ingredient that has antiinflammatory properties (Duwiejua, 1994).
- **Neem** *(Azadirachta indica):* the extracts have been shown to inhibit colonization of tooth surfaces by *Streptococcus* species (Wolinsky, 1996).
- **Myrrh** *(Commiphora myrrha):* a traditional Ayurvedic herb applied topically as a rinse. It may have antiinflammatory and analgesic effects.

Note: Some practitioners have recommended mixing herb extracts with a commercial toothpaste for animals.

Immune modulators

- **Echinacea** *(Echinacea purpurea, E. angustifolia):* anecdotal reports suggest that Echinacea may be helpful in some cats with chronic stomatitis. I (SM) have found this approach to be uniformly unsuccessful.
- **Kampo herbal combinations:** Kakkon-to, Kakkon-oren-ogon-to, Kikyo-to, Haino-to, Haino-san, Mao-to, and Senkinkeimei-san have been used in treating

stomatitis. They all have antiinflammatory properties (Ozaki, 1995).

- *Baccharis trinervis, Eupatorium articulatum,* and *Heisteria acuminata:* inhibited human herpes simplex virus in vitro (Abad, 1999).

Paradigmatic Options

Western Herbs

- Stomatitis is a challenging condition to treat, particularly in cats, and progress in understanding and managing the condition is only beginning to be seen. Alterative formulas recommended in the early Western human medical herbal literature appear to hold out the best hope. One such herbal combination is 6 parts Agrimony and 2 parts Yellow Dock *(Rumex crispus).* A *suggested starting dose* is 0.2 ml per 5 lb of body weight given daily in divided doses. Agrimony helps heal oral ulcers and Yellow Dock helps improve liver function in an attempt to remove the perceived toxic cause of the lesion.
- For more obstinate cases of stomatitis with proliferative oral lesions, equal quantities of Sarsaparilla *(Smilax officinalis)* and Burdock Root *(Arctium lappa)* can be added to the Agrimony and Yellow Dock combination to make up 50% of the total formula. A *suggested starting dose* is 0.2 ml per 5 lb of body weight given daily in divided doses. This recommendation is based on the observed ability of this formula to address mild perioral eosinophilic granuloma lesions and on the recognition that stomatitis in cats frequently has an immune-mediated pathogenesis. For very hot cats with severe stomatitis or eosinophilic granuloma lesions the **Hoxsey Formula** may be employed, using dose ratios discussed in Chapter 13. Agrimony and Yellow Dock may be added to the tincture to enhance its activity against stomatitis.
- Other herbs traditionally recommended for their antimicrobial, astringent, or antiinflammatory properties include Blackberry *(Rubus fructicosis),* Baptisia *(Baptisia tinctoria),* Goldenseal *(Hydrastis canadensis),* Wax Myrtle *(Myrica cerifera),* White Oak Bark *(Quercus alba),* and Sage *(Salvia officinalis).*

Chinese Medicine

- Gingival inflammation is traditionally associated with Stomach Fire in Chinese medicine. Although this may be true for humans, it does not seem to lead to reliable therapies in animals, particularly cats. Nevertheless, some of the formulas that are used to clear Stomach Heat and replenish Stomach Yin include the following:
  - **Tian Wang Bu Xin Dan** (Heavenly Emperor's Nourish the Heart Pill) for Heart Blood and Yin deficiency with Empty Heat that is manifested as insomnia, palpitations, irritability, fatigue, dry stools, stomatitis, a red, dry and tender tongue, and a thin, rapid pulse.
  - **Tiao Wei Cheng Qi Tang** (Regulate the Stomach and Order the Qi Decoction) for excess types of Stomach Heat. Symptoms of this condition are an aversion to all heat, very high thirst, constipation, fullness in the stomach, canker sores, a red or red-purple tongue with a yellow coat, and a slippery, strong, and rapid pulse. This formula is a strong purgative and should never be used in deficient patients.
  - **Qing Wei San** (Clear the Stomach Powder) is commonly indicated in patients with excess Stomach Fire that manifests as painful gingivitis, thirst, dry mouth, fever, constipation, bleeding or ulcerated gums, very bad breath, and tooth pain.
  - **Bai Hu Tang** (White Tiger Decoction) is less specifically oriented toward oral tissues but does address Stomach Fire. Patients that benefit are heat intolerant and often have a high fever, high thirst, a flooding, floating, and rapid pulse, and a red tongue.
  - **Yu Nu Jian** (Fair Maiden Decoction) is used for simple Stomach Yin deficiency, the symptoms of which are bleeding gums, excess hunger, thirst, loose or painful teeth, epistaxis, oral dryness, possible frontal headache or pain, malaise, a red and dry tongue, and a thin, rapid, or floating gigantic pulse.
- The following formulas that clear Damp Heat from the Liver might be more useful in the treatment of gingivitis, given the early indications that alterative formulas seem to help the condition.

- For very hot patients in which consideration might be given to using the Hoxsey Formula, **Long Dan Xie Gan Tang** (Gentian Drain the Liver Decoction) might instead be used. An even more vigorously cooling and drying formula that may be of benefit to constipated cats is **Yin Chen Hao Tang** (Capillaris Decoction). For both formulas the *recommended starting dose* of granular concentrate is ¼ tsp per 10 to 15 lb of body weight, or 60 to 75 mg/kg of body weight, given daily in divided doses.
- **Qing Fei Yi Huo Pian** (Clear the Lung and Eliminate Fire Pills) may be of substantial benefit, given its content of Huang Qin and Da Huang that address liver function and its symptomatic indications of a swollen, painful sore throat, painful mouth or nose, toothache, and bleeding gums. This patent remedy is in a pill form, which promotes ease of administration. A *recommended starting dose* is one tablet per 15 lb of body weight daily in divided doses. As with most of the formulas in this section, this formula is not for use in deficient patients.

AUTHORS' CHOICES:

SM: Alterative formulas; Qing Fei Yi Huo Pian; topical mouthwashes.
SW: Herbal combination mouthwashes, Chinese herbal formulas; Lactoferrin, Propolis.

INFLAMMATORY BOWEL DISEASE

Therapeutic Rationale

- Reduce inflammation.
- Identify triggers.
- Address possible food allergy.

Alternative Options with Conventional Bases

Nutrition

- **Probiotics:** cultures of lactic acid–producing bacteria such as *Lactobacillus salivarius* and other species,

Bifidobacterium longum and other species, *Saccharomyces* spp., and other enteric organisms. Supplementation with viable cultures appears to modulate the host immune response, benefit inflamed intestinal mucosa, inhibit attachment of pathogenic bacteria, and improve diarrhea from a variety of causes, including viral infections. Probiotics may be an important part of inflammatory bowel disease (IBD) treatment (Dunne, 1999; Rolfe, 2000). Unfortunately, it is difficult to ensure that commercially available products contain viable organisms. For that reason we recommend using up to a human dose for a 10-lb animal. If the animal is on an elimination diet, a hypoallergenic probiotic product containing no dairy, wheat, corn, or animal products must be used.

- **Marine fish oil:** has been recommended for treatment of inflammatory bowel disorders but the results of trials are contradictory (Belluzzi, 2000). Fish Oil capsules probably contain fish antigen, which would be a consideration in animals on elimination diets meant to exclude fish. A trial of Fish Oil may be useful; the *recommended dose* is 100 to 200 mg/kg of body weight of ω-3 fatty acid daily.
- **Glutamine:** supports the function of the intestinal mucosa as the primary fuel source for enterocytes, and has been suggested for inflammatory bowel disease (IBD). The clinical benefit is questionable according to results of trials in humans, and glutamine has been associated with side effects in humans with liver-function abnormalities (Buchman, 2001; Reeds, 2001).
- **N-Acetylglucosamine:** provides fuel for synthesis of protective glycosaminoglycans that are lost from the mucosa of inflamed bowel. It may also have a variety of other functions regulating inflammatory pathways intracellularly. In a trial of 12 children with chronic inflammatory bowel disorders, 8 improved when given a total daily dose of 3 to 6 g *N*-acetylglucosamine. An approximate dose of 35 to 75 mg per lb of body weight in dogs and cats would be reasonable based on the findings of this study. No long-term toxicity is expected.

Herbs

- **Fiber supplements:** soluble fiber enhances the production of short chain fatty acids (SCFAs) by intestinal bacteria. In IBD, SCFAs reduce inflammation, normalize mucosal cell proliferation, and increase energy production. The soluble fibers that best support SCFA production are Guar Gum and Citrus Pectin, which can be dosed proportionally to the label suggestions for humans.
- **Peppermint:** appears to have a role in symptom relief in human IBD. It has been shown to possess smooth muscle relaxant properties and to suppress GI motility (Kline, 2001; Micklefield, 2000; Pittler, 1998). Enteric coated capsules may be more effective.
- **Boswellia** *(Boswellia serrata)*: has been effective in reducing bowel inflammation and clinical signs of IBD in both animal models and human trials (Gupta, 1997; Krieglstein, 2001).
- **Mexican Yam** *(Dioscorea villosa)*: is a traditional remedy for inflammatory bowel signs and is popular among some practitioners as a spasmolytic and antiinflammatory agent. It is believed that steroidal saponins in the tuber act as steroids. Yam is, in fact, a source for diosgenin, which is used in the pharmaceutical industry as a precursor for steroid synthesis. However, diosgenin is probably not converted into active steroids in the body. If Yam is effective, it may be for other reasons or because the steroid precursors have antiinflammatory properties. Yams can be fed as part of the diet, or as herbal extracts.
- **Herbs** with less support for use in IBD include Chamomile, Slippery Elm, and Licorice. Licorice is often recommended for IBD on the basis of its potential benefit in peptic ulcer treatment, but since these are rarely seen in dogs and cats, Licorice may work via other mechanisms if effective in bowel disease.

Paradigmatic Options

- Use the appropriate Chinese herbal formula discussed in the preceding sections relating to the patient's dominant symptoms such as vomiting and diarrhea. Some recommendations are:

- **Huang Lian Su Pian** (Coptis Tea Pill) for Damp Heat cases. The signs for its use are the acute onset of foul, yellow, painful diarrhea with small stool volumes that contain blood and mucus, increased thirst, a red or purple-red tongue with perhaps a thick yellow coating, and a rapid, forceful pulse. The pill contains only Huang Lian and is used in humans for bacterial or protozoal dysentery. A recommended dose is one tablet per 15 to 20 lb of body weight daily, in divided doses if possible. This product should never be used in Spleen Qi or Yang deficiency cases.
- **Chuan Xin Lian** (Antiphlogistic Pill) is considered slightly gentler and less cold than Huang Lian Su Pian. Its real advantage may be that it possesses antiviral and antibacterial activity because it contains Chuan Xin Lian, Ban Lan Gen, and Pu Gong Ying. The cautions and dosage recommendations are the same as for Huang Lian Su Pian.
- For inflammatory bowel disease that manifests with Qi and Yin Deficiency, a combination of **Si Jun Zi Tang** (Four Gentlemen Decoction) and **Zhi Bai Di Huang Wan** (Anemarrhena, Phellodendron, and Rehmannia Pill) should be considered. The patient that can benefit from this combination is chronically ill, with small, dark, soft stools that have a slightly foul odor, no mucus or pain on defecation, poor appetite, variable thirst, a pale or red and possibly dry tongue, and a thready, weak pulse. A *recommended starting dose* of granular concentrate is ¼ tsp per 10 to 15 lb of body weight, or 60 to 75 mg/kg of body weight, given daily in divided doses.

AUTHORS' CHOICES:

SM: Appropriate Chinese herbal formula; avoid food allergens.
SW: Elimination diet; probiotics; N-acetylglucosamine; Peppermint; Boswellia; Citrus Pectin; Chinese herbs.

INFECTIOUS ENTERITIS (ALSO SEE DIARRHEA)

Therapeutic Rationale

- Correct bacterial imbalance; eliminate pathogenic organisms.
- Maintain hydration; reduce intestinal fluid loss.
- Maintain electrolyte balance.
- Prolong intestinal transit time.

Alternative Options with Conventional Bases

Nutrition

- **Probiotics:** enhance immune responses and increase resistance to pathogens. In one study, mice whose bacterial populations were disrupted showed corresponding levels of decreased resistance to *Giardia* (Singer, 2000). Probiotics are used in some food animal operations to competitively inhibit attachment of enteropathogens such as *Escherichia coli. Lactobacillus rhamnosus* strain GG may be a preferred species at this time.

Herbs

Antimicrobial herbs

- **Barberry** *(Berberis vulgaris):* see Berberine.
- **Oregon Grape** *(Berberis aquifolium):* see Berberine.
- **Coptis:** see Berberine.
- **Berberine:** exerts an antisecretory effect on the intestinal epithelium, is effective for enterotoxigenic *E. coli* diarrhea in humans, and may slow small intestinal transit time (Rabbani, 1996; Taylor, 1999; Tsai, 1991).

Astringent herbs

- **Raspberry** *(Rubus idaeus):* the leaf is used and contains ellagic acid, as well as benzoic, gallic, lactic, acetic, and other organic acids. Many of these acids have been reported to have antibacterial and antiinflammatory properties (Duke, 1999). The traditional concept is to use these acidic herbs to shrink inflamed tissues and "coagulate" the surface of the inflamed intestinal mucosa.

- **Blackberry:** contains arbutin and hydroquinone as well as lactic, oxalic, ursolic, and malic acids. Many of these acids have been reported to have antibacterial and antiinflammatory properties (Duke, 1999).

Paradigmatic Options

- See sections on Inflammatory Bowel Disease, Diarrhea, and Colitis.

AUTHORS' CHOICES:

SM: Appropriate Chinese herbal formula.
SW: Probiotics; Berberine-containing herbs; Chinese herbal formulas.

MEGACOLON

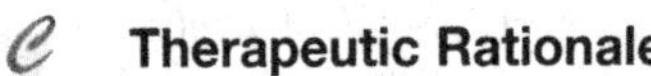

Therapeutic Rationale

- Rule out physical obstruction to defecation such as a stricture.
- Administer enemas as needed to evacuate the colon and avoid distention.
- Administer laxatives.
- Maintain hydration.
- Increase insoluble fiber in diet.
- Enhance colonic motility.

Alternative Options with Conventional Bases

Nutrition

- **5-Hydroxy-L-tryptophan** (5-HTP): different forms of 5HT (serotonin) receptors have been shown to coordinate contraction of canine and human large intestinal muscle as well as stimulate fluid secretion (Gelal, 1998; Prins, 2000). Supplementation of 5-HTP may enhance the contraction of the GI smooth muscle.
- **Melatonin:** induces colonic contraction via specific melatonin receptors (Santagostino-Barbone, 2000). Melatonin is usually supplied as 0.3 mg to 5 mg tablets, and can be administered at approximately 50 µg per lb of body weight bid.

Herbs

- **Cathartic herbs:** see Senna and Cascara in section on Constipation.

Paradigmatic Options

Homeopathy

- **Silica 30C:** may be helpful in cats with a "bashful stool," which is only able to be partly expelled before receding again. The *recommended dose* is once daily for 3 weeks and then as needed.
- **Calcarea carbonica 30C:** the classic remedy indicated for constipation without apparent discomfort or urge to defecate. The *recommended dose* is once daily for 3 weeks and then as needed.
- See the section on Constipation.

Chinese Medicine

- See the section on Constipation.
- Many cases of megacolon seem to arise from Qi deficiency, manifested as poor GI motility, a preference for warmth, a pale, swollen tongue, and a weak pulse. For these cats, 40 g of **Si Jun Zi Tang** (Four Gentlemen Decoction) with about 9 g of Da Huang added has been advocated. The practitioner should also consider the appropriateness of **Ma Zi Ren Wan** and **Dang Gui Cong Rong,** which were discussed in the general section on constipation.
- Acupuncture points that may assist in the management of megacolon include: BL 23, CV 6, BL 20, BL 21, CV 12, ST 36, and LI 4 to address Qi deficiency as a cause of constipation, BL 25, ST 25, SP 6,and ST 37 to move the bowels.
- Consider electrical stimulation of points for added effect.

AUTHORS' CHOICES:

SM: Cascara in Western herbal formula (see section on Constipation); appropriate Chinese herbal formula; Vitamin C and Magnesium (see Constipation); acupuncture.

SW: Electroacupuncture; chiropractic; laxative herbs.

OBESITY

Therapeutic Rationale

- Assess thyroid status to rule out hypothyroidism.
- Manage caloric intake and exercise.
- Review relative fat, protein, and carbohydrate intake.

Alternative Options with Conventional Bases

Nutrition

- **Dehydroepiandrosterone (DHEA):** 25 mg daily (MacEwen, 1991) has been shown to increase weight loss of overweight dogs that are on weight loss diets, but has not gained favor clinically due to apparent lack of efficacy, potential for side effects, and expense.
- **Chromium:** supplementation was shown to enhance loss of fat over nonfat tissue as compared with a placebo in a randomized, placebo-controlled crossover trial in humans (Crawford, 1999). Chromium may be supplied at 50 to 300 mg total dose daily, but it has been associated with side effects in humans when given long term.
- **Conjugated linoleic acid** (CLA): was shown to enhance body fat loss while sparing lean body mass compared to control subjects in a human trial. Up to 3.4 g/day was sufficient to produce a significant effect. CLA may be dosed proportionately on a per-weight basis according to the label directions for humans.
- **Carnitine:** has been shown to accelerate weight loss in obese cats (Center, 2000), as well as reduce fasting ketosis in cats with induced hepatic lipidosis (Blanchard, 2002). The dose used is 250 mg once or twice daily.

Herbs

- *Garcinia camboga:* has been advocated, but clinical experience and the evidence do not support its use.

Paradigmatic Options

Traditional Chinese Medicine

- Much to the chagrin of animal owners, there is no magic pill for obesity. Once predisposing metabolic disorders such as hypothyroidism have been ruled out, the focus should be on regular exercise and, even more important, avoidance of overnutrition. To accomplish this the practitioner should consider putting animals with strong pulses on a raw food or low-carbohydrate diet. Increasing the fiber content of the diet can add bulk and a sense of fullness.

- When animals are chilly, overweight, inappetent, and sluggish in the mornings and have a pale, swollen, moist tongue, and a soft pulse, consideration may be given to formulas that drain Dampness and warm the Yang. Examples include **Shen Qi Wan** (Kidney Qi Pill) for animals with low back stiffness, urinary incontinence, profuse pale urine, and cold intolerance and **Wei Ling Tang** (Decoction to Dispel Dampness in the Spleen and Stomach) for animals with soft, mucoid stools.
- In other animals the very act of eating promotes appetite. The *Nei Jing* describes this as a "form of jaundice," or Damp Heat. Although many herbal formulas may be beneficial in these cases, including **Si Miao San** and **Long Dan Xie Gan Tang,** one formula that has been advocated for obesity in humans with symptoms of Excess Heat is **Fang Feng Tong Sheng San** (Ledebouriella Powder That Sagely Unblocks). Even though it aggressively clears Heat, it does offer some protection to the Spleen Qi and Blood against its cooling and drying effects. The formula also contains Ma Huang (Ephedra), which is used as an appetite suppressant in people. However, unlike with human products there are not likely to be any adverse cardiovascular side effects from the Ma Huang in this formula because of the small amounts that are used.

Homeopathy

- **Calcarea carbonica 30C:** has on occasion been remarkably effective at triggering weight loss. Patients that benefit are typically friendly and often act as nursemaids or peacekeepers among the other members of the household. Dentition may be poor and the teeth inexplicably but heavily eroded. The patient is easily exhausted and either dislikes or is particularly lethargic during cold, damp weather. The *recommended dose* is once daily for 3 to 4 weeks and then as needed.

AUTHORS' CHOICES:

SM: Diet management; Calcarea carbonica; any well-indicated Chinese herbal formula.

SW: Diet changes and calorie counting by increasing protein and decreasing both carbohydrates and fat; exercise; carnitine; CLA.

PANCREATITIS

Therapeutic Rationale

- Maintain proper hydration.
- NPO; avoid oral medication and feeding until vomiting stops.
- Institute parenteral or enteral nutrition as appropriate.
- Decrease inflammation to minimize fibrosis and long-term damage.
- Control pain.
- Control hyperlipidemia in at-risk animals.
- Decrease oxidative damage from free radicals.

Alternative Options with Conventional Bases

- **Outpatient therapy:** mild acute pancreatitis and relapsing episodes of feline pancreatitis may be treated on an outpatient basis. Animals may be treated with daily subcutaneous fluid therapy, liquid enteral feeding every 1 to 2 hours at about 0.5 to 1 ml/kg of body weight via nasoesophageal tube, and antioxidant therapy.
- **Antioxidant therapy:** antioxidant therapy for treatment and prevention of pancreatitis has been studied for many years, but the mechanisms by which it works and which antioxidant is most beneficial are unknown. Certain forms of selenium and ascorbate have proved most promising (McCloy, 1998; Schulz, 1999). Selenious acid at 0.3 mg/kg of body weight IV may be effective in dogs with acute pancreatitis, according to a German trial (Kraft, 1995). I (SW) use a broad-spectrum commercial small animal antioxidant

combination at the dose recommended by the manufacturer.

- **Pancreatic enzymes:** enzyme supplementation is often recommended to reduce pancreatic inflammation. Most studies have shown no beneficial effect on pain after supplementation; however, enzyme therapy has been suggested by some authors to positively influence feedback mechanisms or reduce systemic inflammation.

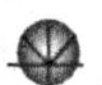

Paradigmatic Options

- See formulas and approaches previously listed in sections on Vomiting, Colitis, and Diarrhea.
- Acupuncture points that have been advocated for pancreatitis include ST 36, PC 6, and GB 34. Acupuncture and administration of herbal formulas as an aqueous enema may be especially beneficial.

Western Herbal Medicine

- **Aqueous decoctions of Fringe Tree Bark** *(Chionanthus virginicus)* appear to rapidly resolve symptoms of pancreatitis and pancreatic enzyme elevations in some cases. It is specifically indicated when liver involvement from local inflammation has resulted in clinical icterus. The mechanism of this effect is unknown. One tablespoon of dried herb is simmered in approximately one cup of water for 15 to 30 minutes, with water added as necessary to achieve a final volume of ⅓ cup. Between 0.5 and 1 ml of this solution per lb of body weight is instilled as a high-retention enema four times daily for 3 days, or until signs resolve. Some claim that Fringe Tree's active ingredients are found only in alcohol extracts, but this form should not be administered rectally.

Homeopathy

- Homeopathy may be particularly attractive for the treatment of pancreatitis, since the remedies are meant to dissolve in the mouth and not stimulate the upper GI tract.
- **Iris versicolor 30C:** to control acute attacks. Guiding symptoms include severe cranial abdominal pain

referable to the pancreas, malaise, constipation, watery and possibly burning stools, and continuous nausea and vomiting. It should be given one to three times daily as needed.

AUTHORS' CHOICES:

SM: Chionanthus via enema; Iris versicolor.
SW: Adequate hydration and parenteral or careful enteral feeding (as outpatient therapy for mild cases); antioxidants for prevention.

PARVOVIRAL ENTERITIS

Therapeutic Rationale

- Maintain hydration and electrolyte status.
- Prevent vomiting to reduce electrolyte loss, reduce risk of aspiration, and provide symptomatic relief.
- Use blood products or colloids to treat anemia or hypoproteinemia.
- Repair intestinal mucosa.
- Supply parenteral nutrition.
- Prevent or treat systemic infection caused by bacterial translocation.
- Support immune function.

Alternative Options with Conventional Bases

- Most herbal and nutraceutical supplements are given orally, which is not useful in vomiting dogs. Enemas containing the supplements listed below may be one option for treatment of vomiting dogs.

Nutrition

- **Glutamine:** oral Glutamine supplementation appears to enhance intestinal villus repair, improve nitrogen balance and protein synthesis, and increase peripheral lymphocyte numbers (Mazzaferro, 2000). Reported oral dose is approximately 0.5 g/kg of body weight. Administration by enema may be more useful in parvovirus-infected dogs with intractable vomiting.

Herbs

- **African plants:** *Bauhinia thonningii, Boswellia dalzielii, Detarium senegalensis,* and *Dichrostachys glomerata* inhibited replication of canine parvovirus in vitro (Kudi, 1999). These plants are not readily available, and dosage guidelines are unknown at this time.

Paradigmatic Options

Homeopathy

- **China 30C:** indicated for patients with abdominal distention, flatulent colic, bloody stools, chills, aversion to touch, and debilitation from loss of fluids.
- **Veratrum album 30C:** potentially a major remedy in the management of parvoviral enteritis. Patients are cold, collapsed, thirsty for water that they vomit immediately after drinking, have copious watery diarrhea reminiscent of cholera, and frequent vomiting. Veratrum should be given four times daily as needed until improvements are maintained, then as needed to maintain improvement.

Chinese Medicine

- Formulas discussed in the sections on Diarrhea and Colitis should be considered. In addition a "CPV formula" (available in the U.S. from Jing Tang Herbal) has been developed with a reported efficacy of 80% in Chinese medical studies on dogs with parvoviral enteritis. It contains the following herbs in undisclosed proportions:

Huang Lian
Huang Qin
Huang Bai
Huang Qi
Cang Zhu
Shan Yao
Zhi Zi
Di Yu
Ban Xia
Zhu Ru
Zhi Qiao
Dang Gui
Mu Xiang
Bai Shao Yao
Gan Cao

The formula does not seem designed for advanced severe cases, which are often purely Qi and Yang deficient. It should probably be used when the patient still has fever and signs of acute external Pathogen invasion. Acupuncture points that are recommended in support of the formula are SP 6, LIV 3, HT 9, ST 25, ST 36, GV 14, BL 17, LI 11, BL 12, and KI 6.

AUTHORS' CHOICES:

SM: Veratrum album; aggressive fluid support; conservative dietary management; appropriate Chinese herbal formula given by enema if necessary.

SW: Fluid support; antimicrobials and parenteral nutrition as needed; Chinese herbs and glutamine by enema.

PARASITES

Therapeutic Rationale

- Eliminate parasites completely, and correct any potential immune deficiency that may predispose to repeated infection.
- Control parasites in environment as needed to prevent reinfection.

Alternative Options with Conventional Bases

Herbs

- **Wormwood** *(Artemisia annua):* an extract of Wormwood reduces lesions associated with *Coccidia* in chickens (Allen, 1998) and some authors have advocated its use in a variety of dog and cat parasites.
- **Berberine-containing herbs** (Goldenseal, Oregon Grape): Berberine inhibits growth of *Giardia* and certain species of amoeba (Kaneda, 1991).
- **Ginger:** has been shown to kill the nematode *Anisakis* that is found in fish, which may be why ginger is traditionally served with sushi (Goto, 1990).
- **Garlic** *(Allium sativum):* whole garlic extract inhibited *Giardia* in vitro with a 50% inhibitory concentration (IC50) of 0.3 mg/ml (Ankri, 1999; Harris, 2000).

- **Turmeric:** Extracts of turmeric have shown activity against some nematodes (Kiuchi, 1993).
- **Pumpkin Seed** *(Cucurbita pepo):* has been used for tapeworms and may have approximately 50% efficacy against some species.
- **Papaya** *(Carica papaya):* Papaya latex has shown activity against helminth infection in mice and against bird ascarids. It exhibited 100% kill of ascarids in pigs at a dose of 8 g/kg of body weight (Satrija, 1994, 1995), and has been suggested to be effective in dogs and cats, although no studies are available in these species.
- **Indian Long Pepper** *(Piper longum):* an Ayurvedic herbal combination containing Long Pepper significantly reduced *Giardia* numbers in stools of human patients and improved clinical signs associated with the infection (Agarwal, 1997).

Paradigmatic Options

Western Herbs

- **Black Walnut:** commonly used by veterinarians as an antiparasitic herb for the intestinal tract. It appears to have a wide spectrum of activity, affecting both helminths and protozoa.

Homeopathy

- **Cina 30C:** used as an antihelminthic by homeopaths. The recommended dose is once daily for 2 weeks.
- **Mercurius solubilis 30C:** can resolve chronic giardiasis. It is used in animals with chronic colitis with tenesmus. Symptoms are usually worse after midnight. One dose is given daily for 10 days and then as needed.

Chinese Medicine

- Use appropriate formulas for the clinical presentation of the case.

AUTHORS' CHOICES:

SM: Given the high safety and efficacy of pharmaceutical dewormers, alternative medicine is seldom necessary. For chronic refractory cases, use appropriate Chinese herbal or homeopathic remedy.

SW: Conventional dewormers.

6 CASE REPORT
Inflammatory Bowel Disease in a Miniature Schnauzer

HISTORY

Bliss, a 2-year-old female spayed Miniature Schnauzer, was seen for treatment of a chief complaint of chronic inflammatory bowel disease of several months' duration. The signs and symptoms included episodes of random vomiting at any time of the day approximately once every 2 weeks. In addition, Bliss exhibited loud borborygmi and had a tendency to yelp when picked up around the middle. Bliss' appetite appeared depraved and she would eat cat and bird feces at every opportunity.

Diagnostic studies included a complete blood count, a serum chemistry panel, and endoscopic examination of the intestinal tract. The chemistry panel indicated elevations in liver enzyme, amylase, and lipase levels, and gastric mucosal biopsies showed lymphocytic plasmacytic inflammatory changes.

Prednisone was administered at a dose of 10 mg once daily. In addition, Bliss was placed on a hypoallergenic fish and potato diet and was given supplements consisting of lecithin, milk thistle extract, and chitin. Lecithin and milk thistle were provided to improve lipid metabolism by the liver and reduce liver inflammation. Chitin was provided as a lipid-chelating agent to reduce lipemic stress on the pancreas, and decreases in serum lipase seemed directly correlated to chitin administration. The prednisone was effective in controlling the vomiting, even if Bliss was weaned off prednisone for months at a time. Eventually, however, the vomiting would start again, and the owner's concern about ongoing prednisone therapy for her young dog led her to seek alternative therapy.

PHYSICAL EXAMINATION

Deep palpation of the abdomen was unremarkable, but light palpation revealed tension of the abdominal wall in the region of the stomach over the CV 12 acupuncture point. In addition, Bliss was markedly tense along the costal arch. This tension appeared related, at least in part, to vertebral fixations in the lower thoracic vertebrae. Additional fixations were found in the upper thoracic and midcervical regions.

Palpation of the pulse for the purposes of TCM diagnosis revealed it to be thin and tense or wiry on the left side and somewhat corpulent or slippery on the right side. Bliss' tongue appeared peeled, pale, and "tender."

ASSESSMENT

Whether pancreatitis or inflammatory bowel disease was Bliss' primary complaint is debatable. From a Chinese medical perspective, upper abdominal disorders invariably involve a disharmony among several organs, and all of them would be expected to show signs of involvement, much like our current concept of triaditis. This was true for Bliss, who showed evidence that the stomach, liver, and pancreas (which approximates the Chinese medical concept of the Spleen) were all affected. Bliss' presentation suggests that she had a "regional condition" of the upper abdomen that Chinese medicine might better be able to address than Western medicine.

From the Chinese medical perspective, Bliss was a classic case of Liver Blood and Yin deficiency with resultant Qi Stagnation. The Liver in Chinese medicine is dependent on an adequate Blood supply to perform its duty of smoothing the flow of Qi in the body. When the Blood, or Yin, of the Liver is inadequate, one of the main locations in which Qi accumulates is the Liver itself. This bottled-up energy is frequently felt as shooting pain along the costal arch in human patients. The tongue becomes somewhat pale and delicate with a mauve center. The pulse becomes thin and taut, reflecting the declining Blood levels and the resultant tension.

Energy cannot be contained for long, and stagnant Liver Qi eventually escapes its normal channels and invades adjacent organs. The two main targets are the Stomach and the Spleen. When Qi invades the Stomach, it suddenly finds an open conduit and follows the path of least resistance up and out of the body. This manifests clinically as vomiting. When Qi invades the Spleen, it interferes with the Spleen's function of transforming food and water into Qi and Blood. This produces elevated pancreatic enzyme levels, pallor, weakness, diarrhea, and a predilection for coprophagy, or the seeking out of other sources of what can best be considered predigested food.

TREATMENT

Yi Guan Jian (One Linking Decoction) is the standard prescription for Bliss' presentation in Chinese medicine. Bliss was prescribed ¼ tsp of granular concentrate of Yi Guan Jian twice daily.

In addition to the herbal therapy, Bliss received a chiropractic treatment to relieve the vertebral fixations that had been noted, and an acupuncture treatment of CV 12, BL 18 through 21, LIV 3, and ST 36.

OUTCOME

Bliss' condition improved immediately, beginning with better tongue and pulse findings immediately after the first appointment. At her first recheck Bliss was already off prednisone and had stopped vomiting. Over the course of the next three visits, spaced anywhere from 3 to 7 weeks apart, her tendencies to coprophagy and borborygmi likewise resolved. Bliss remained asymptomatic as of the last follow-up examination 1 year later, during which all laboratory parameters for Bliss had returned to and had remained within normal levels.

SM

REFERENCES

Abad MJ, Bermejo P, Sanchez Palomino S, Chiriboga X, Carrasco L. Antiviral activity of some South American medicinal plants. *Phytother Res* 13(2):142-146, 1999.

Acupuncture. NIH Consensus Statement. *JAMA* 15(5):1-34, 1997.

Agarwal AK, Tripathi DM, Sahai R, Gupta N, Saxena RP, Puri A, Singh M, Misra RN, Dubey CB, Saxena KC. Management of giardiasis by a herbal drug "Pippali Rasayana": a clinical study. *J Ethnopharmacol* 56(3):233-236, 1997.

Allen PC, Danforth HD, Augustine PC. Dietary modulation of avian coccidiosis. *Int J Parasitol* 28(7):1131-1140, 1998.

Andoh A, Bamba T, Sasaki M. Physiological and anti-inflammatory roles of dietary fiber and butyrate in intestinal functions. *J Parenter Enteral Nutr* 23(5 Suppl):70S-73S, 1999.

Ankri S, Mirelman D. Antimicrobial properties of allicin from garlic. *Microbes Infect* 1(2):125-129, 1999.

Belluzzi A, Boschi S, Brignola C, Munarini A, Cariani G, Miglio F. Polyunsaturated fatty acids and inflammatory bowel disease. *Am J Clin Nutr* 71(1 Suppl):339S-342S, 2000.

Bensoussan A, Talley NJ, Hing M, Menzies R, Guo A, Ngu M. Treatment of irritable bowel syndrome with Chinese herbal medicine: a randomized controlled trial. *J Am Med Assoc* 280(18):1585-1589, 1998.

Beubler E, Kollar G. Stimulation of PGE2 synthesis and water and electrolyte secretion by senna anthraquinones is inhibited by indomethacin. *J Pharm Pharmacol* 37(4):248-251, 1985.

Blanchard G, Paragon BM, Milliat F, Lutton C. Dietary L-carnitine supplementation in obese cats alters carnitine metabolism and decreases ketosis during fasting and induced hepatic lipidosis. *J Nutr* 132(2):204-210, 2002.

Blankson H, Stakkestad JA, Fagertun H, Thom E, Wadstein J, Gudmundsen O. Conjugated linoleic acid reduces body fat mass in overweight and obese humans. *J Nutr* 130(12):2943-2948, 2000.

Braganza JM, Schofield D, Snehalatha C, Mohan V. Micronutrient antioxidant status in tropical compared with temperate-zone chronic pancreatitis. *Scand J Gastroenterol* 28(12):1098-1104, 1993.

Braganza JM, Scott P, Bilton D, Schofield D, Chaloner C, Shiel N, Hunt LP, Bottiglieri T. Evidence for early oxidative stress in acute pancreatitis: Clues for correction. *Int J Pancreatol* 17(1):69-81, 1995.

Brown, MG, Park JF. Control of dental calculus in experimental beagles. *Lab Anim Care* 18(5): 527-535, 1968.

Buchman AL. Glutamine: commercially essential or conditionally essential? A critical appraisal of the human data. *Am J Clin Nutr* 74(1):25-32, 2001.

Center SA, Harte J, Watrous D, Reynolds A, Watson TDG, Markwell PJ, Millinton DS, Wood PA, Yeager AE, Erb HN. The clinical and metabolic effects of rapid weight loss in obese pet cats and the influence of supplemental oral L-carnitine. *J Vet Intern Med* 14(6):598-608, 2000.

Cheng CL, Koo MW. Effects of *Centella asiatica* on ethanol-induced gastric mucosal lesions in rats. *Life Sci* 67(21):2647-2653, 2000.

Crawford V, Scheckenbach R, Preuss HG. Effects of niacin-bound chromium supplementation on body composition in overweight African-American women. *Diabetes Obes Metab* 1(6):331-337, 1999.

Cross ML, Gill HS. Can immunoregulatory lactic acid bacteria be used as dietary supplements to limit allergies? *Int Arch Allergy Immunol* 125(2):112-119, 2001.

Day C. *The Homeopathic Treatment of Small Animals: Principles and Practice.* Saffron Waldon, England, 1990, C.W. Daniel Company.

de Witte P, Lemli L. The metabolism of anthranoid laxatives. *Hepatogastroenterology* 137(6):601-605, 1990.

Duke J. Phytochemical Database, USDA-ARS-NGRL (http://www.ars-grin.gov/duke/), Beltsville Agricultural Research Center, Beltsville, Md, 1999.

Dunne C, Murphy L, Flynn S, O'Mahony L, O'Halloran S, Feeney M, Morrissey D, Thornton G, Fitzgerald G, Daly C, Kiely B, Quigley EM, O'Sullivan GC, Shanahan F, Collins JK. Probiotics: from myth to reality: demonstration of functionality in animal models of disease and in human clinical trials. *Antonie Van Leeuwenhoek* 76(1-4):279-292, 1999 (review).

Duwiejua M, Zeitlin IJ, Waterman PG, Gray AI. Anti-inflammatory activity of *Polygonum bistorta, Guaiacum officinale* and *Hamamelis virginiana* in rats. *J Pharm Pharmacol* 46 (4):286-290, 1994.

Ehling D. *The Chinese Herbalist's Handbook,* revised ed. Santa Fe, NM, 1996, Inword Press.

Erickson KL, Hubbard NE. Probiotic immunomodulation in health and disease. *J Nutr* 130(2S Suppl):403S-409S, 2000.

Ernst E, Pittler MH. Efficacy of ginger for nausea and vomiting: a systematic review of randomized clinical trials. *Br J Anaesth* 84(3):367-371, 2000.

Fernandez-Banares F, Hinojosa J, Sanchez-Lombrana JL, Navarro E, Martinez-Salmeron JF, Garcia-Puges A, Gonzalez-Huix F, Riera J, Gonzalez-Lara V, Dominguez-Abascal F, Gine JJ, Moles J, Gomollon F, Gassull MA. Randomized clinical trial of *Plantago ovata* seeds (dietary fiber) as compared with mesalamine in maintaining remission in ulcerative colitis. Spanish Group for the Study of Crohn's Disease and Ulcerative Colitis (GETECCU). *Am J Gastroenterol* 94(2):427-433, 1999.

Gelal A, Guven H. Characterization of 5-HT receptors in rat proximal colon. *Gen Pharmacol* 30(3):343-346, 1998.

Ginter E, Mikus L. Reduction of gallstone formation by ascorbic acid in hamsters. *Experientia* 33(6):716-777, 1977.

Glowania HJ, Raulin C, Swoboda M. [Effect of chamomile on wound healing—a clinical double-blind study]. *Z Hautkr* 62(17):1262, 1267-1271, 1987.

Goto C, Kasuya S, Koga K, Ohtomo H, Kagei N. Lethal efficacy of extract from *Zingiber officinale* (traditional Chinese medicine) or [6]-shogaol and [6]-gingerol in *Anisakis* larvae in vitro. *Parasitol Res* 76(8):653-656, 1990.

Gupta I, Parihar A, Malhotra P, Singh GB, Ludtke R, Safayhi H, Ammon HP. Effects of *Boswellia serrata* gum resin in patients with ulcerative colitis. *Eur J Med Res* 2(1):37-43, 1997.

Gut A, Shiel N, Kay PM, Segal I, Braganza JM. Heightened free radical activity in blacks with chronic pancreatitis at Johannesburg, South Africa. *Clin Chim Acta* 230(2):189-199, 1994.

Hamasaki N, Ishii E, Tominaga K, Tezuka Y, Nagaoka T, Kadota S, Kuroki T, Yano I. Highly selective antibacterial activity of novel alkyl quinolone alkaloids from a Chinese herbal medicine, Gosyuyu (Wu-Chu-Yu), against *Helicobacter pylori* in vitro. *Microbiol Immunol* 44(1):9-15, 2000.

Hanioka T, Tanaka M, Ojima M, Shizukuishi S, Folkers K. Effect of topical application of coenzyme Q10 on adult periodontitis. *Mol Aspects Med* 15(Suppl): 241S-248S, 1994.

Harkrader RJ, Reinhart PC, Rogers JA, Jones RR, Wylie RE, Lowe BK, McEvoy RM. The history, chemistry and pharmacokinetics of *Sanguinaria* extract. *J Can Dent Assoc* 56(7 Suppl):7-12, 1990.

Harris JC, Plummer S, Turner MP, Lloyd D. The microaerophilic flagellate *Giardia intestinalis*: *Allium sativum* (garlic) is an effective antigiardial. *Microbiology* 146(Pt 12)(10):3119-3127, 2000.

Hawthorn M, Ferrante J, Luchowski E, Rutledge A, Wei XY, Triggle DJ. The actions of peppermint oil and menthol on calcium channel dependent processes in intestinal, neuronal and cardiac preparations. *Aliment Pharmacol Ther* 2(2):101-118, 1988.

Hickman MA. Interventional nutrition for gastrointestinal disease. *Clin Tech Small Anim Pract* 13(4):211-21, 1998.

Hu JP, Takahashi N, Yamada T. *Coptidis rhizoma* inhibits growth and proteases of oral bacteria. *Oral Dis* 6(5):297-302, 2000.

Ishii Y, Tanizawa H, Takino Y. Studies of aloe. V. Mechanism of cathartic effect. *Biol Pharm Bull* 17(5):651-653, 1994.

Izzo AA, Sautebin L, Rombola L, Capasso F. The role of constitutive and inducible nitric oxide synthase in senna- and cascara-induced diarrhoea in the rat. *Eur J Pharmacol* 323(1):93-97, 1997.

Kaneda Y, Torii M, Tanaka T, Aikawa M. In vitro effects of berberine sulphate on the growth and structure of *Entamoeba histolytica, Giardia lamblia and Trichomonas vaginalis*. *Ann Trop Med Parasitol* 85(4):417-425, 1991.

Kase Y, Saitoh K, Makino B, Hashimoto K, Ishige A, Komatsu Y. Relationship between the antidiarrhoeal effects of Hange-Shashin-To and its active components. *Phytother Res* 13(6):468-473, 1999.

Kaya E, Gur ES, Ozguc H, Bayer A, Tokyay R. L-Glutamine enemas attenuate mucosal injury in experimental colitis. *Dis Colon Rectum* 42(9):1209-1215, 1999.

Kiuchi F, Goto Y, Sugimoto N, Akao N, Kondo K, Tsuda Y. Nematocidal activity of turmeric: synergistic action of curcuminoids. *Chem Pharm Bull* (Tokyo) 41(9):1640-1643, 1993.

Kline RM, Kline JJ, Di Palma J, Barbero GJ. Enteric-coated, pH-dependent peppermint oil capsules for the treatment of irritable bowel syndrome in children. *J Pediatr* 138(1):125-128, 2001.

Koo H, Gomes BP, Rosalen PL, Ambrosano GM, Park YK, Cury JA. In vitro antimicrobial activity of propolis and *Arnica montana* against oral pathogens. *Arch Oral Biol* 45(2):141-148, 2000.

Kraft W, Kaimaz A, Kirsch M, Hoerauf A. Behandlung akuter Pankreatiden des Hundes mit Selen. *Kleintierpraxis* 40:35-43, 1995.

Krieglstein CF, Anthoni C, Rijcken EJ, Laukotter M, Spiegel HU, Boden SE, Schweizer S, Safayhi H, Senninger N, Schurmann G. Acetyl-11-keto-beta-boswellic acid, a constituent of a herbal medicine from *Boswellia serrata* resin, attenuates experimental ileitis. *Int J Colorectal Dis* 16(2):88-95, 2001.

Kudi AC, Myint SH. Antiviral activity of some Nigerian medicinal plant extracts. *J Ethnopharmacol* 68(1-3):289-294, 1999.

Kuklinski B, Zimmermann T, Schweder R. [Decreasing mortality in acute pancreatitis with sodium selenite. Clinical results of 4 years antioxidant therapy] Letalitatssenkung der akuten Pankreatitis mit Natriumselenit. Klinische Resultate einer vierjahrigen Antioxidanzientherapie. *Med Klin* 90(1 Suppl)(6):36-41, 1995.

Lal J, Chandra S, Raviprakash V, Sabir M. In vitro anthelmintic action of some indigenous medicinal plants on *Ascardia galli* worms. *Indian J Physiol Pharmacol* 20(2):64-68, 1976.

Magnuson TH, Lillemoe KD, High RC, Pitt HA. Dietary fish oil inhibits cholesterol monohydrate crystal nucleation and gallstone formation in the prairie dog. *Surgery* 118(3):517-523, 1995.

Mazzaferro E, Hackett T, Wingfield W, Ogilive G, Fettman M. Role of glutamine in health and disease. *Compendium* 22(12):1094-1101, 2000.

McCloy R. Chronic pancreatitis at Manchester, UK: focus on antioxidant therapy. *Digestion* 59(4 Suppl)(4):36-48, 1998.

Micklefield GH, Greving I, May B. Effects of peppermint oil and caraway oil on gastroduodenal motility. *Phytother Res* 14(1):20-23, 2000.

Miller MJ, MacNaughton WK, Zhang XJ, Thompson JH, Charbonnet RM, Bobrowski P, Lao J, Trentacosti AM, Sandoval M. Treatment of gastric ulcers and diarrhea with the Amazonian herbal medicine sangre de grado. *Am J Physiol Gastrointest Liver Physiol* 279(1):G192-200, 2000.

Murphy R. *Lotus Materia Medica.* Durango, Colo, 1995, Lotus Star Press.

Naeser MA. *Outline Guide to Chinese Herbal Patent Medicines in Pill Form.* Boston, Mass, 1990, Boston Chinese Medicine.

Ohta Y, Kobayashi T, Nishida K, Sasaki E, Ishiguro I. Preventive effect of Oren-gedoku-to (Huanglian-Jie-Du-Tang) extract on the development of stress-induced acute gastric mucosal lesions in rats. *J Ethnopharmacol* 67(3):377-384, 1999.

Ozaki Y. Studies on antiinflammatory effect of Japanese Oriental medicines (kampo medicines) used to treat inflammatory diseases. *Biol Pharm Bull* 18(4):559-562, 1995.

Pittler MH, Ernst E. Peppermint oil for irritable bowel syndrome: a critical review and metaanalysis. *Am J Gastroenterol* 93(7):1131-1135, 1998.

Phuapradit P, Varavithya W, Vathanophas K, Sangchai R, Podhipak A, Suthutvoravut U, Nopchinda S, Chantraruksa V, Haschke F. Reduction of rotavirus infection in children receiving bifidobacteria-supplemented formula. *J Med Assoc Thai* 82(1 Suppl):S43-48, 1999.

Plotnikov AA, Karnaukhov VK, Ozeretskovskaia NN, Stromskaia TF, Firsova RA. [Clinical trial of cucurbin (a preparation from pumpkin seeds) in cestodiasis] Klinicheskaia ispytaniia kukurbina (preparata iz semian tykvy) pri tsestodozakh. *Med Parazitol* (Mosk) 41(4):407-411, 1972.

Prins NH, Akkermans LM, Lefebvre RA, Schuurkes JA. 5-HT(4) receptors on cholinergic nerves involved in contractility of canine and human large intestine longitudinal muscle. *Br J Pharmacol* 131(5):927-932, 2000.

Prucksunand C, Indrasukhsri B, Leethochawalit M, Hungspreugs K. Phase II clinical trial on effect of the long turmeric *(Curcuma longa* Linn*)* on healing of peptic ulcer. *Southeast Asian J Trop Med Public Health* 32(1):208-215, 2002.

Rabbani GH. Mechanism and treatment of diarrhea due to *Vibrio cholerae* and *Escherichia coli:* roles of drugs and prostaglandins. *Dan Med Bull* 43(2):173-185, 1996.

Rafatullah S, Tariq M, Al-Yahya MA, Mossa JS, Ageel AM. Evaluation of turmeric *(Curcuma longa)* for gastric and duodenal antiulcer activity in rats. *J Ethnopharmacol* 29(1):25-34, 1990.

Reeds PJ, Burrin DG. Glutamine and the bowel. *J Nutr* 131(9 Suppl):2505S-2508S, discussion 2523S-2524S, 2001.

Rees WD, Rhodes J, Wright JE, Stamford LF, Bennett A. Effect of deglycyrrhizinated liquorice on gastric mucosal damage by aspirin. *Scand J Gastroenterol* 14(5):605-607, 1979.

Rolfe RD. The role of probiotic cultures in the control of gastrointestinal health, *J Nutr* 130(2S Suppl):396S-402S, 2000.

Roscoe, JA, Matteson SE. Acupressure and acustimulation bands for control of nausea: a brief review. *Am J Obstet Gynecol* 185(5 suppl):S244-S247, 2002.

Rose P, Fraine E, Hunt LP, Acheson DW, Braganza JM. Dietary antioxidants and chronic pancreatitis. *Hum Nutr Clin Nutr* 40(2):151-164, 1986.

Russell RI, Morgan RJ, Nelson LM. Studies on the protective effect of deglycyrrhinised liquorice against aspirin (ASA) and ASA plus bile acid–induced gastric mucosal damage, and ASA absorption in rats. *Scand J Gastroenterol Suppl* 92:97-100, 1984.

Saeki Y, Ito Y, Shibata M, Sato Y, Okuda K, Takazoe I. Antimicrobial action of natural substances on oral bacteria. *Bull Tokyo Dent Coll* 30(3):129-135, 1989.

Saitoh K, Kase Y, Ishige A, Komatsu Y, Sasaki H, Shibahara N. Effects of Keishi-ka-shakuyaku-to (Gui-Zhi-Jia-Shao-Yao-Tang) on diarrhea and small intestinal movement. *Biol Pharm Bull* 22(1):87-89, 1999.

Santagostino-Barbone MG, Masoero E, Spelta V, Lucchelli A. 2-Phenylmelatonin: a partial agonist at enteric melatonin receptors. *Pharmacol Toxicol* 87(4):156-160, 2000.

Sato R, Inanami O, Tanaka Y, Takase M, Naito Y. Oral administration of bovine lactoferrin for treatment of intractable stomatitis in feline immunodeficiency virus (FIV)-positive and FIV-negative cats. *Am J Vet Res* 57(10):1443-1446, 1996.

Satrija F, Nansen P, Bjorn H, Murtini S, He S. Effect of papaya latex against *Ascaris suum* in naturally infected pigs. *J Helminthol* 68(4):343-346, 1994.

Satrija F, Nansen P, Murtini S, He S. Anthelmintic activity of papaya latex against patent *Heligmosomoides polygyrus* infections in mice. *J Ethnopharmacol* 48(3):161-164, 1995.

Schulz HU, Niederau C, Klonowski-Stumpe H, Halangk W, Luthen R, Lippert H. Oxidative stress in acute pancreatitis. *Hepatogastroenterology* 46(29):2736-2750, 1999.

Scott P, Bruce C, Schofield D, Shiel N, Braganza JM, McCloy RF. Vitamin C status in patients with acute pancreatitis. *Br J Surg* 80(6):750-754, 1993.

Shanahan F. Probiotics and inflammatory bowel disease: is there a scientific rationale? *Inflamm Bowel Dis* 6(2):107-115, 2000.

Shu Q, Lin H, Rutherfurd KJ, Fenwick SG, Prasad J, Gopal PK, Gill HS. Dietary *Bifidobacterium lactis* (HN019) enhances resistance to oral *Salmonella typhimurium* infection in mice. *Microbiol Immunol* 44(4):213-222, 2000.

Siegers CP, von Hertzberg-Lottin E, Otte M, Schneider B. Anthranoid laxative abuse—a risk for colorectal cancer? *Gut* 34(8):1099-1101, 1993.

Singer SM, Nash TE. The role of normal flora in *Giardia lamblia* infections in mice. *J Infect Dis* 181(4):1510-1512, 2000.

Taylor CT, Winter DC, Skelly MM, O'Donoghue DP, O'Sullivan GC, Harvey BJ, Baird AW. Berberine inhibits ion transport in human colonic epithelia. *Eur J Pharmacol* 368(1):111-118, 1999.

Tsai CS, Ochillo RF. Pharmacological effects of berberine on the longitudinal muscle of the guinea-pig isolated ileum. *Arch Int Pharmacodyn Ther* 310:116-131, 1991.

Uden S, Bilton D, Guyan PM, Kay PM, Braganza JM. Rationale for antioxidant therapy in pancreatitis and cystic fibrosis. *Adv Exp Med Biol* 264:555-572, 1990.

Uden S, Bilton D, Nathan L, Hunt LP, Main C, Braganza JM. Antioxidant therapy for recurrent pancreatitis: placebo-controlled trial. *Aliment Pharmacol Ther* 4(4):357-371, 1990.

Uden S, Schofield D, Miller PF, Day JP, Bottiglier T, Braganza JM. Antioxidant therapy for recurrent pancreatitis: biochemical profiles in a placebo-controlled trial. *Aliment Pharmacol Ther* 6(2):229-240, 1992.

Vynograd N, Vynograd I, Sosnowski Z. A comparative multi-centre study of the efficacy of propolis, acyclovir and placebo in the treatment of genital herpes (HSV). *Phytomedicine* 7(1):1-6, 2000.

Wang ZT, Du Q, Xu GJ, Wang RJ, Fu DZ, Ng TB. Investigations on the protective action of *Condonopsis pilosula* (Dangshen) extract on experimentally induced gastric ulcer in rats. *Gen Pharmacol* 28(3):469-473, 1997.

Weese JS. Microbiologic evaluation of commercial probiotics. *J Am Vet Med Assoc* 220(6):794-797, 2002.

Wolinsky LE, Mania S, Nachnani S, Ling S. The inhibiting effect of aqueous *Azadirachta indica* (Neem) extract upon bacterial properties influencing in vitro plaque formation. *J Dent Res* 75(2):816-822, 1996.

Yagi T, Yamauchi K, Kuwano S. The synergistic purgative action of aloe-emodin anthrone and rhein anthrone in mice: synergism in large intestinal propulsion and water secretion. *J Pharm Pharmacol* 49(1):22-25, 1997.

Yeung H. *Handbook of Chinese Herbal Formulas.* Los Angeles, 1995, Self-published.

Yeung H. *Handbook of Chinese Herbs.* Los Angeles, 1996, Self-published.

Zhou H, Mineshita S. The effect of Oren-gedoku-to on experimental colitis in rats. *J Pharm Pharmacol* 51(9):1065-1074, 1999. *Oren-gedoku-to used in a rat model of human Crohn's disease resulted in reduced levels of IL-8, LTB4, PGE-2, a reduction in inflammatory cell infiltrate numbers, and quicker healing of colonic lesions.*

7

Therapies for Ear Disorders

EAR MITES

Therapeutic Rationale

- Eliminate mites.
- Reduce inflammation.

Alternative Options with Conventional Bases

- **Cleaning:** Ear mite eggs hatch every 4 days. Therefore a thorough ear cleaning and treatment repeated every 3 days for three to four times may resolve ear mite infestations. Animal owners should be shown how to thoroughly clean the ears to remove as much debris as possible. Mineral oil or olive oil is used to clean the irritated surfaces of the ears, as the oil may block the spiracles of ear mites causing them to asphyxiate.
- **Essential oils:** One or two drops of an aromatic oil may be added to the oil used for ear cleaning to enhance mite control, relieve itching, and control secondary infections. Practitioners may experiment with small amounts of the following oils, either alone or in combination: Peppermint Oil (has a topical anesthetic effect); Catnip Oil (repels mosquitoes and may be useful in mite control); Tea Tree Oil (may be effective in relieving itch and associated infections); Hypericum Oil (relieves ear pain); Calendula Oil (heals eroded surfaces); or Rosemary Oil (advocated to inhibit ectoparasites). The practitioner should note that Tea Tree Oil is extremely toxic to cats and some small dogs. After 2 weeks of cleaning and treatment every 3 days the ears should be clean and mite free. The only disadvantage to this treatment is the accumulation of oil in the fur

around the ears, which can be removed by bathing at the end of treatment.

AUTHORS' CHOICES:

SM: Thorough ear cleaning with medicated oil every 3 days.
SW: Regular cleaning and oil instillation; ivermectin.

HEMATOMA

Therapeutic Rationale

- Resolve any underlying otitis externa that may lead to excessive head shaking.
- Surgery.

Alternative Options with Conventional Bases

- No suggestions.

Paradigmatic Options

- Bleeding has several different causes in Chinese medicine. Deficient Qi fails to contain the Blood in the vessels. Deficient Blood leads to Blood stasis and the stagnant pools of Blood then passively ooze out of the vessels. Excessive Heat in the Blood agitates the Blood, causing it to "leap" from the vessels. Two of these problems, Blood Heat and Blood deficiency or stasis, are common causes of both otitis externa and skin disease in general.
- Treatment of any associated pathologic conditions of the skin and the ears should thus directly lower the propensity to aural hematomas. See Chapter 5 for more information on cooling, tonifying, and moving Blood in the treatment of otitis externa, dermatitis, and, by extension aural hematomas.
- Once these therapies have been instituted, supplementary treatment with homeopathic remedies or topical agents (see following sections) can be instituted to further address hemorrhage. Alternatively, a Chinese herbal formula to stop bleeding can be instituted along

with a formula to address "constitutional" tendencies to the promotion of bleeding.

- The most popular antihemorrhage Chinese herbal formula among veterinarians is probably **Yunnan Bai Yao** (Yunnan Province White Medicine). This herbal "formula" contains only San Qi (Notoginseng), a Blood-moving herb that shortens clotting times, decreases prothrombin time, and increases platelet counts. It may be taken internally or applied topically. A *suggested internal starting dose* of the patent formula is one capsule or one tablet per 20 lb of body weight once or twice daily, or 250 mg of the powdered form per 20 lb of body weight once or twice daily. If surgical correction is required, the herb may be applied topically to the surgical site to hasten the cessation of postoperative oozing and hemorrhage.

Homeopathy

- **Arnica Montana 30C** or **Hamamelis 30C:** should be considered for simple hematomas that usually have few signs of accompanying ear inflammation. Animals that benefit are often young. These remedies can also be used to help speed resolution of hematomas once specific therapy has been rendered for any accompanying dermatitis and otitis. A *recommended starting dose* is 30C up to twice daily for 1 week, then once a day for 4 to 5 days. Treatment should be stopped if the hematoma continues to enlarge, and surgical correction will be needed. When the hematoma involves less than one third of the pinna and the remedy appears effective, no surgical treatment is likely to be required.

Topical Preparations

- **Arnica:** can also be applied topically to the hematoma as a crude extract or in dermatologic preparations. Arnica should never be applied topically to open wounds. It should be applied three times daily.
- **Hamamelis:** a popular topical treatment for hemorrhoids in humans and may be readily available

in a dermatologic preparation. It is applied three times daily.

AUTHORS' CHOICES:

SM: Arnica 30C in mild or early cases; address underlying skin or ear disease.
SW: Surgery; address underlying ear or skin disease.

OTITIS, GENERAL

Therapeutic Rationale

- Find underlying cause.
- Thoroughly treat primary or secondary infections.

Alternative Options with Conventional Bases

Dietary Support

- **Hypoallergenic diet trials** are critical for dogs with chronic otitis that manifests as inflammation or as repeated infections. After a complete diet history is obtained, a commercial elimination diet or homemade diet may be recommended. Since beef, lamb, pork, chicken, turkey, egg, wheat, corn, rice, milk products, and fish meal are common in commercial pet foods, homemade diets might include goat or game (venison, duck, rabbit, quail) as a meat source, and millet, quinoa, amaranth, or sweet potato as a carbohydrate source. Depending on the animal's diet history, fish and oatmeal are sometimes acceptable as well.

Topical Herbs

- Certain herbs with reputations for antiinflammatory characteristics have been recommended for use in cases of inflamed ears. These include Aloe *(Aloe vera)*, Calendula *(Calendula officinalis)*, and Lavender *(Lavandula angustifolia, L. officinalis)* essential oil. Antiinflammatory herbs may be combined with antimicrobial herbs such as Oregon Grape *(Mahonia aquifolium)*, Thyme *(Thymus vulgaris)*, Garlic *(Allium sativum),* and Sage *(Salvia apiana).* However, these herbs have not been examined experimentally in otitis cases.

- **Sairei-to:** was shown to reduce inflammation of induced otitis media in experimental animal studies (Sugiura, 1997).

Acupuncture

- In a trial of 25 dogs with otitis externa, use of acupuncture every 3 days at TH 17, TH 21, SI 19, GB 20, and LI 4 resulted in faster resolution of pain and secretion compared to dogs receiving sham acupuncture. Both groups received acupuncture in addition to conventional treatment with antibiotics (Sanchez-Araujo, 1997).

Paradigmatic Options

- The external ear is just an extension of the skin and otitis externa that accompanies dermatitis may resolve with successful treatment of the dermatitis. This is especially true for dermatitis that arises from Blood deficiency. The symptoms of Blood deficiency otitis externa are ear redness and scaling without discharge and the ear canal is usually dry and without exudates.
- Although Chapter 5 should be consulted for a complete description of formulas used for treating skin disorders related to Blood deficiency, the typical formula for Blood deficiency that leads to mild-to-moderate and chronic otitis externa and dermatitis is **Si Wu Xiao Feng Yin** (Four Materials Dissipate Wind Beverage). This formula is actually composed of two formulas, **Si Wu Tang** (Four Materials Decoction) and **Xiao Feng San** (Disperse Wind Powder). Si Wu Tang tonifies Blood and Xiao Feng San disperses or dissipates Wind. The latter formula actually has three variations, two of which are commonly applied to skin complaints. **Xiao Feng San II** is the one that is usually combined with Si Wu Tang.
- **Xiao Feng San I** has been advocated for use in otitis externa. This formula, referred to as Tang Kuei and Arctium, or Arctium and Dang Gui Powder, is used for

more pruritic types of weeping skin conditions and rashes. It may be even more effective when the two herbs Shi Gao and Zhi Mu are removed from the formula. This formula can be considered when the patient seems both Damp and Blood deficient, with mild purulent lesions in the ears or on the skin. A *suggested starting dose* for all of the above formulas is ¼ tsp per 15 lb of body weight, or 60 to 75 mg/lb of body weight, divided into two equal portions.

- For cases that are predominantly Damp, skin formulas that focus on Dampness accumulation can be considered. Chapter 5 provides information on identifying and treating Dampness and Damp Heat conditions of the skin. One extreme form of Damp Heat otitis externa that may be encountered is the acutely painful ear with thick yellow exudates, pronounced erythema, a strong odor, and perhaps bleeding. For this problem, **Long Dan Xie Gan Tang** (Gentian Drain the Liver Decoction) can be considered. This is a strong formula that should be reserved for excessive cases. Patients that receive it should have a red to purple tongue and rapid or wiry and forceful pulses. Administration of the formula should be stopped if the patient's appetite becomes suppressed. Acupuncture points that are synergistic with the action of this formula include TH 17, GB 20, GB 41, LR 2, GV 14, and LI 11. TH 17 and GB 20 are local and regional points, respectively, to address the ear. The other four points help to drain Damp and clear Heat from the Gall Bladder meridian, which is the most important meridian penetrating the ear canal. A *suggested starting dose* is ¼ tsp per 15 lb of body weight, or 60 to 75 mg/lb of body weight, divided into two equal portions.
- For less severe or subacute cases of otitis externa that have substantial redness and exudation, **Siler and Coix Decoction** can be considered. This formula contains 3 g each of Chuan Xiong, Bai Zhi, Yi Yi Ren, Huang Qin, Jie Geng, Zhi Zi, and Fang Feng. It also contains 1.5 g each of Jing Jie, Zhi Shi, Huang Lian, Gan Cao, and Bo He. The formula is designed to treat almost any

form of head inflammation (stomatitis, acne, or furuncles) when it is caused by an internal Damp-Heat accumulation. A Wind-Heat component (i.e., sudden onset) to the rash probably also exists in patients for which this formula is especially appropriate. These patients have a wiry and rapid pulse and the tongue is red or purple red and wet. A *suggested starting dose* is ¼ tsp per 15 lb of body weight, or 60 to 75 mg/lb of body weight, divided into two equal portions.

- Two patent remedies to consider are **Lian Qiao Bai Du Pian** (Forsythia Defeat Toxin Pill) and **Bai Fan Ear Drops.** Lian Qiao Bai Du Pian is a milder and more dispersing formula than Siler and Coix Decoction and is used in less severe cases of inflammation and bacterial infection. It can be applied to Wind-Heat skin conditions when they are accompanied by a moderate degree of internal Heat. Patients that benefit have a red tongue and a wiry pulse that may be superficial and somewhat forceful. A *recommended starting dose* is about one tablet per 10 lb of body weight given once or twice daily.
- **Bai Fan Ear Drops** contain Bai Fan (Ming Fan; Potash Alum) and Bing Pian (Borneol) in a flax oil carrier. Some practitioners have found these drops to be effective in obstinate or resistant ear infections such as those caused by *Pseudomonas*. Bai Fan is a cooling, drying, astringent herb that has significant antimicrobial activity against gram-positive flora, *Pseudomonas,* and *Candida.* Bing Pian is an aromatic compound with some antibacterial and analgesic properties. Bai Fan Ear Drops are thus a useful adjunct to treatment of both acute and chronic painful otitis externa when primary or significant secondary infection is evident. A *recommended starting dose* is 2 to 7 drops in each affected ear five to eight times daily for up to 1 month. Internal formulas will be necessary to obtain permanent relief in recurrent cases.
- A less common type of otitis externa may be found in older animals. In these patients the ears are dry and lichenified as they are in Blood-deficient cases. Indeed, Yin-deficient otitis externa may be a late-stage

development in animals with skin and ear lesions that were initially caused by Blood deficiency. Other symptoms exhibited by Yin-deficient animals are possible hearing loss or noise intolerance, low back and hind limb weakness or stiffness, fatigue, restlessness at night, thirst, constipation, and very scanty or no exudates. The tongue is dry and red or "tender," and the pulse is thin and rapid. A formula that has been advocated for these dogs is **Zhi Bai Di Huang Wan** (Anemarrhena, Phellodendron, and Rehmannia Pill). Jin Yin Hua (Lonicera), Ku Shen (Sophora,), Pu Gong Ying (Dandelion Flowers) or Lian Qiao (Forsythia), 9 g of each, may all be considered as possible additives to 100 g of the base formula to help resolve superficial infection of the ear canal. A *suggested starting dose* is ¼ tsp per 15 lb of body weight, or 60 to 75 mg/lb of body weight, divided into two equal portions.

- Acupuncture points that work synergistically with Zhi Bai Di Huang Wan are KI 3 and BL 23 to strengthen the Kidneys, SP 6 to nourish Yin; SP 10 to cool Blood and relieve itch, GV 14 and LI 4 to clear Heat from the head, and TH 21, SI 19, and GB 2 as local points to address the ear complaint.
- One topical preparation that is effective in reducing ear canal thickening and irritation resulting from otitis externa is a 50:50 blend of Thuja Oil and Calendula Oil. It is applied three times daily to affected ears and seems to be effective even in chronic cases of otitis externa of several years' duration. Calendula has mild antifungal and antibacterial properties and may be effective in soothing irritated, inflamed surfaces. Thuja is used topically in human alternative medicine to treat warts of all types. Similarly, it is used in otitis externa cases to reduce proliferative types of skin lesions, such as the gradual canal closure seen in chronic otitis externa. This preparation may be used safely for extended periods.

Dietary Support

- Any condition in which Dampness is confirmed to be present by response to therapy should be evaluated for potential food sensitivities. Diets to consider include low-carbohydrate diets, antigen-elimination diets, and raw food diets for "excessive" cases with Strong pulses. Care should be taken to provide carbohydrates and proteins that are novel to that patient.

- In cases of Damp Heat–otitis externa either carbohydrates or the high bioavailability of commercially processed diets may prove to be the "dampening influence" that overwhelms the Spleen. Alternative health care providers often put human patients with *Candida* overgrowth on "low-yeast" diets. Foods that are typically excluded include many bread products and fermented drinks such as beer. The rationalization behind this practice is vague but centers on eliminating yeast antigens for yeast-sensitive individuals or eliminating exposure to yeast altogether. This reasoning may seem tenuous to conventional practitioners, but the benefit appears to be a result of reducing carbohydrate type or amount in the diet. From a Chinese medical perspective patients with "yeast overgrowth" typically fit the diagnosis of Spleen Qi deficiency with resulting Dampness accumulation. From the Chinese medical perspective elimination of bread and alcohol products is effective in patients with "yeast overgrowth" because carbohydrates are nearly eliminated from the diet. With the dampening influence removed, yeast overgrowth stops as the Dampness disappears and the Spleen and skin "dry out."
- Animals that respond well to Blood-tonifying formulas can be given more "blood-tonifying" foods in their diets, including organ meats and deep leafy greens. For patients demonstrating no evidence of Spleen compromise, in particular a weak pulse, raw food diets may be considered.

AUTHORS' CHOICES:

SM: Appropriate Chinese herbal formula; choose diets based on efficacy of formula (see next two sections on otitis).

SW: Elimination diet trial; appropriately chosen Chinese herbal formulas; appropriate antimicrobial and antiinflammatory drugs.

OTITIS, BACTERIAL

Therapeutic Rationale

- Identify and treat appropriate bacterial pathogens.
- Identify underlying disorders.

Alternative Options with Conventional Bases

- **Combinations of essential oils:** sometimes used in managing otitis. Appropriate dilution of these oils in an inert carrier oil is important. Lemon Grass and Thyme essential oils have shown inhibitory activity against *Staphylococcus aureus, Streptococcus pneumoniae,* and *Streptococcus pyogenes* (Inouye, 2001). Essential oils are diluted at a rate of approximately 10 drops per 8 oz of carrier oil.
- **Herb extracts** (water or alcohol): have been used in managing otitis. Topical applications of Garlic and various extracts of it have shown inhibitory activity against *Pseudomonas* in vitro (Tsao, 2001). Various species of Sage, including *Salvia blepharochlaena, S. apium,* and *S. triloba,* have shown activity against species of bacteria that may contribute to bacterial otitis.

Paradigmatic Options

- Bacterial otitis externa with abundant exudates is often a Damp-Heat condition, especially in its early stages. The previous section on otitis externa will provide help in selecting an appropriate formula. For acute infections the appropriateness of **Long Dan Xie Gan Tang** (Gentian Drain the Liver Decoction), **Siler and Coix Decoction, Lian Qiao Bai Du Pian** (Forsythia Detoxification Pills), and **Bai Fan Ear Drops** should be evaluated.
- When otitis externa is very mild and the ears are largely dry, Yin or Blood deficiency should be ruled out as the underlying condition. The section on otitis externa and Chapter 5 describe identification and treatment of otitis externa caused by Yin and Blood deficiencies. Formulas to consider include **Xiao Feng San I** (Dissipate Wind Powder), **Si Wu Xiao Feng Yin** (Four Materials Dissipate Wind Beverage), and **Zhi Bai Di Huang Wan** (Amenarrhena, Phellodendron, and Rehmannia Pill).

When Blood deficiency is the result of Spleen Qi deficiency **Modified Wei Ling Tang** (Modified Decoction to Dispel Dampness in the Spleen and Stomach) can be considered. More information on these and other formulas to treat skin (and therefore ear) problems caused by Blood deficiency, is given in Chapter 5.

- In addition to these "constitutional approaches" to bacterial otitis externa, several other treatments have been advocated that are more specifically designed to treat acute bacterial infections. One formula some practitioners advocate for acute infections is **Chuan Xin Lian Pian** (Antiphlogistic pills). Although used mainly for acute gastrointestinal, respiratory, and urinary tract infections in China, the medication has substantial heat-dispersing and antimicrobial activity, especially against gram-positive microbes. A *recommended starting dose* is one pill per 15 lb of body weight once or twice daily.
- **Niu Huang Jie Du Pian** (Cow Gallstone Detoxification Tablets) is sometimes used in conjunction with Chuan Xin Lian Pian. Its constituent herbs have strong Heat-clearing properties, and the pills are used in China as a broad-spectrum antibiotic. A *recommended starting dose* is one tablet per 15 to 30 lb of body weight, divided if possible into two doses. These two formulas are contraindicated for patients who do not appear "excessive" with strong, forceful pulses and red tongues because they may cause appetite depression and diarrhea.
- **Bi Yan Wan** (Nose Inflammation Pill) is a popular Chinese herbal formula in veterinary medicine for chronic sinusitis, nasal discharge, and upper respiratory tract infections. Its use has been dubiously broadened to include otitis externa. It is primarily a Wind- and Heat-dispersing formula. A *recommended starting dose* is one tablet per 5 to 10 lb of body weight, divided into two daily doses.

AUTHORS' CHOICES:

SM: Address underlying "constitutional" issues with the appropriate Chinese herbal formula and diet.

SW: Antibiotics and antiinflammatory drugs; investigate role of allergies; appropriately chosen Chinese herbs.

OTITIS, MALASSEZIA

Therapeutic Rationale

- Address underlying allergy or other predisposing cause.
- Suppress yeast growth.

Alternative Options with Conventional Bases

- **Vinegar washes:** have long been used in the management of *Malassezia* otitis. If owners are trained to treat this condition early and on a regular basis, a solution of 50% white vinegar and 50% water is very effective in reducing symptoms and frequency. More established or serious infections are often resistant to this treatment, and the vinegar may be too irritating for highly inflamed or ulcerated ear canals.
- **Tea Tree Oil:** is effective against *Malassezia* species (Nenoff, 1996) and may be used in diluted form to help treat otitis externa caused by yeast. Tea Tree Oil is powerful and should never be used alone to treat ear infections because it may provoke the development of hives or a contact dermatitis when used full strength, and may cause more serious, even fatal, reactions in cats. It should be dissolved in another oil that is used for cleaning the ears, as described in the section on Ear Mites. Topical applications such as ear drops cannot be expected to prevent further outbreaks of yeast otitis, and more systemic treatments are needed to manage predisposing factors such as allergies. Tea Tree and other essential oils are diluted at a rate of approximately 10 drops per 8 oz of carrier oil.
- **Ear drops:** designed for routine use in otitis in humans may be helpful for yeast otitis in animals. These drops typically contain St. John's Wort *(Hypericum perforatum)*, Mullein *(Verbascum thapsus)*, and Garlic. St. John's Wort is used to relieve ear pain and has antimicrobial activity against gram-positive organisms (Reichling, 2001). Mullein is a mucilaginous herb that may have antiinflammatory activity. Garlic has demonstrated significant activity against *Candida* yeast and various gram-positive and gram-negative bacteria.

Only glycerine or oil extracts should be used because alcohol might irritate the ear canal.

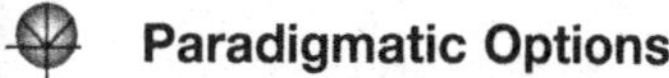

Paradigmatic Options

- Yeast otitis externa is almost always a Damp-Heat condition from a Chinese perspective. The general section on Otitis Externa and Chapter 5 can be consulted for formulas indicated for the treatment of Damp-Heat conditions of the ears and skin. Milder Damp-Heat formulas such as **Modified Wei Ling Tang** (Modified Decoction to Dispel Dampness in the Spleen and Stomach) or **Xiao Feng San II** (Dissipate Wind Powder) will usually be the most appropriate in all but the most severe cases of yeast otitis externa. For very hot dogs, **Si Miao San** (Four Marvels Powder) can be considered.

Dietary Support

- Any condition in which Dampness is confirmed to be present by response to therapy should be evaluated for potential food sensitivities. Diets to consider include low-carbohydrate diets, antigen-elimination diets, and raw food diets for "excessive" cases with strong pulses. Care should be taken to provide novel carbohydrates and proteins. From the Chinese medical perspective elimination of grain-based products is effective in patients with yeast overgrowth because carbohydrates are reduced in the diet. With the dampening influence removed, yeast overgrowth stops as the Dampness disappears and the Spleen and skin "dry out."

AUTHORS' CHOICES:

SM: Appropriate Chinese herbal formula; ear drops with Tea Tree Oil added.

SW: Appropriate Chinese herbal formula; vinegar washes; manage underlying allergies.

7 CASE REPORT
Recurrent Otitis Externa in a Dog

HISTORY

Suzy, a 5-year-old female spayed Shih Tzu, presented with a history of recurrent otitis externa. In the preceding 9 months she had had two episodes of external ear infection and was now in her third. The main symptoms included repeated head shaking, marked redness of the pinnae, and a putrid or rotten odor emanating from the ear canals. Previous treatments included both a preparation of herbal ear drops containing Goldenseal *(Hydrastis canadensis)* and a popular combination antiinflammatory, antifungal, and antibacterial ointment. Both treatments were effective but needed to be given consistently, and during lapses in her treatment the episodes recurred.

Further questioning revealed that Suzy had no history of skin disease, although the owner did complain about her halitosis. She had no history of digestive disorders. On a previous veterinarian's recommendation, Suzy was being fed a commercial diet to prevent uroliths, despite her having no prior history of cystitis or urolithiasis.

PHYSICAL EXAMINATION

Physical examination of the ear canal revealed an accumulation of yellow waxy debris in its vertical portions. The horizontal canal was not visualized. The lining of the canal was mildly reddened and extremely sensitive. The ear had normal skin texture and thickness and typical contours.

Suzy's pulse was rapid, forceful, taut, and floating. The tongue was normal in all respects.

ASSESSMENT

The nature of the discharge and the response both to Goldenseal (which contains the antibacterial compound known as berberine) and to the ear ointment suggested that the otitis was bacterial in origin, although no cultures were done. The lack of chronic inflammatory changes in the external ear spoke to the long-term consistency of previous medications.

Regarding the Chinese medical diagnosis, the superficial and taut nature of Suzy's pulse is typical in humans with an external invasion of Wind. Pathogenic Wind invasions in Chinese medicine are approximately equivalent to simple acute infections without any obvious predisposing factors in conventional medicine. Simple Wind invasions are not a typical cause of otitis in dogs and cats, but the pulse features were unique and compelling enough to support this diagnosis.

TREATMENT

Chai Ge Jie Ji Tang (Bupleurum and Pueraria Combination) was prescribed to treat Suzy's otitis externa. Although this formula is not mentioned in the main body of the text, it is used in humans for external invasions of Wind-Cold or Wind-Heat that are manifested as marked pain and sensitivity of the superficial body layers. It was thus appropriate to Suzy's heightened ear sensitivity, which seemed disproportionate to the level of infection and inflammation visible in her ears. The formula also contains pronounced antibacterial and antiinflammatory activity. Suzy was prescribed an oral dose of ¼ tsp of the granular formula twice daily for 2 weeks. The topical preparations were discontinued.

OUTCOME

Follow-up with the owner 2 weeks later disclosed that Suzy's ear pain that was nonresponsive to the topical preparations had resolved with use of the oral Chinese herbal formula. More than 2 months later, however, Suzy was seen again with a complaint of scratching at her ears of 1 day's duration. This symptom appeared despite the owner's continued use of the Chinese herbal formula and despite topical application of some leftover ear ointment.

Physical examination revealed the ears to be completely normal in appearance. The pulse was wiry and thin. Localized muscle tension and heat were palpable over the BL 10 and GV 14 acupuncture points. Chiropractic evaluation revealed that Suzy had multiple fixations of the cervical and lower lumbar vertebrae. These fixations were adjusted, and Suzy was given a new formula containing the Western herbs *Gelsemium sempervirens, Passiflora incarnata, Valeriana officinalis,* and *Avena sativa,* in a 2:3:3:2 ratio. Suzy was given 1 ml of the alcohol-based tincture twice daily, and acupuncture was administered at BL 10, GV 14, LI 4, and SI 3. Chai Ge Jie Ji Tang and all topical treatments were discontinued. There were no further recurrences of otitis externa or ear irritation as of the last follow-up examination 3 months later.

DISCUSSION

Although not specifically mentioned in the text, the new Western herbal formula seems effective at relaxing the cervical musculature and may be especially useful in relieving obstinate tendencies to vertebral fixations in this area. These vertebral fixations may cause head scratching in dogs and cats that may be mistaken by veterinarians and owners as a sign of otitis. This is especially true for atlantooccipital joint fixations, and the reader is referred to the chapter on musculoskeletal disorders for more information on this condition.

Even though signs of otitis externa were clearly evident on Suzy's first visit, some of the ear sensitivity may even then have been caused by undetected vertebral fixations. Chai Ge Jie Ji Tang may thus have been a good choice for Suzy not only because of its antimicrobial and antiinflammatory constituents but also because it contains several antispasmodic compounds that can help relax the muscle tightness that leads to vertebral fixations. In Suzy's case a formula more specifically directed to the cervical region was sufficient in the end to prevent further recurrences of ear sensitivity.

REFERENCES

Brinker F. *Formulas for Healthful Living.* Sandy, Ore, 1995, Eclectic Medical Publications.

Day C. *The Homeopathic Treatment of Small Animals: Principles and Practice.* Saffron Walden, UK, 1990, C.W. Daniel Company.

Inouye S, Takizawa T, Yamaguchi H. Antibacterial activity of essential oils and their major constituents against respiratory tract pathogens by gaseous contact. *J Antimicrob Chemother* 47(5):565-573, 2001.

Murphy R. *Lotus Materia Medica.* Durango, Colo, 1995, Lotus Star Press.

Naeser MA. *Outline Guide to Chinese Herbal Patent Medicines in Pill Form.* Boston, 1990, Boston Chinese Medicine.

Nenoff P, Haustein UF, Brandt W. Antifungal activity of the essential oil of *Melaleuca alternifolia* (tea tree oil) against pathogenic fungi in vitro. *Skin Pharmacol* 9(6):388-394, 1996.

Sanchez-Araujo M, Puchi A. Acupuncture enhances the efficacy of antibiotics treatment for canine otitis crises. *Acupunt Electrother Res* 22(3-4):191-206, 1997.

Sugiura Y, Ohashi Y, Nakai Y. The herbal medicine, sairei-to, enhances the mucociliary activity of the tubotympanum in the healthy guinea pig. *Acta Otolaryngol Suppl* 531:17-20, 1997.

Tsao S, Yin M. In vitro activity of garlic oil and four diallyl sulphides against antibiotic-resistant *Pseudomonas aeruginosa* and *Klebsiella pneumoniae. J Antimicrob Chemother* 47(5):665-670, 2001.

Yan W. *Practical Therapeutics of Traditional Chinese Medicine.* Brookline, Mass, 1997, Paradigm Publications.
Yeung H. *Handbook of Chinese Herbal Formulas.* Los Angeles, 1995, Self-published.
Yeung H. *Handbook of Chinese Herbs.* Los Angeles, 1996, Self-published.

8

Therapies for Endocrinologic Disorders

DIABETES MELLITUS

Therapeutic Rationale

- Increase carbohydrate, protein, and fat transport into cells and their use by cells.
- Prevent tissue damage from persistent hyperglycemia, electrolyte depletion, metabolic acidosis, and dehydration.

Alternative Options with Conventional Bases

Nutritional Therapies (Box 8-1)

- Even though alternative dietary strategies question the advisability of high-carbohydrate diets for managing diabetic patients, especially cats, a diet containing lower levels of grains that have lower glycemic indices (such as barley and sorghum [Sunvold, 1998]) may be tried. Lower carbohydrate diets sometimes improve weight loss in resistant obese pets. These diets can be formulated with approximately 50% to 70% meat in variety, splitting the rest between a grain (barley, sorghum, or other grain) and vegetables in variety (see the Paleolithic diet in Appendix A). Although the veterinarian should closely monitor clients that prefer homemade foods, the variety and flexibility provided by homemade diets make them safer than many veterinarians have been trained to believe.
- **Meal Feeding:** many veterinarians prefer free choice dry food as a "safer" feeding method for diabetic animals. Meal feeding actually allows the client to monitor the animal's food intake more closely so that insulin can be given only when the animal has been observed to eat a meal.

- **Dietary fiber:** has been shown to reduce glucose absorption from the gut, which increases glycemic control. Insoluble fiber (in the form of 12% cellulose incorporated into the diet) has been shown to reduce glucose absorption in cats (Chastain, 2000) and dogs (Nelson, 1998) in randomized, crossover trials. Another study in dogs with insulin-dependent diabetes compared the fiber content of several diets and its effect on insulin dosage and blood glucose concentrations. Dogs were randomly assigned a low-fiber diet, a high–insoluble fiber diet, or a high–soluble fiber diet. While no significant difference in insulin requirements was found among the three groups, the insoluble-fiber diet resulted in significantly lower blood glucose concentrations compared with the low-fiber and soluble-fiber diets (Kimmel, 2000). Although most fiber food sources contain both insoluble and soluble types, insoluble fiber may be preferable for diabetic animals and can be supplied in homemade diets by the inclusion of vegetables and whole grains.
- **Vanadium:** appears to have insulin-like effects both in people and in experimental animals. Vanadium may be of most use in type 2 diabetes because it is thought to activate tyrosine kinase intracellularly to act as an insulin cofactor. In one study, vanadium as an adjunct to protamine zinc insulin (PZI) therapy resulted in lower insulin doses, lower serum fructosamine values, and fewer clinical signs, including polyuria and polydipsia in diabetic cats (Greco, 1999). Vanadium is usually given at a dosage of 0.2 mg/kg qd or as vanadyl sulfate at 1 mg/kg qd.
- **Chromium:** thought to increase receptor number, receptor sensitivity, and receptor phosphorylation even though most reports have not shown significant benefit from chromium supplementation. In a study on nondiabetic obese and nonobese cats the animals were given supplements of 100 μg of elemental chromium daily for 6 weeks. Intravenous glucose tolerance tests were administered before supplementation and at the end of the test period. Chromium supplementation did not affect glucose tolerance in either group (Cohn,1999).

In a study of seven obese diabetic cats, six diabetic normal-weight cats, and six nondiabetic normal-weight cats, supplementation of 100 μg of chromium as picolinate did not result in clinically significant changes (Chastain, 2000). Another study examined the effects of supplementation of up to 400 μg twice daily (20 to 60 μg/kg/day) for 3 months to dogs with naturally occurring diabetes. In this study there were no differences in serum fructosamine, blood glycated hemoglobin concentration, body weight, insulin dosage, 10-hour mean blood glucose concentration, or daily caloric intake when dogs were given chromium plus insulin versus insulin alone (Schachter, 2001).

- **Antioxidants:** diabetes imposes oxidative stress on many tissues and organs, potentially effecting insulin resistance and beta cell destruction (Bonnefont-Rousselot, 2000). The effects of oxidative stress and endothelial dysfunction are more evident in human conditions such as peripheral vascular disease and diabetic nephropathy, but it is likely that oxidative stress affects veterinary diabetic patients as well. Supplementation of various antioxidants, including Vitamins C and E, has support in human medical literature (Cunningham, 1998). Vitamin E improves vascular reactivity and oxidative stress indices in human diabetics (Paolisso, 2000), and Vitamin C reduces plasma free radicals and insulin levels in human patients with type 2 diabetes (Paolisso, 1995).
- **Alpha-lipoic acid:** has been shown to improve neuropathic deficits of diabetes in humans (Ziegler, 1999) but its efficacy in feline diabetic neuropathy has been questionable in practice. Caution should be advised with this nutrient, however, because unpublished research from the University of California at Davis has shown that cats may demonstrate signs of neurologic toxicity when doses exceed 25 mg/day (Hill, 2000). Dogs may be given up to 200 mg daily for giant breeds and cats no more than 25 mg once daily.
- **Marine Fish Oil:** as a source of the ω-3 fatty acids eicosapentanoic acid (EPA) and docosahexanoic acid (DHA), Fish Oil may increase insulin sensitivity, which

reduces insulin resistance (Mori, 1999). It has been suggested as a treatment for diabetic neuropathy as well (Okuda, 1996; Podolin, 1998). Possible ways that Fish Oil exerts these effects may be via changes in cell membrane composition or transmembrane ion transport (Gerbi, 1999; Stiefel, 1999). Because cats are more prone to type 2 diabetes and diabetic neuropathy than dogs, Fish Oil seems especially appropriate as a supplement for feline diabetes mellitus. The *dose* is one regular-strength capsule per 5 to 10 lb of body weight once or divided daily (regular-strength capsules contain approximately 180 mg of EPA and 120 mg of DHA).

- **Glandular therapy:** administration of an extract of a specific organ or gland given to support that organ's function in the patient. For example, pancreatic glandular extracts contain freeze-dried pancreatic tissue and small amounts of pancreatic enzymes. Recent research has led to the investigation of "oral tolerization" (the induction of immune tolerance) in the treatment of autoimmune disease, including diabetes in humans (Krause, 2000). The specific mechanism of action is unknown but may involve deletion, anergy, or active suppression of T-lymphocytes that initiate immune destruction of target tissues. Since 40% to 50% of dogs have autoantibodies to islet cell antigens, administration of pancreatic glandular extracts may be a rational approach in this species. Questions recently have arisen regarding the safety of glandular therapy because attempts at oral tolerization may exacerbate the immune response to autoantigens instead of tolerizing T-lymphocytes (Hanninen, 2000). Glandular therapy is best used soon after the onset of the disease to decrease destruction of pancreatic beta cells. I (SW) have observed few positive results using glandular therapy.

Herbs

- **Gymnema** *(Gymnema sylvestre):* numerous case series reports indicate that Gymnema improves glucose tolerance and clinical status in human diabetics. Gymnema extract was shown to increase insulin secretion in pancreatic beta cell lines by increasing

BOX 8-1 Herbs and Nutraceuticals for Diabetes Mellitus

Regulators of glucose absorption
Insoluble fiber
Soluble fiber

Regulators of insulin availability or release
Gymnema sylvestre
Momordica charantia
Trigonella foenum-graecum
Panax ginseng
Panax quinquefolius

Regulators of receptor and postreceptor effects
Vanadium
Chromium

Regulators of systemic effects of hyperglycemia
Antioxidants, especially alpha-lipoic acid
Marine fish oil

membrane permeability (Persaud, 1999). Administration of Gymnema extract was observed to increase serum insulin levels as well as the absolute number of pancreatic islet cells in streptozocin-treated rats. The same group showed that Gymnema improved glucose uptake in target tissues (Shanmugasundaram, 1983, 1990). Clinical use suggests that Gymnema must be administered for 2 to 3 months for maximum effect. Although the herb is available alone, it is more often combined with other herbs traditionally used in the treatment of diabetes, including Bitter Melon *(Momordica charantia)*, Fenugreek *(Trigonella foenum-graecum)*, and Ginseng *(Panax ginseng, P. quinquefolius)*.

- **Bitter Melon:** a traditional Ayurvedic herb often included in combinations for diabetes. Animal studies have yielded conflicting results (Day, 1990; Khanna, 1981; Sarkar, 1996; Shibib, 1993). The hypoglycemic effects of this plant may involve increased glucose utilization by the liver (Sarkar, 1996); decreased glucose synthesis by depression of the two key gluconeogenic enzymes glucose-6-phosphatase and fructose-1,6-biphosphatase; and enhancement of glucose oxidation through the shunt pathway via activation of glucose-6-phosphate dehydrogenase (Shibib, 1993).
- **Fenugreek:** has been shown to lower blood glucose in both humans and dogs (Ribes, 1986). Fenugreek seeds contain fiber thought to slow glucose absorption from

the gut, but it may work by a number of mechanisms. In a study of rats given alloxan to induce diabetes, both water and alcohol extracts of Fenugreek had some hypoglycemic activity (Abdel-Barry, 1997). Since alloxan destroys pancreatic beta cells it was presumed that Fenugreek either stimulated insulin release from remaining beta cells or had insulin-receptor activity.

- **Ginseng:** two species of Ginseng, Chinese or Korean *(P. ginseng)* and American *(P. quinquefolius)*, have shown promise in managing diabetes. Both have been shown to reduce hyperglycemia in human patients with type 2 diabetes (Sotaniemi, 1995; Vuksan, 2000). Exactly how Ginseng works against diabetes is unknown but effects on insulin secretion and receptor sensitivity have been suggested (Vuksan, 2000).
- **Rehmannia** *(Rehmannia glutinosa):* a component of Chinese herbal formulas commonly used to treat diabetes. Rhemannia is thought to be a primary active ingredient of a formula that proved to reduce blood sugar in mice with diabetes (Miura, 1997).
- **Antidiabetis:** a patented combination of the herbs Bilberry *(Vaccinium myrtillus)*, Dandelion *(Taraxacum officinale)*, Chicory *(Cichorium intybus)*, Juniper *(Juniperus communis)*, Centaury *(Centaurium umbellatum)*, Bean Pod *(Phaseolus vulgaris)*, Yarrow *(Achillea millefolium)*, Mulberry *(Morus nigra)*, Valerian *(Valeriana officinalis)*, and Nettles *(Urtica dioica)*. This formula was shown to reduce serum glucose and fructosamine in a mouse model of diabetes (Petlevski, 2001).
- **Other herbs** that have shown some effect in laboratory animal studies are Agaricus mushroom *(Agaricus blazei)* and *Ilex guyausa* (Swanston, 1989), *Pterocarpus marsupium* (Manickam, 1997), *Pterocarpus santalinus* (Kameswara, 2001), Eucalyptus *(Eucalyptus globulus)* (Gray, 1998), Madagascar Periwinkle *(Catharanthus roseus)* (Chattopadhyay, 1999), and Neem *(Azadirachta indica)* (Chattopadhyay, 1999).

Acupuncture

- Acupuncture has been studied in Russia and China for many years, mostly as an approach to limiting the secondary complications from diabetes seen in human patients. In a rat model of diabetes, electroacupuncture at a point equivalent to Zhong Wan (CV 12) resulted in transient decreases in blood glucose. This decrease was observed in normal rats and those with type 2 diabetes, but not in rats with type 1 diabetes, and was thought to be mediated through beta-endorphin release (Chang, 1999).

Paradigmatic Options

- Although Chinese herbal formulas are not to be considered a substitute for insulin in the management of diabetes mellitus, the properly chosen formula can be expected to reduce insulin resistance and therefore the required dose of insulin. Appropriately chosen herbal formulas and diets eventually may lead to complete restoration of glucose tolerance and sometimes eliminate the need for insulin. However, patients with uncontrolled diabetes should first be given insulin.
- As with much of Chinese medicine, the prevailing view of diabetes mellitus in humans has been assumed to be directly applicable to animals. Particularly in endocrine disorders, however, quite different treatment strategies may be needed for humans and animals. This is especially true for diabetes mellitus in my opinion (SM).
- The prevailing human perspective is that diabetes mellitus is a Yin deficiency syndrome that leads to Empty Fire and consumptive Heat. This Yin deficiency can exist in the upper, middle, and lower jiaos, or levels, of the body. As Yin deficiency becomes more severe it works its way deeper into the lower jiao and a change in symptoms results. Symptomatic differences between involvement at different levels can be subtle, however, and difficult to distinguish.
- In the upper jiao Yin deficiency produces Lung Heat with injury to lung fluids. This stage is marked by extreme thirst. Formulas used to address Yin deficiency at this level include the following:
  - **Bai Hu Jia Ren Shen Tang** (White Tiger with Ginseng Decoction) for patients with a superficial, rapid, forceful pulse, heat intolerance, red dry tongue, excessive thirst, and severe Heat.

- **Er Dong Tang** (Ophiopogon and Asparagus Decoction) for patients with a rapid, forceless pulse, excessive thirst, lassitude, and frequent urination. This formula nourishes Yin, tonifies Qi, and clears Heat from the upper body.
- **Xiao Ke Fang** (Wasting Thirst Formula) clears Heat, strongly nourishes Yin, and relieves thirst in patients with excessive thirst, dry mouth, frequent urination, excessive hunger, and a rapid pulse.
- When Yin deficiency affects the middle jiao it causes profuse Stomach Fire that results in extreme appetite. It is treated with **Yu Nu Jian** (Jade Lady Brew) to which 6 g of Huang Lian and 9 g of Shan Zhi Zi may be added to 75 g of the base formula. Other symptoms include emaciation, dry stools, constipation, thirst, a large, floating, forceful, full pulse, and a red tongue.
- When Yin deficiency affects the lower jiao, or the Kidney, profuse urination becomes a predominant feature of the case. It is treated with one of several formulas:
- **Liu Wei Di Huang Wan** (Six Flavor Rehmannia Pill) is used when the patient has frequent urination, a dry mouth, thirst, weak back and knees, deafness, a dry coat (fine dander), a thready, rapid, floating pulse, and a red or tender-looking and dry tongue. Some practitioners suggest using a version of the formula that contains large amounts of Shan Zhu Yu and Shan Yao to enhance its effectiveness in the management of diabetes mellitus. If incontinence has become prominent, Ze Xie is omitted from the formula and about 9 g each of Yi Zhi Ren, Sang Piao Xiao, and Wu Wei Zi is added to 90 g of formula.
- **Zhi Bai Di Huang Wan** (Anemarrhena, Phellodendron and Rehmannia Pill) is made by adding 9 g of Zhi Mu and 6 g of Huang Bai to 75 g of Liu Wei Di Huang Wan. It is used in cases of Kidney Yin deficiency that show more symptomatic evidence of Heat such as insomnia or nocturnal restlessness, heat intolerance, itch, and increased thirst.
- For chilly animals in which Kidney Yin deficiency has resulted in a decline of Kidney Yang, **Shen Qi Wan**

(Kidney Qi Pill) can be considered. The patient that would benefit exhibits cold intolerance, profuse urination, a pale tongue, weak pulses, hind limb weakness, and deafness. Some authors advocate the addition of Fu Pen Zi, Jin Ying Zi, and Sang Piao Xiao to help relieve urinary incontinence in these animals.

- For all of the preceding formulas, a *suggested starting dose* of granular concentrate is ¼ tsp per 10 to 15 lb of body weight, or 60 to 75 mg/kg of body weight, divided into two daily doses.
- In my (SM) experience, clinical results using the Yin tonification approach to diabetes in animals are frequently poor except in the most advanced cases. Interpretation of the history and signs of diabetic animals according to their pulse and tongue findings often suggests that diabetes mellitus is a Damp-Heat condition. Although this theory is the polar opposite of the theory that diabetic animals are Yin deficient, it is completely in accord with earliest theories surrounding diabetes recorded in the *Nei Jing Su Wen* about two millennia ago.
- The *Nei Jing*, the seminal classic of Chinese medicine, consistently describes diabetes mellitus as arising from a Spleen deficiency caused by the excessive intake of fatty and sweet foods. As described by this early text the overwhelming of the Spleen by dietary overload leads to "digestive heat," "internal heat," and chest and abdominal fullness. One of the few references the *Nei Jing* makes to herbal medicine is in the recommendation of Euphorbia *(Euphorbia pekinensis)* for this condition. Unlike the formulas discussed previously, Euphorbia has no Yin-tonifying effects. Instead it strongly drains Dampness and is a purgative. **Wu Ling San** (Powder of Five Drugs with Poria), a diuretic Dampness-draining formula, was also advocated for use in diabetes in early Chinese medical works, although this use has largely been forgotten.
- Research supporting the effectiveness of Bitter Melon (described earlier) in diabetes management is consistent with the theory that diabetes is a

Damp-Heat disorder. In subtropical regions of China, Bitter Melon is consumed at the end of meals during the summer months to prevent the generation of Damp Heat by the richer foods that have been consumed.

- If the practitioner subscribes to this theory, consideration of other formulas becomes important in the management of diabetes in animals. **Wei Ling Tang** is a combination, both in name and in content, of two smaller formulas, **Ping Wei San** (Harmonize the Stomach Powder) and **Wu Ling San** (Powder of Five Drugs with Poria). Ping Wei San is the main formula in modern herbalism for addressing the abdominal fullness, nausea, vomiting, heaviness, and malaise that were noted in the *Nei Jing's* discussion of diabetes. It strengthens Spleen Qi, descends Stomach Qi, and harmonizes the Stomach. The Wu Ling San in the formula drains obstructing accumulations of Dampness. Animals that may benefit from Wei Ling Tang have any or all of the following symptoms: greasy coat; pale tongue; soft pulses; tendency to weight gain; alternating preferences for warmth and cold; lassitude; soft stools or diarrhea; undigested food in the stool; increased thirst and decreased appetite or increased appetite and decreased thirst. A *recommended starting dose* is ¼ tsp per 10 to 15 lb of body weight per day. The dosage may be safely doubled or tripled and should be administered in divided doses twice daily.
- For animals that appear "hotter" but still exhibit prominent Dampness symptoms **Si Miao San** (Four Marvels Powder) can be considered. A *recommended starting dose* is ¼ tsp per 10 to 15 lb of body weight per day. The dosage may be safely doubled or tripled and should be administered in divided doses twice daily.
- Consideration may be given to adding two herbs, Da Ji *(Euphorbia pekinensis)* and Yu Mi Xu *(Zea mays)* to each of the above formulas. Yu Mi Xu is made from the stamen of corn silk and is credited with diuretic and hypoglycemic properties. It is a mild herb and

may be given in large amounts to patients with diabetes. Da Ji is a strong purgative. It is probably best used in excessive cases such as patients receiving **Si Miao San**. Both herbs are credited with Damp Heat–draining properties.

- The Damp Heat theory of pathogenesis of diabetes mellitus in animals is in accord with the occasionally impressive benefits seen when carbohydrates are eliminated from diabetic animals' diets. Carbohydrates are credited with a "sweet" taste, and excessive carbohydrate intake can injure the Spleen. The definition of what is considered excessive carbohydrates probably varies with the species under consideration, but dogs and especially cats appear to be adapted to diets with few or no digestible carbohydrates. Response in animals placed on a diet with a low glycemic index can be dramatic enough to suggest that diabetes mellitus may well be considered a manifestation of carbohydrate sensitivity in many animals.
- In my practice, I (SM) use a Western herbal combination that has shown significant ability to stabilize blood glucose levels in animals, and even reverse early type 2 diabetes mellitus in many human patients. It contains the following ingredients:
  - 30 ml Corn Silk (stigma and style)
  - 30 ml Bilberry
  - 40 ml Gymnema

  Although not previously mentioned, Bilberry contains bioflavonoids that are thought to help preserve retinal vasculature. This formula is safe, mild, and suitable for extended use. A recommended starting dose is 0.2 ml per 5 lb of body weight, three times daily. Practitioners should be aware that this formula can markedly enhance an animal's response to insulin, and reductions in insulin dosage may be periodically required as determined by regular blood glucose testing. "Equal parts of Corn Silk and Gymnema can be used without Bilberry as an effective tincture for the management of diabetes mellitus."

AUTHORS' CHOICES:

SM: Low-carbohydrate diets; formulas to clear Damp Heat; insulin and monitoring as needed; Western herb compounds affecting insulin dynamics.

SW: Cats—glucose monitoring and insulin as needed; low-carbohydrate, high protein diets; Fish Oil; antioxidants; vanadium.

Dogs—insulin and glucose monitoring; Gymnema; Ginseng in formulas with other herbs; antioxidants; Fish Oil, low-carbohydrate diets.

HYPERADRENOCORTICISM

Therapeutic Rationale

- Reduce production of glucocorticoids.

Alternative Options with Conventional Bases

Herbs

- **Ginkgo** *(Ginkgo biloba):* has been shown to reduce corticosterone secretion, and reduce corticotropin-releasing hormone (CRH) expression and secretion. It is a monoamine oxidase (MAO) inhibitor (like L-deprenyl) (Amri, 1997; Marcilhac, 1998; Sloley, 2000).

Paradigmatic Options

- The use of Chinese herbal medicine to treat hyperadrenocorticism consistently relieves symptoms and improves laboratory values without the use of pharmaceuticals. In my (SM) experience hyperadrenocorticism represents an accumulation of a Yang pathogen that appears to be, as in many endocrine disorders, Damp Heat. A formula that is particularly useful in clearing Damp Heat is **Long Dan Xie Gan Tang** (Gentian Drain the Liver Decoction). Patients that benefit are usually heat intolerant, weak but agitated and restless, and thirsty. They have increased appetite and urine production. Their pulses are rapid or wiry, and they have a deep- or purple-red tongue with a frothy coating. When animals appear cushingoid but hyperadrenocorticism cannot be definitively diagnosed with low-dose dexamethasone and adrenocorticotropic hormone (ACTH) stimulation tests, they often benefit from this formula. A *suggested starting dose* of granular concentrate is ¼ tsp per 10 to 15 lb of body weight, or 60 to 75 mg/kg of body weight, divided into two daily doses.

- In older, weaker animals, tonifying formulas may be necessary once the excess Yang pathogen has been eliminated. Such formulas should be chosen on the basis of pulse and tongue findings and the signs of the patient. One formula that has been advocated is **Mai Men Dong Tang** (Decoction of Ophiopogon Root). Although traditionally used for Lung and Stomach dryness it may be given to cushingoid animals with polyphagia, dry hair and skin, thin or alopecic coat, excessive thirst and urination, panting especially at night, a dry, red tongue, and a thready, rapid pulse.
- The notion that a Yang pathogen may underlie hyperadrenocorticism is sensible. In Chinese medicine Yang energy is stored in the Kidneys and is the basis for metabolism. In modern medicine the adrenal glands are the basis for metabolism and are intimately associated with the kidneys. A clear correlation between the adrenal glands and Yang energy thus seems to exist.

AUTHORS' CHOICES:

SM: Long Dan Xie Gan Tang.
SW: Gingko; Chinese herbal formulas; Lysodren.

HYPOADRENOCORTICISM (ADDISON'S DISEASE)

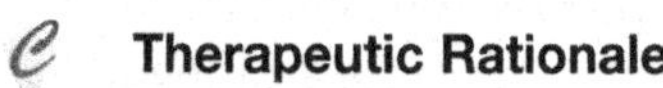

Therapeutic Rationale

- Correct electrolyte abnormalities.
- Supply corticoids.

Alternative Options with Conventional Bases

Herbs

- **Licorice** *(Glycyrrhiza glabra):* has often been recommended in the treatment of Addison's disease. Licorice inhibits the action of an enzyme that inactivates cortisol, and this leads to the retention of cortisol and the activation of mineralocorticoid receptors in the kidneys to cause sodium retention. Licorice is thought to counteract the Addisonian signs of hyperkalemia and steroid insufficiency. However, the mechanisms attributed to Licorice depend on the presence of some degree of steroid production, so Licorice may be of limited usefulness in hypoadrenocorticism. Licorice also interacts adversely with the prednisone that is usually a daily treatment for these patients.
- **Other herbs** that have been reported to elevate corticosteroid levels are Ashwaganda *(Withania somnifera)* and Ginseng (Buffi, 1993; Singh, 2000). These studies involved normal, stressed animals or other models in which applicability to hypoadrenal animals is doubtful.
- **Adrenal glandular extracts:** may prove beneficial in early cases of Addison's disease. Hypoadrenocorticism may involve autoimmune destruction of the adrenal cortex, and glandular extracts are thought to act via immune tolerization. Adrenal glandular extracts may also play a supportive role in treatment by providing adrenal factors other than steroids. Products that have the best clinical efficacy retain their cortisol activity, and excessive doses of these cortisol-containing glandular extracts may produce hyperadrenocortical signs. I (SM) use a starting dose of one tablet of Drenatrophin per 15 lb of body weight daily, given in divided doses if possible.

Paradigmatic Options

- The close association between the adrenal glands and the kidneys is echoed in the Chinese herbal formulas commonly recommended for hypoadrenocorticism. Patients may have deficient Kidney Yin or a more fundamental deficiency of Kidney Jing.

- Formulas for deficient Kidney Yin that manifests as hypoadrenocorticism include **Da Bu Yin Wan** (Great Nourish the Yin Pill) and **Liu Wei Di Huang Wan** (Six Flavor Rehmannia Pill). Da Bu Yin Wan is used when the patient exhibits signs of severe Empty Heat caused by Yin deficiency, including heat intolerance, a forceful, rapid pulse, a red, dry tongue, restlessness, thirst, and agitation. Liu Wei Di Huang Wan is used for patients with milder Yin deficiency that manifests as weakness, mild heat intolerance, thirst, a dry coat and powdery dander, a thready, rapid pulse, and a tender tongue.
- Formulas for more urgent cases of deficient Kidney Yin include **Zuo Gui Wan** (Replenish the Left Pill) and **Zuo Gui Yin** (Replenish the Left Beverage). Zuo Gui Wan is much the stronger of the two because of its antler and turtle shell content. Symptoms indicating the use of these formulas are similar to those calling for Liu Wei Di Huang Wan.
- **Zuo Gui Wan** is sometimes combined with **You Gui Wan** (Replenish the Right Pill). This is done by adding Rou Gui, Dang Gui, Fu Zi, and Du Zhong to Zuo Gui Wan, which produces a formula that tonifies both Yin and Yang. It is thus suited to Kidney Jing deficiency, since Jing is considered by many to be the combined form of Yin and Yang that is stored in the Kidneys. Signs calling for the use of this formula include weakness, anorexia, excessive thirst and urination, vomiting, diarrhea, a pale, flabby, swollen tongue that may be moist or dry, and a deep, slow pulse.
- For all of the these formulas, a *suggested starting dose* of granular concentrate is ¼ tsp per 10 to 15 lb of body weight, or 60 to 75 mg/kg of body weight, divided into two daily doses.

AUTHORS' CHOICES:

SM: Drenatrophin; Licorice.
SW: Conventional treatments with herbal and nutritional support.

HYPERTHYROIDISM

Therapeutic Rationale

- Reduce thyroxine (T_4) and triiodothyronine (T_3) levels.
- Suppress damage at target tissues.

Alternative Options with Conventional Bases

Nutritional Therapies

- **Carnitine:** a peripheral receptor antagonist of thyroxine in some tissues. In a clinical trial using up to 4 g of Carnitine daily in hyperthyroid women symptoms of hyperthyroidism were either prevented or reversed as compared with placebo (Benvenga, 2001). Since hyperthyroidism depletes the body of carnitine stores, supplementation appears advisable in any case. A *recommended starting dose* of carnitine for cats is 250 to 500 mg divided daily.

Herbs

- **Bugleweed** *(Lycopus europeus)* in alcohol extract only: plant extract given orally to rats caused prolonged (more than 24 hours) decrease in T_3 levels, possibly attributable to reduced peripheral T_4 deiodination. A pronounced reduction of T_4 and thyroid-stimulating hormone (TSH) concentrations was observed 24 hours after administration (Winterhoff, 1994). Anecdotal reports of use in hyperthyroid cats have been promising and suggest that a combination of Melissa and Bugleweed normalizes T_4 levels and may extend life without conventional treatment. No adverse effects have yet been reported.
- **Melissa** *(Melissa officinalis):* has not been studied as much as Bugleweed but was shown in one study to reduce human immunoglobulin binding to TSH receptors (Auf'mkolk, 1985). This finding is not relevant to hyperthryoid disease in cats, but Melissa is found in common formulas for hyperthyroidism that are used, apparently successfully, in cats.

Paradigmatic Options

- The current approach in the treatment of hyperthyroidism in humans focuses on quenching Liver Fire, the blazing of which acts to dry up Yin. This theory of Yin deficiency with floating Yang has its adherents in the treatment of feline hyperthyroidism as well. For these cases a proprietary formula known as **Hyper Jia Bing** (Jing Tang Herbs, Reddick, Florida) has been recommended. Patients that may benefit have a thyroid nodule, weight loss, irritability, hyperactivity or restlessness, palpitations or arrhythmias, insomnia, polyphagia, fatigue, loose stools, tachycardia, warm paws, a red, dry tongue, and a rapid, wiry, floating, thin pulse. The formula contains Shu Di Huang, Shan Yao, Shan Zhu Yu, Bai Shao Yao, Ze Xie, Mu Li, Long Gu, Xiang Fu, and Chai Hu.

- Another favored approach in the treatment of human hyperthyroidism focuses on providing sources of organic iodine to the patient. Such sources include shellfish and seaweed, and many experts in Chinese veterinary medicine advocate this simple approach to the treatment of hyperthyroidism in animals. **Hai Zao Yu Hu Tang** (Sargassum Jade Pot Decoction) is the usual prescription and acts to soften and transform Phlegm accumulations in the throat. Some traditional Chinese medicine (TCM) authors credit it with the ability to move stagnant Liver Qi and Blood and prescribe it when the patient exhibits irritability, anxiety, depression, aversion to palpation in the cranial abdomen, a bluish, dark-red tongue with a thin white coat, and a wiry, slippery pulse.
- Iodine supplementation to suppress metabolism of the thyroid gland is one of the original conventional treatments for hyperthyroidism in humans, but long-term efficacy of iodine supplementation is poor and "thyroid storms" have been triggered by this practice.
- Another approach to feline hyperthyroidism I (SM) have developed appears to be effective and does not require the administration of iodine-containing herbs. This approach assumes that hyperthyroidism arises as a result of Phlegm-Fire. This unusual ability of Phlegm, a Dampness pathogen, to induce a pathologic Fire is conferred when it accumulates in the San Jiao, or Triple Burner. The congesting effect of Phlegm in such a Qi-abundant area of the body appears to release a massive

amount of Heat in the same way that grabbing onto a rope generates a "rope-burn." This theory fits well with the progression of symptoms in hyperthyroid cats and is verified by the apparent effectiveness of herbal formulas based on this premise in my practice. The precise formula used depends on the stage of hyperthyroidism present in the patient.

- For all of the formulas in this section a *suggested starting dose* of granular concentrate is ¼ tsp per 10 to 15 lb of body weight, or 60 to 75 mg/kg of body weight, divided into two daily doses.

Phase I—accumulation of Dampness and Phlegm

- Feline hyperthyroidism starts with the insidious accumulation of Dampness that arises from impairment of the Spleen's ability to completely transform food into Qi and usable body fluids. Dampness is a nonusable fluid, and its accumulation further impairs Spleen function, resulting in a vicious cycle. Signs and symptoms of this stage include abdominal distention, vomiting of a slimy vomitus after meals, minimal thirst, poor appetite, excessive appetite (from Damp Heat), weight gain, lethargy, worsening of symptoms in damp or humid weather, mucus in the stool, profuse watery urine, and straining to pass urine or stool. The tongue is swollen, wet, and scalloped from teeth imprints, and there are strings of saliva in the mouth. The pulse is slippery or, in an obese cat, thin.
- The formula to address this phase is **Tao Hong Er Chen Tang** (Decoction of Two Herbs with Carthamus and Persica). The formula consists of 45 g of **Er Chen Tang** with 12 g of Tao Ren and 9 g of Hong Hua added. Use of this formula often halts the progression of the disease into the next three stages and will reduce recurrence of thyroid tumors after surgical excision. At this stage a thyroid tumor is barely palpable and is usually an incidental finding when a cat is brought in for chronic vomiting.
- Any appropriate Spleen-tonifying formula may be effective in reversing hyperthyroidism in Phase I.

Phase II—accumulation of Phlegm-Heat in the San Jiao

- In Phase II Dampness has begun to accumulate and congeal in the Qi-rich Triple Burner and is obstructing the flow of Qi and generating Heat. Thyroid tumors are clinically evident, thyroid hormone levels are elevated, and there are persistent signs of Dampness. Signs of Heat and Qi stagnation are appearing, including irritability, heat intolerance, and increased heart rate, appetite, and thirst. The pulse is slippery, wiry, and rapid. The tongue is swollen and wet, red or lavender, and scalloped. Strings of saliva are present.
- The formula to treat this phase is **Wen Dan Tang** (Warm the Gallbladder Decoction with Coptis) that has been modified by adding 6 g of Huang Lian, 12 g of Tao Ren, 12 g of Hong Hua, 6 g of Zhi Zi, 12 g of Lian Qiao, 9 g of Gua Luo, 9 g of Zhe Bei Mu, 12 g of Mu Li, and 9 g of Jiang Can to about 60 g of the base formula. This formula clears Heat, moves Blood, dissolves Phlegm, drains Damp, and moves Qi.
- **Zhe Bei Mu** and **Mu Li** are paired in another small formula known as **Xiao Luo Wan,** which is used to treat human hyperthyroidism. Mu Li contains significant quantities of iodine, given its marine origins. The use of iodine-containing herbs to suppress thyroid activity is a main initial strategy in human hyperthyroidism but is ineffective as a long-term solution. Emphasis of iodine-containing herbs as part of a "pharmacologic" approach is similarly unrewarding in the long-term treatment of feline hyperthyroidism

Phase III—consumption of Kidney Yin, leading to Empty Heat and Fire

- Any prolonged Heat condition in the body will eventually injure the Yin. Depletion of Kidney Yin stores leads to the development of Empty Heat that further aggravates Heat tendencies. This abundance of Heat congeals Dampness almost completely into Phlegm, and the Phlegm itself is parched into a scanty, tough residue. At this stage the role of Dampness, Phlegm, and Qi stagnation in the pathogenesis of the condition is obscured by overwhelming signs of Heat and Dryness. Signs exhibited by the patient include emaciation, thirst, excessive appetite, agitation, irritability, restless sleep, excessive dreaming, and dry hair and skin. The pulse is rapid, flooding, and wiry, although some slipperiness may still be detected. The tongue is red, dry, and coarse and may appear small.

- Therapeutic intervention in Phase III must be aimed at stabilization by clearing Heat and nourishing Yin. An ideal formula for this is **Zhi Bai Di Huang Wan** (Anemarrhena, Phellodendron, and Rehmannia Pill), which contains 12 g of Zhi Mu and 9 g of Huang Bai added to 60 g of **Liu Wei Di Huang Wan** (Six Flavor Rehmannia Pill).
- Once Empty Heat and Fire have been cleared and adequate Yin has been restored, Phlegm-Heat signs such as a slippery pulse and a red, wet swollen tongue should again be detectable. At this point the practitioner can again use modified **Wen Dan Tang** (see Phase II section) to treat the patient.

Phase IV—Kidney Yin and Yang deficiency with Empty Heat and Fire

- In the endless cycle of Yin and Yang, Yang always arises from Yin. Since Yin must be present before Yang can arise, depletion of Kidney Yin by unrelenting Heat leads to depletion of Kidney Yang. Yang deficiency and excess Heat occur together in the final stage of feline hyperthyroidism and present what seems at first a contradictory clinical picture of Heat signs and cold intolerance. Signs include progressive emaciation, excessive thirst, appetite, and urination, irritability, extreme chilliness, restlessness, exhaustion, and weakness. The pulse is flooding, rapid, and wiry but may become minute in the very late stages of the disease. The tongue is red, dry, and small. It may be pale and small in the very late stages.
- Chronic renal insufficiency or failure is usually demonstrable on serum chemistry panels at this point in the development of feline hyperthyroidism. Even at this late stage, however, Chinese herbs can be used to stabilize the condition of patients and reverse both azotemia and impaired urinary concentrating ability. The appropriate formula for this stage is **Er Xian Tang** (Decoction of Curculigo and Epimedium). Once the patient's condition

has been stabilized, the practitioner can consider the use of **Wen Dan Tang** if Phlegm-Heat recurs.

Dietary Support of Chinese Herbal Treatment

- The high occurrence of hyperthyroidism in cats exhibiting chronic vomiting and the efficacy in hyperthyroidism of formulas that reduce the formation of Phlegm by increasing efficiency of Spleen function imply that feline hyperthyroidism is essentially a digestive disorder in TCM. It commonly arises in animals that have other forms of inflammatory bowel disease (IBD) and seems to become more clinically evident as signs of GI disturbance increase. Similarly, when IBD is successfully controlled through dietary intervention, signs of hyperthyroidism often spontaneously regress to the point that Chinese herbal treatment may be at least temporarily discontinued. Dietary approaches include avoidance of known food allergens. Carbohydrate avoidance may also prove to be a key factor in preventing feline hyperthyroidism.
- As previously mentioned, the Western herb Bugleweed has the reputation of possessing antithyroid activity that can augment the activity of antithyroid drugs such as methimazole. One herb in common use in Chinese medicine that I (SM) have found possesses this same property is Zi Cao *(Lithospermum erythrorhizon)*.
- Zi Cao appears to share the antithyroid properties of its Western cousin Common Gromwell *(Lithospermum officinale)*. The antithyroid properties of *Lithospermum* in cats are probably due to inhibition of the iodide pump by which the thyroid gland takes up iodide from the blood stream, and to inhibition of iodothyronine deiodinase by which T_4 is converted into metabolically active T_3.
- Other antithyroid effects of Western *Lithospermum* include inhibition of TSH and interference with antithyroid immunoglobulin G (IgG), but these are less likely to be helpful in feline hyperthyroidism.
- Despite this apparent antithyroid activity, Zi Cao has never appeared in Chinese herbal formulas used to treat hyperthyroidism in humans. Similarly, I (SM) have not yet investigated it as a component to enhance

the effects of the formulas previously described in the treatment of feline hyperthyroidism. However, clinical experience with the herb commonly demonstrates a reduction in the required dose of methimazole in feline hyperthyroidism by approximately 50% to 75%, thus circumventing the side effects of anorexia, nausea, and vomiting that are frequently associated with the initial use of this drug. *Lithospermum* also seems to reduce the time necessary for methimazole to take effect after treatment is started. Zi Cao does not appear to reduce the drug eruptions and autoimmune reactions that are sometimes seen with the use of methimazole and appears to be ineffective when used alone.

AUTHORS' CHOICES:

SM: Phase I through IV—Chinese herbal formulas; food allergy avoidance.
SW: Bugleweed and Melissa combinations; Carnitine.

HYPOTHYROIDISM

Therapeutic Rationale

- Correct deficiency of thyroid hormone.

Alternative Options with Conventional Bases

Herbs

- **Kelp** ***(Alaria esculenta)*** **and other seaweeds:** are often recommended as adjunct treatment for hypothyroidism because they are a source of iodine. However, 50% to 95% of cases in dogs are due to immune-mediated destruction, so whether additional iodine will help when insufficient T_3 and T_4 can be produced is questionable. Furthermore, iodine appears to enhance the immune-mediated destruction of thyroid cells (Rose, 1999). Therefore, if Kelp contains consistently high levels of iodine, it would appear to be *contraindicated* in the treatment of canine hypothyroidism.

Paradigmatic Options

- Human hypothyroidism is considered in Chinese medicine to arise from Kidney Yang deficiency. The mainstay of treatment is **Shen Qi Wan** (Kidney Qi Pill; Rehmannia 8; Ba Wei Di Huang Wan) and it has been adapted for use in animals. Patients that benefit most are fatigued and chilly, have difficulty rising in the morning, and have a dry, scaly coat. They may have some water retention or edema, a pale tongue with white coating, and a thready and weak pulse. Foods with warming energies that have been advocated for these patients are chicken, chicken liver, lamb, beef, tuna, salmon, herring, mussels, brown rice, corn, potatoes, squash, kale, garlic, ginger, saffron, rosemary, cayenne, cinnamon, and sweet basil.
- Another formula that has been advocated for hypothyroidism is **Sheng Mai San** (Generate the Pulse Powder). This formula is a simple but strong Qi and Yin tonic. Patients that benefit have an aversion to cold, cold extremities, a cold and sore back, reduced libido, loose teeth, deafness, copious clear urine, urinary incontinence, lethargy, exercise intolerance, dry flaky skin, shedding, bilaterally symmetric hair loss, weight gain, a weak voice, and a weak, deep pulse.
- Some authors have taken the same approach to canine hypothyroidism as they do to feline hyperthyroidism. That is, marine origin herbs with high iodine content are selected, in this case to strengthen thyroid function, not to suppress it. From a Chinese medical perspective the marine origin herbs were ostensibly chosen because their salty taste strengthens Kidney function, which is the source of all metabolic drive. The constituent herbs are not known as Kidney tonics, however, but act to transform Phlegm-Heat.
- A family of proprietary formulas has been developed to support this approach. For simple goiter dissolution, which is seldom an issue in canine hypothyroidism, **Si Hai Su Yu Wan** is used. This formula contains 20 g of Mu Xiang, 20 g of Chen Pi, and 12 g each of Hai Dai, Hai Ge Ke, Hai Zao, Hai Piao Xiao, and Kun Bu. The guiding symptoms for

which this formula is thought to work best are irritability, emotional stress, a slightly red tongue, and a wiry or taut pulse.

- For patients with more obvious signs of Kidney Yang and Yin deficiency 18 g of Tu Si Zi, 18 g of Rou Cong Rong, 12 g of He Shou Wu, 12 g of Xuan Shen, and 8 g each of Hai Dai, Hai Ge Ke, Hai Zao, and Hai Piao Xiao are added to the base formula to make **Xiao Ying San.**
- The core formula is likewise modified to suit the dog with Qi, Blood, and Yin deficiencies with the addition of Huang Qi, Dang Shen, He Shou Wu, Shu Di Huang, Shan Yao, and Bai Shao. Other herbs are included because of their goiter-resolving properties and iodine content. This formula is marketed as **Jia Bing Fang.** The exact herb amounts are 30 g each of Xia Ku Cao and Huang Qi; 20 g of Dang Shen; 12 g each of He Shou Wu, Shu Di Huang, Bai Shao, Shan Yao, Xiang Fu, and Chai Hu; and 10 g each of Hai Zao and Kun Bu.
- A *suggested starting dose* of granular concentrate for all of these formulas is ¼ tsp per 10 to 15 lb of body weight, or 60 to 75 mg/kg of body weight daily, divided into two doses.
- Not all hypothyroid patients manifest the classical clinical picture of coldness, lethargy, hair loss, inexplicable weight gains and bradycardia. Such symptoms are frequently poorly developed or absent, and the diagnosis is made in many clinics simply on the basis of low circulating thyroid hormone levels. Such a diagnosis should always be confirmed, ideally with a complete thyroid profile. Such profiles often assess not only T4 but also Free T4, T3, TSH, TgAA and anti-thyroid antibody levels. Concomittant assessment of Free T4 and TSH is a simpler but more crude screening test, with low Free T4 and high TSH levels suggesting hypothyroidism. As many as 20 to 40 percent of animals with low Free T4 and low TSH levels may also be genuinely hypothyroid, making this approach to testing less specific. In the remaining 60 to 80 percent of animals, low TSH with low T4 levels

suggest the hypothyroid state can be considered an adaptive response to a co-existing ailment.

- Adaptive hypothyroidism may be considered tantamount to taking one's foot off the gas pedal when a rattle is heard in the car. That is, reduction of metabolic rates by a reduction of circulating thyroid hormone levels in a disease state may help minimize cellular damage until the disorder is resolved. Clinical experience with Chinese medicine repeatedly suggests that the hypothyroid state in such cases can be spontaneously reversed without employing formulas for hypothyroidism per se. Instead, the improvements come when the underlying disorder from a Chinese medical perspective is successfully treated.
- In many dogs, the disorder associated with adaptive hypothyroidism is Liver Blood Deficiency. Various manifestations of this disorder include chronic active hepatitis, allergic dermatitis, hyperlipidemia, recurrent mast cell tumors, and inflammatory conditions of the gastric mucosa, just to name a few. Liver Blood deficiencies are correctly identified and treated with the appropriate herbal formula, animals receiving supplementation may suddenly become hyperthyroid, and need their thyroxine dose radically reduced or even discontinued.
- Sometimes a low level of thyroid hormone supplementation must be continued, and true hypothyroidism from lymphocytic of the thyroid is suspected to also be present. Consideration should be given to discontinuing vaccination in these animals, as links are increasingly made between the use of polyvalent vaccines and autoimmune inflammation of the thyroid gland.

AUTHORS' CHOICES:

SM: Address underlying conditions; use thyroid hormone supplementation only in truly hypothyroid cases.
SW: Thyroxine supplementation.

8 CASE REPORT

Hyperthyroidism in a Cat

HISTORY

Amadeus, a 7-year-old, neutered male Domestic shorthaired cat, presented with a chief complaint of early hyperthyroidism. His thyroxine levels were elevated at 3.3 (normal range is 0.8 to 2.6).

The problem was detected during a routine chemistry screen that was performed because of Amadeus's history of chronic vomiting. He would vomit at a variety of times, such as after defecation and after eating. The vomitus generally contained undigested food or food mixed with hair. A slimy fluid was also often present.

Minimal other laboratory abnormalities were present. His urine specific gravity level was adequate at 1.035, and his mean blood pressure was well within normal limits.

Mild clinical signs of hyperthyroidism were beginning to manifest themselves. Amadeus had an increased appetite that caused him to steal food from the other cats in the household and to become very agitated at meal times. Despite this Amadeus had lost a small but undetermined amount of weight, possibly because the owner had been trying to reduce his food intake. Amadeus was also making more frequent trips to the litter box to urinate, although the owner had not noticed an appreciable increase in water intake. Amadeus was also slightly irritable and aloof toward the other cats, and he exhibited a preference for cool places to rest.

His past medical history included a peripheral vestibular disturbance characterized by anisocoria, a head tilt to the right, atlantooccipital fixation, and possibly mild otitis. This condition resolved slowly over time with chiropractic support. Amadeus also had a small cataract in his left eye.

PHYSICAL EXAMINATION

Palpation of Amadeus's throat region in the region of the thyroid gland on the right side revealed a small mass perhaps 5 mm in diameter. His tongue was moist, pale, swollen and flabby with teeth imprints visible along its sides, and his pulses were slippery. Amadeus's heart rate was normal and varied between 150 and 192 beats per minute. He weighed 13 pounds and 10 ounces.

ASSESSMENT

From a conventional medical perspective, Amadeus was assessed as being in the very early stages of feline hyperthyroidism. From a Chinese medical perspective, Amadeus was considered to be in the first phase of feline hyperthyroidism. As outlined in the text, this is the phase associated with the initial accumulation of Dampness and Phlegm. Phlegm accumulation in the Stomach produces Stomach Qi rebellion, which results in chronic vomiting, often of a slimy material. As mentioned in Chapter 14, Phlegm accumulation in the Stomach is also considered an important cause of vestibular disorders, which had previously affected Amadeus. This Dampness accumulation was reflected in Amadeus by his swollen tongue and slippery pulses, and turbid Phlegm accumulations are thought to be a major cause of cataracts in small animals. When Phlegm accumulates in the Qi-rich Triple Burner channels, it produces a Phlegm-Fire that creates both the Heat signs of hyperthyroidism and a lump in the ventral or ventrolateral aspect of the neck.

TREATMENT

Amadeus was prescribed ¼ tsp of **Tao Hong Er Chen Tang** twice daily. No other treatment was provided. A follow-up examination was scheduled for 3 weeks later.

OUTCOME

After 3 weeks, Amadeus's thyroxine levels were within normal limits at 2.3.

After 7 weeks, Amadeus's thyroxine levels were still normal and the nodule on the right side in the region of the thyroid gland was no longer palpable. He had stopped vomiting, and it did not recur. His tongue remained pale and slightly swollen, but it was no longer moist. At this point Amadeus was prescribed Er Chen Tang, the base formula of Tao Hong Er Chen Tang. The formula was administered for 3 months.

Sixteen months after his initial visit, at the time of the last follow-up evaluation, Amadeus remained clinically normal.

DISCUSSION

This case illustrates a common clinical association between chronic vomiting and hyperthyroidism. Chinese herbal medicine allows prompt treatment of hyperthyroidism, while it is still in its earliest stages. Tao Hong Er Chen Tang seemed to halt progression of feline hyperthyroidism in this case so that the more advanced stage never developed. The formula seems to promote the regression of small thyroid tumors in some cats so that thyroid levels return to normal, and this should be subjected to further investigation.

SM

REFERENCES

Abdel-Barry JA, Abdel-Hassan IA, Al-Hakiem MH. Hypoglycaemic and antihyperglycaemic effects of *Trigonella foenum-graecum* leaf in normal and alloxan induced diabetic rats. *J Ethnopharmacol* 58:149-155, 1997.

Amri H, Drieu K, Papadopoulos V. Ex vivo regulation of adrenal cortical cell steroid and protein synthesis, in response to adrenocorticotropic hormone stimulation, by the *Ginkgo biloba* extract EGb 761 and isolated ginkgolide B. *Endocrinology* 138(12):5415-5426, 1997.

Auf'mkolk M, Ingbar JC, Kubota K, Amir SM, Ingbar SH. Extracts and auto-oxidized constituents of certain plants inhibit the receptor-binding and the biological activity of Graves' immunoglobulins. *Endocrinology* 116(5):1687-1693, 1985.

Bensky D, Gamble A. *Chinese Herbal Medicine Materia Medica,* revised ed. Seattle, 1993, Eastland Press.

Benvenga S, Ruggeri RM, Russo A, Lapa D, Campenni A, Trimarchi F. Usefulness of L-carnitine, a naturally occurring peripheral antagonist of thyroid hormone action, in iatrogenic hyperthyroidism: a randomized, double-blind, placebo-controlled clinical trial. *Clin Endocrinol Metab* 86(8):3579-3594, 2001.

Bonnefont-Rousselot D, Bastard JP, Jaudon MC, Delattre J. Consequences of the diabetic status on the oxidant/antioxidant balance. *Diabetes Metab* 26:163-176, 2000.

Brinker, F. Inhibition of endocrine runction by botanical agents, part I. *J Nat Med* 1:10-18, 1990.

Buffi O, Ciaroni S, Guidi L, Cecchini T, Bombardelli E. Morphological analysis on the adrenal zona fasciculata of Ginseng, Ginsenoside Rb1 and Ginsenoside Rg1 treated mice. *Boll Soc Ital Biol Sper* 69(12):791-797, 1993.

Chang SL, Lin JG, Chi TC, Liu IM, Cheng JT. An insulin-dependent hypoglycaemia induced by electroacupuncture at the Zhongwan (CV12) acupoint in diabetic rats. *Diabetologia* 42(2):250-255, 1999.

Chastain CB, Panciera D, Waters C. Effect of dietary insoluble fiber on control of glycemia in cats with naturally acquired diabetes mellitus. *Sm Anim Clin Endocrinol* 10:17, 2000.

Chattopadhyay RR. A comparative evaluation of some blood sugar lowering agents of plant origin. *J Ethnopharmacol* 67(3):367-372, 1999.

Cohn LA, Dodam JR, McCaw DL, Tate DJ. Effects of chromium supplementation on glucose tolerance in obese and nonobese cats. *Am J Vet Res* 60:1360-1363, 1999.

Cunningham JJ. Micronutrients as nutriceutical interventions in diabetes mellitus. *J Am Coll Nutr* 17:7-10, 1998.

Day C, Cartwright T, Provost J, Bailey CJ. Hypoglycaemic effect of *Momordica charantia* extracts. *Planta Med* 56:426-429, 1990.

Gerber H, Peter H, Ferguson PC, Peterson ME. Etiopathology of feline toxic nodular goitre. *Vet Clin North Am* 24:541-565, 1994.

Gerbi A, Maixent JM, Ansaldi JL, Pierlovisi M, Coste T, Pelissier JF, Vague D, Raccah D. Fish oil supplementation prevents diabetes-induced nerve conduction velocity and neuroanatomical changes in rats. *J Nutr* 129:207-213, 1999.

Gray AM, Flatt PR. Antihyperglycemic actions of *Eucalyptus globulus* (Eucalyptus) are associated with pancreatic and extra-pancreatic effects in mice. *J Nutr* 128(12):2319-2323, 1998.

Greco DS. *Treatment of feline diabetes mellitus (DM) with PZI and transition metals.* Presented at the American Association of Feline Practitioners Fall Meeting, Nashville, Tenn, October 16-19, 1999.

Hanninen A. Prevention of autoimmune type 1 diabetes via mucosal tolerance: is mucosal autoantigen administration as safe and effective as it should be? *Scand J Immunol* 52:217-225, 2000.

Hill A. Personal communication. School of Veterinary Medicine, University of California, Davis, 2000.

Kameswara Rao B, Giri R, Kesavulu MM, Apparao C. Effect of oral administration of bark extracts of *Pterocarpus santalinus* L. on blood glucose level in experimental animals. *J Ethnopharmacol* 74(1):69-74, 2001.

Khanna P, Jain SC, Panagariya A, Dixit VP. Hypoglycemic activity of polypeptide-p from a plant source. *J Nat Prod* 44:648-655, 1981.

Kimmel SE, Michel KE, Hess RS, Ward CR. Effects of insoluble and soluble dietary fiber on glycemic control in dogs with naturally occurring insulin-dependent diabetes mellitus. *J Am Vet Med Assoc* 216:1076-1081, 2000.

Krause I, Blank M, Shoenfeld Y. Immunomodulation of experimental autoimmune diseases via oral tolerance. *Crit Rev Immunol* 20:1-16, 2000.

Manickam M, Ramanathan M, Jahromi MA, Chansouria JP, Ray AB. Antihyperglycemic activity of phenolics from *Pterocarpus marsupium*. *J Nat Prod* 60(6):609-610, 1997.

Marcilhac A, Dakine N, Bourhim N, Guillaume V, Grino M, Drieu K, Oliver C. Effect of chronic administration of *Ginkgo biloba* extract or Ginkgolide on the hypothalamic-pituitary-adrenal axis in the rat. *Life Sci* 62(25):2329-2340, 1998.

Miura T, Kako M, Ishihara E, Usami M, Yano H, Tanigawa K, Sudo K, Seino Y. Antidiabetic effect of seishin-kanro-to in KK-Ay mice. *Planta Med* 63(4):320-322, 1997.

Mori Y, Murakawa Y, Yokoyama J, Tajima N, Ikeda Y, Nobukata H, Ishikawa T, Shibutani Y. Effect of highly purified eicosapentaenoic acid ethyl ester on insulin resistance and hypertension in Dahl salt-sensitive rats. *Metabolism* 48:1089-1095, 1999.

Nelson RW, Duesberg CA, Ford SL, Feldman EC, Davenport DJ, Keirnan C, Neal L. Effect of dietary insoluble fiber on control of glycemia in dogs with naturally acquired diabetes mellitus. *J Am Vet Med Assoc* 212:380-386, 1998.

Okuda Y, Mizutani M, Ogawa M, Sone H, Asano M, Asakura Y, Isaka M, Suzuki S, Kawakami Y, Field JB, Yamashita K. Long-term effects of eicosapentaenoic acid on diabetic peripheral neuropathy and serum lipids in patients with type II diabetes mellitus. *J Diabetes Complications* 10:280-287, 1996.

Paolisso G, Tagliamonte MR, Barbieri M, Zito GA, Gambardella A, Varricchio G, Ragno E, Varricchio M. Chronic vitamin E administration improves brachial reactivity and increases intracellular magnesium concentration in type II diabetic patients. *J Clin Endocrinol Metab* 85:109-115, 2000.

Paolisso G, Balbi V, Volpe C, Varricchio G, Gambardella A, Saccomanno F, Ammendola S, Varricchio M, D'Onofrio F. Metabolic benefits deriving from chronic vitamin C supplementation in aged non-insulin dependent diabetics. *J Am Coll Nutr* 14:387-392, 1995.

Persaud SJ, Al-Majed H, Raman A, Jones PM. *Gymnema sylvestre* stimulates insulin release in vitro by increased membrane permeability. *J Endocrinol* 163:207-212, 1999.

Petlevski R, Hadzija M, Slijepcevic M, Juretic D. Effect of "antidiabetis" herbal preparation on serum glucose and fructosamine in NOD mice. *J Ethnopharmacol* 75(2-3):181-184, 2001.

Podolin DA, Gayles EC, Wei Y, Thresher JS, Pagliassotti MJ. Menhaden oil prevents but does not reverse sucrose-induced insulin resistance in rats. *Am J Physiol* 274:R840-R848, 1998.

Ribes G, Sauvaire Y, Da Costa C, Baccou JC, Loubatieres-Mariani MM. Antidiabetic effects of subfractions from fenugreek seeds in diabetic dogs. *Proc Soc Exp Biol Med* 182:159-166, 1986.

Rose NR, Rasooly L, Saboori AM, Burek CL. Linking iodine with autoimmune thyroiditis. *Environ Health Perspect* 107 (Suppl 5):749-752, 1999.

Sarkar S, Pravana M, Marita R. Demonstration of the hypoglycemic action of *Momordica charantia* in a validated animal model of diabetes. *Pharmacol Res* 33:1-4, 1996.

Schachter S, Nelson RW, Kirk CA. Oral chromium picolinate and control of glycemia in insulin-treated diabetic dogs. *J Vet Intern Med* 15:379-384, 2001.

Shanmugasundaram ER, Gopinath KL, Radha Shanmugasundaram KR, Rajendran VM. Possible regeneration of the islets of Langerhans in streptozotocin-diabetic rats given *Gymnema sylvestre* leaf extracts. *J Ethnopharmacol* 30:265-279, 1990.

Shanmugasundaram KR, Panneerselvam C, Samudram P, Shanmugasundaram ER. Enzyme changes and glucose utilisation in diabetic rabbits: the effect of *Gymnema sylvestre*, R.Br. *J Ethnopharmacol* 7:205-234, 1983.

Shibib BA, Khan LA, Rahman R. Hypoglycemic activity of *Coccinia indica* and *Momordica charantia* in diabetic rats: depression of the hepatic gluconeogenic enzymes glucose-6-phosphatase and fructose-1,6-bisphosphatase and elevation of both liver and red-cell shunt enzyme glucose-6-phosphate dehydrogenase. *Biochem J* 292:267-270, 1993.

Singh A, Saxena E, Bhutani KK. Adrenocorticosterone alterations in male, albino mice treated with *Trichopus zeylanicus, Withania somnifera* and *Panax ginseng* preparations. *Phytother Res* 14(2):122-125, 2000.

Sloley BD, Urichuk LJ, Morley P, Durkin J, Shan JJ, Pang PK, Coutts RT. Identification of kaempferol as a monoamine oxidase inhibitor and potential neuroprotectant in extracts of *Ginkgo biloba* leaves. *J Pharm Pharmacol* 52(4):451-459, 2000.

Sotaniemi EA, Haapakoski E, Rautio A. Ginseng therapy in non-insulin-dependent diabetic patients. *Diabetes Care* 18:1373-1375, 1995.

Stiefel P, Ruiz-Gutierrez V, Gajon E, Acosta D, Garcia-Donas MA, Madrazo J, Villar J, Carneado J. Sodium transport kinetics, cell membrane lipid composition, neural conduction and metabolic control in type 1 diabetic patients: changes after a low-dose n-3 fatty acid dietary interventions. *Ann Nutr Metab* 43:113-120, 1999.

Sunvold GD, Bouchard GF. Assessment of obesity and associated metabolic disorders. In *Recent Advances in Canine and Feline Nutrition Volume II*. Wilmington, Ohio, 1998, Orange Frazer Press.

Swanston-Flatt SK, Day C, Flatt PR, Gould BJ, Bailey CJ. Glycaemic effects of traditional European plant treatments for diabetes: studies in normal and streptozotocin diabetic mice. *Diabetes Res* (2):69-73, 1989.

Vuksan V, Stavro MP, Sievenpiper JL, Beljan-Zdravkovic U, Leiter LA, Josse RG, Xu A. Similar postprandial glycemic reductions with escalation of dose and administration time of American ginseng in type 2 diabetes. *Diabetes Care* 23:1221-1226, 2000.

Winterhoff H, Gumbinger HG, Vahlensieck U, Kemper FH, Schmitz H, Behnke B. Endocrine effects of *Lycopus europaeus* L. following oral application. *Arzneimittelforschung* 44(1):41-45, 1994.

Yan W. *Practical Therapeutics of Traditional Chinese Medicine*. Brookline, Mass, 1997, Paradigm Publications.

Yeung H. *Handbook of Chinese Herbal Formulas*. Los Angeles, 1995, Self-published.

Yeung H. *Handbook of Chinese Herbs*. Los Angeles, 1996, Self-published.

Ziegler D, Hanefeld M, Ruhnau KJ, Hasche H, Lobisch M, Schutte K, Kerum G, Malessa R. Treatment of symptomatic diabetic polyneuropathy with the antioxidant alpha-lipoic acid: a 7-month multicenter randomized controlled trial (ALADIN III Study). ALADIN III Study Group. Alpha-Lipoic Acid in Diabetic Neuropathy. *Diabetes Care* 22:1296-1301, 1999.

9

Therapies for Hematologic and Immunologic Disorders

ANEMIA (INCLUDING AUTOIMMUNE HEMOLYTIC ANEMIA)

Therapeutic Rationale

- Reduce immune-mediated or other destruction if it is present.
- Identify other disorders that have indirect effects on hemopoiesis, such as kidney disease or chronic disorders.
- Supplement deficient iron.
- Stimulate hemopoiesis.

Alternative Options with Conventional Bases

- **Dehydroepiandrosterone (DHEA)** levels are reduced in many autoimmune diseases (de la Torre, 1995), and DHEA is thought to be beneficial as an adjunct in managing autoimmune diseases such as lupus and rheumatoid arthritis. It may also reduce the adverse effects of glucocorticoid administration (Robinzon, 1999).
- **Dang Qui** *(Angelica sinensis):* a traditional Chinese Blood-tonic herb. A case report in a human kidney patient with anemia who was resistant to erythropoietin treatment indicated that treatment with this herb improved hematologic measures (Bradley, 1999).
- **Ten Significant Tonic Decoction (Shi Quan Da Bu Tang):** has been shown to stimulate hemopoietic factors in animal and clinical studies (Zee-Cheng, 1992).
- **Sheng Mai San,** a formula containing Ginseng *(Panax ginseng)*, Ophiopogon *(Ophiopogon japonicus)*, and

Schisandra *(Schisandra chinensis)* was administered by injection to mice with induced aplastic anemia. This combination of Chinese herbs increased erythroid progenitor cells in injected mice when compared with control mice (Liu, 2001).

Paradigmatic Options

- Anemia often manifests as either primary or secondary Blood deficiency during Chinese medical evaluations of affected patients. Primary Blood deficiency is more common in animals that are dependent on a heavy blood supply, such as canines, and a large number of chronic canine health problems that are of great concern to veterinary practitioners can be successfully treated with formulas that nourish Blood.
- Secondary Blood deficiency is more common in felines than primary Blood deficiency, and it is also commonly encountered in dogs. It arises when the Spleen Qi that is needed to manufacture Blood is deficient. Adequate Spleen function is dependent on adequate Kidney function, since the Kidney acts as the "fire" under the "cooking pot" of the Spleen. Thus both Spleen Qi and Kidney Qi tonics can be used to correct anemia caused by Qi deficiency.
- Chinese medicine is replete with formulas that nourish Qi and Blood. There are far too many to review comprehensively in this chapter, but a handful seem of particular importance in the daily practice of veterinary medicine and are reviewed below. A *suggested starting dose* of granular concentrate of all the formulas listed below is ¼ tsp per 10 to 15 lb of body weight, or 60 to 75 mg/kg of body weight, divided into two daily doses.

Blood Tonic Formulas

- Most Blood tonic formulas contain or are based on a small formula known as **Si Wu Tang** (Four Materials Decoction). Its four constituent herbs, Bai Shao, Chuan Xiong, Shu Di Huang, and Dang Gui, act together to nourish and move Blood. A more comprehensive formula to nourish Blood and Yin is **Bu Gan Tang**

(Nourish the Liver Decoction). The Liver is the main Blood-storage organ in Chinese medicine. Either of these formulas may be used for simple Blood-deficiency anemia, although Bu Gan Tang has more specific symptomatic indications for its use, including muscle stiffness and spasm and insomnia. Both formulas address the usual picture of Blood deficiency in dogs, including fear aggression, a dry lusterless coat, poor hair regrowth, fine, powdery dander, a thin, wiry pulse, and a pale or lavender tongue.

- **Yi Guan Jian** (One Linking Decoction) is a milder formula to nourish Liver Blood and Yin. It was originally developed to address Liver-Stomach disharmonies, but its use has been widened to include almost any Blood deficiency syndrome when Dampness is not present. Significant amounts of Dampness in a patient preclude use of stronger Blood tonic formulas unless Dampness-draining herbs are added. Yi Guan Jian might be a more appropriate Blood tonic for patients that show evidence of Yin deficiency and Empty Heat such as age-related symptoms, thirst, nighttime restlessness, a tendency to lose weight, poor appetite, dry coat, eating grass, hind end weakness, chronic vomiting, and heat intolerance. When Dampness is suspected but not confirmed, Yi Guan Jian is slightly less likely to produce side effects than Bu Gan Tang.

Spleen Qi Tonic Formulas

- When Spleen Qi deficiency is suspected to have caused Liver Blood deficiency, perhaps manifesting with chronic active hepatitis, skin dryness, eructation, undigested food in the stool, poor appetite, soft pulses, and a pale or lavender tongue, **Xiao Yao San** (Rambling Ease Powder) can be considered.
- The preeminent formula to nourish Blood through Qi tonification is **Dang Gui Bu Xue Tang** (Angelica Nourish Blood Decoction). The name of the formula notwithstanding, the chief ingredient is Huang Qi or Astragalus, which is a Spleen tonic that is used in a 5:1 ratio with Dang Gui. This formula is called for when

signs of Liver involvement are not as evident as in cases calling for Xiao Yao San. Guiding symptoms include fatigue, pallor, a tendency to recurrent infections, a pale tongue, and a soft or otherwise feeble pulse. Adding the Blood tonics Shu Di Huang, He Shou Wu, Sang Ji Sheng, and Bai Shao Yao can enhance the formula's action against anemia.

- Several formulas incorporate **Dang Gui Bu Xue Tang's** dynamic within them, including **Gui Pi Tang** (Restore the Spleen Decoction) and **Bu Zhong Yi Qi Tang** (Nourish the Center and Raise the Qi Decoction). Gui Pi Tang is more suited to patients that exhibit evidence of an agitated Heart secondary to Blood and Yin deficiency such as insomnia, vivid dreaming, and anxiety, and that also show signs of Spleen deficiency such as a pale tongue and soft, weak pulses. Bu Zhong Yi Qi Tang is of more benefit to the patient with a typical case of anemia from a conventional point of view. Symptoms of this condition are shortness of breath, fatigue, chills, poor appetite, a pale tongue, and a feeble, soft, or spreading pulse. There may also be indications of organ prolapse or Qi collapse such as perineal hernias, flaccid abdominal distention, and urinary incontinence.

Kidney Tonic Formulas

- Kidney Essence is the foundation of all fluid reserves in the body, including Blood. When the depletion of Kidney Yin and Essence results in anemia in an aged animal with thirst, nighttime restlessness, hind limb weakness, cognitive deficiencies, a tendency to lose weight, deafness, dryness, and heat intolerance, **Zuo Gui Wan** (Restore the Left Pill) can be considered. The animal has a thready and rapid pulse, and the tongue may appear tender, dry, and red.
- When Kidney Qi deficiency manifests with chilliness, profuse, clear urine, renal azotemia, hind limb weakness, deafness, and anemia associated with reduced renal erythropoietin synthesis, **Shen Qi Wan** (Kidney Qi Pill) can be used.
- When there is evidence of Qi, Blood, and Yang deficiency in roughly equal portions, **Shi Quan Da Bu**

Tang (Decoction of Ten Ingredients for Complete Tonification) can be considered. Guiding symptoms include a weak pulse, a pale tongue, fatigue, cold intolerance, shortness of breath, undigested food in the stool, poor appetite, and anemia.

- **Sheng Mai San** (Generate the Pulse Powder) is advocated for cases of Qi and Yin deficiency. Guiding symptoms include a dry tongue, a feeble, weak pulse, fatigue, thirst, heat intolerance, poor appetite, and chilliness. This formula is an "emergency formula," available in China in injectable form for use in crises and in patients after a severe febrile episode has passed.

Acupuncture

- Points to directly nourish Liver Blood include LIV 3, BL 17, BL 18, and SP 6. Points to nourish Blood through tonification of Spleen Qi include ST 36, LI 4, CV 12, and BL 20. Points to nourish Blood through Kidney Qi tonification include KI 3, BL 23, and CV 4. Indirect moxa can be used to warm all of these points.

Western Herbs

- **Yellow Dock** *(Rumex crispus):* has a reputation as an iron source of high bioavailability.
- **New Jersey Tea** *(Ceanothus americanus):* is reputed to reduce splenomegaly associated with hemolytic anemia.
- **Barberry** *(Berberis vulgaris):* may induce splenic contraction and thereby increase platelet counts.

Cautions

- If immunosuppressive therapy is used for an autoimmune cause, it is theoretically best to avoid immunostimulants such as Ginseng, Astragalus *(Astragalus membranaceus)*, and medicinal Mushrooms *(Ganoderma lucidum, Grifola frondosa,* and others). These herbs may be part of well-indicated Chinese herbal formulas, however, so the animal's clinical condition and need for adjunctive treatments must be carefully weighed in deciding to use them.

AUTHORS' CHOICES:

SM: Identify causes of occult blood loss; use appropriate herbal formula.
SW: Identify causes and treat conventionally when appropriate; Angelica sinensis or well-chosen Chinese herbal combinations.

AUTOIMMUNE DISORDERS, GENERAL

Therapeutic Rationale

- Reduce inflammation and tissue destruction at target organs.
- Modulate the inappropriate immune response.

Alternative Options with Conventional Bases

Nutritional Therapies

- **Restricted protein and calories:** patients with autoimmune disease may benefit from restrictions in protein and calories (Keen, 1991; Leiba, 2001). On the other hand, anecdotal reports of improvement when dogs or cats are given homemade diets with higher meat contents are also encouraging. Lipid restriction has also been recommended; however, investigators are focusing increasingly on fatty acid type and balance (see paragraph on fatty acids below).
- **Hypoallergenic diets:** often recommended in managing autoimmune and immune-mediated disease. This is not because of a belief that these diseases are allergic in origin but is rather based on a theory called Leaky Gut Syndrome. In Leaky Gut the mucosal lining of the gut is made hyperpermeable through a number of mechanisms, including the administration of drugs that cause gastrointestinal (GI) inflammation (nonsteroidal antiinflammatory drugs, prednisone, etc.), chronic toxin ingestion, or true food allergy. An inflamed gut is theoretically incapable of maintaining normal active transport mechanisms because carrier proteins and cellular pumps may be damaged. Hyperpermeability of gap junctions also allows abnormal absorption of

macromolecules such as proteins, glycoproteins, polysaccharides, and even microorganisms that are highly allergenic. These molecules may be absorbed systemically and contribute to immune reactivity and deposition of immune complexes. Since food proteins may be part of the problem in Leaky Gut, using hypoallergenic diets may help reduce generalized immune activation and, consequently, clinical signs.

- **Probiotics:** beneficial bacteria that have been shown to modulate immune responses in laboratory animals and people. Some advocates believe that administration of probiotics can dampen the inflammatory processes in autoimmune disease in particular (Maassen, 1998; Matsuzaki, 2000). Most studies involve a variety of *Lactobacillus* spp., and a few involve *Streptococcus, Bifidobacteria, and Saccharomyces* spp. The optimal species and dose for influencing immune responses in companion animals are unknown. We recommend high doses (a human dose for a 20-lb dog, for instance) because of the uneven quality control in this group of supplements. A recent study analyzing label claims for products found that very few contained what their labels claimed; one product that fulfilled its label's claims for activity was Culturelle (http://www.culturelle.com) (Weese, 2002). This product has been used with good results in my (SW) practice.
- **Antioxidants:** may help reduce inflammation in immune-mediated disease and are frequently used as part of a treatment protocol. The role of reactive oxygen species (free radicals) in the generation and maintenance of autoimmune disease is unknown (Bauer, 1999), but they are suspected to contribute to pathologic conditions.
- **Fatty acid supplementation:** diets low in fat or high in fish oils increase survival and reduce severity in spontaneous autoantibody-mediated disease. Diets rich in linoleic acid (an ω-6 fatty acid) appear to augment severity in antibody-mediated autoimmune diseases. In T-cell–mediated autoimmune disease, diets supplemented with ω-3 fatty acids increase disease symptoms, whereas ω-6 fatty acids prevent or reduce the severity of symptoms (Harbige, 1998). Fish Oil may

have other beneficial effects because it tends to block production of inflammatory cytokines. In summary, evidence at present appears to support supplements of ω-6 fatty acids for autoimmune disease characterized by cell-mediated pathology, and supplements of ω-3 fatty acids when antibody-mediated pathology predominates.

Other

- **DHEA** levels are reduced in many autoimmune diseases (de la Torre, 1995), and DHEA is thought to be beneficial as an adjunct in managing autoimmune diseases such as lupus and rheumatoid arthritis. It may also reduce the adverse effects of glucocorticoid administration (Robinzon, 1999).

Paradigmatic Options

- See Chapter 5 for information on Pemphigus Foliaceus.
- Autoimmune hemolytic anemia (AIHA) remains a challenge to Chinese medical veterinary practitioners. No formula has been identified that will consistently stop and prevent hemolytic crises. At this time comanagement with prednisone, at least in the acute stages and until the patient is stable, is the most prudent recommendation.
- Some progress has been made in understanding the pathogenesis of AIHA from a Chinese medical perspective. The condition is complex and multifactorial, but appears to be a Damp-Heat condition compounded by latent tendencies to Blood stasis and Blood deficiency. Dampness accumulations obstruct blood flow, producing organomegaly. Blood deficiency increases the tendency of Blood to "pool," which leads to Blood stasis. Vaccines and various drugs that seem to act as Damp- or Toxic-Heat pathogens in the body directly contribute to and trigger episodes of Blood stasis and Damp-Heat accumulation. Blood stasis aggravates Blood deficiency and the patient enters a self-perpetuating state of anemic crisis.
- Some new formulas are proposed here for experimental use in treating AIHA based on the preceding theory of pathogenesis. A potentially valuable formula can be made from **Xi Jiao Di Huang Tang** (Decoction

of Rhinoceros Horn and Rehmannia). The practitioner combines 100 g of this formula with 12 to 15 g each of Da Huang and Huang Qin. Rhinoceros Horn is never used in modern versions of the formula but is replaced by Shui Niu Jiao (Water Buffalo Horn) obtained from a domesticated species. Alternatively, Bai Mao Gen (*Imperata* spp.) is used if Shui Niu Jiao is unavailable. Bai Mao Gen should make up 30% of the formula by weight. Xi Jiao Di Huang Tang acts to clear pathogenic Heat from the Blood and cools and moves Blood. Da Huang moves Blood and clears Damp Heat and Toxic Heat. It may also have a protective effect against further hemolysis, since Da Huang is known to interfere with immune-mediated cross-reactions against the major human blood group antigens. Huang Qin aids in the clearing of Damp Heat and Toxic Heat. One caution is that addition of Da Huang to the formula may produce diarrhea. A *suggested starting dose* of granular concentrate is a minimum of ¼ tsp per 10 to 15 lb of body weight, or 60 to 75 mg/kg of body weight, given at least once daily. This formula may be very difficult to obtain in North America.

- A formula that is similar to Xi Jiao Di Huang Tang but is broader in impact is **Qing Ying Tang** (Clear the Nutritive Level Decoction). This formula may be the overall best choice for managing acute AIHA. This formula normally contains Rhinoceros Horn or Water Buffalo Horn. Since both of these are not readily available in North America, Bai Mao Gen *(Imperata)* may be safely substituted. The ingredients of the formula I use in my (SM) clinic are listed below. Da Huang and Zi Cao Gen are added to cool and move Blood and clear Toxic Heat.

  30 g Bai Mao Gen
  12 g Sheng Di Huang
  6 g Mai Men Dong
  9 g Huang Lian
  9 g Xuan Shen
  9 g Dan Zhu Ye
  9 g Lian Qiao
  9 g Dan Shen
  9 g Jin Yin Hua

15 g Da Huang
15 g Zi Cao Gen

My early experience with this formula suggests that it can rapidly stabilize AIHA patients, minimizing required steroid use to just the first day or two, and promoting more rapid and complete rises in the hematocrit values in recovering patients. In addition, the particulars of its complex design suggest that it may be of particular value in vaccine-induced hemolytic crises. A suggested starting dose of granular concentrate is a minimum of b tsp per 10 to 15 lb of body weight, or 60 to 75 mg/kg of body weight, given three times daily.

- Another formula that may be considered in acute outbreaks when signs of jaundice, debility, and fever are more prominent than signs of anemia is **An Gong Niu Huang Wan** (Bezoar Resurrection Pills). This formula is also especially appropriate for the early stages of vaccine- and drug-induced cases. The Niu Huang in the formula increases red blood cell count and mean cell hemoglobin concentration, but the mercury compounds and gold salts the formula contains make it potentially toxic. The formula is very strong and should be used only in peracute cases. Da Huang may be added to the formula to enhance its Heat-clearing and erythrocyte-protective effects. Versions of the formula in which Xi Jiao has not been replaced with Shui Niu Jiao or Bai Mao Gen should be avoided. A *suggested starting dose* is one pill daily for a 20-lb dog, two pills daily for a 60-lb dog, and three pills daily for a 100-lb dog. This formula may be very difficult to obtain in North America.
- Once a hemolytic crisis has passed, formulas and preventive measures should be used to reduce latent levels of Damp Heat in the body and ensure that Blood deficiency and stasis are not apparent. Raw food diets in animals with moderate to strong pulses should be considered provided the diet is not allergenic for the animal. Restriction of carbohydrates should be contemplated because of their dampening influence. All food allergens should be avoided because they frequently manifest as Dampness and Phlegm accumulations.

- One formula to consider between bouts is **Yin Chen Wu Ling San** (Capillaris and Five Ingredient Powder with Poria). The practitioner can add 6 g of Da Huang and 9 g each of Dang Gui, Bai Shao, and Chuan Xiong to 70 g of the base formula to create a formula that also embodies and improves on **Dang Gui Shao Yao San** (Angelica and Peony Powder), which showed early promise in my practice (SM) in resolving subacute and chronic cases but was not powerful enough to prevent further relapses. A *suggested starting dose* of granular concentrate is ¼ tsp per 10 to 15 lb of body weight, or 60 to 75 mg/kg of body weight, given at least once daily.
- A final but important note: herbs high in saponin content may theoretically cause hemolysis if large amounts of saponins are absorbed from the GI tract. This risk has not yet been documented to our knowledge. Some such herbs are San Qi *(Panax notoginseng)*, Astragalus, Black Cohosh *(Actea racemosa)*, Licorice *(Glycyrrhiza glabra)*, Ginseng, and Pokeroot *(Phytolacca americana)*.

Acupuncture

- Acupuncture points to support cooling the Blood and clearing of Damp Heat in affected animals are GV 14, LI 4, BL 40, LI 11, SP 9, BL 22, CV 3, and BL 25. Blood tonification points in chronic cases include BL 17, BL 18, BL 20, SP 10, ST 36, LI 4, CV 12, CV 6, LIV 3, and SP 6.

Cautions

- Immunostimulating herbs such as Ginseng, Mushrooms, Echinacea *(Echinacea* spp.), and Astragalus should be used with caution if immunosuppressant therapy is being administered.

AUTHORS' CHOICES:

SM: Chinese herbal formulas; avoid food allergens; cease vaccination; avoid pharmaceuticals known to trigger AIHA; concurrent use of immunosuppressives when necessary.

SW: Hypoallergenic diet; cease vaccination; probiotic; antioxidants; fish oil; appropriately chosen Chinese herbs and acupuncture; immunosuppressive therapy when necessary.

COAGULOPATHY

Therapeutic Rationale

- Identify specific clotting defect and treat accordingly.

Alternative Options with Conventional Bases

- **Yunnan Bai Yao** (White Medicine from Yunnan Province): the most popular Chinese herbal formula in veterinary medicine for the control of hemorrhage. The "formula" contains only San Qi *(Panax notoginseng)*, an herb that has a reputation for being able to stop bleeding anywhere in the body. Yunnan Bai Yao has been shown to decrease both clotting times and prothrombin times (Ogle, 1977) and to initiate platelet release (Chew, 1977). It should be administered in heavy doses of 75 to 100 mg/kg of body weight daily of granular concentrate, given in divided doses, or as one tablet per 10 lb of body weight daily, given in divided doses if possible.

Paradigmatic Options

- The comments below on coagulopathies also apply to immune-mediated thrombocytopenia (ITP). Additional comments on ITP are included in a separate section later in the chapter.
- Formulas to address bleeding in specific organs are discussed in the chapters addressing each organ system. In addition, some formulas for bleeding in specific locations are mentioned below. A *suggested starting dose* of granular concentrate for all of these formulas is ¼ tsp per 10 to 15 lb of body weight, or 60 to 75 mg/kg of body weight, given at least once daily.
- For hematuria caused by Damp Heat in the bladder, **Xiao Ji Yin Zi** (Cephalanoplos Beverage) may be used. This formula cools Blood and Heart Fire, clears Damp Heat in the bladder, and stops bleeding.
- **Ning Xue Tang** (Quiet the Blood Decoction) can be used for hemorrhage in the anterior chamber of the eye. This formula may be slightly more appropriate in animals with Empty Heat conditions, but it is basically a hemostatic.

- **Si Sheng Wan** (Four Fresh Herbs Pill) can be used for epistaxis. This formula cools Blood and stops bleeding, especially in the upper body.
- For gastrointestinal hemorrhage associated with Damp Heat accumulation, **Di Yu San** (Sanguisorba Powder) can be considered. The formula is vigorously cooling and should be used only for excess conditions. It is a good formula for GI ulceration.
- Formulas to address systemic tendencies to bleeding that may be manifested in any organ fall into three types: those that address hemorrhage caused by Excess Heat agitating the blood, those that address hemorrhage that arises from Blood stasis, and those that address bleeding caused by a failure of Spleen Qi to hold blood in the vessels.
- For bleeding associated with Empty Fire, **Da Bu Yin Wan** (Great Nourish the Yin Decoction) can be considered. This formula strongly nourishes Yin and clears Empty Heat. Huang Bai provides much of the cooling action and has been credited with a protective effect on platelet integrity.
- For bleeding associated with Heat in the Blood that shows no evidence of Damp Heat and only a mild suggestion of Empty Heat, **Xi Jiao Di Huang Tang** (Decoction of Rhinoceros Horn and Rehmannia) can be considered. Rhinoceros Horn is never used in modern versions of the formula but is replaced by Shui Niu Jiao (Water Buffalo Horn) obtained from a domesticated species. Xi Jiao Di Huang Tang acts to clear pathogenic Heat from the Blood and to cool and move Blood. This formula may be very difficult to obtain in North America.
- For coagulopathies arising from Blood stasis, caution is needed in using typical Blood movers. Formulas with significant quantities of Bai Shao, Dan Shen, and Chuan Xiong should be avoided because these three herbs inhibit platelet aggregation. Dang Gui is a hemostatic and Blood mover and should be safe to use. Yunnan Bai Yao has mild Blood-moving properties and is suited to these cases.
- **Bu Zhong Yi Qi Tang** (Tonify the Center to Boost the Qi Decoction) is the main formula to arrest bleeding caused by Spleen Qi deficiency.

Western Herbs

- **Liquid extracts** of the following herbs can be used to create a formula to control gastrointestinal hemorrhage: 15 ml Agrimony *(Agrimonia eupatoria)*, 15 ml Cranesbill *(Geranium maculatum)*, 10 ml Prickly Ash Bark *(Xanthoxylum* spp., especially *X. americanum)*, and 10 ml Marshmallow *(Althaea officinalis)*.
- **Nettles** (*Urtica dioica*): have historically been used for Damp Heat that causes epistaxis or dysentery.
- **Yarrow** *(Achillea millefolium)*: has a reputation as a hemostatic in conditions of Blood stasis.
- For all of these herbs a *suggested starting dose* is 0.2 ml of liquid extract per 5 lb of body weight given at least once daily.

AUTHORS' CHOICES:

SM: Western formula for GI hemorrhage; San Qi; Dang Gui; Da Bu Yin Wan in appropriate cases.
SW: Yunnan Bai Yao; other herbs as appropriate for system-specific signs.

HYPERLIPIDEMIA

Therapeutic Rationale

- Identify predisposing factors such as endocrinologic disorders, liver disease, and pancreatitis.
- Reduce dietary fat.
- Clear excess serum lipids.

Alternative Options with Conventional Bases

Nutritional Therapies

- **Marine Fish Oil:** epidemiologic and some experimental evidence in humans shows that ω-3 polyunsaturated fatty acids reduce triglyceride and cholesterol levels. The dose used in people is 3.6 g of total fatty acids composed of eicosapentaenoic acid (EPA) and docosahexanoic acid (DHA). This is equivalent to approximately 100 mg/kg of body weight of total fatty acids (not Fish Oil) for dogs.

- **Niacin:** reduces triglyceride levels in people (Tavintharan, 2001) but is not without side effects. The dose used in people is 1.5 to 6 g daily in divided doses. The dose equivalent for dogs is approximately 15 to 75 mg/lb of body weight in divided doses daily.

Herbs

- **Garlic** *(Allium sativum):* has shown modest efficacy in lowering cholesterol and triglyceride levels in laboratory animals and people (Ackermann, 2001). Garlic has potential for causing Heinz-body anemia in dogs and especially in cats. Many veterinarians use garlic for their patients and monitor blood parameters. Garlic therapy can be attempted at a dose of one clove per 40 lb of animal, or 10 to 30 mg/lb of body weight of the common brand Kyolic.
- **Red Yeast Rice** *(Monascus purpureus):* has been shown to reduce cholesterol and triacylglycerol concentrations in controlled trials in humans (Heber, 1999). The calculated proportional *dose* for dogs is 30 mg/lb once daily.
- **Guggulipid** *(Commiphora mukul):* contains resins that have been shown to have cholesterol- and triglyceride-lowering activity in humans (Singh, 1994) and laboratory animals. However, the overall effect is mild to moderate compared with cholesterol-lowering drugs used in people (Caron, 2001). The calculated *dose* based on recommendations for humans is approximately 0.2 to 0.3 mg/lb tid.

Paradigmatic Options

- Hyperlipidemia is commonly associated with an underlying Blood deficiency in Chinese medicine. There is also an associated Dampness that suggests a Liver-Spleen disharmony in which the Liver impairs normal production of Blood and Fluids by the Spleen. **Dang Gui Shao Yao San** (Angelica and Peony Powder) addresses this dynamic well in the majority of cases. The ability of the formula to specifically address hyperlipidemia and hypercholesterolemia is endowed by its content of Ze Xie and can be enhanced by adding any or all of Shan Zha, Dan Shen, and Chai Hu. Each additive should make up no more than 10% to 15% of the final formula. These herbs assist the main body of the formula in nourishing Blood and soothing the Blood-impoverished Liver, and they have a documented ability to lower blood cholesterol. Patients that benefit from this formula may have soft, slippery, or wiry pulses, a pale tongue, anxiety, a greasy coat, alopecia or poor hair regrowth, elevated liver and pancreatic enzyme levels, poor appetite, mucoid stools, and undigested food in the stool. A *suggested starting dose* is 60 to 75 mg/kg of body weight daily in divided doses.

- Individual herbs that can be "woven" into other formulas to help reduce blood cholesterol and lipid levels include He Shou Wu, Shan Zha, Ze Xie, Da Huang, Jue Ming Zi, Chai Hu, and Dan Shen. He Shou Wu and Dan Shen are used by themselves as small formulas in Chinese medicine and are available as **Shou Wu Pian** and **Dan Shen Pian,** respectively. Shan Zha is Hawthorn *(Crataegus oxycantha)* and is used by itself at times in Western herbal medicine. Ze Xie, Da Huang, and Chai Hu are too strong to be prudently used alone. A *suggested starting dose* is one tablet per 10 lb of body weight, divided into two daily doses.
- It is conceivable that a purely Damp Heat case of hyperlipidemia may be encountered that shows no evidence of Blood deficiency. In such a case **Yin Chen Wu Ling San** (Capillaris and Five Herbs with Poria Powder) might be appropriate. This formula contains Yin Chen Hao and Ze Xie, both of which lower serum lipids and cholesterol. A *suggested starting dose* is 60 to 70 mg/kg of body weight daily in divided doses.

Cautions

- Herbs and nutritional supplements may have additive effects with lipid-lowering drugs.

AUTHORS' CHOICES:

SM: Dang Gui Shao Yao San with Chai Hu and Shan Zha added.
SW: Niacin, Fish Oil, Guggulipid; Red Yeast Rice.

IMMUNOSUPPRESSION

Therapeutic Rationale

- Identify causative factors (e.g., retroviral or other chronic disorders).

Alternative Options with Conventional Bases

- Immunodeficiency syndromes are associated with retroviral infections such as feline immunodeficiency virus (FIV), feline leukemia virus (FeLV), demodectic mange, and other chronic disorders. In some cases these syndromes may reflect a disturbance in the balance of immune function rather than a deficiency of all functions. We do not understand enough of the immune milieu to address individual mechanisms, so some caution is advised with wholesale immunostimulation.

Nutritional Therapies

- **Vitamin A:** deficiency is associated with immune function defects. Supplementation enhances immune responses in a variety of clinical trial situations in people and may beneficially influence cell-mediated immune function (Semba, 1999).
- **Vitamin E:** supplementation has improved humoral and cellular immune function in a variety of trials in people (Moriguchi, 2000).
- **Vitamin C:** deficiencies are associated with depressed nonspecific immunity. Supplementation improves humoral and cellular responses in many animal species.
- **Minerals:** supplementation of zinc and selenium improves response to vaccination and may reduce infection rates.
- **Carotenoids:** lutein increases delayed-type hypersensitivity response to specific and nonspecific antigens in cats and dogs (Kim, 1999, 2000). Beta-carotene enhances cell-mediated and humoral immune responses in dogs (Chew, 2000).
- **Amino acids:** arginine and possibly glutamine are associated with improved immune function and lower infection rates (Field, 2000; Heyland, 2001).

- **Conjugated linolenic acid:** increases interleukin (IL-2) and T-lymphocyte activity, decreases immunoglobulin E levels, and increases immunoglobulin G levels in a few laboratory animal and in vitro studies.

Herbs

- **Immunostimulant herbs:** include Echinacea *(Echinacea purpurea, E. angustifolia, E. pallida)*, Astragalus, Ginseng *(Panax* spp.), and medicinal fungi including Reishi mushroom *(Ganoderma lucidum)*, Maitake mushroom *(Grifola frondosa)*, Shiitake mushroom *(Lentinus edodes)*, Turkey Tail *(Trametes versicolor)*, and Cordyceps fungus *(Cordyceps sinensis)*.
- **Echinacea:** extracts have been shown to increase phagocytic activity in human peripheral monocytic cells, increase production of various cytokines, and increase natural killer cell function, all of which are parts of the innate immune system as opposed to specific, antigen-mediated processes. Most clinical studies in humans have involved upper respiratory infections, and Echinacea appears to shorten the duration of the common cold (Percival, 2000). A blend of different Echinacea species is advisable at this time, since each possesses different antimicrobial and immune-stimulating properties. Echinacea is often recommended for chronic recurrent viral upper respiratory infections in cats, and some practitioners use Echinacea in retroviral infections. Although some practitioners caution against long-term use of Echinacea because toxicity or autoimmune conditions may result, this concern is not well documented. However, immunostimulants are probably best used as pulsed treatments, since full response to treatment is probably reached in a few weeks and does not continue to increase. Short-term (2- to 4-week), on-off administration is most sensible.
- **Astragalus:** a traditional Chinese herb that has been shown to increase T-cell–mediated immune functions in vitro, in mice, and in uncontrolled trials in humans (Sun, 1983; Yoshida, 1997; Zhao, 1990). It has also been shown to enhance phagocytosis, increase macrophage numbers, and enhance humoral immunity (Yeung, 1996).

- **Ginseng** polysaccharides and saponins: have shown immunostimulating capacity in vitro and in animal models (Kitts, 2000). In one study, rats with chronic *Pseudomonas aeruginosa* lung infections were administered extracts of *Panax ginseng* and the treated group exhibited higher bacterial clearance and lower serum immunoglobulin levels than the untreated group, which suggests enhancement of cell-mediated immunity (Song, 1998).
- **Medicinal fungi:** Reishi, Maitake, Shiitake, Cordyceps, and Turkey Tail are likely to show similar pharmacologic activities. All contain polysaccharide complexes and sterols that appear to enhance cell-mediated immune functions and that may have antitumor activity as well (Ooi, 2000; Wasser, 1999; Zhu, 1998). As a rule, polysaccharide complexes such as are found in some species of Echinacea and in medicinal fungi are more likely to be completely extracted in aqueous or dried preparations than in alcohol extracts.
- **Sterols/sterolins:** According to a preliminary study of FIV-infected cats these may improve TH1/TH2 ratio and they have been shown to improve neurokinin (NK) and T-cell function (Bouic, 1997). TH1 cells are a subset of T-helper (CD4+) lymphocytes that participate in the cellular immune response, and TH2 cells are the subset that support antibody-mediated immune responses.

Paradigmatic Options

- The holistic practitioner is commonly requested to stimulate the immune system of animals that have generalized demodicosis and recurrent superficial pyoderma. Consult Chapter 5 for information about these problems. Most of them are referable to conditions of Blood deficiency and will be corrected when the appropriate formula is selected to address the Blood deficiency.
- In cats affected with immunodeficiency viruses the distinction must be made between cats that are truly deficient and those that suffer signs of "toxicity." In other words, a diagnosis of immune deficiency does not necessarily imply a diagnosis of deficiency from a Chinese medical perspective. For immune-deficient

cats with excess patterns from a Chinese perspective (e.g., purulent nasal discharges, chronic colitis, and severe stomatitis), the reader should consult the appropriate section in the book dealing with the animals' signs and treat appropriately.

- Immune-deficient animals that are also deficient from a Chinese medical perspective tend to lack Qi and Blood, and several options exist to correct these deficiencies.
- **Ling Zhi Feng Wang Jiang** (Ganoderma Royal Jelly Essence) contains Reishi, Royal Jelly, the Spleen tonic Dang Shen *(Codonopsis pilulosa)*, and Gou Qi Zi (Wolfberry Fruit, *Lycium barbarum)*. It is a strong Qi and Blood tonic and is especially useful in consumptive disorders accompanied by weakness, a pale tongue, feeble pulses, and weight loss. A *suggested starting dose* is 1 ml per 10 to 15 lb of body weight given once daily.
- A related product is **Shuang Bao Su Kou Fu Ye** (Double Precious Extract Drink), which consists of Ginseng and Royal Jelly. It is likewise used only for truly Qi- and Blood-deficient weakened patients. A *suggested starting dose* is one capsule daily per 10 lb of body weight.
- **Wu Jia Pi** *(Acanthopanax spinosus)* is used as a single herb to strengthen the immune system. Its actions against fatigue are considered stronger than those of Ginseng. It may be especially useful in Kidney-deficient patients with joint stiffness and pain, in cancer patients, and in animals that are diabetic. Wu Jia Pi has been ascribed antitumor, antiinflammatory, and hypoglycemic properties.
- In the treatment of Qi and Blood deficiency in immune-deficient patients formulas containing Astragalus once again assume importance. The section on Anemia earlier in this chapter provides more information on these formulas, which include **Dang Gui Bu Xue Tang** (Angelica Nourish Blood Decoction), **Bu Zhong Yi Qi Tang** (Nourish the Center and Raise the Qi Decoction), and **Gui Pi Tang** (Replenish the Spleen Decoction).

Western Herbs

- From an energetic perspective, Echinacea appears to act to transform Phlegm. It may be most useful as an immunostimulant in patients with abundant mucus and phlegm production.

AUTHORS' CHOICES:

SM: Appropriate Chinese herbal formula.
SW: Attention to improving diet; a combination of antioxidant vitamins, minerals and amino acids; medicinal mushrooms; plant sterols; Chinese herbs as appropriate.

THROMBOCYTOPENIA

Therapeutic Rationale

- Identify platelet pathology.
- Suppress immune-mediated damage if it is autoimmune in origin (most common in dogs).
- Give blood or platelet transfusions.
- Administer anabolics to enhance regeneration.

Alternative Options with Conventional Bases

- **See section on Autoimmune Diseases** for general recommendations on immune-mediated disease.
- **Vitamin C:** has been recommended on the basis of case reports. Studies in which Vitamin C was given alone in the treatment of ITP have shown conflicting results, but if Vitamin C is given in combination with conventional treatments, it may improve outcomes (Jubelirer, 1993; Masugi, 1994).
- **Melatonin:** has recently been recognized as an important modulator of blood and platelet production and maintenance. In a clinical case series of humans with thrombocytopenia from different causes melatonin was thought to improve outcomes (Lissoni, 1996). The dose used in that report was 20 mg once in the evening for 2 months in humans. Doses used in dogs and cats range up to 6 mg tid.
- **Yunnan Bai Yao** (see entry under Coagulopathy): the "formula" contains only San Qi *(Panax notoginseng)*, an herb that has a reputation for being able to stop

bleeding anywhere in the body. Yunnan Bai Yao has been shown to decrease clotting times (Ogle, 1977) and initiate platelet release (Chew, 1977). It should be administered in heavy doses of 75 to 100 mg/kg of body weight daily of granular concentrate, given in divided doses, or as one tablet per 10 lb of body weight daily, given in divided doses if possible.
- **Jia Wei Gui Pi Tang** (Kami-kihi-to): appeared to increase platelet count and decrease autoantibodies in a case series of 10 human patients with thrombocytopenic purpura (Yamaguchi, 1993).

Paradigmatic Options
- See the section on Clotting Disorders earlier in the chapter for information about the Chinese medical treatment of ITP.
- A few comments are worth underscoring about ITP:
  - Formulas with Huang Bai seem to have a greater ability to halt platelet destruction. Huang Bai is contained in formulas that clear Empty Heat and Damp Heat from the lower body. **Da Bu Yin Wan** (Great Tonify Yin Pill) and **Si Miao San** (Four Marvels Powder) are prominent examples of formulas containing Huang Bai. They can be used when other signs and symptoms of the patient agree with the general thrust of these formulas.
  - Blood-moving herbs such as Dan Shen, Bai Shao, and Chuan Xiong have antiplatelet effects. Their use should be avoided in ITP cases if possible.

Western Herbs
- **New Jersey Tea:** has a reputation for reducing splenomegaly associated with hemolytic anemia and perhaps ITP.
- **Barberry:** may induce splenic contraction thereby increasing platelet counts.

Cautions
- Fish Oil has long been thought to alter platelet function and prevent blood hypercoagulability in humans and laboratory animals. In cats given 2.6 g of ω-3 fatty acids daily (a very high dose), no effect on platelet function was noted (Bright,

1994). In a trial using ω-3-enriched diets (ω-6:ω-3 ratio of 1.3:1), cats developed increased bleeding time, decreased platelet activation, and decreased platelet aggregation at 112 days (Saker, 1998). Other researchers have noted that canine cancer patients fed a diet high in ω-3 fatty acids showed no clotting or platelet abnormalities (McNiel, 1999).

- Other natural substances with possible anticoagulant effects include Ginkgo *(Ginkgo biloba)*, Garlic, Bromelain, Papain, Feverfew *(Tanacetum parthenium)*, and Cayenne *(Capsicum frutescens, Capsicum* spp.).

AUTHORS' CHOICES:

SM: Use the appropriate Chinese herbal formula; also consider formulas in the section on blood-clotting disorders.
SW: Identify allergies or other sources of nonspecific inflammation; melatonin; conventional treatments where effective.

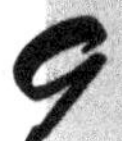

CASE REPORT

Immune-Mediated Thrombocytopenia in a Dog

HISTORY

Didgeree, a 10-year-old, neutered, male Maltese terrier, presented with a chief complaint of immune-mediated thrombocytopenia of 1 month's duration. The condition had first been discovered approximately 1 month earlier after cuts the dog received during grooming were observed to ooze pale, thin, watery blood for the next 4 days.

Didgeree's local veterinarian initially assessed and treated the bleeding disorder. Didgeree's past medical history at that time included normal blood counts but elevated alanine amino transferase (ALT) and alkaline phosphatase (ALP) levels, which had been noted 9 months earlier during a routine preanesthetic chemistry screen, and hypothyroidism that had been diagnosed on the basis of low serum T_4 levels accompanying lethargy, depression, and weight gains. Didgeree was receiving thyroid hormone supplementation at the time he developed ITP, but despite its use his current physical complaints still included lethargy, nighttime vomiting, and a progressive degree of constipation.

Physical examination by the referring veterinarian revealed petechiae of the gums and ears, ecchymoses of the skin, and hemorrhage and bruising of the preputial area. A peripheral blood smear revealed a platelet count of 9×10^9 per liter (normal: 170 to 400×10^9 per liter). Laboratory testing ruled out any abnormalities in the intrinsic and extrinsic clotting cascades. Red and white blood cell numbers were otherwise normal, ruling out bone marrow failure. A tentative diagnosis of immune-mediated thrombocytopenia was made. The dog was discharged the next day with instructions to the owner to administer 10 mg of prednisone orally twice daily. Vitamin K_1 was also prescribed along with cage rest and soft food. Over the next few days the owner observed that the physical evidence of hemorrhage improved, but the lethargy, vomiting, and constipation persisted.

The incomplete nature of the dog's improvement prompted the owner to consult with a local herbal practitioner for humans. Didgeree was prescribed two mild patented Chinese herbal tonic formulas, neither of which is described in this chapter. The herbalist recommended that the owner stop thyroid supplementation, which the owner felt was at too high a dose because of the dog's incessant panting and high heart rate.

One month later the owner brought Didgeree to the veterinary hospital for reevaluation of his platelet and liver enzyme levels. Despite continued use of the prednisone and herbs, the platelet count had failed to improve and now rested at 6×10^9 per liter and his liver enzyme level elevations were higher than 9 months previously. His blood urea nitrogen and creatinine levels were also mildly elevated. He had gained more weight and was now at 20 pounds. Vomiting, constipation, and lethargy were still present. Thyroid hormone was again prescribed and the owner advised to seek alternative health care from a veterinarian experienced in the practice of alternative medicine. Because of the poor response to immunosuppressive therapy, a guarded prognosis was given for resolution of the ITP and the conventional treatment was discontinued. The patented Chinese herbs were also discontinued at this time, not because of any suspected adverse effects on Didgeree's platelets but because of their apparent ineffectiveness.

When Didgeree was brought to the referral clinic several days later, he was being fed various brands of kibble supplemented by a home-cooked diet of ground beef, liver, rice, chicken broth, and raw carrots. He was very lethargic and seemed constipated. Thyroid hormone was once again being administered. The owner complained of filmy mucous accumulations in the dog's eyes and labored breathing by Didgeree after even mild exercise that precluded all but the shortest walks. He showed a tendency to snap at small children and other dogs, had gained even more weight, and had a tendency to snoring and apparent sleep apnea.

PHYSICAL EXAMINATION

On physical examination, Didgeree was largely moribund. He had a red tongue with a brick-red tip, as well as thin, wiry pulses. Didgeree's abdomen was bulging, round, and firm. Acupuncture points that were warm, thick, or bulging included GV 14, SP 9, LI 11, CV 6, and BL 24. His platelet count was 6×10^9 per liter, but there was no evidence of petechiae, bruising, or hemorrhage.

Additional laboratory testing was not performed because of financial considerations.

ASSESSMENT

From a Chinese medical perspective, Didgeree's hemorrhagic tendencies were perceived metaphorically to be arising from three main pathways: Spleen Qi deficiency, Excess Heat in the Blood, and Blood stasis.

Spleen Qi deficiency was suggested by the watery and passively oozing nature of the hemorrhage first noted after grooming. Declining Spleen Qi can also lead to constipation, since Spleen and Stomach Qi is considered in Chinese medicine to supply the motive force of intestinal peristalsis. Decreased Spleen Qi also causes the accumulation of Dampness, which was manifested in this case as vomiting, mucoid accumulations in the eyes, a tendency to easy weight gain, lethargy, and congestive swelling of the throat that resulted in a tendency to snore.

When Dampness is present for extended periods, it turns to Damp Heat. Signs of Damp Heat here included panting and tachycardia in response to routine thyroid supplementation, a brick-red tongue and a wiry pulse, increasing irritability, and a tendency for the blood to become agitated by the accumulating Heat, culminating in its "leaping" from the vessels as hemorrhage.

Deep purple bruises and ecchymoses suggest a clear tendency to Blood stagnation. When Blood stagnates, it is considered more likely to extravasate in an attempt to flow around the obstruction. Blood deficiency is usually manifested in dogs as a thin, wiry pulse and is considered more likely to predispose to Blood stagnation in the same way a river does not flow as quickly when its level drops.

Treatment goals were to tonify the Spleen, drain Damp, clear Heat, and nourish and move Blood. Although acupuncture was not used to achieve these goals because of the risk of hemorrhage, "active points" still have diagnostic value. BL 24 and CV 6 tonify Qi. SP 9, LI 11, and GV 14 clear Heat, especially Damp Heat.

TREATMENT

Although there were multiple objectives to be addressed in Didgeree's condition, a relatively simple formula was employed to treat him. I (SM) combined 8 g of Dang Gui *(Angelica sinensis)* granules with 30 g of **Si Miao San** (Four Marvels Powder) granules. Si Miao San contains four herbs: Cang Zhu (Red Atractylodes), Huai Niu Xi (Achryanthes), Yi Yi Ren (Coix), and Huang Bai (Phellodendron). The formula was administered at a dose of ¼ tsp twice daily. Milk thistle glycerite was also prescribed at a dose of 2 ml twice daily to protect and stabilize hepatocytes. A follow-up appointment was scheduled for 1 month later. No diet changes were prescribed, and existing thyroid supplementation was continued.

OUTCOME

At the follow-up appointment Didgeree showed many improvements. He was now active and playful and able to go for extended walks. He seemed less hot and had exhibited no episodes of bleeding or bruising. Constipation and vomiting had resolved. He was still irritable to other dogs but no longer snapped at them. Eye discharge was minimal, as was the occurrence of snoring and sleep apnea. He had lost approximately 24 ounces of body weight. Didgeree's platelet count was now over $300{,}000 \times 10^9$ per liter. Because of his excellent progress, the owner was reluctant to reevaluate Didgeree for elevations in liver enzyme, BUN, and creatinine levels. Several months later, at the last follow-up examination, Didgeree's improvements had been maintained.

DISCUSSION

As mentioned in the text, formulas containing Huang Bai (Phellodendron) have a significant ability to halt platelet destruction. Like other Damp Heat–clearing herbs, Huang Bai possesses significant antiinflammatory activity, but it excels over the others in its ability to halt ITP.

It is important to ensure that formulas used in holistic medicine are both metaphorically and pharmacologically appropriate. When a formula is appropriate from both a traditional and a pharmacologic perspective, it has a greater chance of being effective. Si Miao San was appropriate for Didgeree from a Chinese medical perspective because it is one of the main formulas for use in Spleen-deficient animals that have excessive accumulations of Damp Heat.

Blood-moving herbs in Chinese medicine are often anticoagulant, the exception being Dang Gui *(Angelica sinensis)*, which is hemostatic. Dang Gui was also selected for use in Didgeree because of these hemostatic properties and because it has traditionally been used to modify Si Miao San to address Blood stasis. It also has Blood-tonifying properties, thus helping to address Didgeree's Blood deficiency.

Long-term care of Didgeree involved weaning him from Si Miao San and Dang Gui at the same time as a "nondampening" raw food diet free of carbohydrates was used to replace his home-cooked diet and kibble.

SM

REFERENCES

Ackermann RT, Mulrow CD, Ramirez G, Gardner CD, Morbidoni L, Lawrence VA. Garlic shows promise for improving some cardiovascular risk factors. *Arch Intern Med* 161(6):813-824, 2001.

Bauer V, Bauer F. Reactive oxygen species as mediators of tissue protection and injury. *Gen Physiol Biophys* 18 Spec No.:7-14, 1999.

Bensky D, Barolet R. *Chinese Herbal Medicine Formulas and Strategies.* Seattle, 1990, Eastland Press.

Bensky D, Gamble A. *Chinese Herbal Medicine Materia Medica*, revised ed. Seattle, 1993, Eastland Press.

Bouic PJD. Immunomodulation in HIV/AIDS: the Tygerberg/Stellenbosch University Experience. *AIDS Bull* 6:18-20, 1997.

Bradley RR, Cunniff PJ, Pereira BJ, Jaber BL. Hematopoietic effect of *Radix angelicae sinensis* in a hemodialysis patient. *Am J Kidney Dis* 34(2):349-354, 1999.

Bright JM, Sullivan PS, Melton SL, Schneider JF, McDonald TP. The effects of n-3 fatty acid supplementation on bleeding time, plasma fatty acid composition, and in vitro platelet aggregation in cats. *J Vet Intern Med* 8(4):247-252, 1994.

Caron ME, White CM. Evaluation of the antihyperlipidemic properties of dietary supplements. *Pharmacotherapy* 21(4):481-487, 2001.

Chew BP, Park JS, Wong TS, Kim HW, Weng BB, Byrne KM, Hayek MG, Reinhart GA. Dietary beta-carotene stimulates cell-mediated and humoral immune response in dogs. *J Nutr* 130(8):1910-1913, 2000.

Chew EC. Yunnan Bai Yao–induced platelet release in suspensions of washed platelets. *Comp Med East West* 5(3-4):271-274, 1977.

de la Torre B, Fransson J, Scheynius A. Blood dehydroepiandrosterone sulphate (DHEAS) levels in pemphigoid/pemphigus and psoriasis. *Clin Exp Rheumatol* 13(3):345-348, 1995.

Ehling D. *The Chinese Herbalist's Handbook*, revised ed. Santa Fe, NM, 1996, Inword Press.

Field CJ, Johnson I, Pratt VC. Glutamine and arginine: immunonutrients for improved health. *Med Sci Sports Exerc* 32(7 Suppl):S377-S388, 2000.

Harbige LS. Dietary n-6 and n-3 fatty acids in immunity and autoimmune disease. *Proc Nutr Soc* 57(4):555-562, 1998.

Heber D, Yip I, Ashley JM, Elashoff DA, Elashoff RM, Go VL. Cholesterol-lowering effects of a proprietary Chinese red-yeast-rice dietary supplement. *Am J Clin Nutr* 69(2):231-236, 1999.

Heyland DK, Novak F, Drover JW, Jain M, Su X, Suchner U. Should immunonutrition become routine in critically ill patients? A systematic review of the evidence. *J Am Med Assoc* 286(8):944-953, 2001.

Jubelirer SJ. Pilot study of ascorbic acid for the treatment of refractory immune thrombocytopenic purpura. *Am J Hematol* 43(1):44-46, 1993.

Keen CL, German BJ, Mareschi JP, Gershwin ME. Nutritional modulation of murine models of autoimmunity. *Rheum Dis Clin North Am* 17(2): 223-234, 1991.

Kitts D, Hu C. Efficacy and safety of ginseng. *Public Health Nutr* 3(4A): 473-485, 2000.

Leiba A, Amital H, Gershwin ME, Shoenfeld Y. Diet and lupus. *Lupus* 10(3):246-248, 2001.

Lissoni P, Tancini G, Barni S, Paolorossi F, Rossini F, Maffe P, Di Bella L. The pineal hormone melatonin in hematology and its potential efficacy in the treatment of thrombocytopenia. *Recent Prog Med* 87(12):582-585, 1996.

Liu LP, Liu JF, Lu YQ. Effects of Sheng-Mai injection on the PRPP synthetase activity in BFU-es and CFU-es from bone marrows of mice with benzene-induced aplastic anemia. *Life Sci* 69(12):1373-1379, 2001.

Maassen CB, van Holten JC, Balk F, Heijne den Bak-Glashouwer MJ, Leer R, Laman JD, Boersma WJ, Claassen E. Orally administered *Lactobacillus* strains differentially affect the direction and efficacy of the immune response. *Vet Q* 20:S81-S83, 1998.

McNiel EA, Ogilvie GK, Mallinckrodt C, Richardson K, Fettman MJ. Platelet function in dogs treated for lymphoma and hemangiosarcoma and supplemented with dietary n-3 fatty acids. *J Vet Intern Med* 113(6):574-580, 1999.

Masugi J, Iwai M, Kimura S, Ochi F, Suzuki K, Nakano O, Sakamoto T, Fukunaga H, Amano M, Fukuda T. Combination of ascorbic acid and methylprednisolone pulse therapy in the treatment of idiopathic thrombocytopenic purpura. *Intern Med* 33(3):165-166, 1994.

Matsuzaki T, Chin J. Modulating immune responses with probiotic bacteria. *Immunol Cell Biol* 78(1):67-73, 2000.

Mills S, Bone K. *Principles and Practice of Phytotherapy: Modern Herbal Medicine.* London, 2000, Churchill Livingstone.

Mitchell W. *Plant Medicine: The Bastyr Years.* Bastyr University, Seattle, 1999, Self-published.

Moriguchi S, Muraga M. Vitamin E and immunity. *Vitam Horm* 59:305-336, 2000.

Naeser MA. *Outline Guide to Chinese Herbal Patent Medicines in Pill Form.* Boston, Mass, 1990, Boston Chinese Medicine.

Ogle CW, Dai S, Cho CH. The hemostatic effects of orally administered Yunnan Bai Yao in rats and rabbits. *Comp Med East West* 5(2):155-160, 1977.

Ooi VE, Liu F. Immunomodulation and anti-cancer activity of polysaccharide-protein complexes. *Curr Med Chem* 7(7):715-729, 2000.

Percival SS. Use of echinacea in medicine. *Biochem Pharmacol* 60:155-158, 2000.

Robinzon B, Cutolo M. Should dehydroepiandrosterone replacement therapy be provided with glucocorticoids? *Rheumatology* (Oxford) 38(6): 488-495, 1999.

Saker KE, Eddy AL, Thatcher CD, Kalnitsky J. Manipulation of dietary (n-6) and (n-3) fatty acids alters platelet function in cats. *J Nutr* 128(12 Suppl):2645S-2647S, 1998.

Semba RD. Vitamin A and immunity to viral, bacterial and protozoan infections. *Proc Nutr Soc* 58(3):719-727, 1999.

Singh RB, Niaz MA, Ghosh S. Hypolipidemic and antioxidant effects of *Commiphora mukul* as an adjunct to dietary therapy in patients with hypercholesterolemia. *Cardiovasc Drugs Ther* 8(4):659-664, 1994.

Song Z, Kharazmi A, Wu H, Faber V, Moser C, Krogh HK, Rygaard J, Hoiby N. Effects of ginseng treatment on neutrophil chemiluminescence and immunoglobulin G subclasses in a rat model of chronic *Pseudomonas aeruginosa* pneumonia. *Clin Diagn Lab Immunol* 5(6):882-887, 1998.

Sun Y, Hersh EM, Talpaz M, Lee SL, Wong W, Loo TL, Mavligit GM. Immune restoration and/or augmentation of local graft versus host reaction by traditional Chinese medicinal herbs. *Cancer* 52(1):70-73, 1983.

Tavintharan S, Kashyap ML. The benefits of niacin in atherosclerosis. *Curr Atheroscler Rep* 3(1):74-82, 2001.

Wasser SP, Weis AL. Therapeutic effects of substances occurring in higher *Basidiomycetes* mushrooms: a modern perspective. *Crit Rev Immunol* 19(1):65-96, 1999.

Weese JS. Microbiologic evaluation of commercial probiotics. *J Am Vet Med Assoc* 220(6):794-797, 2002.

Yamaguchi K, Kido H, Kawakatsu T, Fukuroi T, Suzuki M, Yanabu M, Nomura S, Kokawa T, Yasunaga K. Effects of kami-kihi-to (jia-wei-gui-pi-tang) on autoantibodies in patients with chronic immune thrombocytopenic purpura. *Am J Chin Med* 21(3-4):251-255, 1993.

Yeung H. *Handbook of Chinese Herbal Formulas.* Los Angeles, Calif, 1995, Self-published.

Yeung H. *Handbook of Chinese Herbs.* Los Angeles, Calif, 1996, Self-published.

Yoshida Y, Wang MQ, Liu JN, Shan BE, Yamashita U. Immunomodulating activity of Chinese medicinal herbs and *Oldenlandia diffusa* in particular. *Int J Immunopharmacol* 19(7):359-370, 1997.

Zee-Cheng RK. Shi-quan-da-bu-tang (ten significant tonic decoction), SQT: a potent Chinese biological response modifier in cancer immunotherapy, potentiation and detoxification of anticancer drugs. *Methods Find Exp Clin Pharmacol* 14(9):725-736, 1992.

Zhao KS, Mancini C, Doria G. Enhancement of the immune response in mice by *Astragalus membranaceus* extracts. *Immunopharmacology* 20(3):225-233, 1990.

Zhu JS, Halpern GM, Jones K. The scientific rediscovery of a precious ancient Chinese herbal regimen: *Cordyceps sinensis*. II. *J Altern Complement Med* 4(4):429-457, 1998.

10

Therapies for Infectious Diseases

BACTERIAL INFECTIONS, GENERAL

Therapeutic Rationale

- Kill or suppress bacterial growth.
- Enhance host defense mechanisms if patient has recurrent or chronic infections.

Alternative Options with Conventional Bases

Immunostimulants

- See discussion in Chapter 9 under Immunosuppressive Disorders.

Antibacterial Herbs

- **Boneset** *(Eupatorium perfoliatum):* has long been used for infections in humans. One study found a weak antibacterial effect against gram-positive organisms (Habtemariam, 2000).
- **Goldenseal** *(Hydrastis canadensis):* also a traditional antimicrobial. Some evidence supports this use against *Staphylococcus* spp., *Streptococcus* spp., *Escherichia coli,* and *Pseudomonas aeruginosa* (Scazzocchio, 2001). Other berberine-containing plants such as Coptis *(Coptis chinensis),* Barberry *(Berberis vulgaris),* and Oregon Grape *(Mahonia aquifolium)* have shown activity against a variety of bacteria (Sun, Abraham, 1988; Sun, Courtney, 1988).
- ***Salvia* spp.**: have demonstrated antibacterial activity. Extracts from the traditional Chinese herb called Dan Shen *(Salvia miltorrhiza)* have shown activity against a range of gram-positive bacteria in vitro (Lee, 1999). Other *Salvia* species extracts that appear to have antibacterial activity against a variety of bacteria are

S. blepharochlaena, S. ringens, S. viridis, S. leriaefolia, and *S. palaestina.*

- **Thymus spp.**: the essential oil of Oregano *(Thymus origanum)* is highly inhibitory to a variety of bacteria including *E. coli, Staphylococcus aureus,* and *P. aeruginosa* (Elgayyar, 2001). Thyme extracts *(Thymus vulgaris),* usually tested as the essential oil, have shown activity against *Streptococcus* species, *Staphylococcus* species, and *Haemophilus* species (Dorman, 2000; Inouye, 2001; Kulevanova, 2000).
- **St. John's Wort** *(Hypericum perforatum):* has shown activity against resistant strains of *S. aureus* and *Helicobacter pylori* (Reichling, 2001).
- **Papaya** *(Carica papaya):* has shown some activity against *Salmonella typhi, E. coli, S. aureus, P. aeruginosa,* and other bacteria when the meat, seed, and pulp of the unripe fruit were used (Osato, 1993).
- **Cordyceps** *(Cordyceps sinensis):* an extract of *Cordyceps,* Cordycepin, appears to selectively inhibit growth of *Clostridium* species, including *C. perfringens* (Ahn, 2000; Rabbani, 1987).

Paradigmatic Options

- The herbs possessing documented antibacterial properties in Chinese medicine number in the hundreds. Many of these herbs, such as Huang Bai, Huang Lian, Da Huang, Ban Lan Gen, Yin Chen Hao, and Huang Qin, are Heat clearing and downward draining. Some of them such as Pu Gong Ying, Jin Yin Hua, and Lian Qiao are pungent and disperse Heat from the superficial layers of the body, which makes them more suited for superficial infections. Some such as Bo He are antibacterial because of their volatile oil content. Another commonly used herb that possesses antibacterial properties is Chai Hu.
- All of these herbs have the potential for side effects and should be used only when also appropriate from a Chinese medical perspective. Use of herbs according to their individual pharmacologic ingredients without regard for their general appropriateness tends to reduce their efficacy and can lead to undesirable results.

- The best holistic medical approach to dealing with an infection is to identify the pattern of disease according to Chinese medical thinking and select acupuncture points and herbs appropriate for the treatment of that pattern. If the formula is well suited to the patient and contains antimicrobial herbs, the chances of a favorable outcome are increased.
- A formula that has antibiotic properties but is ill matched to the patient from a Chinese medical perspective is generally unlikely to be effective and may be detrimental. This is particularly true when bitter antimicrobial herbs are selected for treatment of infections in Qi-, Yin-, or Blood-deficient patients. The most expedient route to resolving infections in these patients probably is to correct their deficiencies.

Cautions

- Goldenseal is said to counteract anticoagulants, which may be important for cats receiving aspirin therapy.

AUTHORS' CHOICES:

SM: Treat infections holistically; resist selecting herbs in holistic medicine solely because of the action of an individual ingredient and focus on using herbs and formulas because of their appropriateness as a whole.

SW: Antibiotics based on culture and sensitivity; herbs recommended only as an adjunct or for chronic or resistant infections; in these circumstances, refer to the appropriate systems-based chapter in addition to this section and administer combinations of Thyme, Salvia, berberine-containing herbs, and system-specific or Chinese herbal combinations.

FUNGAL INFECTIONS, GENERAL

Therapeutic Rationale

- Suppress fungal growth and replication.
- Remove locally invasive foci of organisms.

Alternative Options with Conventional Bases

- **Berberine-containing herbs,** including Goldenseal, Barberry, Oregon Grape, Coptis, and Gold Thread *(Xanthorrhiza simplicissima)*: have shown activity against some fungi. The berberine component of Gold Thread has shown activity against *Candida albicans, Cryptococcus neoformans,* intracellular mycobacteria, and other fungal pathogens (Okunade, 1994).
- **Garlic** *(Allium sativum)*: has shown activity as a topical agent against common dermatophytes (Venugopal, 1995). The usual warnings apply against use of high oral doses of garlic in dogs and cats, but low doses can often be used safely; the practitioner should regularly monitor the blood counts of patients being treated with garlic.
- **Essential oils:** Eucalyptus *(Eucalyptus globulus)* Oil has shown good efficacy against common dermatophytes, including *Microsporum canis, M. gypseum,* and *Trichophyton mentagrophytes* (Shahi, 2000). Unfortunately, Eucalyptus is extremely toxic and death may result if animals lick topically applied Eucalyptus. Similarly, Tea Tree *(Melaleuca alternifolia)* Oil is somewhat effective against dermatophytes (Nenoff, 1996) but deadly to cats (Bischoff, 1998).
- Brinker (Brinker, 1995) summarizes the antifungal action of several common Western herbs. Yerba Mansa *(Anemopsis californica)* contains methyleugenol, which has shown moderate activity against yeast and fungi. Black Walnut *(Juglans nigra)* contains juglone, which has shown significant antifungal activity against *Aspergillus* (Mahoney, 2000). Pau d'arco *(Tabebuia impestignosa, T.* spp.) is popular for yeast overgrowth. Usnea *(Usnea barbata)* is a lichen that contains usnic acid, which has shown antifungal activity (Broksa, 1996). I (SM) have combined the four herbs for use topically for superficial dermatophyte and fungal infections.
- **Plantain** *(Plantago* sp.): can be considered for treatment of topical fungal infections. It contains benzoic acid (Mitchell, 1999), which has been credited with action against dermatophytes by Chinese medicine (Naeser, 1996). It is a very mild herb that is unlikely to have

significant activity on its own but can be used topically or taken internally.

Paradigmatic Options

Chinese Herbs

- Many dermatophyte infections eventually resolve as the patient develops immunity to them; therefore enhancing the immune response is presumed to help resolve dermatophytosis more quickly. Approaches to improving immune response are discussed in Chapter 9. In addition, improved immune response within the skin can be achieved with Blood-tonifying formulas. Consult Chapter 5 to select the formula that appears most appropriate.
- Most yeast infections in otitis externa seem secondary to an underlying condition of Dampness and Damp-Heat accumulation. Consult Chapters 5 and 7 for Chinese herbal formulas that can reduce the Dampness of the skin and ears in patients with yeast infections and help them develop greater resistance to these infections.

AUTHORS' CHOICES:

SM: Diluted Tea Tree Oil; Garlic; appropriate Chinese herbal formula.
SW: Diet and immunomodulation; topical Oregon Grape; Goldenseal; Garlic; diluted Tea Tree Oil.

VIRAL INFECTIONS

Therapeutic Rationale

- Suppress viral growth and replication.
- Control secondary infections.
- Control inflammation caused by immunopathologic processes.

Alternative Options with Conventional Bases

- **Immunomodulation** in viral diseases may be helpful. See Chapter 9 for more information, especially on antioxidants, bioflavonoids, and plant sterols.

- **Herbs that reduce clinical signs** of the "common cold" include Echinacea *(Echinacea purpurea, E. angustifolia)* (Percival, 2000) and Andrographis *(Andrographis paniculata)* (Caceres, 1999). These effects are probably due to enhancement of the immune response rather than a direct antiviral effect, at least in the case of Echinacea. Echinacea is reported anecdotally to help reduce symptoms in some cats with viral upper respiratory tract infections.
- **Herbs or their extracts** reported to have activity against human herpes simplex virus type 1 (HSV-1) in vitro or in laboratory animals include Clove *(Syzygium aromaticum)* (Kurokawa, 1998) and *Stephania cepharantha* (Nawawi, 1999). However, these herbs have not been tested against feline herpesviruses. Tetrandine, an extract of *Stephania tetranda*, inhibited development of keratitis by modulating the immune-inflammatory response in mice infected with HSV-1 (Hu, 1997). Stephania is not generally used alone. Rosemarinic acid, which is found in Rosemary, is also present in Lemon Balm *(Melissa officinalis)* (Brinker, 1995). This may account for its widespread use in the treatment of herpesvirus in humans. Caffeic acid in Lemon Balm also contributes to these antiviral effects.
- **Herbal combinations** that enhance survival through immunologic mechanisms in laboratory animals infected with herpes simplex virus (HSV) include Si Ni Tang (Ikemoto, 1994) and Ge Gen Tang (Nagasaka, 1995).
- **Herbs or their extracts that inhibit HIV** in vitro include Rosemary *(Rosmarinus officinalis)* (Aruoma, 1996), Andrographis (Chang, 1991), the combination Xiao Chai Hu Tang (Buimovici-Klein, 1990), Prunella *(Prunella vulgaris)* (Tabba, 1989), and Chinese Skullcap *(Scutellaria baicalensis)* (Li, 1993).
- **Lomatium** *(Lomatium dissectum):* has a reputation for efficacy in the treatment of influenza (Brinker, 1995), possibly because of the tetronic acid it contains. It is a mainstay of treatment of human upper respiratory disorders by modern herbalists.

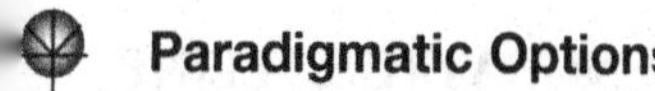

Paradigmatic Options

- There are dozens of antiviral herbs used in Chinese medicine. Long Dan Cao is perhaps the most popular herb for the treatment of viral-induced shingles. Ban Lan Gen is arguably the most popular herb for addressing upper respiratory viral infections. It is included in the formula **Pu Ji Xiao Du Yin** (Universal Antiphlogistic Decoction), a time-honored prescription for acute epidemic viral infections affecting the head and neck of humans, including, most notably, mumps.
- The same comments apply here for the treatment of viral infections as those for bacterial infections. The best holistic medical approach to dealing with an infection is to identify the pattern of disease according to Chinese medical thinking and select acupuncture points and herbs appropriate for the treatment of this pattern. If the formula is well suited to the patient and contains antiviral herbs, the chances of a favorable outcome are increased.
- A formula that has antiviral properties but is ill matched to the patient from a Chinese medical perspective is generally unlikely to be effective and may be detrimental. This is particularly true when bitter herbs are selected for treatment of infections in Qi-, Yin-, or Blood-deficient patients. The most expedient route to resolving viral infections in these patients probably is to correct their deficiencies.

AUTHORS' CHOICES:

SM: Select an appropriate Chinese herbal formula based on the animal's clinical presentation.
SW: Diet improvement; well-chosen Chinese or Western herbal combinations.

FELINE IMMUNODEFICIENCY VIRUS/FELINE LEUKEMIA VIRUS

Therapeutic Rationale

- Control secondary infections.
- Immunomodulation.
- Administer antiviral therapy such as interferon.

Alternative Options with Conventional Bases

- **Immunostimulants:** often recommended for treatment of feline immunodeficiency virus (FIV). We would submit clinical experience that such herbs as Reishi *(Ganoderma lucidum)*, Maitake *(Grifola frondosa)*, Turkey Tail *(Trametes versicolor)*, Cordyceps *(Cordyceps sinensis)*, and Echinacea species are good for episodes of opportunistic infections but do little to change life expectancy or well being in asymptomatic cats. Also, most immunostimulants such as Echinacea should be used only for short periods of time, since it has been suggested that long-term use results in tolerance by the immune system. Therapy should focus on supporting patients with recurrent opportunistic infections or clear weakness and suppressing viral replication when the therapies to do so become available.

Nutrition

- **Antioxidants:** include Vitamin C, Vitamin E, Selenium, and *N*-acetylcysteine (NAC). NAC and Vitamin C were administered to eight patients infected with human immunodeficiency virus (HIV) in one study. In those with the most advanced disease supplementation led to increases in $CD4^+$ lymphocyte count, increases in $CD4^+$ intracellular glutathione, and a reduction of HIV plasma RNA (Muller, 2000). Vitamin C inactivates HIV in vitro (Harakeh, 1990; Rawal, 1995), and can be administered to cats at 250 to 500 mg daily. NAC and alpha-lipoic acid inhibit HIV activation mechanisms in vitro (Shoji, 1994). NAC should be given with food at approximately 25 mg tid. Alpha-lipoic acid should be administered to cats at no more than 25 mg daily.

- **B vitamins:** cobalamin (Weinberg, 1998), nicotinamide (Murray, 1995), and thiamine disulfide (Shoji, 1994) have anti-HIV activity in vitro.

Herbs

- **Herbs or their extracts that inhibit HIV** in vitro include Rosemary (Aruoma, 1996), Andrographis (Chang, 1991), the combination Sho Saiko To (Buimovici-Klein, 1990), Prunella (Tabba, 1989), and Chinese Skullcap (Li, 1993).
- **Plant flavonoids:** inhibit activation of latent HIV in vitro (Critchfield, 1996).
- **Plant sterols:** may improve TH1/TH2 ratio and neurokinin (NK) and T-cell function. In a clinical trial of FIV-infected cats, supplementation with Moducare resulted in enhanced survival times (Bouic, 1997).
- **St. John's Wort:** has shown some activity against HIV in vitro (Takahashi, 1989). However, it is not used to treat infected humans because it interferes with the efficacy of antivirals used to treat AIDS.

Paradigmatic Options

- Substantial relief can be achieved for cats affected with FeLV and FIV by evaluating the patient's clinical presentation in light of Chinese medical thinking. The animals often will appear Qi or Blood deficient, and formulas can be chosen that enhance the immune response of the animal. See Chapter 9 for more information on these formulas and their indications.
- For emaciation, chronic respiratory infections, and hind limb weakness, **Dong Chong Xia Cao** *(Cordyceps)* is used as a single herb in HIV-infected patients in Africa. A *suggested starting dose* is ¼ tsp per 15 lb of body weight, or 60 to 75 mg/kg of body weight, divided into two daily doses. Seafoods have also been advocated for use in the treatment of HIV because of their Yin tonification effects.
- For tonification of cats with chronic diarrhea, poor appetite, and restlessness, Lian Zi (Lotus Seed) can be administered as a single herb. This should be given only to deficient patients. The dose should be the same as for Dong Chong Xia Cao.

- A significant number of FeLV- and FIV-positive cats have signs of a pathologic excess of Damp Heat. These cats should not be given tonifying formulas despite their perceived deficiency from a conventional perspective. Consult the chapter that covers the symptomatic presentation of the patient to find out which Damp Heat–clearing formulas or approaches are most appropriate for the patient.
- One example of a Damp Heat–clearing formula that is of reputed efficacy in the treatment of HIV is **Gan Lu Xiao Du Dan** (Antiphlogistic Pills of Dew). This formula is especially appropriate for patients exhibiting fever, malaise, jaundice, thirst, nausea, vomiting, and diarrhea. The pulse is soft and rapid, and the tongue is coated. Once the excess pathogen is removed, **Yi Guan Jian** (One-Linking Decoction) may be used to address any newly exposed condition of Yin deficiency. A *suggested starting dose* of granular concentrate for both formulas is ¼ tsp per 10 to 15 lb of body weight, or 60 to 75 mg/kg of body weight, divided into two daily doses.
- When Dampness is manifested as lower limb edema, cold limbs, cold intolerance, poor appetite, malaise, and decreased urination, **Shi Pi Yin** (Bolster the Spleen Beverage) is used for the treatment of HIV. The pulse of patients that benefit is deep, slow, or thin, and the tongue is pale and sticky. A *suggested starting dose* of granular concentrate is ¼ tsp per 10 to 15 lb of body weight, or 60 to 75 mg/kg of body weight, divided into two daily doses.
- For Dampness manifested as dysenteric stools **Xiang Lian Wan** (Saussurea and Coptis Pill) can be considered. The specific dynamic this formula addresses is Damp Heat that has been generated by a coldness of the Spleen and Stomach. Alternatively, it has been used in patients with Stomach Fire secondary to Liver Qi Stagnation. The patient may seek warmth despite obvious Heat signs in the stools such as yellow mucus or bright red blood. Elevated thirst, halitosis, stomatitis, and vomiting may also be present, and diarrhea may be worse in the morning. A *suggested starting dose* of granular concentrate is ¼ tsp per 10 to 15 lb of body weight, or 60 to 75 mg/kg of body weight, divided into two daily doses.

- For Dampness and Toxicity that manifests as acute throat inflammation and infection with swelling, purulent lesions, pain, and difficulty swallowing, **Liu Shen Wan** (Six Spirits Pill) can be administered. This is a strongly pungent Heat-clearing formula not for use in deficient patients. Patients that benefit have a red tongue with a yellow coating, and the pulse is rapid and forceful. A *suggested starting dose* is one tablet daily.

AUTHORS' CHOICES:

SM: Appropriate Chinese herbal formula based on clinical presentation.
SW: Improved diet; Vitamin C in combination with other antioxidants; N-acetylcysteine; Moducare; well-chosen Chinese herbal combinations.

FELINE VIRAL UPPER RESPIRATORY INFECTION

Therapeutic Rationale

- Maintain food intake.
- Maintain hydration.
- Treat secondary bacterial infection.

Alternative Options with Conventional Bases

- Control keratitis with topical antiviral and antibacterial preparations.

Nutrition

- **Lysine:** has been shown to reduce herpesvirus replication in vitro in cell cultures containing low arginine levels. Clinical experience suggests that Lysine supplementation at 250 to 500 mg bid reduces herpes recrudescence. It is often necessary to give Lysine long term even though the long-term safety of high levels of lysine is unknown. In a placebo-controlled trial of eight cats, those receiving 500 mg L-lysine bid had less severe conjunctivitis and higher blood lysine levels after infection with herpesvirus (Stiles, 2002).

- **Vitamin C:** as ascorbate, both alone and in combination with copper, inactivated herpes simplex virus in vitro (Sagripanti, 1997), but whether this is relevant for feline herpesvirus strains is unknown. Vitamin C is one of the most popular alternative treatments for herpesvirus infection in cats, but it has not been investigated in clinical trials. Cats usually tolerate a dose of 250 mg daily well; overdose may lead to diarrhea.

Herbs

- **Echinacea:** has been examined extensively in the prevention and treatment of acute viral respiratory disease in humans, and it is thought to act on the innate immune system to activate mononuclear cells. Studies (all published in German) reporting on a total of 910 human subjects appear to suggest that Echinacea significantly shortens the severity and duration of upper respiratory symptoms. If used preventively, it may enhance the immunopathologic action that accounts for some of the symptoms of viral upper respiratory infection (URI) (Percival, 2000). Echinacea has not been examined in cats, but is popular among cat owners as a home remedy for feline "colds." The literature on Echinacea consistently warns against use of the herb for longer than 2 weeks. This is less a warning about toxicity than it is a guideline for effective use because Echinacea exerts its full effect on mononuclear cell production of cytokines within 2 weeks. Longer use will not likely have additional benefit, and it has been suggested to result in induction of tolerance by the system.
- **Lemon Balm:** has shown activity against HSV-1 in vitro (Dimitrova, 1993). The dose is 500 mg to 1 g daily mixed in food.
- **Other herbs or their extracts** reported to have activity against human HSV-1 in vitro or in laboratory animals, but which have not been tested against feline herpesviruses, include Clove (Kurokawa, 1998) and *Stephania cepharantha* (Nawawi, 1999). Tetrandine, an extract of *Stephania tetranda,* inhibited development of keratitis in mice infected with HSV-1 by modulating the immune-inflammatory response (Hu, 1997). Herbal combinations

that enhance survival through immunologic mechanisms in laboratory animals infected with HSV include Si Ni Tang (Ikemoto, 1994) and Ge Gen Tang (Nagasaka, 1995).

Paradigmatic Options

Homeopathy

- The remedy should be selected based on the signs of the patient. The following are some candidates for consideration:
  - **Eyebright** *(Euphrasia officinalis):* in either tincture or homeopathic form, seems effective for chronic herpesvirus infection of the upper respiratory tract and eyes. Guiding symptoms include photophobia and relatively abundant but irritating eye discharge, often resulting in excoriations in the medial canthi. A *suggested starting dose* of tincture is 0.2 ml per 5 lb of body weight twice daily or a single dose of 30C homeopathic pellets once daily, for 1 to 2 weeks.
  - **Homeopathic *Allium cepa:*** seems appropriate for many cats with chronic upper respiratory tract infections. It is especially applicable in cats in which sneezing produces copious, irritating, watery nasal discharges. As with cats that benefit from Euphrasia, these cats often are sensitive to light and have a tendency to squint, and they may be hoarse. A *suggested starting dose* is one to three doses of 30C potency for up to 1 week. It can be used prophylactically in catteries to reduce morbidity from epidemics.
  - When differentiation of symptoms is difficult some practitioners prescribe both *Euphrasia and Allium* simultaneously with apparent effectiveness.

Chinese Medicine

- Select an appropriate formula from Chapter 16.

AUTHORS' CHOICES:

SM: Euphrasia; Allium cepa.
SW: Attention to diet; Lysine; Lemon Balm.

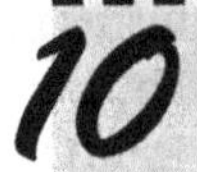

CASE REPORT

Feline Conjunctivitis and Respiratory Disease Complex

HISTORY

Heidi, a 12-year-old, female, spayed Domestic long-haired cat, presented with a chief complaint of eye pain, redness, and discharge of just over 1 year's duration. The condition began as an acute conjunctivitis with blepharospasm and yellow discharge. A conjunctival scraping at that time revealed no evidence of viral or chlamydial infection. A topical preparation containing triple antibiotic and dexamethasone was given three times daily for 10 days, but no improvement was noted. A topical preparation containing tetracycline was then given three times daily for 10 days to address presumptive chlamydial infection, but again no improvements were noted.

Heidi's owner consulted a different practitioner 1 week later. At this time, Heidi's eye was still painful, but the discharge had changed from purulent to serous. Severe gingivitis with dental tartar accumulation was also noted. Based on the serous nature of the discharge and the poor response to previous antimicrobial and antiinflammatory therapy the veterinarian suspected a chronic herpes viral infection. L-Lysine was prescribed at a dose of 250 mg every 12 hours for the next 2 months. Interferon was also prescribed at a dose of 30 IU orally once daily for 1 week. A routine dental scaling and polishing was performed 1 month later. No note was made of the condition of the eye at that time. Two upper incisors and one molar were extracted, and nine other teeth were found to be missing.

Heidi's eye condition worsened over the next 10 months. The owner elected to explore alternative therapies and consulted me (SM). At the time of evaluation, Heidi had not been given therapy of any type for several months. She spent most of her time in the dark, presumably because of severe photophobia. Heidi showed no evidence of pruritus and no respiratory symptoms. Heidi was still eating and had a tendency to gain weight. She was reasonably affectionate despite her discomfort.

PHYSICAL EXAMINATION

Heidi's physical examination revealed copious bilateral epiphora and an accumulation of red mucus that covered a mild superficial excoriation in both medial canthi. Her right eye was painful to the touch, although no corneal abrasions or lacerations were present. Its conjunctiva was markedly inflamed and showed follicular hyperplasia. Other physical examination findings were normal. Laboratory studies were not performed at this time.

ASSESSMENT

The cause of Heidi's chronic conjunctivitis was unknown. In routine clinical practice a specific etiologic diagnosis for feline conjunctivitis and respiratory disease complex is often not pursued beyond the steps taken with this case. Chronic follicular conjunctivitis with no associated symptoms is consistent with feline pneumonitis *(Chlamydia psittaci)*, although Heidi's level of discomfort was unusually severe for chlamydial infection. Feline pneumonitis could not be confirmed because of Heidi's lack of response to the topical tetracycline preparation and the absence of elementary bodies on both conjunctival smears. Chronic herpesvirus infection was possible, indicated by the chronic recurrent nature of the pathologic signs. Severe gingivitis, such as was noted in Heidi, can be caused by calicivirus.

TREATMENT

Heidi was given Homeopathic Euphrasia officinalis 30C orally once daily for 1 week. Euphrasia was selected because of her chronic conjunctivitis, canthal excoriations, and photophobia.

OUTCOME

Three weeks later the owner reported that the homeopathic remedy appeared to be helping. Heidi was exhibiting less photophobia, was hiding less, and was more active. The ocular discharge was serous and reduced in volume. The owner was instructed to resume giving Euphrasia 30C for another week to see if further improvements could be noted.

Heidi was brought for follow-up evaluation 4 weeks later. At this time the owner was still administering Euphrasia 30C. The owner reported Heidi exhibited only slight squinting and eye discharge, and she was no longer hiding. Although the conjunctiva of the right eye was no longer reddened, follicular conjunctivitis was still pronounced. A conjunctival scraping of the right eye revealed mucus strands, amorphous pigmented epithelial cells, and lymphocytes. No eosinophils were observed. Euphrasia 30C was discontinued in case overuse of the remedy was creating a mild aggravation of symptoms. A subcutaneous injection containing 75,000 IU of Vitamin A and 12,500 IU of Vitamin D was administered to reduce the hyperplastic epithelial changes, boost the immune response, and improve conjunctival integrity.

The next follow-up was 5 months later, when the owner reported that Heidi's eye complaints had resolved. When any eye discharge was noted, the owner administered Euphrasia 30C once daily for a few days until it resolved. Three years later, at the time of the last follow-up, the condition had not recurred.

COMMENTS

It is not known whether the Vitamin A injection had any benefit in Heidi's case. Although not discussed in the text, Vitamin A helps promote cell differentiation and keratinization of epithelial cells, including the conjunctiva. It is commonly used in tandem with Vitamin C for human patients with viral conjunctivitis to enhance conjunctival integrity to better resist pathogenic invasion. Vitamin A supplementation above recommended daily allowances also has been shown to enhance humoral and cellular immunity in human viral infections. Despite these potential benefits, Heidi's improvement may have stemmed from the discontinuation of the Euphrasia, or from a natural waning of the infection.

The greatest problem with homeopathic remedies in veterinary clinical practice is their overuse by owners. Some practitioners view homeopathics as behaving more like stimulants than pharmaceuticals. They are envisioned as stimulating recovery in weak areas in a patient, the same way that weight training is used to stimulate weak muscles to become stronger. If not too heavy a weight is used and if rests are provided between sessions, the muscle grows in strength. Similarly, if the right potency, and frequency of administration are used in homeopathy, the patient becomes stronger. If, however, too high or low a potency or too frequent doses are used, the homeopathic remedy may aggravate the patient's weakness and cause a resurgence of symptoms, the same way an overtrained muscle loses strength and becomes weaker.

SM

REFERENCES

Ahn YJ, Park SJ, Lee SG, Shin SC, Choi DH. Cordycepin: selective growth inhibitor derived from liquid culture of *Cordyceps militaris* against *Clostridium* spp. *J Agric Food Chem* 48(7):2744-2748, 2000.

Aruoma OI, Spencer JP, Rossi R, Aeschbach R, Khan A, Mahmood N, Munoz A, Murcia A, Butler J, Halliwell B. An evaluation of the antioxidant and antiviral action of extracts of rosemary and Provencal herbs. *Food Chem Toxicol* 34(5):449-456, 1996.

Bensky D, Barolet R. *Chinese Herbal Medicine Formulas and Strategies.* Seattle, 1990, Eastland Press.

Bischoff K, Guale F. Australian tea tree *(Melaleuca alternifolia)* oil poisoning in three purebred cats. *J Vet Diagn Invest* 10(2):208-210, 1998.

Boericke W. *Materia Medica with Repertory,* ed 9. Santa Rosa, Calif, 1927, Boericke & Tafel.

Bouic PJD. Immunomodulation in HIV/AIDS: the Tygerberg/Stellenbosch University experience. *AIDS Bull* 6:18-20, 1997.

Brinker F. *Formulas for Healthful Living.* Sandy, Ore, 1995, Eclectic Medical Publications.

Broksa B, Sturdikova M, Pronayova N, Liptaj T. (-)- Usnic acid and its derivatives: their inhibition of fungal growth and enzyme activity. *Pharmazie* 51(3):195-196, 1996.

Buimovici-Klein E, Mohan V, Lange M, Fenamore E, Inada Y, Cooper LZ. Inhibition of HIV replication in lymphocyte cultures of virus-positive subjects in the presence of sho-saiko-to, an oriental plant extract. *Antiviral Res* 14(4-5):279-286, 1990.

Caceres DD, Hancke JL, Burgos RA, Sandberg F, Wikman GK. Use of visual analogue scale measurements (VAS) to assess the effectiveness of standardized *Andrographis paniculata* extract SHA-10 in reducing the symptoms of common cold: a randomized double blind-placebo study. *Phytomedicine* 6(4):217-223, 1999.

Chang RS, Ding L, Chen GQ, Pan QC, Zhao ZL, Smith KM. Dehydroandrographolide succinic acid monoester as an inhibitor against the human immunodeficiency virus. *Proc Soc Exp Biol Med* 197(1):59-66, 1991.

Critchfield JW, Butera ST, Folks TM. Inhibition of HIV activation in latently infected cells by flavonoid compounds. *AIDS Res Hum Retroviruses* 12(1):39-46, 1996.

Dimitrova Z, Dimov B, Manolova N, Pancheva S, Ilieva D, Shishkov S. Antiherpes effect of *Melissa officinalis* L. extracts. *Acta Microbiol Bulg* 29:65-72, 1993.

Dorman HJ, Deans SG. Antimicrobial agents from plants: antibacterial activity of plant volatile oils. *J Appl Microbiol* 88(2):308-316, 2000.

Ehling D. *The Chinese Herbalist's Handbook,* revised ed. Santa Fe, NM, 1996, Inword Press.

Elgayyar M, Draughon FA, Golden DA, Mount JR. Antimicrobial activity of essential oils from plants against selected pathogenic and saprophytic microorganisms. *J Food Prot* 64(7):1019-1024, 2001.

Habtemariam S, Macpherson AM. Cytotoxicity and antibacterial activity of ethanol extract from leaves of a herbal drug, boneset *(Eupatorium perfoliatum). Phytother Res* 14(7):575-577, 2000.

Harakeh S, Jariwalla RJ, Pauling L. Suppression of human immunodeficiency virus replication by ascorbate in chronically and acutely infected cells. *Proc Natl Acad Sci USA* 87(18):7245-7249, 1990.

Hu S, Dutt J, Zhao T, Foster CS. Tetrandrine potently inhibits herpes simplex virus type-1-induced keratitis in BALB/c mice. *Ocul Immunol Inflamm* (3):173-180, 1997.

Ikemoto K, Utsunomiya T, Ball MA, Kobayashi M, Pollard RB, Suzuki F. Protective effect of shigyaku-to, a traditional Chinese herbal medicine, on the infection of herpes simplex virus type 1 (HSV-1) in mice. *Experientia* 50(5):456-460, 1994.

Inouye S, Takizawa T, Yamaguchi H. Antibacterial activity of essential oils and their major constituents against respiratory tract pathogens by gaseous contact. *J Antimicrob Chemother* 47(5):565-573, 2001.

Kulevanova S, Kaftandzieva A, Dimitrovska A, Stefkov G, Grdanoska T, Panovski N. Investigation of antimicrobial activity of essential oils of several Macedonian *Thymus* L. species (Lamiaceae). *Boll Chim Farm* 139(6):276-280, 2000.

Kurokawa M, Hozumi T, Basnet P, Nakano M, Kadota S, Namba T, Kawana T, Shiraki K. Purification and characterization of eugeniin as an anti-herpesvirus compound from *Geum japonicum* and *Syzygium aromaticum*. *J Pharmacol Exp Ther* 284(2):728-735, 1998.

Lee DS, Lee SH, Noh JG, Hong SD. Antibacterial activities of cryptotanshinone and dihydrotanshinone I from a medicinal herb, *Salvia miltiorrhiza* Bunge. *Biosci Biotechnol Biochem* 63(12):2236-2239, 1999.

Li BQ, Fu T, Yan YD, Baylor NW, Ruscetti FW, Kung HF. Inhibition of HIV infection by baicalin—a flavonoid compound purified from Chinese herbal medicine. *Cell Mol Biol Res* 39(2):119-124, 1993.

Mahoney N, Molyneux RJ, Campbell BC. Regulation of aflatoxin production by naphthoquinones of walnut *(Juglans regia)*. *J Agric Food Chem* 48(9): 4418-4421, 2000.

Mitchell W. *Plant Medicine: The Bastyr Years.* Bastyr University, Seattle, 1999, Self-published.

Muller F, Svardal AM, Nordoy I, Berge RK, Aukrust P, Froland SS. Virological and immunological effects of antioxidant treatment in patients with HIV infection. *Eur J Clin Invest* (10):905-914, 2000.

Murray MF, Srinivasan A. Nicotinamide inhibits HIV-1 in both acute and chronic in vitro infection. *Biochem Biophys Res Commun* 210(3):954-959, 1995.

Naeser MA. *Outline Guide to Chinese Herbal Patent Medicines in Pill Form.* Boston, Mass, 1990, Boston Chinese Medicine.

Nagasaka K, Kurokawa M, Imakita M, Terasawa K, Shiraki K. Efficacy of kakkon-to, a traditional herb medicine, in herpes simplex virus type 1 infection in mice. *J Med Virol* 46(1):28-34, 1995.

Nawawi A, Ma C, Nakamura N, Hattori M, Kurokawa M, Shiraki K, Kashiwaba N, Ono M. Anti-herpes simplex virus activity of alkaloids isolated from *Stephania cepharantha. Biol Pharm Bull* 22(3):268-274, 1999.

Nenoff P, Haustein UF, Brandt W. Antifungal activity of the essential oil of *Melaleuca alternifolia* (tea tree oil) against pathogenic fungi in vitro. *Skin Pharmacol* 9(6):388-394, 1996.

Okunade AL, Hufford CD, Richardson MD, Peterson JR, Clark AM. Antimicrobial properties of alkaloids from *Xanthorhiza simplicissima. J Pharm Sci* 83(3):404-406, 1994.

Osato JA, Santiago LA, Remo GM, Cuadra MS, Mori A. Antimicrobial and antioxidant activities of unripe papaya. *Life Sci* 53(17):1383-1389, 1993.

Ozturk F, Kurt E, Cerci M, Emiroglu L, Inan U, Turker M, Ilker S. The effect of propolis extract in experimental chemical corneal injury. *Ophthalmic Res* 32 (1):13-18, 2000.

Percival SS: Use of Echinacea in medicine. *Biochem Pharmacol* 60(2):155-158, 2000.

Rabbani GH, Butler T, Knight J, Sanyal SC, Alam K. Randomized controlled trial of berberine sulfate therapy for diarrhea due to enterotoxigenic *Escherichia coli* and *Vibrio cholerae. J Infect Dis* 155(5):979-984, 1987.

Rawal BD, Bartolini F, Vyas GN. In vitro inactivation of human immunodeficiency virus by ascorbic acid. *Biologicals* 23(1):75-81, 1995.

Reichling J, Weseler A, Saller R. A current review of the antimicrobial activity of *Hypericum perforatum* L. *Pharmacopsychiatry* 34:S116-S118, 2001.

Scazzocchio F, Cometa MF, Tomassini L, Palmery M. Antibacterial activity of *Hydrastis canadensis* extract and its major isolated alkaloids. *Planta Med* 67(6):561-564, 2001.

Shahi SK, Shukla AC, Bajaj AK, Banerjee U, Rimek D, Midgely G, Dikshit A. Broad spectrum herbal therapy against superficial fungal infections. *Skin Pharmacol Appl Skin Physiol* 13(1):60-64, 2000.

Shoji S, Furuishi K, Misumi S, Miyazaki T, Kino M, Yamataka K. Thiamine disulfide as a potent inhibitor of human immunodeficiency virus (type-1) production. *Biochem Biophys Res Commun* 205(1):967-975, 1994.

Sun D, Courtney HS, Beachey EH. Berberine sulfate blocks adherence of *Streptococcus pyogenes* to epithelial cells, fibronectin, and hexadecane. *Antimicrob Agents Chemother* 32(9):1370-1374, 1988.

Stiles J, Townsend WM, Rogers QR, Krohne SG. Effect of oral administration of L-lysine on conjunctivitis caused by feline herpesvirus in cats. *Am J Vet Res* 63(1):99-103, 2002.

Sun D, Abraham SN, Beachey EH. Influence of berberine sulfate on synthesis and expression of Pap fimbrial adhesin in uropathogenic *Escherichia coli. Antimicrob Agents Chemother* 32(8):1274-1277, 1988.

Tabba HD, Chang RS, Smith KM. Isolation, purification, and partial characterization of prunellin, an anti-HIV component from aqueous extracts of *Prunella vulgaris. Antiviral Res* 11(5-6):263-273, 1989.

Takahashi I, Nakanishi S, Kobayashi E, Nakano H, Suzuki K, Tamaoki T. Hypericin and pseudohypericin specifically inhibit protein kinase C: possible relation to their antiretroviral activity. *Biochem Biophys Res Commun* 165(3):1207-1212, 1989.

Venugopal PV, Venugopal TV. Antidermatophytic activity of garlic *(Allium sativum)* in vitro. *Int J Dermatol* 34(4):278-279, 1995.

Vynograd N, Vynograd I, Sosnowski Z. A comparative multi-centre study of the efficacy of propolis, acyclovir and placebo in the treatment of genital herpes (HSV). *Phytomedicine* 7(1):1-6, 2000.

Weinberg JB, Shugars DC, Sherman PA, Sauls DL, Fyfe JA. Cobalamin inhibition of HIV-1 integrase and integration of HIV-1 DNA into cellular DNA. *Biochem Biophys Res Commun* 246(2):393-397, 1998.

Yeung H. *Handbook of Chinese Herbal Formulas*. Los Angeles, 1995, Self-published.

Yeung H. *Handbook of Chinese Herbs*. Los Angeles, 1996, Self-published.

11

Therapies for Liver Disorders

ASCITES

Therapeutic Rationale

- Decrease sodium intake.
- Administer intermittent diuretic therapy.

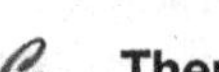

Paradigmatic Options

- Laboratory evaluation can be of great help to the practitioner in the determination of the correct Chinese medical approach to reducing ascites. When fluid accumulation is due to low albumin levels, a Spleen tonification approach must be used. Use of the typically aggressive diuretic formulas described in the following paragraphs should be avoided unless severe or life-threatening edema is present. For cases that are not immediately life threatening, **Wei Ling Tang** (Decoction to Dispel Dampness in the Spleen and Stomach) is one formula that tonifies the Spleen to nourish the Liver, indirectly producing Blood and albumin, and that has a mild but significant diuretic action. Guiding signs and symptoms to its use include abdominal fullness and distention, edema, poor appetite, diarrhea, a soft pulse, and a swollen or wet and pale tongue. A *suggested starting dose* of granular concentrate is ¼ tsp per 10 to 15 lb of body weight, or 60 to 75 mg/kg of body weight, divided into two daily doses.
- **Xiao Yao San** (Rambling Ease Powder) also is useful in addressing Spleen deficiency leading to Liver Blood deficiency when hypoalbuminemia and anemia are present. This formula has no diuretic function. A *suggested starting dose* of granular concentrate is ¼ tsp

per 10 to 15 lb of body weight, or 60 to 75 mg/kg of body weight, divided into two daily doses. This is a good finishing formula for a patient with ascites that has resolved with Wei Ling Tang, but in which albumin levels are still low. Its Chai Hu component acts to stimulate RNA synthesis in hepatocytes, and this may lead to increased albumin production.

- Acupuncture points that help support the Liver by supporting the Spleen include CV 6, CV 12, ST 36, LI 4, BL 20, and BL 21. Points that directly nourish Blood include LIV 3, SP 6, and BL 17.
- Chinese herbal formulas generally induce catharsis, diuresis, or both to eliminate severe ascites. This approach is used in strong excessive patients only, and is achieved by the formulas below:
  - **Yu Gong San** can be considered for mild ascites with constipation. This formula contains the strong diuretic and cathartic Qian Niu Zi and the antispasmodic Xiao Hui Xiang (Fennel). Fennel counteracts the forcefulness of the large intestinal contractions induced by Qian Niu Zi. A *suggested starting dose* of granular concentrate is no more than ¼ tsp per 10 to 15 lb of body weight, or 60 to 75 mg/kg of body weight, divided into two daily doses. Once the ascites accumulation has been drained, use of the formula should end and underlying problems be addressed.
  - **Fen Shui Dan** contains Gan Cao and Gan Sui in a 5:1 ratio. Gan Sui induces catharsis, and Gan Cao guards against severe abdominal pain associated with the forceful contractions of the large intestine. A *suggested starting dose* of granular concentrate is no more than ¼ tsp per 10 to 15 lb of body weight, or 60 to 75 mg/kg of body weight, divided into two daily doses. Once the ascites accumulation has been drained, use of the formula should end and underlying problems be addressed.
  - Another formula is essentially a combination of **Fen Shui Dan** and **Yu Gong San** in that it contains both Gan Sui and Qian Niu Zi. It also contains Da Huang and Bing Lang as additional purgatives and Lai Fu Zi and Chen Pi to reduce the severity of intestinal

contractions. All herbs are present in equal ratios except Gan Sui, which should be one third the amount of each of the other constituents. A *suggested starting dose* of granular concentrate is no more than ¼ tsp per 10 to 15 lb of body weight, or 60 to 75 mg/kg of body weight, divided into two daily doses. Stop formula use and address underlying problems once the ascites accumulation has been drained.

- Since ascites is a type of Yin accumulation, an excessively Yin nature of the body can foster its development. Yang deficiency is the usual mechanism by which Yin excess develops. A formula to address Spleen and Kidney Yang deficiency that results in the accumulation of pathologic water is **Fu Gui Li Zhong Tang** (Warm the Center Decoction with added Aconite and Ginger) combined with the **Yu Gong San** previously described. Signs and symptoms suggesting the appropriateness of this formula include fatigue, edema, low back stiffness and pain, coldness over the low back and extremities, a pale, swollen, wet tongue, and a deep, weak pulse. A *suggested starting dose* of granular concentrate is ¼ tsp per 10 to 15 lb of body weight, or 60 to 75 mg/kg of body weight, divided into two daily doses.
- Deficient Damp patients with jaundice for which a milder diuretic is sought may benefit from **Yin Chen Wu Ling San** (Capillaris and Five Herbs with Poria Powder). This formula is not cathartic or particularly Spleen tonifying, but is a surprisingly potent diuretic. Patients that benefit have edema, diarrhea, vomiting, dysuria, jaundice, a pale, wet tongue, and a soft or slippery pulse. A *suggested starting dose* of granular concentrate is ¼ tsp per 10 to 15 lb of body weight, or 60 to 75 mg/kg of body weight, divided into two daily doses.
- When jaundice is not present, Yin Chen Hao is omitted from Yin Chen Wu Ling San and the base formula known as **Wu Ling San** (Five Herbs with Poria Powder) is used. Indications for its use include substantial edema accumulations and slippery pulses. It may be useful for reducing edema in patients with congestive

heart failure that respond poorly to furosemide. A *suggested starting dose* of granular concentrate is ¼ tsp per 10 to 15 lb of body weight, or 60 to 75 mg/kg of body weight, divided into two daily doses.

- For all cases of ascites useful acupuncture points include BL 22, BL 39, and CV 9. These points have a diuretic effect and drain the three burners in which the fluid builds up. For Yang-deficient patients add BL 23, KI 3, or CV 4.
- A more common presentation of ascites is its development secondary to hepatomegaly and cirrhotic changes. The formula **Hua Yu Fang** is recommended in these cases to move the stagnant Blood causing the hepatomegaly. The constituents are listed as Tao Ren 9 g, Hong Hua 9 g, Tu Bie Chong 9 g, Dan Shen 15 g, Chi Shao 15 g, Yu Jin 9 g, Dang Gui 15 g, Mu Li 30 g, Chai Hu 9 g, Chuan Lian Zi 12 g, Jie Geng 9 g, Zi Wan 9 g, Ting Li Zi 9 g, and Jiao Mu 9 g. Only the last two herbs are diuretics, and most of this formula is directed at softening the liver enlargement. A *suggested starting dose* of granular concentrate is ¼ tsp per 10 to 15 lb of body weight, or 60 to 75 mg/kg of body weight, divided into two daily doses. Acupuncture points that supplement the action of this formula are ST 37, ST 39, BL 11, BL 17, BL 22, SP 6, and CV 9.

Western Herbs

- Two Western herbs that have been advocated as diuretics are Dandelion *(Taraxacum officinale)* and Parsley *(Petroselinum crispum)*. Dandelion was specifically recommended in the early Western herbal literature as a diuretic to consider in ascites secondary to liver failure. Unfortunately, my (SM) initial clinical experience with Dandelion in such cases has been disappointing. A suggested starting dose of liquid extract of either of these herbs is 0.2 ml per 5 lb of body weight divided into two doses.
- **Milk Thistle** *(Silybum marianum):* may stimulate the activity of RNA polymerase in hepatocytes, leading to increased albumin synthesis. Evidence also supports its function as an anticirrhotic. Milk Thistle may therefore

be valuable in the management of Ascites secondary to liver failure. A suggested starting dose of liquid extract is 0.2 ml per 5 lb of body weight given two to three times daily. Milk Thistle appears to have a high therapeutic index and is generally regarded as safe for prolonged use. It is also indicated for ascites arising from hepatic cirrhosis.

AUTHORS' CHOICES:

SM: Appropriate Chinese herbal formula.
SW: Appropriate Chinese herbal formula; acupuncture.

CANINE CHRONIC HEPATITIS

Therapeutic Rationale

- Remove or treat underlying cause.
- Slow the inflammatory process.
- Attempt to stop fibrotic change.

Alternative Options with Conventional Bases

- See the section on General Hepatitis.

Paradigmatic Options

- See the section on General Hepatitis for a list of formulas useful in canine hepatitis. Give special consideration to formulas dealing with Liver Blood deficiency, which is arguably the most common cause of chronic active hepatitis in the dog.
- **Long Dan Xie Gan Tang** (Gentian Drain the Liver Decoction) can be considered for excessive patients with wiry, forceful pulses, a red or yellow tongue, icterus, irritability, red eyes, and lethargy. This formula may be used in dogs or cats, but is particularly relevant for the treatment of dogs. A formula that has been advocated for cats in particular but is probably also suitable for dogs with this condition is **Yin Chen Hao Plus** (Capillaris Plus). Some herb companies may sell this formula under the name **Artemisia**

Formula or **Li Dan Pian.** The constituents of the formula are 20 g of Yin Chen Hao; 12 g each of Mu Dan Pi and Sheng Di Huang; 11 g of Huang Lian; 10 g each of Zhi Zi, Chi Shao, Fu Ling, Zhu Ling, and Ze Xie; and 5 g of Da Huang. This formula probably has stronger jaundice-clearing effects than **Long Dan Xie Gan Tang** does. Neither of these formulas should be used for weak patients with feeble pulses and a pale tongue.

AUTHORS' CHOICES:

SM: Appropriate Chinese herbal formula.
SW: Milk Thistle; SAMe; Vitamin E; Turmeric; Chinese herbs.

COPPER-ASSOCIATED HEPATOPATHY

Therapeutic Rationale

- Decrease copper absorption by decreasing copper in diet and using drugs to prevent absorption.
- Increase excretion (copper chelators).

Alternative Options with Conventional Bases

- **Homemade diets:** concentrate on low-copper foods such as fruits, vegetables, eggs, fish, beef, pork, or poultry if a homemade diet is recommended. Avoid shellfish, organ meat, white flour, white rice, and dairy products.
- **Consider distilled or bottled water** depending on the mineral levels in the household water.
- **Antioxidants:** are increasingly recognized as important to mitigating the damage in copper storage disease (Sokol, 1996). Vitamin C in a dose of 250 to 1000 mg per day has been recommended to augment excretion and decrease absorption, but it has a prooxidant effect in the presence of metals and should probably be avoided. Vitamin E is the preferred antioxidant.
- **Zinc:** a recognized treatment for copper hepatopathy, it is used as a chelator to decrease copper absorption.

Elemental zinc should be administered at 200 mg in divided doses on an empty stomach to double serum zinc, then decrease to 50 to 100 mg per day. Supplement as acetate, sulfate, or methionine at 2 to 3 mg/kg of body weight daily. The goal is to maintain serum zinc at 200 to 300 μg/ml. Zinc methionine (Pala-Z, Z-Bec) may be better tolerated than other supplement forms.

Paradigmatic Options

- The signs exhibited by the patient should be matched to the most appropriate Chinese herbal formula in the General Hepatitis section of this chapter. The practitioner should also consider hepatoprotective antioxidant herbs such as Milk Thistle.

AUTHORS' CHOICES:

SM: Zinc and Vitamin E supplementation; Milk Thistle; appropriate Chinese herbal formula.
SW: Zinc; Vitamin E; Milk Thistle; appropriate Chinese herbal formula.

FELINE CHOLANGIOHEPATITIS COMPLEX (SUPPURATIVE AND NONSUPPURATIVE)

Therapeutic Rationale

- See the section on General Hepatitis.

Alternative Options with Conventional Bases

- See the section on General Hepatitis.

Paradigmatic Options

- See the comments and formula recommendations in the section on General Hepatitis. **Long Dan Xie Gan Tang** (Gentian Drain the Liver Decoction) can be considered for cats that have wiry, forceful pulses, a red or yellow tongue, icterus, irritability, red eyes, and lethargy. **Yin Chen Hao Plus** (Capillaris Plus) also has been advocated for cats with this condition. Herb companies may sell this formula under the name **Artemisia Formula** or **Li Dan Pian.** The constituents of the formula are 20 g of Yin Chen Hao, 12 g each of Mu Dan Pi and Sheng Di Huang, 11 g of Huang Lian, 10 g each of Zhi Zi, Chi Shao, Fu Ling, Zhu Ling, and Ze Xie, and 5 g of Da Huang. This formula probably has stronger jaundice-clearing effects than **Long Dan Xie Gan Tang.** Neither of these formulas should be used for weak patients with feeble pulses and a pale tongue.

AUTHORS' CHOICES:

SM: Appropriate Chinese herbal formula.
SW: Milk Thistle; SAMe; Vitamin E; Carnitine; Arginine; Phosphatidylcholine; Turmeric; appropriate Chinese herbal formula.

HEPATIC ENCEPHALOPATHY

Therapeutic Rationale

- Feed frequently to prevent hypoglycemia.
- Avoid use of short-chain fatty acids and aromatic amino acids.
- Reduce hyperammonemia by lowering colon pH.

Alternative Options with Conventional Bases

- **Soluble fiber in a low-protein diet:** soluble fiber such as psyllium and oat bran traps ammonia in the colon as NH_4^+, which effectively acidifies the colon and systemically reduces hyperammonemia.
- **Arginine:** experimentally induced arginine deficiency produces hepatic encephalopathy in cats (Taboada, 1995). Whether supplementation is needed above and beyond that included in a balanced diet is unknown, but might be considered at 250 to 500 mg bid.

Paradigmatic Options

- Hepatic encephalopathy seems to be a relatively severe form of Damp Heat accumulation. The abruptness and severity of symptoms suggest that strong formulas are needed. Many patients exhibit signs of Heat, including heat intolerance or a preference for cool areas or heat radiating from the area of GV 14 at the dorsal base of the neck and from the Gall Bladder channel on the head. Acupuncture points to address hepatic encephalopathy include GB 41 and GB 43 to drain Heat pathogens from the Gall Bladder channel and GV 14 to clear excessive Heat from the body.

- Herbal treatment seems to be more important than acupuncture in producing long-term improvements in patients affected by hepatic encephalopathy. **Long Dan Xie Gan Tang** (Gentian Drain the Liver Decoction) might be considered when symptoms include seizures or abrupt blindness and when Heat symptoms abound. A *suggested starting dose* of granular concentrate is ¼ tsp per 10 to 15 lb of body weight, or 60 to 75 mg/kg of body weight, divided into two daily doses. Acupuncture points to support the action of this formula include KI 1, LIV 2, GB 41, GB 43, GV 20, and GV 14.
- Strong detoxifying Western herbal formulas, including the **Hoxsey Formula,** might be beneficial in hepatic encephalopathy. For further information on this formula see Chapter 13. A *suggested starting dose* is 0.2 ml per 5 lb of body weight daily in divided doses.
- Lipotropic herb complexes, such as are discussed in the section on Hepatic Lipidosis, may help in the management of hepatic encephalopathy, particularly if they contain Oregon Grape *(Mahonia aquifolium).*

AUTHORS' CHOICES:

SM: Low-protein diet supplemented with soluble fiber; Long Dan Xie Gan Tang; Oregon Grape.
SW: Low-protein diet supplemented with soluble fiber; Chinese herbs.

HEPATIC LIPIDOSIS

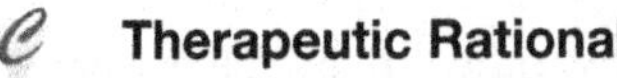

Therapeutic Rationale

- Maintain or stimulate appetite and reduce hepatic fat stores.

Alternative Options with Conventional Bases

- **Carnitine** (Carroll, 2001): it has been suggested that cats with hepatic lipidosis (HL) may have carnitine deficiency, since this can result in hepatic fat accumulation and overt disease. Whether or not this is true, the accumulation of fat deposited in the liver may overwhelm the normal Carnitine function in metabolizing fatty acids and worsen the problem. Reports of hastened recovery when carnitine is supplemented have fueled greater interest in carnitine as a treatment, and it is currently being investigated. It does appear that choline should be coadministered with carnitine, since choline is apparently necessary for hepatic uptake and transport of carnitine. The *dose* for cats is 250 to 500 mg per day.
- **Choline** (Carroll, 2001): required for hepatic uptake of carnitine. The supplementation of choline by administering lecithin reversed HL in human patients in a controlled trial (Buchman, 1992). Lecithin contains large amounts of phosphatidylcholine and the *suggested dose* is 1 g per 20 lb of body weight. Choline is also available as choline bitartrate and phosphatidylcholine. The *dose* for animals as calculated from human doses is about 10 to 15 mg per lb of body weight daily.
- **Arginine:** a deficiency of arginine may be associated with HL, either as a relative cause or because of the decreased food intake that precedes clinical signs. Arginine can be supplemented at a dose of 250 to 500 mg twice daily.
- **Betaine:** protected rats against carbon tetrachloride–induced fatty lipidosis (Junnila, 1998). Betaine has not yet been suggested as a treatment for HL in cats.
- **Vitamin B_{12}:** a deficiency possibly exists in cats with HL (Center, 1998). Supplementation is nontoxic and should be part of the treatment regimen.
- **Taurine:** supports bile acid conjugation in cats and may modify damage from bile acids in addition to enhancing their excretion (Center, 1998).

Paradigmatic Options

- Although Blood deficiency is the major bane of canine health, the main pathophysiologic mechanism underlying most feline disorders is Spleen Qi deficiency with the resultant elaboration of Phlegm and Dampness. Some of the most tangible manifestations of Dampness are lipid deposits. Even though lipid deposits are viewed as a normal body tissue in conventional medicine, most holistic paradigms see excess adipose as contributing little to the health of the organism or presenting a burden. Naturopathic medicine traditionally described excess adipose deposits as "morbid encumbrances." Similarly, the very connotation of the word Dampness in Chinese medicine is "an unusable tenacious substance."

- Several sequelae can result from Dampness accumulation including loss of appetite and jaundice. Indeed, jaundice is considered in Chinese medicine to be a form of Damp Heat or a stagnant accumulation of Dampness that has simply "composted" or become hot. In naturopathic medicine, lipid deposits are thought to serve as storage depots for various toxins, both ingested and autogenously produced. The natural decline in appetite accompanying obesity is thought to potentially result in these toxins becoming mobilized along with fat reserves. Once they enter the circulation, the toxins are perceived to damage the liver or interfere with liver metabolism, creating hyperlipidosis and jaundice.
- Naturopathic treatments of hepatic lipidosis use "lipotropic" herbs to counter tendencies to liver failure and jaundice by boosting bile production in hepatocytes. These herbs also contain other bitter principles that stimulate gastric secretion, peristalsis, and appetite. Many products combine lipotropic herbs with hepatoprotective plants such as Milk Thistle. Lipotropic products may be delivered by enema in anorexic cats that do not have a feeding tube in place. See the section on Nonsuppurative Hepatitis for further discussion on the usefulness of administering hepatic herbs via enema.
- Scientific investigation has confirmed the benefits of lipotropic herbs on increasing bile production. Oregon Grape stimulates the liver and gall bladder and increases production and secretion of bile by as much as threefold. Yellow Dock *(Rumex crispus)* similarly

promotes production and secretion of bile. Celandine *(Chelidonium majus)* causes the liver to secrete less viscous and more profuse bile and prevents formation of biliary calculi. It also has a spasmolytic effect on the bile ducts. Fringe Tree Bark *(Chionanthus virginicus)* promotes normal liver and pancreatic metabolism and enhances the clearing of jaundice.

Chinese Herbs

- The therapeutic goals in hepatic lipidosis in cats from the Chinese medical perspective are to drain Damp, clear Heat, and tonify the Spleen Qi. A formula that fulfills these goals is **Si Miao San** (Four Marvels Powder). Cats that benefit from this formula have a pale or yellow-coated tongue that is either small or swollen and wet, a soft, rapid pulse, poor appetite, possible elevated thirst, jaundice, colitis, and vomiting.
- An even more important formula to consider is **Yin Chen Wu Ling San** (Capillaris and Five Herbs with Poria Combination) since it contains Yin Chen Hao, which has long been used in Chinese medicine to eliminate jaundice. Patients benefiting from this formula might appar chilly, more mildly jaundiced, less thirsty, and more weakened and emiciated than patients benefiting from Si Miao San. Consider this formula also for patients that are not adequately responding to Si Miao San.
- Once jaundice has been largely cleared in an affected animal, a formula more directed at simply supporting the Spleen to improve appetite such as **Wei Ling Tang** (Decoction to Dispel Dampness in the Spleen and Stomach) can be used. Patients that benefit have abdominal fullness, loss of appetite, and loose stools.
- Another formula that has been suggested to support the Spleen in hepatic lipidosis cats is **Ping Wei Er Chen Tang** (Harmonize the Stomach Plus Two Herbs Decoction). This formula is made by combining **Ping Wei San** with the herbs Ban Xia and Fu Ling. These herbs figure prominently in **Er Chen Tang** (Two Herbs Decoction), and their addition to Ping Wei San allows more Dampness to be drained and more Phlegm to be transformed than with Ping Wei San alone. Guiding

symptoms to the use of Ping Wei Er Chen Tang are marked weight loss, anorexia, lethargy, vomiting, diarrhea, and salivation. The tongue is pale or pale yellow and wet, and the pulse is weak and wiry.

- Neither **Ping Wei Er Chen Tang** nor **Wei Ling Tang** have herbs to clear jaundice. The addition of 12 g of Yin Chen Hao and 9 g of Ban Xia to Wei Ling Tang corrects this shortfall and produces a formula that includes Ping Wei Er Chen Tang. This combination is probably the single best Chinese herbal formula for hepatic lipidosis in cats that have a poor appetite, vomiting, diarrhea, salivation, a pale tongue, soft and rapid or wiry pulses, and low-grade jaundice. Regardless which of the above formulas are used, a *suggested starting dose* of granular concentrate is ¼ tsp per 10 to 15 lb of body weight, or 60 to 75 mg/kg of body weight, divided into two daily doses.

AUTHORS' CHOICES:

SM: Wei Ling Tang with Yin Chen Hao and Ban Xia; lipotropic herbs with Carnitine, Taurine, and Phosphatidylcholine; give formulas in large doses by enema.

SW: Carnatine; Phosphatidylcholine; B-complex, Arginine; Taurine; Vitamin B_{12} injections.

HEPATITIS, GENERAL NONSUPPURATIVE

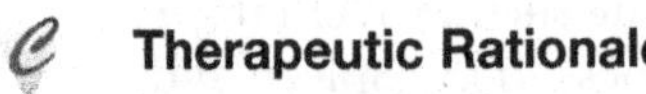

Therapeutic Rationale

- Rule out infectious or toxic causes.
- Reduce inflammation and fibrosis.

Alternative Options with Conventional Bases

Nutrition

- **Homemade diet:** there is growing belief that commercial diets may have excessive amounts of iron. Archived liver histopathology samples from dogs show increasing hepatic iron stores (Twedt, 2001, TNAVC lecture). Vegetable and dairy proteins should constitute the greater part of the protein in cases of chronic hepatitis.

- ***S*-Adenosylmethionine (SAMe):** a potent antioxidant that detoxifies free radicals and regenerates intracellular glutathione. Controlled trials in humans have found SAMe effective in a number of different diseases (Coltorti, 1990; Mato, 1999). The *dose* for animals is approximately 20 mg/kg of body weight daily.
- **Antioxidant vitamins:** Vitamin E may reduce the toxicity of bile acids to hepatocytes. Use of only the d-alpha form is recommended, since it may be more available and active in the liver (Stocker, 2000). The *dose* for animals is 10 IU per lb of body weight. Vitamin C has been recommended; however, it has a prooxidant effect in the presence of metals and is therefore not recommended in copper accumulation hepatitis.
- ***N*-Acetylcysteine:** has been investigated in human liver disease models with variable results.
- **Liver:** addition of liver to the diet or supplementation with liver glandulars has been recommended for many types of liver disease. Liver is a concentrated source of vitamins, minerals, amino acids, and other nutrients. Japanese studies have documented improvements in various types of liver disease or injury following administration of a liver hydrolysate (Fukuda, 1999; Washizuka, 1998). Supplementation with liver is probably contraindicated in copper storage disease.

Herbs

- **Milk Thistle:** appears to act as an antioxidant that reduces inflammation and stabilizes hepatic cell membranes (Flora, 1998). The most important reported use for Milk Thistle is to reduce damage from toxic insults. Trials in dogs poisoned with *Amanita* mushrooms showed that Milk Thistle greatly improved survival, liver function tests, and histopathology compared with dogs that received only supportive care (Floersheim, 1978; Vogel, 1984).
- **Artichoke Leaf** *(Cynara scolymus):* a traditional remedy for liver disease that exhibits protectant and antioxidant effects on hepatocytes in vitro (Gebhardt, 1997).
- ***Phyllanthus amarus:*** primarily used in human medicine to control viral growth and pathologic abnormalities of

the liver caused by hepatitis B infection. It is of questionable benefit in canine and perhaps feline hepatitis unless a viral connection is established.

- **Schisandra** *(Schisandra chinensis)*: a traditional Chinese herb that has been shown in animal studies to protect the liver from toxin damage (Ip, 1996).
- **Licorice** *(Glycyrrhiza glabra, G. uralensis)*: extracts may have some hepatoprotective properties (Shim, 2000). However, Licorice also may affect hepatic drug metabolism enzymes and should be administered with care if other drugs are being used (Paolini, 1998).
- **Turmeric** *(Curcuma longa)*: a powerful antioxidant and extracts of it have been demonstrated to inhibit hepatocellular carcinogenesis as well as toxin-induced damage to the liver (Chuang, 2000; Reddy, 1996; Soni, 1992).
- Many of these herbs are included in lipotropic herbal compounds manufactured to protect hepatocytes against damage and enhance bile production and secretion.

Paradigmatic Options

- One of the fastest ways to gain control of hepatitis is to deliver the appropriate herb or herbal formula by enema. The goal is to provide a retention enema that will allow herbal constituents to bypass any dysfunction in the upper gastrointestinal tract and enter the liver through the portal system that drains the large intestinal mucosa. The ability to deliver doses several times greater than those that can be reasonably given orally compensates for any reduced absorption of herbal constituents across the large intestinal mucosa. Clinical experience with the use of herbal enemas as a delivery system for hepatic herbs has been very encouraging and is probably the best strategy in critical cases until parenteral preparations become more available. An aqueous preparation is made by adding the desired dose of dried herb or granular concentrate to about ¼ to ½ ml of warm water per lb of body weight. Alcohol extracts are never used for retention enemas, since they tend to irritate the large intestinal mucosa and promote peristalsis, which limits their absorption. The enema is instilled as high in the colon as possible. This is repeated three times daily, or more often in severe or acute cases. No risk of hyperosmotic diarrhea appears to be present with this technique. Side effects are extremely rare if the herbs used in the enema are appropriate to the case, even with massive doses of 6 to 10 times larger than those that would normally be given.

Liver Blood Deficiency

- Blood deficiency plays a major role in canine low-grade asymptomatic or chronic hepatitis that is detected through routine chemistry panels. As discussed in other chapters there are many clinical manifestations of Blood deficiency in dogs. An appropriate Blood tonic formula to address the particular case will also usually lower liver enzymes. Individual herbs supportive of Blood tonification such as Milk Thistle or Wu Wei Zi (Schisandra) may be included to increase benefits to the liver. They may also be used when hepatitis is the presenting complaint.
- One of the major causes of Liver Blood deficiency is Spleen Qi deficiency. The Spleen generates Blood for the entire body, but the Liver exhibits a particular dependence on the Spleen because of its proximity to the Spleen and the generally interdependent relationship of the two organs in Chinese medicine. A formula that assists the Spleen in manufacturing Blood for the Liver is **Xiao Yao San** (Rambling Ease Powder). Guiding symptoms to the use of this formula include a poor appetite, a pale or lavender tongue, soft or thin, wiry pulses, anemia, lassitude, chronic vomiting, and chilliness. A *suggested starting dose* of granular formula is ¼ tsp per 10 to 15 lb of body weight, or 60 to 75 mg/kg of body weight, divided into two daily doses. This formula contains a substantial amount of Chai Hu (Bupleurum), which has major benefits in hepatitis. Research indicates that the herb has a significant choleretic action that lowers blood cholesterol and acts to decrease aspartate aminotransferase (AST) and

alanine aminotransferase (ALT) levels. It also increases the synthesis of glycogen and RNA in the hepatocytes, which makes Chai Hu of particular interest in hypoalbuminemia cases.

- Because Chai Hu is useful in combating hepatitis, I (SM) recommend adding it to any Liver Blood–deficiency formulas when the patient is also exhibiting some degree of Qi stagnation. One such formula is **Dang Gui Shao Yao San** (Angelica and Peony Powder). This formula is used when Liver Blood deficiency and Dampness accumulation are evident and Spleen Qi–deficiency signs are not prominent. Guiding symptoms to the use of this formula include slippery and wiry pulses, a frothy or slightly swollen lavender or pale tongue, anemia, mild ascites, poor appetite, vomiting, mucoid stools, hyperlipidemia, crystalluria, and cystitis. Add about 9 g of Chai Hu per 50 g of base formula. A *suggested starting dose* of granular concentrate is ¼ tsp per 10 to 15 lb of body weight, or 60 to 75 mg/kg of body weight, divided into two daily doses.
- When Blood deficiency exists without any evidence of Dampness or Spleen Qi deficiency, **Bu Gan Tang** (Nourish the Liver Decoction) can be used with the addition of about 12 g Chai Hu to 70 g of the base formula. Guiding symptoms to the use of this formula include fear aggression, a tendency to muscle spasms or stiffness, a dry coat, a thin, wiry pulse, and a pale-lavender tongue. A *suggested starting dose* of granular concentrate is ¼ tsp per 10 to 15 lb of body weight, or 60 to 75 mg/kg of body weight, divided into two daily doses.
- Milk Thistle, although a Western herb, embodies the energetic of a Blood-moving herb in my opinion (SM). One indication of the herb's Blood-moving ability is Milk Thistle's documented anticirrhotic activity. Milk Thistle also stimulates RNA polymerase activity in the liver, which makes it, like Chai Hu, of particular potential benefit in hypoalbuminemia. The herb may be used in addition to the above formulas when Blood stasis appears to be present. A suggested starting dose for Milk Thistle is 0.2 ml per 5 lb of

body weight twice daily. Milk Thistle is generally safe and may be used at twice this dose if necessary.

- Acupuncture points that help support the Liver by supporting the Spleen include CV 6, CV 12, ST 36, LI 4, BL 20, and BL 21. Points that directly nourish Blood include LIV 3, SP 6, and BL 17.
- Other authors do not emphasize Blood tonic formulas in their treatment of hepatitis. They instead identify the following five types of hepatitis from a Chinese medical perspective.

Liver Qi Stagnation

- Guiding symptoms include flank pain, irritability or depression, belching, vomiting, diarrhea, anorexia, increased ALT, a red or purple-red tongue, and a wiry pulse. One formula that has been advocated to address this problem is **Chai Hu Shu Gan San** (Bupleurum Ease the Liver Decoction). This formula makes heavy use of Bupleurum and contains the ingredients of the preeminent formula to move Liver Qi, **Si Ni San** (Four Cold Extremities Powder). Chai Hu Shu Gan San also contains Xiang Fu and Chuan Xiong, which are added to reduce abdominal pain and move Blood, respectively. A *suggested starting dose* of granular concentrate is ¼ tsp per 10 to 15 lb of body weight, or 60 to 75 mg/kg of body weight, divided into two daily doses.
- The foremost acupuncture point combination to move stagnant Liver Qi is LIV 3 and LI 4, also known as the Four Gates.

Damp Heat in the Liver

- The hallmark of Damp Heat is icterus. Accompanying signs and symptoms include dry stools, colitis, anorexia, dark, scanty urine, thirst, abdominal distention, a red tongue that may have a yellow coating, and a rapid, wiry pulse. **Yin Chen Hao Tang** (Capillaris Decoction) is the main formula used to treat severe acute excessive cases of hepatitis with associated jaundice. Various herbs, including Chai Hu and Yu Jin, can be added to increase the effect of the formula against hepatitis and to help move Qi and clear jaundice. Never use this formula in obviously deficient patients, since it may depress appetite and cause diarrhea. A *suggested starting dose* of granular concentrate is ¼ tsp per 10 to 15 lb of body weight, or 60 to 75 mg/kg of body weight, divided into two daily doses.

- When acute hepatitis is characterized by heat intolerance, inguinal rashes, aggression, scleral congestion, and thirst, **Long Dan Xie Gan Tang** (Gentian Drain the Liver Decoction) can be considered. This formula should never be used in a deficient patient, since it may cause depression, weakness, loss of appetite, and diarrhea. A *suggested starting dose* of granular concentrate is ¼ tsp per 10 to 15 lb of body weight, or 60 to 75 mg/kg of body weight, divided into two daily doses.
- When acute hepatitis has a prominent Spleen Qi–deficiency component that is manifested as marked jaundice, soft pulses, a pale tongue, vomiting, diarrhea, poor appetite, and weight loss, **Si Miao San** (Four Marvels Powder) can be used. **Yin Chen Wu Ling San** (Capillaris and Five Herbs with Poria) can also be considered for patients that respond poorly to Si Miao San or that are especially weak and chilly. A *suggested starting dose* of granular concentrate for both of these formulas is ¼ tsp per 10 to 15 lb of body weight, or 60 to 75 mg/kg of body weight, divided into two daily doses.
- **Ji Gu Cao Wan** (Abri Pill) is used for acute hepatitis when there is a suggestion of Blood deficiency or Blood stasis. A *suggested starting dose* is one tablet per 10 lb of body weight per day, divided into two or three doses if possible.

Liver Blood Stagnation

- When Liver Blood stagnation is more fully developed, it is manifested as hepatomegaly, abdominal distention, flank pain, weight loss, anorexia, exercise intolerance, depression, belching, a pale or purple tongue, and a weak or wiry pulse. The formula recommended for this condition is **Fu Yuan Huo Xue Tang** (Revive Health by Invigorating the Blood Decoction), and it is particularly recommended for treatment of subacute hepatic abscesses. Mild jaundice may be cleared with this formula even though its focus is on moving Blood. A *suggested starting dose* of granular concentrate is ¼ tsp per 10 to 15 lb of body weight, or 60 to 75 mg/kg of body weight, divided into two daily doses.

Liver Yin Deficiency

- There are milder or more chronic cases of hepatitis that are characterized by flank pain, red dry eyes, itching, vomiting, a red, dry tongue, thirst, a dry coat, poor appetite, and a rapid, thin, floating pulse. The main formula for this condition is **Yi Guan Jian** (One Linking Decoction). A *suggested starting dose* of granular concentrate is ¼ tsp per 10 to 15 lb of body weight, or 60 to 75 mg/kg of body weight, divided into two daily doses.

Qi and Blood Deficiency

- Patients with chronic hepatitis that is manifested as chills, fatigue, exercise intolerance, a pale tongue, and a frail pulse can be treated with **Shi Quan Da Bu Tang** (Ten Great Tonifiers Decoction). A *suggested starting dose* of granular concentrate is ¼ tsp per 10 to 15 lb of body weight, or 60 to 75 mg/kg of body weight, divided into two daily doses.

Cautions

- There are case reports of hepatitis caused by various herbs. These include Kava Kava *(Piper methysticum)*, Celandine *(Chelidonium majus)*, Comfrey *(Symphytum officinale)*, Chaparral *(Larrea tridentata)*, Germander *(Teucrium chamaedrys)*, Sassafras *(Sassafras albidum)*, and others. None of these except for Celandine has been advocated for treatment of liver disease. In addition, the Chinese herbal formulas **Xiao Chai Hu Tang** and **Jin Bu Huan** have been associated with liver damage.

AUTHORS' CHOICES:

SM: Appropriate Chinese herbal formula.
SW: SAMe; Vitamin E; N-Acetylcysteine; Milk Thistle; Turmeric.

HEPATOMEGALY

Therapeutic Rationale

- Identify the cause.

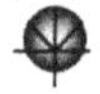

Paradigmatic Options

- Historically, Chinese medicine was fairly literal in its interpretation of pathologic conditions. An enlarged, deep-red organ would represent an accumulation of Blood, or Blood stasis. A series of formulas were developed about 200 years ago to address Blood stasis in various parts of the body. They are exceedingly helpful in many animal conditions and include **Xue Fu Zhu Yu Tang** (Drive Out Stasis from the Mansion of Blood) and **Shao Fu Zhu Yu Tang** (Drive Out Stasis from the Lower Abdomen Decoction), both of which are discussed in detail elsewhere in this text.
- The classic formula to address hepatomegaly is **Ge Xia Zhu Yu Tang** (Drive Out Stasis from Below the Diaphragm Decoction). A patient that may benefit has a wiry or choppy pulse, a lavender or purple tongue, upper abdominal pain, palpable abdominal masses, irritability, and poor appetite. This formula deals strictly with Blood stasis and may be of exceptional value in the treatment of hepatic neoplasia.
- Several modern formulas have been developed to address hepatomegaly (Pang, 1991). **Hardness Softening Powder** is recommended for cases of active hepatitis, icterus, a red tongue, and a rapid, forceful pulse. It contains 10 g each of San Leng, E Zhu, Pu Huang, Wu Ling Zhi, and Chi Shao to move Blood, 15 g each of Kun Bu, Hai Zao, and Bie Jia (Turtle Shell) and 30 g of Xia Ku Cao to soften masses, 30 g each of Pu Gong Ying and Yin Chen Hao to remove jaundice, and10 g of Huai Jiao to cool Liver fire. The formula also appears to contain 10 g of Xuan Fu Hua to help transform the Phlegm that obstructs both Blood flow and the normal descent of Qi through the diaphragm past the Liver. A *suggested starting dose* of granular concentrate is ¼ tsp per 10 to 15 lb of body weight, or 60 to 75 mg/kg of body weight, divided into two daily doses.

- **Jiang Chun Hua Fang** is recommended for Liver Blood Stasis with Qi deficiency (Chen Jun, 1987). However, this formula contains anteater scales and turtle shell, which may be objectionable to some practitioners. The formula contains 9 g each of Tao Ren, Tu Bie Chong, Chuan Shan Jia, and Dan Shen to soften masses and move Blood, 9 g of Da Huang to move Blood and address jaundice, and 12 g of Bie Jia to soften the Liver mass. The formula also contains 20 g of Huang Qi, 30 g of Bai Zhu, and 9 g of Dang Shen. These herbs are Qi tonics and are included in the formula to increase strength, Blood formation, and appetite. The anteater scales (Chuan Shan Jia) can be substituted with Zao Jiao Ci (Locust Fruit Spine).
- A variation of **Jiang Chun Hua Fang** has been created for patients with mild Yin deficiency. Patients that benefit from this formula exhibit mild heat intolerance, thirst, restlessness, weight loss, and thin, wiry pulses. The herbal additives are 15 g of Sheng Di Huang and 10 g each of Di Gu Pi, Mai Men Dong, and Xuan Shen.
- A third version of **Jiang Chun Hua Fang** addresses Yang-deficient patients by including 3 g of Fu Zi, 12 g of Gui Zhi, and 9 g each of Yi Zhi Ren and Gan Jiang. Patients that benefit are older and chilly, with stiff backs and perhaps urinary incontinence.
- **Gan Ying Hua Wan** has also been advocated for Liver Blood Stasis accompanied by Qi and Blood deficiency. Patients benefiting from this formula are chronically affected and have a poor appetite, thin, wiry pulses, a pale-lavender tongue, chilliness, weakness, and upper abdominal pain. The formula contains 60 g each of Zhi Shi, Shao Yao, Bai Zhu, and Fu Ling, 45 g of Chai Hu, 30 g each of San Leng, E Zhu, Tao Ren, Di Long, Xue Jie, Mu Dan Pi, Bing Lang, Wu Yao, Chuan Lian Zi, Dang Gui, Chuan Xiong, Yu Jin, Ren Shen, Cang Zhu, Hou Pu, Qian Niu Zi, Ban Xia, and Hou Po, 15 g of Che Pi, Qing Pi, Mu Xiang, and Rou Gui, and 5 g of Sha Ren.
- A *suggested starting dose* for all of these formulas is ¼ tsp of granular concentrate per 10 to 15 lb of body

weight, or 60 to 75 mg/kg of body weight, divided into two daily doses.

AUTHORS' CHOICES:

SM: Ge Xia Zhu Ye Tang.
SW: Treat according to biopsy results.

---

11 CASE REPORT
Liver Failure in a Dog

HISTORY

Josh, an 8-year-old, male, neutered Yorkshire terrier, was brought to his local veterinarian with acute onset of polyuria and polydipsia and distention of the chest and abdomen. Clear fluid was aspirated from the chest and abdomen. The results of a complete blood count and serum chemistry profile showed low albumin of 1.09 g/dL (normal is 2.7 to 3.8 g/dL), low total bilirubin level, and a mildly reduced packed cell volume (PCV) of 34.7%. Abdominal ultrasound showed the liver to be hypoechoic and the bowel walls to be thickened, presumably with edema. Both preprandial and postprandial bile acid levels were elevated. Despite evidence to suggest pathologic abnormalities in the liver (abnormal bile acids, severe hypoalbuminemia, a hypoechoic liver, and hypobilirubinemia), lymphangiectasia was diagnosed as the cause of the severe edema accumulations.

Josh was prescribed a low-fiber and low-residue commercial dog food, which he found unpalatable. He was also prescribed furosemide to reduce edema accumulations. Twice the normal dose seemed to be required to provide adequate control and any reduction in the dose of the diuretic resulted in an immediate recurrence of ascites. This prompted the owner to seek out therapeutic alternatives that might have a more enduring effect.

My (SM) questioning of the owner revealed that Josh had persistent mucoid diarrhea despite the diet that had been prescribed. There was no evidence of blood in the stool or straining during defecation. In addition, the owner complained that Josh's body smelled like rotten eggs and that he had severe halitosis. Josh snored loudly when sleeping and often gagged and coughed.

When asked about Josh's general behavior, the owner remarked that Josh exhibited a poor appetite and seemed to be losing muscle mass. He was especially inappetant in hot weather, but ordinarily sought the comfort of heat. He dreamed often and was slow to wake in the morning.

PHYSICAL EXAMINATION

Josh's physical examination revealed loud borborygmi, normal lung sounds, fetid breath, tightness of the flanks but an otherwise normal abdomen on palpation, a pale, delicate tongue, and slow, soft, and slippery pulses. Acupuncture points that seemed particularly warm or turgid included BL 20 and 25 and CV 4.

ASSESSMENT

Despite the absence of any elevation in liver enzyme levels, sufficient evidence seemed present to suspect liver failure as the cause of Josh's accumulations of edema. Although elevations in liver enzyme levels are commonly called "liver function tests," this phrase is probably best reserved for true products of liver metabolism, such as BUN, cholesterol, albumin, and bilirubin. A depression of two or more of these values seems to be a reliable indicator of depressed liver function, especially when supported by other evidence such as a hypoechoic or "underfed" liver.

In Chinese medicine, impoverishment of the liver immediately implies that a Spleen-tonifying formula may be indicated. In Josh's case, this was supported by abundant evidence of Spleen deficiency with resultant Dampness, namely, chronic mucoid diarrhea, foul body odors, poor appetite, low energy, soft pulses, pharyngeal congestion that caused snoring, and accumulations of edema. Josh's declining muscle mass was a direct indicator of Spleen deficiency as was the activity felt at the acupuncture points BL 20 (a Spleen-tonification point), BL 25, which often becomes active when Damp-Heat accumulations are present in the body, and CV 4, which is an important point to stoke the fire under the cooking pot of the Spleen.

Josh's tongue pallor suggested the exact manner in which his Liver had become impoverished; Spleen deficiency had led to Liver Blood deficiency. In both Chinese and conventional medicine an adequate Blood supply is imperative to normal liver function.

TREATMENT

Therapeutic goals for Josh were to tonify the Spleen, to drain Dampness, and to nourish Liver Blood. A formula that fulfills these objectives and has significant diuretic action to physically reduce edema accumulations is **Wei Ling Tang** (Decoction to Dispel Dampness in the Spleen and Stomach). Josh was given ⅛ tsp twice daily. Furosemide was continued until laboratory evidence indicated that it was no longer needed. He was provided a home-cooked diet that he would find palatable to ensure that adequate nutrition was available to support albumin generation.

OUTCOME

Within 1 month Josh no longer needed diuretics and had gained so much weight that his edema was initially assessed as unchanged. However, laboratory tests showed his albumin level to have more than doubled and his PCV to be well within normal limits. In addition, Josh's stool had become formed and contained no mucus. Ascites was absent, his tongue was a normal pink color, and his pulses were moderate. His halitosis and body odor were much reduced, and he no longer sought heat. To consolidate these improvements Josh was prescribed **Xiao Yao San** (Rambling Ease Powder). As noted in the text, its content of Chai Hu (Bupleurum) stimulates RNA synthesis, which may result in increased albumin production in hepatocytes. Administration of furosemide was discontinued, and no further recurrences of edema were noted.

COMMENT

Possibly the single most important reason for investigation of therapeutic alternatives in veterinary medicine is the presence of drugs in plants for which we have no equivalent in conventional medicine. These include chemical compounds to improve renal perfusion, stabilize specific membranes in the body, and induce normal liver metabolism. The absence of these compounds in "pill form" does not imply that they are ineffective, but rather that it has been impossible to create a product that improves on them.

SM

REFERENCES

Bensky D, Gamble A. *Chinese Herbal Medicine Materia Medica,* revised ed. Seattle, 1993, Eastland Press.

Buchman AL, Dubin M, Jenden D, Moukarzel A, Roch MH, Rice K, Gornbein J, Ament ME, Eckhert CD. Lecithin increases plasma free choline and decreases hepatic steatosis in long-term total parenteral nutrition patients. *Gastroenterology* 102(4 Pt 1):1363-1370, 1992.

Carroll MC, Cote E. Carnitine: a review. *Compendium* 23(1):45-51, 2001.

Center SA, Warner K. Feline hepatic lipidosis: better defining the syndrome and its management. In the proceedings of the 16th Annual American College of Veterinary Internal Medicine Forum, San Diego, 1998, pp 56-58.

Chuang SE, Cheng AL, Lin JK, Kuo ML. Inhibition by curcumin of diethylnitrosamine-induced hepatic hyperplasia, inflammation, cellular gene products and cell-cycle-related proteins in rats. *Food Chem Toxicol* 38(11):991-995, 2000.

Coltorti M, Bortolini M, Di Padova C. A review of the studies on the clinical use of S-adenosylmethionine (SAMe) for the symptomatic treatment of intrahepatic cholestasis. *Methods Find Exp Clin Pharmacol* 12(1):69-78, 1990.

Floersheim GL, Eberhard M, Tschumi P, Duckert F. Effects of penicillin and silymarin on liver enzymes and blood clotting factors in dogs given a boiled preparation of *Amanita phalloides*. *Toxicol Appl Pharmacol* 46(2):455-462, 1978.

Flora K, Hahn M, Rosen H, Benner K. Milk Thistle *(Silybum marianum)* for the therapy of liver disease. *Am J Gastroenterol* 93(2):139-143, 1998.

Fukuda Y, Sawata M, Washizuka M, Higashino R, Fukuta Y, Tanaka Y, Takei M. [Effect of liver hydrolysate on hepatic proliferation in regenerating rat liver.] *Nippon Yakurigaku Zasshi* 114(4):233-238, 1999.

Gebhardt R. Antioxidative and protective properties of extracts from leaves of the artichoke *(Cynara scolymus* L.) against hydroperoxide-induced oxidative stress in cultured rat hepatocytes. *Toxicol Appl Pharmacol* 144(2):279-286, 1997.

Guoming Pang, editor. *1000 Most Effective Chinese Herbal Formulas from the Modern TCM Experts.* Beijing, China, 1991, China TCM Press.

Ip SP, Mak DH, Li PC, Poon MK, Ko KM. Effect of a lignan-enriched extract of *Schisandra chinensis* on aflatoxin B1 and cadmium chloride–induced hepatotoxicity in rats. *Pharmacol Toxicol* 78(6):413-416, 1996.

Jun C. *Pattern Identification for Tough Cases.* Shanghai, China, 1987, Shanghai Science and Technology Press.

Junnila M, Barak AJ, Beckenhauer HC, Rahko T. Betaine reduces hepatic lipidosis induced by carbon tetrachloride in Sprague-Dawley rats. *Vet Hum Toxicol* 40(5):263-266, 1998.

Mato JM, Camara J, Fernandez de Paz J, Caballeria L, Coll S, Caballero A, Garcia-Buey L, Beltran J, Benita V, Caballeria J, Sola R, Moreno-Otero R, Barrao F, Martin-Duce A, Correa JA, Pares A, Barrao E, Garcia-Magaz I, Puerta JL, Moreno J, Boissard G, Ortiz P, Rodes J. S-Adenosylmethionine in alcoholic liver cirrhosis: a randomized, placebo-controlled, double-blind, multicenter clinical trial. *J Hepatol* 30(6):1081-1089, 1999.

Naeser MA. *Outline Guide to Chinese Herbal Patent Medicines in Pill Form.* Boston, 1990, Boston Chinese Medicine.

Paolini M, Pozzetti L, Sapone A, Cantelli-Forti G. Effect of licorice and glycyrrhizin on murine liver CYP-dependent monooxygenases. *Life Sci* 62(6):571-582, 1998.

Reddy AC, Lokesh BR. Effect of curcumin and eugenol on iron-induced hepatic toxicity in rats. *Toxicology* 107(1):39-45, 1996.

Shim SB, Kim NJ, Kim DH. Beta-glucuronidase inhibitory activity and hepatoprotective effect of 18 beta-glycyrrhetinic acid from the rhizomes of *Glycyrrhiza uralensis. Planta Med* 66(1):40-43, 2000.

Sokol RJ. Antioxidant defenses in metal-induced liver damage. *Semin Liver Dis* 16(1):39-46 1996.

Soni KB, Rajan A, Kuttan R. Reversal of aflatoxin induced liver damage by turmeric and curcumin. *Cancer Lett* 66(2):115-121, 1992.

Stocker A, Azzi A. Tocopherol-binding proteins: their function and physiological significance. *Antioxid Redox Signal* 2(3):397-404, 2000.

Taboada J, Dimski D. Hepatic encephalopathy: clinical signs, pathogenesis, and treatment. *Vet Clin North Am* 25(2):337-355, 1995.

Vogel G, Tuchweber B, Trost W, Mengs U. Protection by silibinin against *Amanita phalloides* intoxication in beagles. *Toxicol Appl Pharmacol* 73(3):355-362, 1984.

Washizuka M, Hiraga Y, Furuichi H, Izumi J, Yoshinaga K, Abe T, Tanaka Y, Tamaki H. [Effect of liver hydrolysate on ethanol- and acetaldehyde-induced deficiencies.] *Nippon Yakurigaku Zasshi* 111(2):117-125, 1998.

Yeung H. *Handbook of Chinese Herbal Formulas.* Los Angeles, 1995, Self-published.

Yeung H. *Handbook of Chinese Herbs.* Los Angeles, 1996, Self-published.

12

Therapies for Musculoskeletal Disorders

MUSCULOSKELETAL PAIN—GENERAL CONSIDERATIONS

Alternative Options with Conventional Bases

Antiinflammatory Agents

- **Glycosaminoglycans** (GAGs) such as glucosamine appear to have mild antiinflammatory effects along with their more pronounced chondroprotective effects (Creamer, 2000). Glucosamine has been shown to be as effective as ibuprofen in well-designed human clinical trials and is safer than nonsteroidal antiinflammatory drugs (NSAIDs) (Qiu, 1998). Glucosamine HCl is better absorbed than glucosamine sulfate although we do not know if there is a clinical difference in dogs. Glucosamine or combined glucosamine and chondroitin are given at 20 to 50 mg/kg of body weight daily in divided doses.
- **Methylsulfonylmethane** (MSM): is an oxidation product of dimethyl sulfoxide (DMSO) and is sometimes considered a nutraceutical. It is found in plants such as Horsetail *(Equisetum arvense)*, fruits, vegetables, and grains and provides a sulfur source for methionine. MSM is said to reduce inflammation by acting as an antioxidant, but the antiinflammatory effects have not been substantiated. No toxicity has been reported, and clinical reports of efficacy against osteoarthritic pain continue to be encouraging. Practitioners administer MSM at 100 to 1000 mg per day, based on the animal's weight.
- **S-Adenosylmethionine** (SAMe): has been used in human medicine for depression, liver disease, and

arthritis. Laboratory animal studies suggest that SAMe has some chondroprotective function, and human clinical trials indicate that it may be as effective as NSAIDs and have fewer side effects. The *dose* for SAMe is 20 mg/kg of body weight per day.

- **Proteolytic enzymes:** have been used as anti-inflammatory pain agents because of their inhibition of proinflammatory compounds and fibrinolytic activity. In a randomized double-blind study comparing a combination enzyme product (bromelain, trypsin, and rutin) to diclofenac, the enzyme produced equivalent improvements in pain indices (Klein, 2000). Although that product is not available in the United States, a similar product, Wobenzym, is used in my (SW) practice at doses proportional to the human label dose.
- **Cetyl myristolate** (CMO): has apparent anti-inflammatory actions (Diehl, 1994), although it is not well studied. It is being used by some practitioners at a dose of 250 mg sid to 1155 mg bid. One potential advantage to using CMO is that its use is recommended for 2 to 4 weeks and then stopped indefinitely as opposed to the constant use required by most other nutritional supplements for osteoarthritis.
- **Evening Primrose Oil**, **Black Currant Oil**, and **Borage Oil:** all sources of γ-linolenic acid; they have been recommended for treatment of osteoarthritis in humans. In an excellent controlled study in people by Belch (1988), Evening Primrose Oil did not reduce morning stiffness, grip strength, joint tenderness, or debility test scores, but did allow a reduction in the use of NSAIDs. Leventhal (1994) examined Black Currant Oil and found that a daily dose of 15 capsules reduced some symptoms but did not produce an overall better response than in control groups. The large dose may be a deterrent to clinical use even if it does show better efficacy in future trials. Leventhal (1993) and Zurier (1993) conducted controlled trials comparing Borage Seed Oil to Cottonseed or Safflower Oil controls in clinical trials of 37 and 56 people, respectively. Borage Oil

appeared to lead to significant improvement in clinical signs with negligible side effects. The dose in Zurier's trial was 4 capsules bid.

- **Fish Oil:** although ω-3 fatty acids are potentially useful for their antiinflammatory effects, work to date suggests only that Fish Oil is effective for induced and immune-mediated arthritides.
- **Devil's Claw** *(Harpagophytum procumbens):* a plant used in traditional African medicine for arthritis. In two large trials totaling 315 human patients by Chrubasik (described in Ernst, 2000), Devil's Claw treatment at doses of 600 to 1600 mg per day resulted in more pain-free patients at the end of the trial.
- **Willow Bark** *(Salix alba):* two studies reviewed in Ernst, 2000, suggest that Willow Bark significantly decreases pain. Willow Bark is a source of salicin and might be expected to exert its effects through salicylate mechanisms. The usual caution veterinarians exercise in administering salicylate drugs in animals should be extended to the use of Willow Bark, Poplar *(Poplar* spp.), Sweet Birch *(Betula lenta),* and related plant species in veterinary medicine.
- **Feverfew** *(Tanacetum parthenium):* an herb with potential use in migraine headaches. In one trial detailed in Ernst, 2000, Feverfew was not effective in reducing pain in patients with arthritis.
- **Nettles** *(Urtica dioca):* in his review Ernst describes unpublished data from a randomized controlled trial in which a stew of aerial parts of the plant was effective for pain, but a concentrated juice containing 10 times more of the presumed active ingredient (lipoxygenase inhibitor caffeoyl malic acid) was not.
- **Ginger** *(Zingiber officinalis):* has been recommended for antiinflammatory effects through eicosanoid modulation. The few studies done may suggest some such activity (Bliddall, 2000).
- **Boswellia** *(Boswellia serrata):* may reduce pain and inflammation through its activity as a lipoxygenase inhibitor. It is commonly combined with Curcumin (an extract of Turmeric) in Ayurvedic arthritis remedies. In a single study on 37 patients with rheumatoid arthritis,

Boswellia extract was indistinguishable from placebo treatment in terms of reduction of NSAID use and subjective, clinical, or laboratory measures (Sander, 1998). One study demonstrated improvements in pain and disability in 42 human patients with osteoarthritis using a formula of Boswellia, Curcumin, Ashwaganda, and zinc compared with placebo (Kulkarni, 1993). In bovine serum albumin–induced arthritis, boswellic acids reduced inflammatory cell infiltrates (Sharma, 1989).

- **Yucca** *(Yucca schidigera):* popular but not well studied. One proposed mechanism of action involves the suppression of gut bacterial endotoxin production by saponins, which thus removes a supposed suppressor of proteoglycan synthesis.
- **Wild Yam** or **Mexican Yam** *(Dioscorea villosa):* traditionally used for pain control. It contains diosgenin, which has been used as a precursor in the manufacture of commercial corticosteroids. However, diosgenin does not appear to be converted to glucocorticoid by mammalian systems so the efficacy of Yam in treating arthritis is still questionable.

Analgesics

- **DLPA** (dl-phenylalanine): a precursor to L-dopa, norepinephrine, and epinephrine. It appears to inhibit decarboxylation of endogenous opioids (Budd, 1983; Kitade, 1988), and anecdotal reports of pain relief in some cases of osteoarthritis are encouraging.
- ***Corydalis yanhusuo, C. turtschaninovii, C. decumbens,*** and ***C. incisa:*** part of traditional Chinese herbal combinations for pain. Although a specific mechanism of action has not been well described, authorities state that continued use will lead to tolerance and to cross-tolerance with opioids.

Other Treatments

- **Massage and trigger point therapy:** dogs with chronic painful disorders often have accompanying painful muscular spasms and trigger points. Regular massage provides clear relief to many of these animals, and owners can be taught to identify problem areas and to

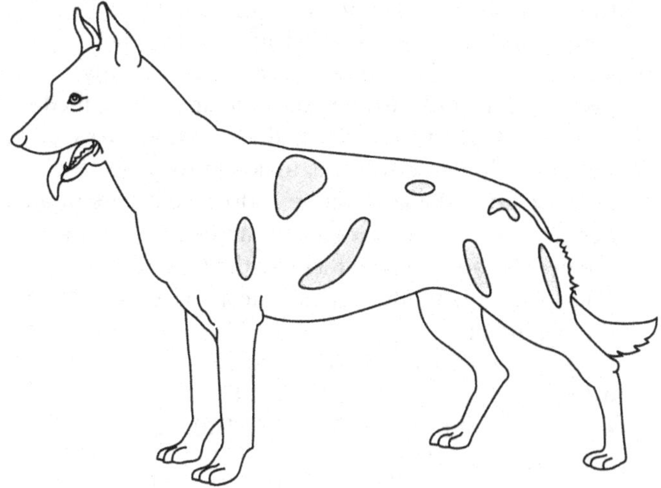

Fig. 12-1 Pain zone map. These are common zones that should be examined for trigger points and other painful muscular problems.

provide treatment at home. Owners may also consult licensed massage therapists for guidance. Figure 12-1 shows common zones that should be examined for trigger points and other painful muscular problems.

- Acupuncture has been shown useful in management of pain in osteoarthritis and other sources of musculoskeletal pain, either as a primary or adjunct intervention (Acupuncture, 1997; Ezzo, 2001; Green, 2002).
- Before treatment of musculoskeletal pain begins, referred pain from an internal organ problem should be ruled out. For example, chronic severe cystitis may produce substantial back pain that can only be resolved successfully by addressing the bladder inflammation.

Paradigmatic Options

Acupuncture

- Following is a list of suggested local or regional acupuncture points for the relief of localized pain. Not all of the points are taught in standard veterinary acupuncture courses, but it is reasonable to attempt to transpose the location of a human point to its corresponding position on an animal, especially if the area with which the point is associated is focally painful, hot, cold, swollen, or nodular. As described in Chapter 14, massage and moxibustion may prove to be valuable adjunct techniques to acupuncture for the relief of pain. Massage can be performed before or after needle insertion. Indirect moxa can be used to warm the needles and thereby increase the stimulation of the point and potentially enhance the analgesic effects of the treatment.

- Shoulder pain: LI 15, TH 14, SI 10
- Scapular pain: SI 11, SI 12, SI 14
- Elbow pain: LI 11, LU 5, LI 4, TH 10, TH 5
- Carpal pain: TH 4, LI 5, TH 5
- Lumbar pain: any or all of BL 23 through BL 27, BL 40 (Wei Zhong), GB 30, BL 59, BL 58
- Hip pain: GB 30, GB 29, GB 39, GB 34
- Knee pain: ST 35, GB 34, ST 34, SP 9, ST 36
- Tarsal pain: BL 62, KI 6, ST 41, BL 60, KI 3, GB 40

- Acupuncture points for the relief of pain in general and that may be combined with the local points are listed below. Specific indications for the points are listed. These points either have major influence over broad regions of the body or treat the root cause of the pain.
  - SI 3: relief of pain anywhere along the spine (the master point of the Du Mai or Governing Vessel) and relief of muscle spasm tendencies along the path of the small intestine channel, which includes the posterolateral aspects of the neck and shoulder joints and the maxillary region of the face. This point may be especially useful for Blood-deficient dogs that have thin pulses, a pale or lavender tongue, fine dander with a dull coat, and poor hair regrowth. They are itchy but have minimal skin lesions, are fearful or timid, and have dream-filled sleep.
  - GB 34: frequently indicated in Blood-deficient dogs as described under SI 3. As the Influential point for the Sinews, GB 34 is indicated in muscle spasm conditions anywhere in the body but especially along the lateral aspects of the body. The name of

this point can be translated as "Yang Mound Spring," which suggests that this point should be considered whenever Yang energy is required to mobilize the legs.

- LI 11: relief of pain that appears to be caused by the accumulation of Dampness pathogens, such as Damp Heat. Pulses may be fast, wiry, or slippery, and the tongue is often red to brick-red or purple-red. Past medical history may include colitis or cystitis. Musculoskeletal complaints may worsen in damp weather. The animal may seek cool places and show an increased appetite with low thirst or increased thirst with low appetite. Greasy skin complaints, moist pyoderma, and otitis externa with copious exudates are common.
- LI 4: relief of facial pain and all facial conditions. It is often combined with LIV 3 to make up "the Four Gates" when pain is arising from Qi stagnation. Guiding symptoms for pain caused by Qi stagnation include sudden temporary pain, shooting pain, a distending pain sensation, and pain improved by movement. Since animals cannot comment on the sensations attending pain, tongue and pulse diagnosis becomes especially important. The pulse is wiry, and the tongue is purple to lavender. LI 4 is also an important point to clear Heat from the body and it can play an important role in treating Heat Bi.
- LIV 3 (see LI 4): an important point for pain caused by Blood deficiency. Blood deficiency injures the Liver and hampers its ability to smoothly move Qi, which leads to pain. The tendency for Blood deficiency to "dry out the tendons" leads to muscle spasms. LIV 3 is the Source point for the Liver and it can nourish vacuities of the Liver including deficiencies of Blood and Yin. See SI 3 for symptoms of Blood deficiency.
- BL 17: for relief of pain caused by Blood deficiency. See LIV 3, SI 3, and GB 34 for more information. BL 17 is the Influential point for Blood.
- TH 5: an extremely important point for pain and stiffness involving the lateral aspects of the head and

neck. Its effects may be enhanced by combining it with GB 41.

- GB 30: perhaps the most important point for pain associated with the hind limb. Since opinions vary as to the exact location of this point, practitioners should carefully palpate the regions dorsal, posterior, and craniodorsal to the trochanter to determine the most advantageous point to place the needle. For some practitioners the optimum site will be the point they learned as GB 29, and for others it will be BL 54. The optimum site for the needle is often the center of the area that feels warmest when the palm of the hand is held ½ to ¾ inch above the skin overlying the hip. This may be interpreted in Chinese medicine as a location where Qi is not flowing. A return of radiant heat to the area after needling is attended by relief of pain.
- GB 39: As the lower uniting point of the three Yang channels of the leg, this point is theoretically of tremendous importance in relieving pain in the back, side, or front of the leg. In practice the point is not as useful as one might expect, but it is highly effective in certain cases. A guiding symptom to its use is the presence of swelling or distention in the region of the point.
- BL 40: relieves pain along the entire back, since it is the Command point for the back.
- SP 10: an important point to move and cool Blood. Blood stasis is a frequent complication of obstructed circulation that in Chinese medicine is the main cause of musculoskeletal pain.

- Acupuncture can be combined with a number of Chinese herbal formulas to treat musculoskeletal pain. Chronic pain in Chinese medicine is termed "Bi Syndrome," in which "Bi" means obstruction or blockage. The blockage is of Qi and Blood, which are normally viewed to flow over the surface of the body like a river within the "banks" of the twelve regular channels and the eight extraordinary vessels.
- When the flow of Qi and Blood is smooth and even, it produces no sensation. When a slight obstruction is present, it interferes with the flow of Qi first,

producing symptoms of fleeting, temporary, or shifting pains that are sometimes severe. Symptoms of Qi stagnation often improve with movement and sometimes with warmth.

- As the obstruction worsens, it increasingly interferes with circulation on a physical level and Blood stasis eventually develops. Symptoms of Blood stasis include stabbing, persistent, localized pain, a purple tongue, and a wiry or irregular pulse. Bruising or varicosities may be observed.
- The obstructions themselves are often considered to "invade" from the exterior. As they become more entrenched, more Blood stasis develops. An inherent general predisposition to internally accumulate the "pathogen" that invades externally is often present. For example, an animal prone to Dampness will be more prone to the invasion of Wind Damp and develop Damp Bi. The main types of Bi Syndrome are Wind Bi, Cold Bi, Damp Bi, Heat Bi, and Bony Bi.

Chinese Herbal Medicine

- Although each type of Bi Syndrome is treated with a distinct herbal formula, the formulas themselves share several similarities. Most of the formulas contain warm, pungent herbs to expel the pathogen, herbs to regulate the movement of Qi and Blood, and herbs to clear Heat, drain Damp, and warm the Yang. The different types of Bi Syndrome, the formulas to address them, and the Western diseases and conditions to which they roughly correspond are discussed below.
- **Wind Bi:** Wind Bi refers to pain syndromes that are fairly mild and not yet fully developed. The hallmark of these syndromes is a tendency for the pain to shift from one joint or meridian to another. Onset is often acute or rapid, and the pain may worsen with exposure to drafts or wind. The tongue is largely normal, but the pulse is often floating and tight. Herbal formulas classically indicated for this condition include **Fang Feng Tang** (Ledebouriella Decoction) and **Gui Zhi Shao Yao Zhi Mu Tang** (Cinnamon Twig, Peony, and Anemarrhena Decoction). Fang Feng Tang is somewhat

of an all-purpose formula in the sense that it disperses Wind, drains Damp, moves Blood, and is mildly cooling. When Wind or Dampness Invasion, Blood stasis, and Heat all seem to be present in a mild case of shifting lameness, this formula is indicated. The *recommended starting dose* of granular concentrate is approximately 60 mg per lb of body weight, or approximately ¼ tsp per 15 lb of body weight.

- **Gui Zhi Shao Yao Zhi Mu Tang** is a simpler formula to be used when Heat signs are mild but in evidence, as in patients with early rheumatoid arthritis. In particular, the affected joints may feel hot and be more painful at night even though they may act chilly overall. The *recommended starting dose* of granular concentrate is approximately 60 mg per lb of body weight, or approximately ¼ tsp per 15 lb of body weight.
- **Cold Bi:** Cold Bi is characterized by severe pain of the joints and limbs. Older animals are often affected, especially during winter. The pain is fixed, lessens with the application of heat, and worsens in cold weather. The patient has stiff limbs, a taut, wiry pulse, and a pale to normal tongue with a thin white coating. There may be an underlying weakness. Acupuncture points to aid this patient include warming points such as CV 4, GV 4, GV 14, CV 6, BL 23, Bai Hui (located between L7 and S1 on the midline), and KI 7. Indirect moxibustion around inserted needles is highly appropriate. The main herbal formula to manage this condition is **Wu Tou Tang** (Aconite Main Tuber Decoction). This formula contains Aconite and is potentially toxic with long-term use. The *recommended starting dose* of granular concentrate is approximately 60 mg per lb of body weight, or approximately ¼ tsp per 15 lb of body weight.
- **Du Huo Ji Sheng Tang** (Du Huo and Mistletoe Decoction) can be considered for the chilly deficient patient such as the older dog or cat. This formula treats pain arising from Liver and Kidney vacuity accompanied by depletion of Qi and Blood. From the modern Western medical perspective it is for chronic hind limb and low back pain in the old, feeble patient. Patients that benefit

often have a weak, thready pulse and a pale tongue. Alternatively, the pulse may be forceful and wiry, which reflects the struggle of the healthy Qi in the body against pathogenic Qi that is invading as a result of the patient's weakened status. A *recommended starting dose* of granular concentrate is approximately 60 mg per lb of body weight, or approximately ¼ tsp per 15 lb of body weight.

- **Damp Bi:** Signs of Damp Bi are heaviness and aching of the joints and limbs, fluid accumulations that cause distention and swelling of joints, or fixed pain that worsens during damp weather. The patient may also exhibit mental dullness or anxiety and have a slimy pale or lavender tongue and a slippery or wiry pulse. Damp Bi Syndrome may be more common in cases in which a link has been established between arthropathies and food allergies or sensitivities. The formula for Damp Bi Syndrome is **Yi Yi Ren Tang** (Coix Decoction), and patients with early rheumatoid arthritis may benefit from it. This formula moves Blood, warms and releases the exterior, dispels Wind Damp, drains Dampness, and tonifies the Spleen to reduce Dampness production. A *recommended starting dose* of granular concentrate is approximately 60 mg per lb of body weight, or approximately ¼ tsp per 15 lb of body weight.
- In cases in which it is difficult to determine whether the patient is affected by Wind, Cold, or Damp Bi, **Juan Bi Tang** (Bi Alleviating Decoction) can be considered. This all-purpose formula mainly addresses Qi and Blood stasis, or what is known as Fixed Bi. There are two versions of this formula. **Juan Bi Tang II** is probably a more powerful analgesic, but both versions of the formula have a similar thrust. The *recommended starting dose* of granular concentrate is approximately 60 mg per lb of body weight, or approximately ¼ tsp per 15 lb of body weight.
- Useful acupuncture points for Damp Bi patients, in addition to those summarized previously, include CV 6, ST 36, and SP 9.
- **Heat Bi:** Heat Bi is characterized by severe pain, local heat, redness and swelling of affected joints, difficulty

moving, fever, sore throat, irritability, and dark, scanty urine. Affected animals with the diagnosis may have a more advanced form of rheumatoid arthritis from a Western perspective. **Si Miao San** (Four Marvels Powder) is one formula for this condition. Animals that may especially benefit from this formula have an accumulation of Damp Heat in the lower burner that is manifested as lower limb swelling, cystitis, or colitis. They may have a red, wet, or yellow-coated tongue and a pulse that is soft, wiry, or slippery, and rapid. For these patients the practitioner should consider adding 9 g each of Mu Tong, Fang Ji (Stephania; currently under scrutiny; may be hard to obtain), Bi Xie, and Hai Tong Pi to 40 g of the base formula. These herbs will enhance the pain-relieving properties of the formula and aid in the drainage of obstructing Dampness. The *recommended starting dose* of granular concentrate is approximately 60 mg per lb of body weight, or approximately ¼ tsp per 15 lb of body weight. If acupuncture is used in the treatment of these patients, benefit should be seen from acupuncture at SP 9, ST 36, LI 11, BL 39, BL 40, LI 4, and CV 3.

- Other authors have suggested the use of **Bai Hu Jia Gui Zhi Tang** (Cinnamon Twig and White Tiger Decoction) for Heat Bi. Patients that benefit from this formula will commonly have systemic febrile illness, and it is more appropriate for severe immune-mediated arthritides. The *recommended starting dose* of granular concentrate is approximately 60 mg per lb of body weight, or approximately ¼ tsp per 15 lb of body weight. Acupuncture points for this presentation of Bi Syndrome include GV 14, ST 44, BL 40, LI 4, and LI 11.
- **Bony Bi:** Other classifications of Bi Syndrome include those that affect each of the various body tissues such as tendons, muscles, vessels, and bones. Bony Bi is relatively common in veterinary practice and results in bony deformities such as bone spurs, spondylosis deformans, and osteophyte production.
- Bony Bi is associated with deficient Kidney Yin or Yang, since the Kidneys are responsible for bone growth and integrity. Typical symptoms of the Kidney

Yang-deficient patient with Bony Bi are difficulty in rising and walking, coldness in the back and extremities, lameness that is worse in cold, damp weather, soft stools, and a desire to seek heat. The tongue is pale or pink, and the pulse typically weak and deep, although it may be forceful and wiry in some patients. An herbal formula to treat this syndrome is the previously mentioned **Du Huo Ji Sheng Tang** (Angelica and Loranthus Decoction). The *recommended starting dose* of granular concentrate is approximately 60 mg per lb of body weight, or approximately ¼ tsp per 15 lb of body weight. Acupuncture points to support Kidney Yang are BL 23, KI 7, and KI 3. Key points to relieve pain include BL 40, BL 60, GB 34, and GB 39. Other points that benefit patients affected with Bony Bi are BL 11, which is the Influential point of the Bones, Bai Hui, which is a meeting point of the three Yang channels of the leg, BL 17, and BL 24.

- Some practitioners advocate the patent remedy **Kang Gu Zeng Sheng Pian** (Against Bone Hyperplasia Tablets) for patients with Bony Bi. Although it is potentially useful, the formula unfortunately contains ground tiger bone. Its use cannot therefore be advocated here given the tiger's endangered status. Some preparations simply substitute bone from other sources, but the interchangeability in efficacy between tiger bone and the bones of other species is questionable.
- **Yin-deficient Bony Bi:** refers to conditions with such extreme Yin deficiency and Empty Fire that heat is felt to be steaming from the bones of the patient. The patient may have a host of Yin-deficient symptoms such as dry cough, weight loss, nighttime restlessness, thirst, heat intolerance, and weakness. Occasionally, the Yin-deficient patient attempts to immerse his or her limbs in cool water and may be found standing in the water dish or a swimming pool. Pulses are typically rapid and thin, and the tongue is red or tender and possibly small and dry. Acupuncture points to relieve this Bony Bi are KI 2, KI 3, LIV 3, SP 6, LI 11, and ST 36. An herbal formula for this condition is **Di Gu Pi Yin** (Lycium Root Bark Decoction). The *recommended*

starting dose of granular concentrate is approximately 60 mg per lb of body weight, or approximately ¼ tsp per 15 lb of body weight.

- **Wan Bi:** Another type of Bi Syndrome is Wan Bi, or Stubborn Obstruction, which may give rise to joint deformities. The main formula to treat Wan Bi is **Tao Hong Yin** (Peach Kernel and Carthamus Beverage). This formula addresses the Blood stasis and Phlegm accumulation that are the two main processes by which obstinate growths develop. The formula is not limited to pain in a particular location but can be used for localized persistent pain of any joint. Patients who will benefit from this formula typically have a dark or purple tongue and slippery, wiry, or erratic pulses. Tao Hong Yin's action against Phlegm may be made more powerful by the addition of 12 g each of Dan Nan Xing and Di Long to 75 g of base formula. A *recommended starting dose* of granular concentrate is approximately 60 mg per lb of body weight, or approximately ¼ tsp per 15 lb of body weight.
- A similarly designed formula is **Xiao Huo Luo Dan** (Minor Invigorate the Collaterals Pills). This formula not only deals with Blood stasis and Phlegm accumulation, but also warms the channels to both invigorate Qi and Blood and dispel Cold. It should not be used for extended periods because of the potential risk of Aconite toxicity, but it is otherwise a profoundly useful formula in veterinary practice. A *recommended starting dose* of granular concentrate is approximately 60 mg per lb of body weight, or approximately ¼ tsp per 15 lb of body weight.
- **Bu Gan Tang** (Nourish the Liver Decoction) is an aggressive Yin and Blood tonic and should not be used in cases in which Dampness symptoms are prominent (e.g., mucoid stools, weight gains, greasy coats, copious exudates, moist pyoderma, deep, dreamless sleep, and mental dullness). The formula's specific use is in cases of pure Blood deficiency with muscle spasms and tightness. Other guiding symptoms include thin, dry, powdery skin, dull and alopecic hair, thin, wiry pulses, pale to lavender tongue, fearfulness, irritability or fear aggression, and

low-grade skin allergies. The *recommended starting dose* of granular concentrate is approximately 60 mg per lb of body weight, or approximately ¼ tsp per 15 lb of body weight, divided into two doses.

- **Xue Fu Zhu Ye Tang** (Drive Out Stasis in the Mansion of Blood Decoction) can be used for less severe cases of pain caused by Blood deficiency. Lameness without obvious spasm may be present along with other typical Blood deficiency symptoms. This is an extremely useful formula in veterinary medicine. The *recommended starting dose* of granular concentrate is approximately 60 mg per lb of body weight, or approximately ¼ tsp per 15 lb of body weight.

Western Herbs

- In early Western herbalism the origin of chronic joint problems was commonly considered to be a form of autogenous intoxication by metabolites that were not properly cleared by normal body detoxification mechanisms. Skin disorders were thought to share the same pathophysiology, and the same herbs were often used to treat both joint and skin problems. Later Western herbal approaches to musculoskeletal disorders were very similar to approaches used in Chinese herbalism. That is, formulas often contained herbs that can be considered to move Qi and Blood, drain Dampness, transform Phlegm, and warm the circulation. Herbs from both Western and Chinese herbalism are useful today in veterinary practice and are listed below along with their proposed action according to Chinese medicine.
- **Qi-moving herbs:** Queen's Root *(Stillingia sylvitica)*, Black Cohosh *(Actea racemosa)*, Yellow Jasmine *(Gelsemium sempervirens)*, St. John's Wort *(Hypericum perforatum)*, Valerian Root *(Valeriana officinalis)*, and Kava-Kava *(Piper methysticum)*. Note that Gelsemium is potentially toxic and should constitute no more than 20% of a larger formula to address stiffness and pain. Gelsemium may be especially beneficial in relieving chronic tendencies to cervical vertebra fixation, including atlantooccipital joint fixation. See the section

on Chiropractic later in this chapter for further information on this disorder. St. John's Wort is specifically indicated for pain arising from nerve root compression caused by vertebral fixations.
- **Blood-moving herbs:** Prickly Ash Bark *(Xanthoxylum* spp.).
- **Warming or diffusive herbs:** Ginger *(Zingiber officinalis)*, Prickly Ash Bark *(Xanthoxylum* sp.), Pleurisy Root *(Asclepias tuberosa)*, Juniper *(Juniperus communis)*, Kava-Kava.
- **Phlegm-transforming herbs:** Sarsaparilla *(Smilax officinalis)*, Yucca, Burdock *(Arctium lappa)*, Pokeroot *(Phytolacca decandra)*. Note that Pokeroot is toxic.
- **Dampness-draining herbs:** Cleavers *(Galium aparine)*.

Useful Herbal Formulas

- For rheumatic complaints in chilly animals aggravated by damp weather: 25 ml Yucca, 25 ml Prickly Ash Bark, 25 ml Kava-Kava, 12.5 ml Black Cohosh, 12.5 ml Ginger. (Yucca has a tendency to cause diarrhea unless combined with Prickly Ash Bark.) The *suggested starting dose* is 0.1 ml per 2½ lb of body weight in two divided doses. Dose may need to be doubled.
- For obese, hot, painful, sluggish animals: 35 ml Cleavers, 20 ml Queen's Root, 20 ml Prickly Ash Bark, and 25 ml Burdock. The *suggested starting dose* is 0.1 ml per 2½ lb of body weight in two divided doses. Dose may need to be doubled. Animals that respond to this formula should be evaluated according to traditional naturopathic theory for problems in the eliminative and digestive systems that lead to "autointoxication." One such problem is Leaky Gut Syndrome. See the section on Osteoarthritis for further information.

Chiropractic

- Vertebral fixations are a common cause of lameness and weakness in dogs and cats. Fixations may occur at any vertebra, with the signs of the fixations dependent on where the spinal column is affected. Fixations of the lower lumbar and sacral vertebrae typically produce hind limb weakness and are especially common in cases with spondylosis deformans. In cats such fixations are associated with kidney failure or may be traumatically induced. See the section on Spondylosis Deformans for more information.

- Chiropractic recognizes that fixations in one part of the spine may produce fixations in another area, which may either be adjacent to the region of fixation or be some distance away. Lumbosacral fixations are frequently associated with problems in the atlantooccipital joint at the opposite end of the spinal column.
- Although it is not discussed in conventional veterinary textbooks, atlantooccipital joint fixation appears to be a well-defined clinical syndrome of dogs and cats. Following are my (SM) observations regarding this chiropractic condition.
- Causes of atlantooccipital fixation include lumbosacral fixation and traumatic injury. One additional situation in which the joint may become fixed is during dentistry procedures performed under general anesthesia when the animal's head may be inadvertently placed in an extreme of rotation, flexion, or extension to expose a particular tooth. Animals with an atlas fixation from dental procedures may also exhibit ataxia and imbalance upon suddenly turning their head. Veterinarians who provide chiropractic services to animals should routinely examine their patients after dentistry procedures to ensure that the atlas bone and adjacent cervical vertebrae are in normal alignment and exhibit a normal range of motion.
- In humans over half of the normal range of cervical flexion and extension is conferred by the atlantooccipital joint. The joint probably assumes similar importance in dogs and cats. Affected animals may resist extension of the neck during grooming or when eating, and owners often have to place food dishes on raised platforms in order to encourage affected animals to eat. Similarly, an animal may resist pronounced flexion and may also consistently hang its head off the edge of the bed during sleep. A tendency to wake up screaming in the middle of the night is virtually pathognomonic for atlantooccipital joint dysfunction, particularly in dogs. This probably occurs when the animal inadvertently overextends or

flexes its neck during the normal unconscious body movements of sleep.

- A diagnosis of atlantooccipital joint fixation is easily confirmed with careful palpation of the joint. The entire spine should be palpated and any fixations found elsewhere addressed. The diagnosis of atlantooccipital joint dysfunction can be confirmed by radiography when an obvious difference in the size of the gap between the atlas and occiput on one side versus the other is easily seen. In true atlantooccipital joint dysfunction this gap is independent of patient positioning during radiography.
- Response to chiropractic treatment of atlantooccipital joint fixations in dogs and cats is usually immediate, although long-standing fixations have a tendency to recur. Such recurrence is generally assumed to arise from muscle spasms secondary to nerve root impingement, or lingering fixations of adjacent cervical vertebrae or at the lumbosacral junction.

Cautions

- Herbs with corticoid-like activity (Licorice) may reduce blood salicylate concentration if being used with aspirin or with herbs that contain salicylate (Willow Bark, Meadowsweet, Birch, Poplar, Black Cohosh). Licorice may offer some protection against gastrointestinal (GI) irritation from salicylates.
- Licorice's corticoid activity may enhance the effects of concurrently administered glucocorticoids. Other studies suggest that Licorice increases the half-life of corticosteroids but reduces their immune-modulating effects.
- GAGs may affect clotting mechanisms, although studies have not verified these effects as clinically significant. If NSAIDS are being used, GAGs or herbs that have potential anticoagulant activity (*Gingko biloba,* Ginger, Ginseng, Garlic) may enhance the potential for bleeding. Blood-moving herbs in Chinese medicine frequently reduce platelet aggregation tendencies as well.
- Salicylate-containing herbs (Meadowsweet, Willow, Poplar, Birch, Black Cohosh) may interact with other NSAIDs.
- Devil's Claw has theoretical interactions with antiarrhythmic drugs.

AUTHORS' CHOICES:

SM: Acupuncture; chiropractic; Chinese herbal medicine appropriate to the presentation of the patient.
SW: Massage; acupuncture; GAGs; combinations of antiinflammatory herbs such as Devil's Claw; analgesic herbs such as Corydalis combinations for more severe, end-stage conditions.

CRANIAL CRUCIATE LIGAMENT RUPTURE

Therapeutic Rationale

- Stabilize joint.
- Minimize degenerative changes.
- Control pain.
- **Note**: A complete rupture of the ligament will probably require surgery for best results. Partial tears or instability may respond to conservative management with alternative medicine and physical therapy. These improvements are a double-edged sword, in that reduction in pain makes the animal more vulnerable to complete ligament rupture from leg overuse until the ligament has had adequate time to heal if healing is possible. Owners should always be warned of the possibility of rupture if the patient's activity is not controlled, even in animals that have responded well to alternative treatment.

Alternative Options with Conventional Bases

- See Musculoskeletal Pain section for a review of antiinflammatory herbs. Best choices may be Ginger, White Willow, and Devil's Claw.
- **GAGs:** are being investigated for their use in reducing degenerative changes following surgery. Although changes in joint glycosaminoglycan content have been observed, the clinical significance is yet unclear. However, there is a rational basis for use in preventing degenerative changes so we regularly use GAGs in managing the aftermath of cruciate ligament disease.
- **Prolotherapy:** the injection of sterile, irritating solutions around joints. These solutions include 50% dextrose, hypertonic saline, sodium morrhuate,

lidocaine, procaine, and pitcher plant extracts. The ensuing inflammation causes scar formation around injured or weakened ligaments that is thought to stabilize joints. It is important *not* to limit physical activity during the healing phase (up to 6 to 12 weeks after injection) so that the developing scar allows proper mobility with organized scar tissue.

Paradigmatic Options

Homeopathy

- *Ruta graveolens*: for ligamentous and periosteal injury. Patients are restless after prolonged immobility and have pain that worsens when motion is initiated and when the joint is used to excess. A specific symptom suggesting the usefulness of *Ruta graveolens* is an abrupt giving way of the limb during normal movement despite the absence of lower lumbar vertebral fixations. A *recommended starting dose* is 30C three times daily, tapering as improvements allow to one daily dose. Discontinuation of the remedy may be possible.
- ***Rhus toxicodendron:*** for discomfort that is worse on rising and is evident again following rest after heavy exercise. Patients that benefit are frequently Blood deficient from a Chinese medical perspective. Some patients benefiting from *Rhus toxicodendron* have pain aggravated by damp weather. This remedy may be used after *Ruta* if the response to *Ruta* is incomplete. A *recommended starting dose* is 30C three times daily, tapering as improvements allow to one daily dose. Discontinuation of the remedy may be possible.
- ***Lycopodium:*** has many of the modalities of *Rhus toxicodendron,* in that it addresses lameness that is worse on rising and better with continued motion. It may help in chronic cases in which *Rhus toxicodendron* was initially effective but later was not. Patients are often Blood deficient from a Chinese medical perspective and often exhibit either bullying or fear aggressive behavior. Overuse of *Lycopodium* 30C may produce malaise. A *recommended starting dose* is 30C once daily, tapering as improvements allow to the lowest effective dose.

- **Colchicum autumnale:** for advanced degenerative changes that result in pronounced crepitance and aggravation from motion. There may be irritability and aggravation in damp weather. The patient may be especially uncomfortable in the evening and at night. A *recommended starting dose* is 30C three times daily, tapering as improvements allow to one daily dose. Discontinuation of the remedy may be possible.

Traditional Chinese Medicine

- Ligamentous integrity is associated with adequate Liver function in Chinese medicine. Inadequacies of the Liver in dogs in Chinese medicine are almost always associated with Blood deficiency either as a primary problem or arising from poor Spleen function. The association of adequate connective tissue integrity with adequate Liver Blood is underscored by the use of compounds of connective tissue extracts, such as Donkey Hide Gelatin (E Jiao), as Blood tonics in Chinese medicine. This association puts a new light on the use of GAGs for osteoarthritic conditions in dogs, since it suggests that these compounds may be acting as Blood tonics from a Chinese medical perspective. This association also suggests that other Blood-tonifying herbs may be of benefit. A formula that contains both Blood-tonic herbs and E Jiao is **Jiao Ai Tang** (Donkey-Hide and Mugwort Decoction). Although it was developed to address problems associated with excessive uterine bleeding in women, the formula may be of benefit for truly Blood-deficient dogs. These dogs do not have any significant suggestion of Spleen deficiency or Dampness, and have pale tongues and thin, wiry pulses. Limb pain may be significant and may be especially aggravated on first motion and after exposure to cold. The *recommended starting dose* of granular concentrate is approximately 60 mg per lb of body weight, or approximately ¼ tsp per 15 lb of body weight per day, divided into two doses.
- For older, weaker Yin- and Blood-deficient animals that have some Dampness signs, the more complex **Jia Wei Si Wu Tang** (Augmented Four Materials Decoction) can

be tried. Patients that benefit will have muscle atrophy or weakness, particularly in the hind limbs, and experience difficulty walking. The tongue may be pale and coated and the pulse both thin and slippery. *Recommended starting dose* of granular concentrate is approximately 60 mg per lb of body weight, or approximately ¼ tsp per 15 lb of body weight per day, divided into two doses.

Acupuncture

- Acupuncture points commonly used for treatment of ligament problems include GB 34, GB 39, GB 30, ST 36, SP 6, LIV 3, and BL 17. See the general section on Musculoskeletal Pain for more information on the energetics of these points and further point suggestions.

AUTHORS' CHOICES:

SM: Acupuncture; appropriate homeopathic remedies.
SW: Surgery when appropriate; GAGs; acupuncture; physical therapy.

LUXATING PATELLA

Therapeutic Rationale

- Identify concurrent problems such as cruciate ligament rupture or hip laxity.
- Reduce degenerative changes.
- ◆ Control weight.
- Stabilize patella and correct other joint deformities.

Alternative Options with Conventional Bases

- **Conservative management:** appropriate if grade I and possibly grade II patellar luxation is asymptomatic and detected only on physical examination or if luxations produce only infrequent and very temporary "skipping" of the affected hind leg.
- **GAGs:** supplementation may help support cartilage repair and reduce inflammation. Starting dose is approximately 10 to 30 mg per lb of body weight.

Paradigmatic Options

Homeopathy

- ***Ledum palustre:*** for acute onset of knee pain that is worse during the night and with movement, and improves with the application of warmth or heat. The animal may have had recent trauma to the limb. A *recommended starting dose* is 30C three times daily, tapering as improvements allow to one daily dose. If pain does not resolve, *Ruta* may be required to "finish the case."
- ***Ruta graveolens:*** for subacute and chronic knee pain. Patients are restless after prolonged immobility, and have pain that worsens when motion is initiated and when the joint is used to excess. A *recommended starting dose* is 30C three times daily to start, tapering as improvements allow to one daily dose. Discontinuation of the remedy may be possible.

Acupuncture

- Key points to relieve pain include ST 35, Xi Yan (on either side of the patellar tendon between the tibial tuberosity and the inferior border of the patella; needle insertion is into the joint), ST 34, ST 36, LIV 7, and LIV 8. In addition, when it is suspected that weakness of the vastus medialis is contributing to poor patellar tracking, apply acupuncture at SP 10, KI 3, KI 10, and SP 6.

AUTHORS' CHOICES:

SM: Glucosamine; homeopathy; acupuncture.
SW: GAGs; surgery when necessary.

MYASTHENIA GRAVIS

Therapeutic Rationale

- Administer anticholinesterase drugs.
- Administer immunosuppressive drugs.
- Give supportive care.

Alternative Options with Conventional Bases

- In China herbs have been investigated for their effects on acetylcholine (ACh) receptors and ACh receptor antibodies. Astragalus *(Astragalus membranaceus)* and the Chinese herbal formula Bu Zhong Yi Qi Tang had encouraging effects in ex vivo systems from human patients with myasthenia (Tu, 1994).

Paradigmatic Options

Traditional Chinese Medicine

- The hallmark of myasthenia gravis is weakness or collapse after brief periods of muscular use. In Chinese medicine such a patient is considered to be depleting reserves of Qi or Yin, which results in the temporary inability to move until these reserves are restored.
- Depletion of Qi: signs include muscular flaccidity and weakness, general fatigue, poor appetite, loose stools, shortness of breath, and perhaps cold intolerance. The pulse is soft, thready, and weak. The tongue is pale and perhaps has a thin white coating. Appropriate acupuncture points for this condition include CV 12, SP 6, BL 20, ST 36, and SP 3. Indirect moxa can be applied to all of these points. Herbal formulas to consider include **Bu Zhong Yi Qi Tang** (Supplement the Center to Boost Qi Decoction), **Shen Ling Bai Zhu San** (Ginseng, Poria, and Atractylodes Decoction), and **Liu Jun Zi Tang** (Six Gentlemen Decoction). Shen Ling Bai Zhu San can be used if there is significant painless watery diarrhea. Bu Zhong Yi Qi Tang can be used if there is any tendency to ptosis, prolapse, perineal herniation, or abdominal distention. Liu Jun Zi Tang can be used if diarrhea, ptosis, prolapse, or abdominal distention is not present. Bu Zhong Yi Qi Tang is the standard prescription in China for myasthenia gravis caused by Spleen Qi deficiency. The *recommended starting dose* of granular concentrate for all of these formulas is approximately 60 mg per lb of body weight, or approximately ¼ tsp per 15 lb of body weight, divided into two daily doses.
- Depletion of Yin: Yin deficiency with Empty Heat is indicated by heat intolerance, weakness, restlessness at

night, thirst, heat at the crown of the head, weight loss, thin, rapid, floating pulses, and a red or dry tongue. **Zhi Bai Di Huang Wan** (Amenarrhena, Phellodendron, and Rehmannia Pill) is used to clear Empty Heat and generally nourish Yin. The practitioner may add 12 g Huang Qi, 9 g Dang Shen, 9 g Dang Gui, and 12 g Ji Xue Teng to 100 g of base formula to help nourish patients who are also Qi and Blood deficient. Acupuncture points that may be used to augment the effectiveness of the herbal formula include BL 18, BL 23, GB 39, and GB 34.

- When Yin deficiency has resulted in a failure to nourish the tendons, **Hu Qian Wan** (Hidden Tiger Pill) can be used. This formula is probably even more important than Zhi Bai Di Huang Wan for musculoskeletal weakness in Yin-deficiency cases. This formula should not be used in its traditional form, since it contains ground tiger bone and tigers are an endangered species. The versions that contain ground pork bone as a substitute for tiger bone are acceptable. If Huai Niu Xi is not present in the formula, it should be added to make up 15% of the total formula. The *recommended starting dose* of granular concentrate is approximately 60 mg per lb of body weight, or approximately ¼ tsp per 15 lb of body weight, divided into two daily doses.
- Damp Heat: A form of Spleen deficiency in which Damp Heat has accumulated and is causing particular weakness of the hind limbs in dogs with red, wet tongues and slippery or wiry pulses can be treated with **Jia Wei Er Miao San** (Four Marvels Powder). The *recommended starting dose* of granular concentrate is approximately 60 mg per lb of body weight, or approximately ¼ tsp per 15 lb of body weight, divided into two daily doses. Acupuncture points to treat this condition include SP 9, BL 20, BL 22, BL 39, BL 40, and LI 11.

AUTHORS' CHOICES:

SM: Chinese herbs and acupuncture.
SW: Conventional treatment; Chinese herbs and acupuncture.

MYOPATHY

Therapeutic Rationale

- Reduce inflammation in inflammatory diseases.

Alternative Options with Conventional Bases

- **Carnitine:** has proved helpful in some forms of human myopathy and is recommended for many cases of myopathy in small animals.
- **Antioxidants,** especially Vitamin E and Selenium, may be of benefit in myopathies in a variety of animals. A therapeutic trial of an antioxidant combination is generally safe.

Paradigmatic Options

Traditional Chinese Medicine

- Myopathy often represents a deficiency of Liver Blood from a Chinese medical perspective. This is especially true when the clinical presentation includes tight, fibrotic, fasciculating muscles on palpation and other evidence of Blood deficiency, including a pale tongue, thin, wiry pulses, fine dander, timidity or fear aggression, low-grade itch, mild allergic dermatitis or otitis externa with minimal discharge, ear margin dermatosis, and mild hypertension.
- Masticatory myositis: one myopathy that often appears to be caused by Blood deficiency is masticatory myositis. An herbal formula that can be used for these cases is **Bu Gan Tang** (Nourish the Liver Decoction). Patients that benefit usually have minimal or no evidence of Spleen compromise or Dampness changes (e.g., mucoid stools, extreme flatulence, moist skin or ear lesions, slippery pulses, and a wet, red tongue).
- The acute phase of inflammation in some dogs with masticatory myositis resembles an external invasion of Wind-Damp that manifests as painful facial swelling and edema. The channels of the face may be more vulnerable to invasion if they are deficient in Wei Qi and Blood. Resolving the problem requires dispelling pathogenic Wind, tonifying Qi, and nourishing and moving Blood in the head. A formula combination that

can be used for this purpose is 80 g **Bu Yang Huan Wu Tang** (Tonify the Yang to Restore Five-Tenths Decoction) and 30 g **Fang Ji Huang Qi Tang** (Stephania and Astragalus Decoction). Dogs that may benefit have dry coats, timidity, choppy pulses, and pale tongues.

- The *recommended starting dose* of granular concentrate for both of these formulas is approximately 60 mg per lb of body weight, or approximately ¼ tsp per 15 lb of body weight, divided into two daily doses.
- Acupuncture is an important part of treatment of masticatory myositis. Points to consider include LIV 3 and SP 6 to nourish Blood and Yin, LI 4 to regulate the face, ST 6 (in the center of the masseter muscle), and BL 7 (alongside the prominence of the sagittal crest). The practitioner should consider BL 17, BL 18, ST 36, and CV 12 to help engender Liver Blood. Other useful points are ST 7 and ST 10.
- General myopathy causing hind limb weakness: for older, weaker Yin- and Blood-deficient animals that have some Dampness signs, the more complex **Jia Wei Si Wu Tang** (Augmented Four Materials Decoction) can be used. Patients that benefit have evidence of muscle atrophy or weakness, particularly in the hind limbs, and experience difficulty walking. The tongue may be pale and coated, and the pulse thin and slippery. The *recommended starting dose* of granular concentrate is approximately 60 mg per lb of body weight, or approximately ¼ tsp per 15 lb of body weight, divided into two daily doses.
- Some cases of myopathy may well have Dampness or Damp Heat as the main cause. Patients may have swollen limbs, a rapid, slippery, or wiry pulse, and a red tongue. **Si Miao San** (Four Marvels Powder) should be considered for these cases. The *recommended starting dose* of granular concentrate is approximately 60 mg per lb of body weight, or approximately ¼ tsp per 15 lb of body weight, divided into two daily doses.

AUTHORS' CHOICES:

SM: Bu Gan Tang and acupuncture for masticatory myositis.
SW: Acupuncture; Chinese herbs; Carnitine.

OSTEOARTHRITIS

Therapeutic Rationale

- Slow degenerative damage.
- Stabilize unstable joints if possible.
- Reduce inflammation.
- Control pain.

Alternative Options with Conventional Bases

Nutritional Therapies

Basic diet

- Leaky Gut is a theoretical situation in which mucosal inflammation (caused by food allergy, intolerance to other dietary factors or toxins, or nonsteroidal or other drugs that induce inflammation in the gut) leads to systemic absorption of substances normally sequestered in the gut. This increased permeability allows abnormally large and potentially immunogenic food proteins and microbial elements systemic access, which potentially exacerbates inflammation elsewhere in the body. Elimination diets, glutamine, fiber, and probiotics are often recommended for this diagnosis. Whether or not Leaky Gut is a real diagnosis, many affected dogs experience less inflammation and pain when they are switched to a limited diet of fresh foods. Some practitioners believe that the preparation and cooking of commercial diets changes proteins sufficiently that switching to whole food versions of the same ingredients essentially changes the food antigens presented at the gut. It is also possible that fresh foods provide sources of phytoantioxidants, MSM, and other nutrients useful for the relief of arthritis. Homemade diets are also generally composed of fewer and better defined ingredients, in most cases, than poorer commercial diets.

Glycosaminoglycans

- **Complex sugars** used for treatment of osteoarthritis include polysulfated glycosaminoglycan (Adequan), pentosan polysulfate (Elmiron), glucosamine or chondroitin sulfate or combinations (Cosequin, Osteocare, Promotion, Arthroplex, and many others), or the sea organisms Green-Lipped Mussel *(Perna canaliculus)* and Sea Cucumber *(Stichopus chloronotus, S. variegatus, S. japonicus,* and other related species in the family Holothurioidea) (a possible source of chondroitin plus other components of the organism). Clinical impression tends to support the use of these supplements as early in the disease as possible.

- **Glucosamine:** probably the most popular of glycosaminoglycans (GAGs) administered orally for arthritis. In patients with osteoarthritis the body's demand for proteoglycan precursors exceeds the supply because of increased destruction of joint cartilage and oral administration of glucosamine may support greater synthesis of GAGs, proteoglycans, and collagen. In addition, glucosamine may act as a cyclooxygenase-independent antiinflammatory agent. Concerns have been raised regarding GI absorption of glucosamine; in one study 87% of orally administered glucosamine was absorbed in the GI tract (Setnikar, 1991).
- **Chondroitin sulfate:** a related compound that is often combined with glucosamine. It is also relatively well absorbed: 62% of orally administered chondroitin, in one study (Conte, 1995). Chondroitin sulfate probably has similar antiinflammatory and stimulatory properties that result in decreased cartilage destruction. Chondroitin sulfate is much more expensive than plain glucosamine. Since glucosamine is a precursor molecule for chondroitin, glucosamine alone may provide clinical effects and cost less to use. The best studied product is Cosequin, a combination of glucosamine, chondroitin, magnesium, and ascorbate.

Antioxidants

- **Vitamin C** (ascorbate): functions in collagen synthesis by reducing prolyl hydroxylase and lysyl hydroxylase, which are catalysts in the formation of hydroxyproline and hydroxylysine. In one study (Berge, 1990), 100 dogs with osteoarthritis were given polyascorbate (calcium ascorbate plus ascorbate metabolites, a pH-neutral form of ascorbate that is thought to be better absorbed than other forms). The dose was 30 mg tid po for 6 months.

Diagnosis was based on lameness, decrease in mobility, pain, physical examinations, and in some cases radiography. There were no control subjects in this study. Outcomes were based on owner reports and physical examination results at 7 days, 6 weeks, and 6 months. After 1 week 71% of dogs with hip dysplasia were judged to have good improvement or were symptom free. Another 28% were judged to have shown small improvement. Of dogs with spondylosis and disk disease, 76% were judged to have shown good improvement and 24% small improvement. No side effects were reported. The author also conducted a very small crossover trial in which six of the dogs with chronic arthritis were examined. Three were given the polyascorbate product and three were given placebo. After a washout phase of 4 weeks, the groups were crossed over with similar results: those given the polyascorbate improved while those given placebo did not.

- **Vitamin E:** appeared to show benefit in one study in dogs (Impellizeri, 1998). The *recommended dose* is approximately 10 IU per lb of body weight.
- Other antioxidant micronutrients have proved helpful in people (McAlindon, 1996; Sowers, 1999). In practice, many practitioners find that antioxidant combinations are more beneficial than choosing selected antioxidant vitamins and veterinary products can be supplied at label doses. Antioxidant enzymes, particularly superoxide dismutase, have also been used in the treatment of osteoarthritis and may be found in veterinary products designed for osteoarthritis treatment. Studies suggest but do not show conclusively that superoxide dismutase is of therapeutic aid.
- **Essential fatty acids:** appear to act as anti-inflammatories. See the previous discussion under Musculoskeletal Pain for more information.
- **DLPA:** an analgesic. See the discussion in the Musculoskeletal Pain section. The dose is variable at 250 to 500 mg bid.

Herbs

- **Antiinflammatory herbs:** as described in the section on Musculoskeletal Pain they are frequently used for osteoarthritis. The most popular are Boswellia, Ginger, Devil's Claw, and Yucca.

- **One Chinese herbal combination** tested in dogs appeared effective (Bonnett, 1996). In a study of 143 clinical canine patients, a Chinese herbal combination was compared with Devil's Claw combination, aspirin, and placebo. The Chinese herbal prescription contained White Peony, Licorice, Epimedium, Oyster Shell, Reishi Mushroom, Isatidis, and Corydalis. The Chinese herbal combination and aspirin produced significant improvement according to owner and veterinary evaluation, whereas the response to Devil's Claw combination was equivalent to the placebo response (Bonnett, 1996). This Chinese herbal combination is not commercially available to my (SW) knowledge, but it can be formulated on request by reputable Chinese pharmacies (such as Brion, Mayway, or Jing Tang) or naturopathic pharmacies.

Paradigmatic Options

Chinese Herbal Medicine

- Osteoarthritis should be treated with the most appropriate acupuncture points and Chinese herbal formula for the case as outlined in the general section on Musculoskeletal Pain. In general, relatively mild formulas will probably be more appropriate for osteoarthritis. Specifically, the practitioner might consider the following formulas:
  - **Fang Feng Tang** (Ledebouriella Decoction) for patients with shifting lameness, acute episodes of lameness, and aggravation from exposure to cold. The tongue is largely normal, and the pulse is floating and perhaps tight. *The recommended starting dose* of granular concentrate is approximately 60 mg per lb of body weight, or approximately ¼ tsp per 15 lb of body weight, divided into two doses.
  - For dogs with localized lameness accompanied by hot joints and restlessness, particularly at night, **Gui Zhi Shao Yao Zhi Mu Tang** (Cinnamon Twigs, Peony, and Anemarrhena Decoction) can be used. The *recommended starting dose* of granular concentrate is

approximately 60 mg per lb of body weight, or approximately ¼ tsp per 15 lb of body weight, divided into two doses.

- For chilly older animals with hind limb or low back weakness and lameness, **Du Huo Ji Sheng Tang** (Angelica and Loranthus Decoction) may be considered. The patient may have difficulty rising in the morning, but improve with heat applications. The condition is aggravated by exposure to any cold and even moderate exercise. The tongue is often pale, and the pulse wiry. This formula is less effective for lameness in the forelimbs. The *recommended starting dose* of granular concentrate is approximately 60 mg per lb of body weight, or approximately ¼ tsp per 15 lb of body weight, divided into two doses.
- For cold painful animals that resent the slightest touch, **Wu Tou Tang** (Aconite Decoction) should be considered. This formula is for short-term use of a few months' duration at most. After that, one of the other formulas should be evaluated for appropriateness. The *recommended starting dose* of granular concentrate is approximately 60 mg per lb of body weight, or approximately ¼ tsp per 15 lb of body weight per day, divided into two doses.
- For cases with mild joint swelling or a history of Dampness-related complaints, **Yi Yi Ren Tang** (Coix Decoction) may be used. The symptoms of patients who benefit will often be worse in damp or humid weather. The *recommended starting dose* of granular concentrate is approximately 60 mg per lb of body weight, or approximately ¼ tsp per 15 lb of body weight, divided into two doses.
- For hot, panting, thirsty, or excessively hungry dogs with a history of cystitis and colitis, **Si Miao San** (Four Marvels Powder) can be considered. Dogs that benefit often have a history of hind limb and low back weakness and lameness. The *recommended starting dose* of granular concentrate is approximately 60 mg per lb of body weight, or approximately ¼ tsp per 15 lb of body weight, divided into two doses.

- **Bai Hu Jia Gui Zhi Tang** (White Tiger with Cinnamon Twigs Decoction) should be considered if fevers are prominent in the clinical history. The *recommended starting dose* of granular concentrate is approximately 60 mg per lb of body weight, or approximately ¼ tsp per 15 lb of body weight, divided into two doses.
- For nonspecific lameness for which the practitioner cannot find any guiding symptoms or decide on one formula, **Juan Bi Tang II** (Remove Painful Obstruction Decoction) can be used. The *recommended starting dose* of granular concentrate is approximately 60 mg per lb of body weight, or approximately ¼ tsp per 15 lb of body weight, divided into two doses.
- For obstinate pain aggravated by exposure to cold, **Xiao Huo Luo Dan** (Minor Invigorate the Collaterals Pill) can be considered. The *recommended starting dose* of granular concentrate is approximately 60 mg per lb of body weight, or approximately ¼ tsp per 15 lb of body weight, divided into two doses. If this formula is effective, the practitioner should eventually switch to **Tao Hong Yin** (Peach Kernel and Carthamus Beverage) because of concern about extended use of Aconite.

Acupuncture

- Once an herbal approach has been selected, the general section on Musculoskeletal Pain can be consulted for advice on acupuncture points appropriate to that formula. (Also see the general point recommendations in the general section.)

Homeopathy

- *Rhus toxicodendron* 30C: for lameness that is aggravated in cold, damp weather, is worse on initial movement, but improves with sustained movement. Overexertion severely aggravates the condition, and the patient may be restless when at rest. The patient may appear Blood deficient from a Chinese perspective. The minimum required dose should be used, but it can be given up to three times daily in initial case management.

- *Lycopodium:* has many of the modalities of *Rhus toxicodendron,* in that it is useful for lameness that is worse on rising and improves with continued motion. *Lycopodium* may help in chronic cases in which *Rhus toxicodendron* worked initially, but was less effective later. Patients are often Blood deficient from a Chinese medical perspective and exhibit either bullying or fear aggressive behavior. Overuse of *Lycopodium* may produce malaise. A *recommended starting dose* is 30C once daily, tapering as improvements allow to the lowest effective dose.
- **Colchicum autumnale**: for advanced degenerative changes that result in pronounced crepitance and aggravation from motion. There may be irritability and aggravation in damp weather. The patient may be especially uncomfortable in the evening and at night. A *recommended starting dose* is 30C three times daily to start, tapering as improvements allow to one daily dose. Discontinuation of the remedy may be possible.

Cautions

- Herbs with corticoid-like activity (Licorice) may reduce blood salicylate concentration if used with herbs that contain salicylate (Willow Bark, Meadowsweet, Birch, Poplar, Black Cohosh). Licorice also offers some protection against GI irritation from salicylates.
- Licorice's corticoid activity may enhance the effects of concurrently administered glucocorticoids. Some studies suggest that Licorice increases the half-life of corticosteroids but reduces their immune-modulating effects.
- GAGs may affect clotting mechanisms, although studies have not verified these effects as clinically significant. If NSAIDS are being used, GAGs or herbs that have potential anticoagulant activity (Gingko biloba, Ginger, Ginseng, Garlic) may enhance the potential for bleeding. Blood-moving herbs in Chinese medicine frequently reduce platelet aggregation tendencies as well.
- Salicylate-containing herbs (Meadowsweet, Willow, Poplar, Birch, Black Cohosh) may interact with other NSAIDs.
- Devil's Claw has theoretical interactions with antiarrhythmic drugs.

AUTHORS' CHOICES:

SM: Chinese herbal medicine combined with acupuncture; Rhus toxicodendron 30C.
SW: GAGs; combinations of Boswellia, Ginger, Devil's Claw and other herbs; Chinese herbs; acupuncture.

OSTEOCHONDROSIS

Therapeutic Rationale

- Control nutritional risk factors.
- Avoid hard concussive activity.
- Slow degenerative changes.
- Remove flap where appropriate.

Alternative Options with Conventional Bases

- **GAGs:** are chondroprotective and may limit cartilage degeneration as well as alleviate pain and inflammation (see Musculoskeletal Pain section).

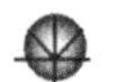

Paradigmatic Options

Traditional Chinese Medicine

- A Chinese herbal formula appropriate to the signs of the patient should be selected. The general section on Musculoskeletal Pain can be consulted for more information. Given the nature of the lesion, formulas to address Fixed Bi or Bony Bi are more likely to be helpful. For older, chilly, weaker animals with long-standing lesions **Du Huo Ji Sheng Tang** (Angelica and Loranthus Decoction) can be considered. For obstinate pain aggravated by cold, **Xiao Huo Luo Dan** (Minor Invigorate the Collaterals Pill) can be used. Patients that respond well to the latter may be given **Tao Hong Yin** (Persica and Carthamus Beverage) on a long-term basis. For clearly Blood-deficient animals with pain aggravated by cold **Jiao Ai Tang** (Donkey Hide and Artemisia Decoction) should be considered. The *recommended starting dose* of granular concentrate for all of these formulas is approximately 60 mg per lb of body weight, or approximately ¼ tsp per 15 lb of body weight, divided into two daily doses.

Acupuncture

- Acupuncture points should be those appropriate for the joint involved, as well as points to address the general pathologic condition involved. The general section on Musculoskeletal Pain can be consulted for more information.

AUTHORS' CHOICES:

SM: Surgery when appropriate; Chinese herbs; acupuncture.
SW: Surgery when appropriate; GAGs; acupuncture.

PANOSTEITIS

Therapeutic Rationale

- Support patient while reducing pain.

Alternative Options with Conventional Bases

- **Acupuncture:** can be very effective in reducing pain.

Paradigmatic Options

Homeopathy

- **Mercurius solubilis:** has proved useful in hastening the improvement of panosteitis and stopping the spread to other limbs. After an initial dosage of 30C three times daily for 4 days the dosage should be tapered to the lowest effective dose, perhaps once daily for an additional 2 weeks.
- ***Eupatorium perfoliatum:*** after an initial dosage of 30C three times daily for 4 days, the dose should be to the lowest effective dose. See the Western Herbs section for further information.

Western Herbs

- **Boneset** *(Eupatorium perfoliatum):* has a long-standing reputation in Western herbalism for relieving deep-seated bone pains of a recurrent nature. It thus seems well suited for use in panosteitis, especially given its apparent clinical usefulness in more severe bone inflammatory conditions such as osteosarcoma. It is a fairly strong herb and should be used as part of another formula. If it is used by itself, a *suggested starting dose* is 0.1 ml of liquid extract per 5 lb of body weight, divided into two doses. Homeopathic versions of the herb may also be helpful.

Traditional Chinese Medicine

- Match the clinical signs of the patient to one of the Chinese herbal formulas and appropriate acupuncture points discussed in the section on the treatment of general musculoskeletal pain. The notorious shifting nature of panosteitis may make it amenable to treatment using **Fang Feng Tang** (Ledebouriella Decoction) or **Gui Zhi Shao Yao Zhi Mu Tang** (Cinnamon Twig, Peony, and Anemarrhena Decoction). The more general pain-relieving formula known as **Juan Bi Tang I or II** (Remove Obstructions Decoction) can also be considered. The *recommended starting dose* of granular concentrate for all of these formulas is approximately 60 mg per lb of body weight, or approximately ¼ tsp per 15 lb of body weight, divided into two daily doses.

AUTHORS' CHOICES:

SM: Mercurius; Eupatorium.
SW: Acupuncture.

RHEUMATOID ARTHRITIS

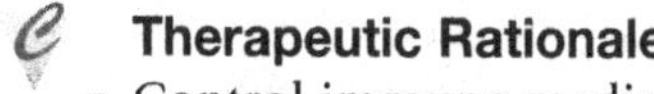

Therapeutic Rationale

- Control immune-mediated damage to joints.

Alternative Options with Conventional Bases

Nutritional Therapies

- **See the section on basic diet** under Osteoarthritis. If Leaky Gut is a real phenomenon, it may play a role in rheumatoid arthritis and elimination diets and probiotics would be recommended.

- **γ-Linolenic acid (GLA):** a fatty acid derived from a number of plant sources, including Evening Primrose Oil, Black Currant Oil, and Borage Seed Oil. It is an ω-6 fatty acid that is a precursor of prostaglandin E_1. GLA has been shown in controlled trials and critical reviews to be effective in reducing signs of rheumatoid arthritis (Darlington, 2001; Little, 2001; Zurier, 1996). Doses used in human trials ranged up to 2800 mg of GLA daily provided as 4 capsules of Borage Seed Oil. Black Currant Oil contains less GLA and may have to be supplemented at 15 to 30 capsules daily at this level. Borage Seed Oil appears to be the best source of GLA.
- **Fish Oil:** contains the antiinflammatory ω-3 fatty acids EPA and DHA and has been recommended for rheumatoid arthritis. In a controlled trial in humans 10 capsules daily of a product containing 171 mg of EPA and 114 mg of DHA per capsule resulted in reduced intake of NSAID to control pain. The effect reached a maximum at 12 months and lasted 15 months (Lau, 1993).
- **GAGs:** have shown significant benefit in humans with rheumatoid arthritis. These compounds modulate inflammation and provide cartilage precursors. An *appropriate starting dose* of glucosamine is approximately 10 to 100 mg per lb of body weight, and an *appropriate starting dose* for mixed glycosaminoglycans is approximately 7 mg per lb of body weight. These compounds are generally believed to be safe, and the practitioner may use higher doses if deemed appropriate.
- **Antioxidants:** see the section on antioxidants under Osteoarthritis. A general antioxidant combination may be helpful.
- **Proteolytic enzymes:** these, particularly Bromelain, have been suggested for treatment of rheumatoid arthritis. See the general section on Musculoskeletal Pain.

Herbs

- As discussed in the section on Musculoskeletal Pain, Boswellia, Ginger, Devil's Claw, and Turmeric may be useful.
- **Keishi-bushi-to,** a Kampo prescription of five herbs: reduced circulating IgG and IgM anti-CII levels in

rats with collagen-induced arthritis (Wakabayashi, 1997).

- *Tripterygium wilfordii:* a Chinese herb that has well-documented antiinflammatory properties and appears well indicated for rheumatoid arthritis. Unfortunately, the herb is potentially very toxic and is not recommended for use.

Paradigmatic Options

Homeopathy

- **Colchicum autumnale:** for advanced degenerative changes that result in pronounced crepitance and aggravation from motion. There may be irritability and aggravation in damp weather. The patient may be especially uncomfortable in the evening and at night. A *recommended starting dose* is 30C three times daily, tapering as improvements allow to one daily dose. Discontinuation of the remedy may be possible.
- ***Rhus toxicodendron*** 30C: for lameness that is aggravated in cold, damp weather, is worse upon initial movement, but improves with sustained movement. Overexertion severely aggravates the condition, and the patient may be restless when at rest. The patient may appear Blood deficient from a Chinese perspective. The minimum required dose should be administered, but it can be given up to three times daily in initial case management.
- ***Lycopodium:*** has many of the modalities of *Rhus toxicodendron,* in that it is useful for lameness that is worse on rising and improves with continued motion. *Lycopodium* may help in chronic cases in which *Rhus toxicodendron* worked initially, but was less effective later. Patients are often Blood deficient from a Chinese medical perspective, and often exhibit either bullying or fear-aggressive behavior. Overuse of *Lycopodium* may produce malaise. A *recommended starting dose* is 30C once daily, tapering as improvements allow to the lowest effective dose.

Traditional Chinese Medicine

- The practitioner should attempt to match the patient with rheumatoid arthritis to the indications for one of the Chinese herbal formulas and acupuncture prescriptions discussed in the general section on Musculoskeletal Pain. Any of the formulas discussed in previous sections may be appropriate. In general, however, stronger Heat-clearing formulas will be called for, including **Bai Hu Jia Gui Zhi Tang** (White Tiger with added Cinnamon Twig Decoction) and **Gui Zhi Shao Yao Zhi Mu Tang** (Cinnamon Twig, Peony, and Anemarrhena Decoction). Damp animals with localized hind limb pain may benefit from **Si Miao San** (Four Marvels Powder), and patients that seem impossible to differentiate may be treated with **Juan Bi Tang I or II** (Remove Painful Obstruction Decoction). **Xiao Huo Luo Dan** (Invigorate the Collaterals Decoction) can be used for obstinate localized and persistent pain, especially in old, weak, and chilly animals. The practitioner should switch to **Tao Hong Yin** (Persica and Carthamus Beverage) for long-term treatment of these patients. For patients whose arthritis is strongly aggravated by cold, **Wu Tou Tang** (Aconite Decoction) can be used on a short-term basis. The *recommended starting dose* of granular concentrate for all of these formulas is approximately 60 mg per lb of body weight, or approximately ¼ tsp per 15 lb of body weight, divided into two daily doses.

Cautions

- Herbs with corticoid-like activity (Licorice) may reduce blood salicylate concentration if being used with aspirin or with herbs that contain salicylate (Willow Bark, Poplar, Birch, Meadowsweet, Black Cohosh). Licorice may offer some protection against GI irritation from salicylates.
- Licorice's corticoid activity may enhance the effects of concurrently administered glucocorticoids. Other studies suggest that Licorice increases the half-life of corticosteroids but reduces their immune-modulating effects.
- GAGs may affect clotting mechanisms, although studies have not verified these effects as clinically significant. If NSAIDS are being used, GAGs or herbs that have potential anticoagulant activity *(Gingko biloba,* Ginger,

Ginseng, Garlic) may enhance the potential for bleeding. Blood-moving herbs in Chinese medicine frequently reduce platelet aggregation tendencies as well.
- Salicylate-containing herbs (Meadowsweet, Willow, Poplar, Birch, Black Cohosh) may interact with other NSAIDs.
- Devil's Claw has theoretical interactions with anti-arrhythmic drugs.

AUTHORS' CHOICES:

SM: Elimination diet; herbal formulas and acupuncture as appropriate to case presentation.
SW: Elimination diet; GLA or Fish Oil; enzymes; herbal combinations; acupuncture.

SPONDYLOSIS DEFORMANS

Therapeutic Rationale

- This condition is generally viewed as asymptomatic.
- Provide pain control for acute fracture of spinous bridges.
- Administer antiinflammatory therapy for neurologic defects.

Alternative Options with Conventional Bases

- Alternative viewpoints tend to consider spondylosis as a pathologic condition that causes pain and decreased mobility. As such, spondylosis may be treated more often with alternative methods than with conventional medicine.
- **GAGs:** see section on Musculoskeletal Pain.
- **Antioxidants:** see section on Musculoskeletal Pain. Whether or not antioxidants have a direct effect on pain caused by spondylosis is unknown; however, many practitioners note that antioxidant supplementation increases activity in older dogs. This may be due to enhanced cognitive ability or better energy level, as opposed to direct pain-relieving effects.

Paradigmatic Options

Chiropractic

- From an alternative medical perspective, a substantial amount of hind-limb weakness and pain in dogs seems to be directly or indirectly related to lower back rigidity possibly caused by the compression of one or more sciatic nerve roots. Even animals with significant hip dysplasia can experience substantial improvement in hind limb weakness and lameness when lower back fixations are released.
- Chiropractic is of major importance in the treatment of spondylosis deformans. It should be performed once weekly until mobility is consistently restored. With the simultaneous use of appropriate systemic therapies, chiropractic therapy should be required for only a few weeks. After this clients are advised to bring patients in because symptoms of low back stiffness recur such as a tendency to repeated stretching and the inability to turn in a tight circle.
- When palpating backs before adjustment, the practitioner must pay special attention to the L7 S1 junction, since motion fixations in this area will often not be obvious. An L7 fixation can be easily detected by static palpation. The sacrum should also be palpated and adjusted if motion restrictions are found. The presence of lumbosacral fixations is often correlated with atlantooccipital joint fixations, and these should be sought out and mobilized.
- Veterinarians unfamiliar with chiropractic may understandably counsel pet owners to shun chiropractic for affected dogs in the mistaken belief that chiropractic adjustments may lead to fractures of bridges between vertebrae. In reality, adjustments are highly unlikely to be forceful enough to compromise bony integrity.
- Some practitioners assert that bony bridges will prevent any degree of mobilization of vertebral segments. This is occasionally true, but a surprising amount of mobility may still be restored even between vertebrae that have been partially fused.
- That some flexibility can be restored between partially fused vertebrae suggests that rigidity is in part caused

by lack of resilience in muscular and connective tissues. This is highly likely given the pathophysiologic mechanism that has been proposed for spondylosis in humans. Degenerative changes in connective tissues of the intervertebral disks and the posterior longitudinal ligament that connects them are perceived to produce corresponding increases in tensile forces. This increase in tension is translated to the tissues into which the ligaments and disks insert, most notably the periosteum of the vertebrae. The periosteum responds to this stimulation by producing more bone, which results in deformities that occur first where tensile forces are greatest, namely, at the convergences of the disks, longitudinal ligaments, and vertebral end plates.

- In the context of the proposed mechanism of pathogenesis the use of connective tissue protomorphogens is indicated, not only as a means of reducing pain, but perhaps also as a source of "building blocks" to restore healthy ligament structure. Other related compounds such as gelatin and the Chinese herb E Jiao (Donkey Hide Gelatin) may also be beneficial. A useful *starting dose* of either type of gelatin might be ¼ tsp per 15 lb of body weight, given once daily in food.

Western Herbs

- **Valerian Root** *(Valeriana* spp.): a very useful herb for releasing muscle spasms that are initially triggered through nerve root compression and subsequently keep the back in a rigid state. The *suggested starting dose* is 0.1 ml per 2½ to 5 lb of body weight, in divided doses. Valerian is a safe herb, and this dose may be increased.

Chinese Herbs

- Enduring flexibility and the cessation of further osteophyte formation seem to be aided by appropriate treatment of any underlying Chinese medical disorders. Several pathologic conditions are thought to lead to low back stiffness, including Blood stasis, Liver Qi stagnation (often caused by Blood deficiency), Kidney

Qi, Yin, or Yang depletion, and Damp Heat in the lower burner. The *recommended starting dose* of granular concentrate for all the formulas in this section is approximately 60 mg per lb of body weight, or approximately ¼ tsp per 15 lb of body weight, divided into two daily doses.

- Liver Qi stagnation/Blood deficiency: **Bu Gan Tang** (Supplement the Liver Decoction) can be used to nourish Blood and relieve muscle spasms. Patients that benefit from this formula have pale tongues and thin and wiry pulses. This formula should not be given to Damp dogs. **Jiao Ai Tang** (Donkey Hide and Artemisia Decoction) may be used for Blood-deficient animals, especially when they have pain that worsens with exposure to cold. For older, weaker Yin- and Blood-deficient animals that have some degree of aggravation from Dampness, the more complex **Jia Wei Si Wu Tang** (Augmented Four Materials Decoction) can be tried. Patients that benefit exhibit evidence of muscle atrophy or weakness, particularly in the hind limbs, and have difficulty walking. The tongue may be pale and coated, and the pulse thin and slippery.
- Kidney deficiency: **Du Huo Ji Sheng Tang** (Angelica and Loranthus Decoction) can be considered for older animals with Kidney, Qi, and Blood deficiency whose condition worsens from exposure to cold. **Zuo Gui Wan** (Restore the Left Kidney Pill) should be considered for aged animals with pure Kidney Yin deficiency accompanied by chronic weakness in the back and hind limbs. These patients will have nighttime restlessness, thirst, and heat intolerance. **Yuo Gui Wan** (Restore the Right Kidney Pill) should be considered for older, chilly animals with Kidney Yang deficiency. Signs are back pain aggravated by exertion and ameliorated by warmth, a pale and wet tongue with a white coating, and a weak, deep pulse. Some patients benefiting from Yuo Gui Wan will have evidence of Empty Heat in the upper jiao, and of Yang deficiency in the lower jiao. Another formula designed specifically for low back pain arising from Kidney Yang deficiency is **Qing E Wan** (Blue Fairy Pills).

- Damp Heat accumulation: **Si Miao San** (Four Marvels Powder) can be used for animals with this condition. The tongue of affected animals is dark red and wet, and the pulse is rapid, slippery, or wiry. There may be a past history of repeated cystitis or colitis. Limbs may be swollen or atrophied, and the patient may have a predisposition to moist pyoderma.
- Blood stasis: for pure Blood stasis caused by trauma, **Shen Tong Zhu Yu Tang** (Drive Out Stasis from a Painful Body) can be used. For Blood stasis that is aggravated by exposure to cold and damp, **Shu Jing Huo Xue Tang** (Relax the Channels and Invigorate the Blood Decoction) should be considered. **Yi Yi Ren Tang** appears to be highly effective for Blood stasis that is aggravated by damp weather. Patients that benefit may exhibit pronounced back stiffness, epaxial muscle spasms, and a pale or purple moist tongue.

Acupuncture

- Acupuncture acts to relax muscle spasms and promote analgesia in dogs with low back stiffness and pain. Useful points include BL 25 through BL 28, GB 30, Bai Hui, and BL 40. BL 23 should be used for Kidney deficiencies. SP 9 and CV 3 should be added for Damp Heat accumulations. GB 34 and LIV 3 should be used in Blood deficiency. Indirect moxa is always appropriate.

AUTHORS' CHOICES:

SM: Chiropractic; acupuncture; Chinese herbs; Valerian.
SW: Chiropractic, acupuncture; GAGs; antioxidants.

TRAUMA

Therapeutic Rationale

- Reduce inflammation.

Alternative Options with Conventional Bases

- **Proteolytic enzymes** such as Bromelain: may be used to curtail inflammation. The general section on

Musculoskeletal Pain can be consulted for further information and dosage recommendations. Proteolytic enzymes for use as an antiinflammatory agent should not be given with food.

Paradigmatic Options

Chiropractic

- The practitioner should rule out fixations, which may frequently arise as a result of trauma. Guiding symptoms are the sudden onset of weakness or lameness.

Homeopathy

- *Arnica montana:* for acute injuries and sprains with passive bleeding, bruising, and pain that worsens with movement. *Arnica* is used in all cases of head and spinal trauma, or when this cannot be ruled out. The *recommended dose* is 30C up to three times daily as needed to relieve pain or 1M once daily.
- *Rhus toxicodendron* 30C: helpful for subacute and chronic nonhealing soft tissue trauma that manifests as pain that is aggravated in cold damp weather, is worse on initial movement, and improves with sustained movement. Overexertion severely aggravates the condition, and restlessness may be seen when the patient is at rest. The patient may appear Blood deficient from a Chinese medicine perspective. The minimum required dose should be used, but it can be given up to three times daily in initial case management.

Western Herbs

- **Topical ointments** containing crude Arnica extract may be applied several times a day. They should never be used in an open wound. Arnica can be toxic if ingested.

AUTHORS' CHOICES:

SM: Arnica; Rhus toxicodendron.
SW: Enzymes.

12 CASE REPORT

Hind Limb Lameness in a Golden Retriever

HISTORY

Murphy, a 9-year-old, female, spayed Golden Retriever presented with a chief complaint of residual lameness after bilateral cranial cruciate ligament rupture and repair. The first injury had occurred 4 years earlier with a partial tear of the cranial cruciate ligament of the left hind leg. Although the owner did not know the method of repair used, surgery was performed immediately after onset of clinical signs.

Several months after surgery, Murphy continued to have a significant amount of lameness, although a cranial drawer test demonstrated no knee instability. Occasional acupuncture treatments provided pain relief for up to 1 year after the date of initial surgical repair. At this point, the owner believed that Murphy reinjured her left hind leg when she was kenneled for an extended period. Although the owner did not know which points were used, additional efforts to provide analgesia for this new injury using acupuncture were unsuccessful.

Approximately 2 years after Murphy's initial injury to her left hind leg, her right cranial cruciate ligament ruptured and was repaired. Pain relief afforded by surgery was once again insufficient.

Murphy was prescribed meloxicam (Metacam) to address the lingering pain in both hind legs. The drug initially appeared to be effective, although the owner could not recall exact doses used. Over the next year, however, the drug's effectiveness against Murphy's pain declined to the point that it eventually merely palliated any pain increases from overexertion. Periodic hyaluronic acid injections were then made into both stifle joints, but no significant benefit was observed. Additional therapies included a patent Chinese herbal formula (Clematis 19; Seven Forest Herbs) and a green-lipped mussel extract. Neither of these products provided relief for Murphy, and almost 4 years after the initial tear in the left cruciate ligament Murphy was brought to my (SM) clinic to explore other therapeutic alternatives for pain relief.

At the time of presentation, Murphy was lame in the hindquarters, and also the right forelimb as indicated by a pronounced head bob. She had difficulty rising, and stiffness was alleviated with gentle continued motion. Her exercise tolerance was poor with her hind limbs becoming incapacitated after even modest exertion.

Past medical complaints included otitis externa of the right ear caused by a recurrent yeast infection. Even after its successful resolution with a topical antifungal medication, Murphy's owners described her as having a perpetual "yeasty" odor from the right ear.

Murphy also had suffered mild skin complaints, including marked pruritus during the summer months after swimming. Occasionally, a pruritic dry rash appeared on the left shoulder that was responsive to topical antiinflammatory sprays. A lipoma was present on the right trunk.

General physical traits of concern to the owners were Murphy's increasing body weight; she now weighed over 80 pounds. She was being fed a commercial "reducing diet" without apparent benefit. Murphy also panted continuously at night, even when the room was cold. No coughing had been observed.

Other physical signs included reduced thirst, an excessive appetite that vanished when Murphy's hind limb pain was aggravated, and a tendency to coprophagy. Murphy was described as friendly and tolerant toward other animals.

PHYSICAL EXAMINATION

Physical examination of Murphy disclosed normal heart and lung sounds and an absence of any cranial drawer response in either leg. Murphy was moderately overweight at 83 pounds. No difference in gait could be discerned between the two hind legs, although there was a pronounced head drop as the left forelimb was placed. The hind legs exhibited a mild to moderate bilateral varus deformity. The right elbow appeared slightly swollen and warm at LI 11, and this point was considered to be active.

Murphy's femoral pulses were thin and weak. Multiple vertebral fixations were found on palpation of the vertebral column. Affected vertebrae included L7, the sacrum, L1 through L3, all cervical vertebrae, and all thoracic vertebrae. Murphy's pulse became more forceful after release of these vertebral fixations. Marked vessel wall tension was felt at the Spleen/Stomach and Kidney/Bladder positions on the distal femoral arteries (see Chapter 2 for further discussion of pulse diagnosis). Palpation of the Kidney, Bladder, and Spleen channels revealed swelling, heat, and thickening at SP 9, BL 22, BL 27, SP 6, and ST 35 on the right hind leg. Murphy's tongue appeared dark pink.

ASSESSMENT

Radiographs of the right elbow were not obtained. Instead, it was decided to observe Murphy's response to alternative medical therapy before further pursuing a conventional medical diagnosis.

From a Chinese medical perspective, Murphy was considered to be suffering from Damp Heat arising from Spleen deficiency. Damp Heat accumulations were considered to be obstructing the flow of Blood to the hind limbs. Murphy thus seemed to be suffering from a combination of Heat Bi and Obstinate or Stubborn Bi Syndrome. Evidence for Dampness was abundant, suggested by the activity at BL 22, Murphy's increased body weight, her yeast otitis externa, her tendency to lipomas, and her pruritus aggravated by getting wet. SP 6 and 9 activity confirmed Spleen deficiency as the source of the Dampness. Murphy's panting at night and the activity noted at LI 11 suggested that the Dampness was generating Damp Heat. The obstruction of Blood flow by an accumulation of Dampness and Phlegm in the channels was suggested by the amelioration of pain by gentle motion; by the increases in pulse force following initiation of therapy; by the congested color of the tongue; and by the varus joint deformities.

TREATMENT

The goals of therapy were to support the Spleen, clear Heat, drain Dampness, and move Blood. The Heat Bi formula **Si Miao San** (Four Marvels Powder) fulfilled most of these objectives and was made appropriate for Wan or Stubborn Bi with the addition of 25 g of Dang Gui Wei to 100 g of base formula. Although not specifically discussed in Chapter 12, Dang Gui is typically added when the patient exhibits Blood deficiency, and Dang Gui Wei is added when the patient exhibits Blood stasis. Murphy was prescribed 3/4 tsp of a granular extract of the formula, to be taken twice daily.

Acupuncture was administered to the active points, and vertebral fixations were released using an Activator (Activator Methods, Phoenix). Murphy was prescribed a commercially prepared, low-carbohydrate raw food diet, consisting of various grated vegetables and ground bones, meat, and organ meat. The guiding philosophy in this choice was that highly processed foods rich in carbohydrates represented a major dampening influence in Murphy's diet.

Given Murphy's poor response to previous therapies, the Metacam and all other supplements were discontinued.

OUTCOME

Murphy was brought for her first follow-up evaluation 9 days later. After her acupuncture and chiropractic treatment, Murphy's hind end weakness and stiffness first increased for a day, then slowly subsided over several days. She was still lame after moderate exercise.

Murphy's forelimb lameness now seemed more pronounced, especially after walks. The owners reported that Murphy occasionally stumbled on her right foreleg, and that her head bob persisted.

Murphy's skin and ears were normal, but she still panted at night. Physical examination revealed fixations of L5 through to the sacrum. Murphy's femoral pulses were strong, and her tongue was unchanged. Her hind limb lameness was assessed as perhaps improved, and her treatment was continued. Acupuncture was performed at SP 6, BL 17, GB 21, and points approximating LI 11, 9, and 17 on the right side. Electroacupuncture was performed at LI 9, LI 17, GB 21, and LI 11. Homeopathic *Rhus toxicodendron* was prescribed at a dose of 30C to be given twice daily for 10 days.

Approximately 2 weeks later, on day 21 of treatment, Murphy was acting more "peppy." She had begun playing with her toys, a behavior that the owners had not seen in several years. Murphy continued to pant all night long. She was less lame in her hindquarters, but still lame in the right forelimb. Lameness of all three limbs was still aggravated by overuse and initial movement.

Active points included BL 17, SP 6, and LI 11 on the right side. The sole vertebral fixation identified was at the level of C2, which indicated that the forelimb lameness was unlikely to be caused by nerve root compression. The activity noted at SP 6 and BL 17 suggested that Blood stasis was becoming more prevalent and that Damp Heat Bi was becoming less prevalent.

The formula **Tao Hong Yin** was prescribed to address Blood stasis arising from Phlegm and Dampness. Tao Hong Yin was thought to be more appropriate as the chief concerns of the case shifted from the hind limbs to the forelimbs, since Si Miao San has a particular effect on hind limb complaints. Di Long was added to the Tao Hong Yin, as described in the text, to increase its action against Dampness and Phlegm. The same dosage was prescribed for Tao Hong Yin as for Si Miao San. Vertebral fixations were relieved, acupuncture was performed on active points.

Two weeks later, on day 34 of treatment, Murphy's owners reported that her hind limb lameness had largely resolved and she was regaining the ability to jump easily onto furniture and into the car. Her forelimb lameness was now less consistent, and her exercise tolerance was increasing. Vertebral fixations and residual stiffness were noted at C2, L6, L7, and the sacrum. Her tongue was still dark pink. After the Si Miao San was stopped, Murphy had had a mild infection of the right ear with the production of dark brown exudates. No treatment had been administered for the otitis.

Vertebral fixations were released, and acupuncture was performed on active points, including BL 17, 19, and 25; GB 29 on the left side; LI 11; and SP 6. The Tao Hong Yin was continued, and 15 g of Chuan Niu Xi was added to 100 g of the base formula to promote lower lumbar relaxation.

One month later, on day 63 of treatment, Murphy continued to improve. The hind limb lameness had resolved, forelimb lameness was only sporadically seen, the ear infection had resolved without treatment, and Murphy no longer seemed hot at night. Murphy had lost 7 pounds on the raw food diet. Vertebral fixations were restricted to L7, and her back seemed to be more supple. Herbal treatment was continued. Acupuncture was performed at the few active points that could be identified, namely, BL 23, SP 6, and GV 14. The fixation at L7 was relieved, and a follow-up examination scheduled for 6 weeks later. Improvements had been sustained up to the date of Murphy's last visit three months later, and over 5 months after her initial presentation.

COMMENTS

In ancient China it was said that before undertaking the study of medicine a person had to learn to play the Qin, one of the oldest stringed instruments in the world. It was felt that learning to play music had many similarities to practicing medicine. The patient's body could be considered analogous to an instrument, and the strings resemble the various modalities and interventions that could be used to act upon it. In this analogy, knowledge of how to pluck and press the strings to create a pleasing melody is akin to deft use of various modalities to restore balance within a body.

In Murphy's case many modalities were brought to bear to achieve the therapeutic goals suggested by the assessment. It is doubtful that any one of them can be considered primarily responsible for Murphy's improvements, and it is likely that all played a part in restoring her quality of life. Just as various themes can be alternately represented within a single piece of music, various formulas and points were used as Murphy progressed in her recovery, in order to render the most individualized treatment possible.

Although improvements are commonly expected in the first 2 weeks of using alternative medicine, the time when improvements will be complete, if it ever arrives, cannot be predicted. As is typical of many lameness problems, even with appropriate therapy it took 2 months and much patience for Murphy's complaints to be largely resolved. Patience was particularly required during the temporary worsening of symptoms that is commonly seen after release of long-standing vertebral fixations. In addition, Murphy's presentation changed over the course of treatment, necessitating reevaluation and adaptation. Murphy's case thus illustrates how success in alternative medicine demands persistent effort both by the owner and by the veterinarian.

SM

REFERENCES

Acupuncture. *NIH Consens Statement JAMA* 15(5):1-34, 1997.

Berge GE. Polyascorbate (C-Flex R) an interesting alternative by problems in the support and movement apparatus in dogs. *Norwegian Vet J* 102: 581-582, 1990.

Bliddal H, Rosetzsky A, Schlichting P, Weidner MS, Anderson LA, Ibfelt HH, Christensen K, Jensen ON, Barsley J. A randomized, placebo-controlled, cross-over study of ginger extracts and ibuprofen in osteoarthritis. *Osteoarthritis Cartilage* 8(1):9-12, 2000.

Bonnett B, Poland C. Preliminary results of a randomized, double blind, multicenter, controlled clinical trial of two herbal therapies, acetylsalicylic acid and placebo for osteoarthritic dogs. Proceedings of the American Holistic Veterinary Medical Association, Burlington, Vt, 1996.

Budd K. Use of D-phenylalanine, an enkephalinase inhibitor, in the treatment of intractable pain. *Ad Pain Res Ther* 5:305-308, 1983.

Cheng X, editor. *Chinese Acupuncture and Moxibustion.* Beijing, China, 1987, Foreign Languages Press.

Creamer P. Osteoarthritis pain and its treatment. *Curr Opin Rheumatol* 12(5):450-455, 2000.

Darlington LG, Stone TW. Antioxidants and fatty acids in the amelioration of rheumatoid arthritis and related disorders. *Br J Nutr* 85(3):251-269, 2001.

Diehl HW, May EL. Cetyl myristoleate isolated from Swiss albino mice: an apparent protective agent against adjuvant arthritis in rats. *J Pharm Sci* 83(3):296-299, 1994.

Ehling D. *The Chinese Herbalist's Handbook*, revised ed. Santa Fe, NM, 1996, Inword Press.

Ernst E, Chrubasik S. Phyto-anti-inflammatories: a systematic review of randomized placebo controlled double blind trials. *Rheumatic Dis Clin North Am* 26(1):13-27, 2000.

Ezzo J, Hadhazy V, Birch S, Lao L, Kaplan G, Hochberg M, Berman B. Acupuncture for osteoarthritis of the knee: a systematic review. *Arthritis Rheum* 44(4):819-825, 2001.

Green S, Buchbinder R, Barnsley L, Hall S, White M, Smidt N, Assendelft W. Acupuncture for lateral elbow pain. *Cochrane Database Cyst Rev* (1):CD003527, 2002.

Impellizeri JA, Lau RE, Azzara FA. Fourteen week clinical evaluation of an oral antioxidant as a treatment for osteoarthritis secondary to canine hip dysplasia. *Vet Q* 20(Suppl 1):S107-S108, 1998.

Kitade T, Odahara Y, Shinohara S, Ikeuchi T, Sakai T, Morikawa K, Minamikawa M, Toyota S, Kawachi A, Hyodo M, et al. Studies on the enhanced effect of acupuncture analgesia and acupuncture anesthesia by D-phenylalanine (first report)—effect on pain threshold and inhibition by naloxone. *Acupunct Electrother Res* 13(2-3):87-97, 1988.

Klein G, Kullich W. Short-term treatment of painful osteoarthritis of the knee with oral enzymes: a randomised, double-blind study versus diclofenac. *Clin Drug Invest* 19(1):15-23, 2000.

Kulkarni RR, Patki PS, Jog VP, Gandage SG, Patwardhan B. Treatment of osteoarthritis with a herbomineral formulation: a double-blind, placebo-controlled, cross-over study. *J Ethnopharmacol* 33(1-2):91-95, 1991.

Lau CS, Morley KD, Belch JJ. Effects of fish oil supplementation on non-steroidal anti-inflammatory drug requirement in patients with mild rheumatoid arthritis—a double-blind placebo controlled study. *Br J Rheumatol* 32(11):982-989, 1993.

Little C, Parsons T. Herbal therapy for treating rheumatoid arthritis (Cochrane Review). *Cochrane Database Syst* Rev 1:CD002948, 2001.

Macioca G. *The Practice of Chinese Medicine.* New York, 1994, Churchill Livingstone.

McAlindon TE, Jacques P, Zhang Y, Hannan MT, Alibadi P, Weissman B, Rush D, Levy D, Felson DT. Do antioxidant micronutrients protect against the development and progression of knee osteoarthritis? *Arthritis Rheum* 39:648, 1996.

Marz RB. *Medical Nutrition from Marz,* ed 2. Portland, Ore, 1997, Omni-Press.

Murphy R. *Lotus Materia Medica.* Pagosa Springs, Colo, 1995, Lotus Star Press.

Naeser MA. *Outline Guide to Chinese Herbal Patent Medicines in Pill Form.* Boston, 1990, Boston Chinese Medicine.

Qiu GX, Gao SN, Giacovelli G, Rovati L, Setnikar I. Efficacy and safety of glucosamine sulfate versus ibuprofen in patients with knee osteoarthritis. *Arzneimittelforschung* 48:469-474, 1998.

Sander O, Herborn G, Rau R. [Is H15 (resin extract of Boswellia serrata, "incense") a useful supplement to established drug therapy of chronic polyarthritis? Results of a double-blind pilot study]. *Z Rheumatol* 57(1):11-16, 1998.

Sharma ML, Bani S, Singh GB. Anti-arthritic activity of boswellic acids in bovine serum albumin (BSA)-induced arthritis. *Int J Immunopharmacol* 11(6):647-652, 1989.

Tu LH, Huang DR, Zhang RQ, Shen Q, Yu YY, Hong YF, Li GH. Regulatory action of *Astragalus* saponins and buzhong yiqi compound on synthesis of nicotinic acetylcholine receptor antibody in vitro for myasthenia gravis. *Chin Med J (Engl)* 107(4):300-303, 1994.

Wakabayashi K, Inoue M, Ogihara Y. The effect of keishi-bushi-to on collagen-induced arthritis. *Biol Pharm Bull* 20(4):376-380, 1997.

Xie H. *Traditional Chinese Veterinary Medicine.* Beijing, China, 1994, Beijing Agricultural University Press.

Yan W. *Practical Therapeutics of Traditional Chinese Medicine.* Brookline, Mass, 1997, Paradigm Publications.

Yeung H. *Handbook of Chinese Herbal Formulas.* Los Angeles, 1995, Self-published.

Yeung H. *Handbook of Chinese Herbs.* Los Angeles, 1996, Self-published.

Zurier RB, Rossetti RG, Jacobson EW, DeMarco DM, Liu NY, Temming JE, White BM, Laposata M. Gamma-linolenic acid treatment of rheumatoid arthritis: a randomized, placebo-controlled trial. *Arthritis Rheum* 39(11):1808-1817, 1996.

13

Therapies for Neoplastic Disorders

CANCER, GENERAL

- It should be understood that different cancer types require different strategies for treatment, and our level of knowledge about the mechanisms of natural treatments is not sufficient to target these different cancer mechanisms. It should also be understood that therapies listed in the Paradigmatic sections have not been researched for the most part. The recommendations in those portions of this chapter are merely the product of early clinical observations. We therefore present an introductory section on general cancer treatment, and when specific protocols or studies exist for individual cancer types, we consider these "add on" treatments.
- According to Boik (2001), there are seven categories of procancer event clusters that may be targets for natural therapy in cancer:
  - Genetic instability
  - Abnormal transcription factor activity
  - Abnormal signal transduction
  - Abnormal cell-to-cell communication
  - Abnormal angiogenesis
  - Invasion and metastasis
  - Abnormal immune function
- Boik recommends large combinations of natural compounds (15 to 18 substances) to increase the practitioner's chances of covering all of these events and to facilitate synergism between the ingredients. According to the many studies cited in Boik's text, many natural compounds have multiple effects that are

important in managing cancer patients. These include but are not limited to:

- **Inducing differentiation:** arctigenin, vitamin A, boswellic acid, flavonoids, emodin (an anthraquinone contained in aloe and some laxative herbs), eicosapentaenoic acid (EPA), docosahexanoic acid (DHA), resveratrol, vitamin D_3.
- **Inducing apoptosis:** Vitamins C, E, D_3, and A, boswellic acid, curcumin (from turmeric), EPA, flavonoids, garlic, resveratrol, selenium.
- **Inhibiting protein kinases:** curcumin, emodin, flavonoids, EPA, DHA.
- **Facilitating cell-to-cell communication:** apigenin, genistein, melatonin, selenium, resveratrol, vitamin D_3.
- **Inhibiting factors that support angiogenesis:** anthocyanidins, boswellic acid, curcumin, EPA, DHA, flavonoids, garlic, glutathione-enhancing agents, melatonin, resveratrol, vitamin E, Siberian ginseng, vitamin C.
- **Inhibiting cancer cell invasion mechanisms:** apigenin, boswellic acids, proanthocyanidins, luteolin, resveratrol, EPA, curcumin, emodin, genistein, quercetin, mushroom polysaccharides, *Panax ginseng*.
- **Inhibiting metastasis mechanisms:** anthocyanidins, astragalus, bromelain, curcumin, emodin, EPA, feverfew, flavonoids, reishi mushroom, garlic, genistein, resveratrol, vitamin E.
- **Enhancing immune function:** astragalus, eleuthero, reishi and other mushroom polysaccharides, *Panax ginseng,* glutamine, most antioxidants, bromelain, melatonin.

Alternative Options with Conventional Bases

Nutrition

- It is hardly fair to attempt to summarize Boik's 500-page text with thousands of references in a few sentences, but suffice it to say here that the evidence in support of antioxidants, flavones and flavonoids, bromelain, turmeric (curcumin), and fish oil is strong enough to recommend their use in most cases of cancer. A review of some of the more popular natural methods used as adjuncts in cancer therapy follows.

- **Low-carbohydrate, moderate- to high-fat and moderate-protein diet:** there is evidence that animals with lymphoma, and probably other cancers, have altered carbohydrate metabolism and that reducing simple carbohydrates in the diet may reduce substrate for cancer cell energy production. Many cancer cells cannot use fat as an energy source, unlike host cells. Since cancer cachexia is a result of both fat and lean body mass loss, fat should be a significant proportion of the dietary energy (Ogilvie, 1998). Although a commercial diet is available that fulfills what we know of the requirements of cancer patients (Hills N/D), some clients and veterinarians prefer homemade foods that are slightly less optimal (inasmuch as they do not have exactly the profile of N/D). We have used a diet of 50% poultry or fish and 50% mixed nonstarchy vegetables for dogs, and 80% poultry and 20% mixed nonstarchy vegetables for cats. These diets are supplemented with high levels of Fish Oil as the fat source (flaxseed oil or olive oil, if necessary), calcium, and a vitamin-mineral supplement.
- **Vitamins and minerals** are best supplemented in combination with each other:
  - **Vitamin A:** has cytotoxic effects and may induce differentiation and apoptosis, as well as having other potential anticancer effects. The *dose* recommended by Boik based on animal and human studies is equivalent to 625 to 7500 IU per lb of body weight per day. High doses of Vitamin A are potentially toxic, especially if given for months at a time; however, most veterinarians are unduly frightened of Vitamin A toxicity. As an example, a toxic dose of Vitamin A for a 30-lb dog is approximately 250,000,000 IU given daily for 3 months.
  - **Vitamin C:** may inhibit cancer cell proliferation by suppressing free radicals. Boik does not recommend Vitamin C as a single therapy because of its documented prooxidant effect when given intravenously at high doses. Vitamin C is best used in combination with other antioxidant vitamins and minerals, at a *dose* of up to 25 mg per lb of body weight.

  - **Vitamin D_3:** may inhibit tumor growth, angiogenesis, and metastasis according to animal studies. The doses used in animal studies are toxic, however, and lead to hypercalcemia. Boik recommends a *dose* of 10 to 30 mg per lb of body weight daily for future investigation, and the veterinarian should be wary of oversupplementation.
  - **Vitamin E:** may inhibit tumor growth in addition to its indirect antioxidant and immune-enhancing activity. The *suggested dose* is approximately 10 IU per lb of body weight daily.
  - **Selenium:** has cytotoxic effects on some cancer cells in addition to its preventive role in cancer development. *Dosage* for use in animals, scaled down from Boik's recommendation for people, is 2 to 5 μg per lb of body weight daily.
- **ω-3 fatty acids:** although ω-6 fatty acids may promote tumor progression in a number of ways, ω-3 fatty acids have a well-established role in cancer management. Dozens of animal studies suggest that they inhibit tumor growth and metastasis, inhibit cachexia, and may increase the effectiveness of some chemotherapy drugs. These studies have investigated EPA and DHA, which are contained in Fish Oil. Other sources of ω-3 fatty acids have been recommended, such as Flaxseed Oil, but these contain alpha-linolenic acid (ALA), which is converted at low efficiency to EPA and DHA by humans and possibly dogs, but probably not converted by cats. The relative proportion of dietary ω-3 to ω-6 fatty acid is critical and difficult to determine in diets other than the defined commercial diet N/D. An empirical *dose* of Fish Oil is approximately 300 mg EPA and 200 mg DHA (contained in a double-strength 1000 mg capsule of Fish Oil) per 10 lb of body weight. If the animal does not tolerate Fish Oil at this high dose, it should be administered to the level possible.
- **Flavonoids (or bioflavonoids):** contained in a wide range of medicinal and food plants. These include flavones (luteolin, apigenin), isoflavones (daidzein, genistein), flavonols (quercetin, kaempferol), flavanols (tea catechins), and anthocyanidins-proanthocyanidins.

The various compounds may have antioxidant, estrogenic, antiestrogenic, antimetastatic, and cytotoxic effects. Proanthocyanidin *dose* is approximately 20 to 60 mg/lb of body weight daily. Flavonol, flavone, and isoflavonoid *doses* range from 15 to 50 mg or more per lb of body weight daily.

Amino Acids

- **Glutathione:** a tripepticle composed of cysteine, glutamine, and glycine that acts as an intracellular antioxidant and detoxifying agent. Low levels of glutathione are associated with increased cancer risk, impaired detoxification, and suppressed immunity. Supplementing glutathione does not increase glutathione levels; however, administration of other antioxidants such as Vitamin E, Vitamin C, alpha-lipoic acid, and melatonin increases plasma and intracellular glutathione levels.
- **Arginine:** appears to enhance immune function and may inhibit the growth of some tumors. The *dose* is approximately 500 to 3000 mg daily.
- **Glutamine:** may inhibit tumor growth and cachexia and is useful for inhibiting the adverse effects of chemotherapy. It also increases glutathione levels. Although in vitro studies suggest that Glutamine serves as a fuel for cancer cells, in vivo studies do not bear this finding out and the value of Glutamine is recognized as an adjunct in cancer treatment. Glutamine should be administered at 0.5 g/kg of body weight daily.
- **Melatonin:** has cytotoxic effects against cancer cells, is an antioxidant, increases efficacy of chemotherapy drugs, and has other potential activity against cancer according to animal and human studies. Boik's proportional *dose* would suggest 0.2 mg/lb of body weight daily for animals.
- **Inositol hexaphosphate** (IP6, phytate): may beneficially alter signal transduction pathways, cell cycle regulatory genes, differentiation genes, oncogenes, and tumor suppressor genes. In vitro and animal studies suggest a role in treatment of various carcinomas and leukemias. Empirical *dose* is 10 to 50 mg/lb of body weight daily.

- **Cartilage:** has been shown to have antiangiogenic properties and has tissue inhibitors of metalloproteinases that inhibit tumor metastasis. However, controlled trials in humans and animals have shown no benefit from administering shark cartilage. Since the wild shark population is being decimated through commercial fishing for meat and cartilage, it makes no sense to use shark cartilage.

Herbs

- **Garlic** *(Allium sativum):* appears to have antioxidant, immune-enhancing, and eicosanoid-mediated mechanisms that are active in treatment of cancer. Because the high doses studied in animal and in vitro reports are likely to be toxic, Boik presumes that garlic must be used in combination with other natural treatments to take advantage of synergism. The toxic dose for garlic is not well established in dogs and cats, although the potential for Heinz body anemia after acute high doses or chronic use is well recognized. There does appear to be an individual susceptibility to garlic toxicity, but veterinarians have used *doses* of approximately one clove per 30 to 50 lb of body weight for dogs, and ⅛ to ¼ clove for cats. Some practitioners use the extract product Kyolic at 10 to 30 mg/lb of body weight daily. Concurrent antioxidant supplementation is potentially protective against the oxidative damage garlic may induce in red blood cells.
- **Mushroom polysaccharides:** Reishi Mushroom *(Ganoderma lucidum),* Shiitake Mushroom *(Lentinus edodes),* Turkey Tail *(Trametes versicolor),* Maitake Mushroom *(Grifola fondosa),* and other mushrooms have established immunostimulating and antitumor activity. Boik suggests a *dose* equivalent to 20 to 100 mg/lb of body weight daily for animals.
- **Curcumin,** a yellow pigment from the spice Turmeric *(Curcuma longa):* inhibits tumor growth and metastasis, reduces the side effects of chemotherapy, and may increase the action of some chemotherapy agents, as well as prevent cancer. The *dose* equivalent suggested by Boik is 15 to 20 mg/lb of body weight daily for animals.

- **Green Tea** *(Camellia sinensis):* may inhibit tumor growth, angiogenesis, and metastasis in addition to preventing cancer. Dried Green Tea can be mixed in food at the highest dose the animal will tolerate. Standardized Green Tea extract contains a constant amount of epigallocatechin gallate, which can be administered at 5 mg/lb of body weight daily.
- **Ginseng** *(Panax ginseng):* appears to decrease cancer growth and metastasis, and to enhance immune function and survival times.
- **Cat's Claw** *(Uncaria tomentosa):* has been advocated for treatment of many cancer types, but no studies are available to judge the advisability of using Cat's Claw.
- **Essiac Tea:** contains a combination of herbs with evidence of biologic activity including antitumor antioxidant, antiestrogenic, and immunostimulant actions, but no studies examining the formula in vitro or in vivo have been published.
- **Hoxsey Formula:** a combination of about nine herbs that each may have cytotoxic and immunostimulating activity. No controlled trials addressing Hoxsey herbal formula therapy are available; however, a case series following 39 patients with advanced cancers over 48 months reported that six were still alive. These survivors had lung, melanoma, recurrent bladder, and labial cancers (Austin, 1994).

Other

- **714-X** (CDNC, Camphor Derivative Nitrogenated Compound): a compound developed by Gaston Naessons. Naessons believes that it disrupts the life cycle of pleomorphic or cell wall–deficient bacteria that he thinks are critical to the development of cancer. 714-X or CDNC is derived from camphor, which is said to have increased affinity for cancer cells. Nitrogen is added to the compound to satisfy the nitrogen requirements of cancer cells, which are said to act as nitrogen traps and deplete the body of needed nitrogen. Ammonium salts are also part of the compound. All in all, Naesson designed the compound to prevent cancer cells from nutritionally depleting immune cells as it stimulates immune function. CDNC is administered as a sterile injection into lymph nodes—probably popliteal nodes in dogs. It has also been administered via nebulization for lung and oronasal cancers. No adverse effects have been reported, although I (SW) observed a single aged dog to have a seizure for the first time after administration of CDNC. It may be available as an investigational drug from Naesson's research center, Centre Expérimental de Recherches Biologiques de l'Estrie, Inc. (CERBE), in Rock Forest, Quebec (http://www.cerbe.com/index.html) (Kaegi, 1998).

- **Hydrazine sulfate:** inhibits gluconeogenesis (when products of anaerobic metabolism are reconstituted into glucose), which is thought by the developer of hydrazine to be a primary metabolic pathway for cancer cells. Hydrazine is thought to reduce cancer-related cachexia and to suppress cancer growth. Hydrazine sulfate is given orally or as an injection. The human dose is 60 mg tid for 30 to 45 days, followed by a resting period of 2 to 6 weeks. This cycle is repeated indefinitely. The drug may be available as an investigational product from the Syracuse Center Research Institute, Syracuse, New York. More information is available from the Center's web site at http://www.ngen.com/hs-cancer (Kaegi, 1998).
- **Escharotic salves:** have been used for centuries to destroy surface tumors (Naiman, 2000). These salves generally contain caustic herbs, especially Bloodroot *(Sanguinaria canadensis)*. The salves are difficult to use for animals because they are potentially dangerous if taken orally and it is not always possible to prevent the animal from licking itself.

Paradigmatic Options

Homeopathy

- Homeopathy cannot be advised as a first line of treatment in small animal neoplasia. Aggravations of tumors are common if the wrong remedy is used or the correct remedy is overused. Although many authors on veterinary homeopathy believe they have good reason to dispute this advice, homeopathic aggravations and the tremendous risks they pose to human cancer patients are well known.

Chinese Medicine

- Cancer is the greatest foe of all medicines. Because the exact means by which some alternative medicines exert their effect is yet unknown, cancer patients and owners of animals that have cancer turn to these therapies in the hope that the therapies "can do something that conventional medicine can't," thus allowing alternative practitioners to perhaps circumvent walls that have so far protected cancer from consistently effective conventional treatment. In short, cancer patients quite understandably hope for a miracle.
- New practitioners of alternative medicine find their clients' and patients' expectations of a miracle weighty, and initially they seem impossible to fulfill. Yet the persistent need of cancer patients for options to toxic therapies has provided the necessity that appears to hold promise of being the mother of invention. Effectiveness against cancer is probably the unofficial high water mark of success for every medical system, and the alternative medical practitioners are quite right to be in awe of every positive cancer outcome they witness in response to alternative therapies. But the cracks in the edifice of cancer these outcomes represent are now appearing a little too regularly for them to still be called miracles. It does indeed appear that alternative medicine has something extremely important to offer cancer management, both in the form of additional tools of intervention and, more important, in the form of a new perspective. It is entirely conceivable that the coming decades will yield demonstrably efficacious cancer protocols that had their germ in alternative medicine.
- Most medical systems in history have been founded on a paradigmatic approach to disease. That is, they looked at a disease in abstract or metaphoric terms, defined a solution in those same terms, and then found real-world tools that seemed appropriate and to metaphorically fit the definition for a solution. It is this

perspective that likewise seems to hold promise for giving birth to effective cancer treatments.

- Two metaphoric pathways so far seem to account for the development of most cases of cancer. Some cases seem to arise from a tangible accumulation of Phlegm that possesses a Toxic Heat that eats its way through a body like a hot ember through fabric. The second mechanism appears to be through increasing sluggishness of the river of circulation to the point that the stagnant pools of Blood effectively congeal into clumps. The two pathways are not mutually exclusive. Accumulations of Phlegm can promote Blood stasis. Heat generated by stagnant Blood may have a corrosive effect on neighboring tissues. In general, this simplistic metaphoric view of cancer pathogenesis seems appropriate to virtually all tumors when cancer patients are evaluated from the Chinese medical perspective.
- The Chinese medical perspective has led over the course of centuries to the identification of therapies that effectively "clear Toxic Heat, transform Phlegm, drain Damp, and move Blood." Many of these alternative therapies have been the subjects of pharmacologic research. Constituents were identified and assessed for antineoplastic activity. Different plants and molecules were found to possess greater anticancer activity than others. Use of these agents in crude or refined form in conventional cancer therapy is not yet widespread, however, in part because of modern medicine's ignorance of their existence but also because the agents do not seem powerful enough compared with existing chemotherapeutics.
- The initial impression of the inferiority of some alternative anticancer therapies is sometimes misleading. These therapies are understood from a metaphoric perspective in the cultures that use them, and they are applied only to tumors for which they are metaphorically appropriate. They are ineffective and thus never used in the management of tumors that have developed through other mechanisms. Therefore a Blood-moving herb might be helpful to address tumors that have developed from Blood stasis but would be

ineffective for those arising from Phlegm accumulations. Unfortunately, conventional and metaphoric understandings of the pathogenesis of a particular type of tumor, such as a mast cell tumor, cannot be perfectly superimposed. That is, some mast cell tumors develop from Blood stasis and some from Phlegm accumulations. A Blood-moving agent used for mast cell tumors arising from Blood stasis that is investigated for efficacy against mast cell tumors of Phlegm origin will be falsely interpreted as ineffective. Future clinical trials examining the effectiveness of alternative therapies against certain tumor types should probably use the expertise of alternative diagnosticians so that patients with a given tumor type can be subdivided into appropriate subgroups according to the metaphoric interpretation of their tumor pathogenesis and be given an appropriate therapy or its corresponding placebo. Only then will the effectiveness, or lack thereof, of the alternative therapy be truly appreciated.

- The ability to be metaphorically classified is not restricted to alternative anticancer therapies. Modern Chinese medicine as practiced in China is usually highly integrated with conventional medicine to the point that certain drugs are commonly incorporated into various Chinese herbal formulas to create a synergistic combination that has greater therapeutic power than either drug or herb has when used alone. Fledgling attempts are being made in the West to similarly classify Western therapeutics according to the Chinese medical paradigm. So far this investigation has largely been limited to Western herbs, but methodologies have been proposed that seem equally able to accurately describe the energetic nature of drugs and nutritional supplements.
- Themes that are emerging from these fledgling energetic descriptions of drugs echo the Chinese medical interpretation of the pathogenesis of cancer. This adds further support to these metaphoric impressions, but the resonance between the energetics of Eastern and Western therapeutics has a much greater importance.

Speculations can now be made as to which alternative and conventional therapeutics may be combined to synergistic advantage to yield greater results than when either therapeutic is used alone. Such synergies might not only assist treatment of the tumor, but also help reduce side effects of conventional therapies. These synergies may exist not only between chemotherapeutics and herbs, but also, for example, between herbs and vitamins, or nutraceuticals and herbs.

- An explosion of possibilities for new cancer therapy protocols seems imminent when consideration is given to the prospect of applying metaphoric thinking to conventional cancer therapeutics. Effective herb-drug or herb-vitamin combinations that result might otherwise take decades to be developed, given the pace and direction of current efforts in botanical medical research. Research is understandably still very much focused on determining the presence and value of individual active ingredients in plants. Observations on how secondary ingredients might interact both within and between plants in herbal formulas to enhance efficacy of the active ingredients are slowly emerging. The variables involved are too complex to make reasonable hypotheses about which plants or compounds might interact favorably. Metaphoric thinking provides a shortcut to identifying candidates for such synergistic reactions and helps to provide fodder for future research.
- The therapeutic combinations that are suggested when we find a common ground for divergent therapies will have the same advantage that a fork has over a knife in chasing a pea on a plate. A single metaphoric classification usually encompasses herbs and drugs with a number of different physiologic effects. When they are combined into a single protocol, these therapies will have the same thrust from a general perspective, but will achieve their effect through a variety of chemical mechanisms. In this way, multiple procancer events can be addressed simultaneously and perhaps in a highly coordinated fashion.

- The current state of development and research of alternative treatments of cancer is not advanced enough to tell us whether the existence and discovery of these synergistic therapeutic possibilities is truly realistic or merely a tantalizing possibility. A promising synergistic combination may already be in the making, however, for the management of cancers arising from the accumulation of Dampness, Phlegm, and Toxic Heat.

Dampness, Phlegm, and Toxic Heat: pathophysiology

- The hallmarks of cancers arising from this pathway are the development of Heat signs and destructive lesions. The lesion usually takes root some time earlier as a benign accumulation of Dampness and Phlegm. Some authors believe that entry of the pathogen is via an acupuncture channel, which makes it an externally derived condition. Others suggest that external pathogen invasion is just a trigger, a final overburdening of a system already encumbered by previous accumulations of the same pathogen.
- The beliefs of Chinese medicine are in striking accord with those generally held by Naturopathic medicine that chronic inflammation that manifests as a tumor arises from a preexisting toxic state in which an external irritant has essentially done nothing more than ignite a previously accumulated toxic tinder pile. For both Chinese and Naturopathic medicine the generation of internal accumulations of Dampness or toxins arises from faulty digestive function.
- Generation of Dampness and Phlegm occurs in Chinese medicine secondary to Spleen Qi deficiency. The organ itself often is not at fault but is simply overwhelmed by an excessive intake of food. Theoretically, "overnutrition" may stem from excessive intake of fat, but the benefit to some animal cancer patients of a diet high in fat as discussed previously seems to contradict this contention. For animals, the excessive dampening influence may be an excessive intake of carbohydrates. High body fat content rather than a high fat content in the diet may be more important in promoting some human cancers. The greatest source of this fat may,

however, be carbohydrates. This is consistent with the Chinese medical dictum that the Spleen is overwhelmed by an excess of the Sweet taste, which is the taste assigned relatively faithfully by Chinese medicine to carbohydrate ingredients. Lowering the carbohydrate content of the diet may make sense from a conventional medical perspective as well, since the metabolism of many tumors appears to rely on anaerobic glycolysis.

Signs

- Specific signs of tumors arising from accumulations of Dampness, Phlegm, and Toxic Heat include the following.
  - Red or purple-red frothy tongue, although some patients' tongues may be paler in color.
  - Inflamed suppurative yellow lesions (yellow is the color of Heat in Chinese medicine).
  - Destructive malignancies.
  - Elevated appetite or thirst, but often not both in skin disease.
  - Preference for cool surfaces (tile, shade, holes dug in the yard, sleeping on the floor rather than the bed, hard surfaces, basements).
  - Skin that is hot to the touch.
  - Exudative or crusting skin lesions.
  - Autoimmune skin disorders.
  - Lesions that bleed and the blood is bright red.
  - Extreme agonizing itch (Heat in the Blood causes an itch according to Chinese medicine).
  - Rapid and forceful, wiry pulses.

Signs of Dampness

- Greasy or "clumped" hair.
- Lichenification and thickening of the skin.
- Large flakes of dander, often tinted; note that they are often dry even though their underlying cause is Dampness.
- Slimy vomitus.
- A tendency to sleep very deeply.
- Reverse sneezing, snoring during sleep.
- Strong skin or ear odor.

- Strong odor to breath or flatus.
- Yeast otitis externa.
- Copious exudates from mucous membranes.
- Aggravation during humid weather.
- Loose or mucoid stools.
- Past medical history of cystitis or colitis.
- Anal gland inflammation, infection, and impaction.

Tumor types with this clinical presentation

- Squamous cell carcinoma.
- Nasal adenocarcinoma.
- Lymphosarcoma.
- Osteosarcoma.
- Fibrosarcoma.
- Some chondrosarcomas.

Treatment protocol

- The general emphasis of this protocol appears to be to increase the rate of cell differentiation in Toxic Heat tumors. My (SM) protocol components are as follows:
  - Vitamin A, 5000 IU sq per lb of body weight every 3 to 4 weeks as needed.
  - Vitamin D, 750 IU sq per lb of body weight every 3 to 4 weeks as needed.
  - DHA, as a component of an ω-3 fatty acid preparation, up to 24 mg per lb of body weight daily.
  - Hoxsey-like formula, using the approximate ratios of herbs described in the following section, at a dose of 0.2 ml per 5 lb of body weight at least once daily.
  - Diet low in carbohydrates and high in Vitamin A and natural carotenes, which often entails providing a home-prepared diet. Raw preparations may contain a higher quantity of antineoplastic nutraceuticals. High levels of organ meat, especially liver, may help boost antioxidant and Vitamin A levels. The recent decline in the use of organ meats in commercial pet foods may play a role in increasing susceptibility to tumor generation.

Treatment rationale

- Many tumors are immature cells, locked in a perpetual state of immaturity, in which normal mechanisms that trigger cell aging, limitations on cell division, and eventually cell death are not yet activated. Vitamin A is a primary agent in the body that promotes cell differentiation in addition to being an antioxidant with the ability to protect regulatory genes from deactivation. From a holistic perspective, Vitamin A appears to promote the clearance of Damp Heat. Concern over the potential toxicity of large doses of Vitamin A has restricted its use in cancer therapy, but the tolerance for large, infrequent doses of Vitamin A in nonpregnant humans and animals may have been underestimated. The dose described in the treatment protocol appears to be well tolerated by dogs and cats, although occasional type I hypersensitivity reactions to preservatives that is manifested chiefly as hives have been observed in some individuals. For these patients, Vitamin A may be administered orally in the same dose as a concentrated emulsion.

- One way to obtain the benefits of Vitamin A in promoting cell differentiation without using toxic doses may be to use Vitamin A in tandem with other agents that either promote cell differentiation by themselves or assist Vitamin A in this action. DHA, commonly found in commercial ω-3 fatty acid preparations for the treatment of skin disease, is known to enhance the cell-differentiating effect of Vitamin A.
- The Hoxsey-like formula in the treatment protocol also contains ingredients that enhance cell differentiation. Berberine is a potent cell differentiator and is contained in one of the main ingredients of the formula, Oregon Grape. Relatively high doses are ordinarily required to achieve this effect, but the herb's ability to promote cell differentiation may be enhanced by using the formula in tandem with the Vitamin A. The Hoxsey-like formula contains the same ingredients as a similar "alterative" formula that preceded development of the Hoxsey Formula. As an alterative the Hoxsey-like formula enhances the detoxifying action of the digestive organs, particularly the liver. It is therefore highly appropriate for use in Damp Heat cases in which initial dampness accumulations are considered to arise from digestive dysfunction. Other anticancer properties have been

identified for both ω-3 fatty acids and the Hoxsey-like formula, as discussed earlier in this chapter.

- The Hoxsey Formula is available only from affiliates of the original formula developer, and knowledge of the exact ratios and ingredients of the formula has been somewhat proprietary. Various Hoxsey-like products are available commercially, but some do not use very large amounts of the ingredients of most interest, Oregon Grape and Burdock, because of palatability concerns (Burdock *[Arctium lappa]*, an important ingredient of the Hoxsey formula, contains components cytotoxic to neoplastic cells). Chinese medical understanding of the actions of the constituent herbs allows us to make an educated guess at appropriate ratios of ingredients. I (SM) suggest the following ratio:

  3 parts Oregon Grape *(Mahonia aquifolium)*
  3 parts Burdock Root *(Arctium lappa)*
  1 part Pokeroot *(Phytolacca americana)*
  1 part Cascara *(Rhamnus purshiana)*
  1 part Buckthorn *(Rhamnus frangula)*
  1 part Licorice *(Glycyrrhiza glabra)*
  1 part Stillingia *(Stillingia sylvatica)*
  2 parts Prickly Ash Bark *(Xanthoxyllum americanum)*
  3 parts Red Clover *(Trifolium pratense)*

  - Depending on the tumor involved and the clinical presentation of the case, other herbs may be considered for addition such as Boneset *(Eupatorium perfoliatum)* to relieve the pain of osteosarcoma, or Agrimony *(Agrimonia eupatoria)* and Yellow Dock *(Rumex crispus)* to heal ulcerations of the oral mucosa. Alfalfa *(Medicago sativa)* may also be added for Yin- or Blood-deficient patients. Any additions should be made carefully to ensure that Oregon Grape, Burdock, and Red Clover remain the chief ingredients. Red Clover contains genistein, another chemical compound with demonstrated anticancer activity through a number of different mechanisms.
  - The Hoxsey-like formula's content of Pokeroot makes it potentially toxic, but toxicity is seldom seen when the formula is given with these ratios at the recommended dose to patients for which it is appropriate.

Extended or inappropriate use of the formula may lead to inappetence or vomiting, in which case the formula should be at least temporarily discontinued.

- I (SM) have not evaluated or made use of other Western herbal formulas developed for the treatment of cancer, but Essiac Tea contains some of the same ingredients and therefore perhaps some of the alterative and cell-differentiating effects of the Hoxsey-like formula.

Other therapies to address Dampness and Phlegm

- **Ban Xia Bai Zhu Tian Ma Tang** (Pinellia, White Atractylodes, and Gastrodia Decoction) has shown potential in ameliorating signs associated with *some brain tumors* in dogs. Twenty grams of Jiang Can is added to 100 g of formula to enhance this effect. Dogs that benefit may exhibit signs reminiscent of headaches or pain and appear depressed and dull. They may have soft or slippery pulses and a pale and swollen tongue with tenacious saliva, may vomit viscid mucus, and may vomit after eating.

Acupuncture

- Controversy exists among veterinary acupuncturists over the appropriateness of acupuncture in the treatment of cancer. Fears center on the possibility of aiding metastasis during the needling process. Needling a tumor directly may not be prudent, but acupuncture treatment of points distant to the tumor to correct the underlying imbalance that gave rise to the tumor appears to be safe and is commonly used in the acupuncture treatment of cancer in humans. Points used to drain Damp, transform Phlegm, and clear Heat include LI 11, BL 22, BL 39, SP 9, ST 40, PC 6, BL 25, CV 3, LI 4, BL 40, CV 12, GB 41, and LR 3. The points that seem palpably "active" on a patient should be used. Consult Appendix E for further information on point action to help refine the point prescription.

Dietetics

- In addition to the previous dietary recommendations, some Chinese medical practitioners recommend eliminating wheat and mucus-forming foods such as dairy products and heating foods such as garlic, spices, and beef. The metaphoric actions of these foods may potentially worsen the conditions thought to lead to the cancer itself.

Blood stasis: pathophysiology

- Blood stasis appears to be the other main avenue of tumor generation, especially in dogs. From a Chinese medical perspective, Blood deficiency often leads to Blood stasis, just as water in a river becomes more stagnant as the level drops. Blood deficiency also aggravates the Liver's ability to regulate the circulation of Qi, which causes Qi stagnation. Since Qi is the motive force of Blood, Qi stagnation leads to Blood stagnation.
- Blood deficiency may arise from inappropriate diets. Raw diets that contain ample organ meat and are low in digestible carbohydrates should be fed to affected animals with strong pulses. Organ meats have long been considered by Chinese medicine to be excellent sources of Blood, and the reduced carbohydrate load will help support Blood production by ensuring that the Spleen is not overwhelmed. Note that these high-protein, high-fat, and low-carbohydrate diet recommendations for cancer patients are similar to those proposed in conventional medicine.

Signs

- Anemia.
- Pale-lavender or purple tongue.
- Thin and possibly tense or taut pulses.
- Very fine, powdery dander.
- Coat dryness or dullness.
- Alopecia; fine coat.
- Failure of hair to grow back after surgery.
- Restless, dream-filled sleep.
- Low-grade skin rashes with pruritus.
- Preponderance of lesions and tumors along the sides of the body, in the axillae, on the pinnae, and in the inguinal region.
- Fear aggression, timidity, and anxieties of all types.

- Keratoconjunctivitis sicca.
- Chronic lameness of soft tissue origin; tendency to muscle spasm.
- The practitioner may have the diagnostic impression that there is reduced immunity in the skin resulting in recurrent pyoderma, generalized demodectic mange, and similar disorders.

Signs when Blood deficiency is secondary to Spleen deficiency

- Soft or slippery pulses.
- Tongue swelling or scalloping; tongue coating.
- Greasy coat and waxy ears.
- Undigested food in the stool.
- Coprophagy; a predilection for consuming rotting (i.e., predigested) debris.
- Episodic diarrhea with pale mucus in the stool.
- Depressed appetite.
- Lethargy.
- Weight gain.

Signs as Blood deficiency turns to Blood stasis

- Purple masses.
- Localized boring or stabbing pain.
- Hepatomegaly and splenomegaly.
- Associated hemorrhage or blood pockets.
- Engorged vessels.
- Varicosities.
- Purple tongue.
- Wiry pulse.
- Choppy pulse.

Treatment options

- Blood-moving formulas seem to be highly effective alone for this type tumor. I typically combine them with the use of Vitamin A, since diets low in Blood-tonifying organ meats might also be presumed to be lacking high levels of Vitamin A.
- Possibly the single most important formula in Chinese veterinary medicine for treating tumors arising from Blood deficiency and Blood stasis is **Xue Fu Zhu Yu Tang** (Drive Out Stasis from the Mansion of Blood

Decoction). To 100 g of this formula, 15 g each of the Blood-moving herbs San Leng and E Zhu is added because they possess significant antineoplastic activity. These two herbs can be omitted when tumors are not present and the formula is being used prophylactically to prevent tumor regrowth after surgical removal.

- Specific indications for the use of **Xue Fu Zhu Yu Tang** are for patients exhibiting signs of Qi stagnation, Blood deficiency, and Blood stasis. The formula contains **Si Ni San** (Four Cold Extremities Powder) and **Si Wu Tang** (Four Materials Decoction). These formulas allow Xue Fu Zhu Yu Tang to address the core issues surrounding the development of Blood stasis, namely, Qi stagnation and Blood deficiency. Signs include a lavender or purple tongue and a wiry or choppy pulse. The formula seems most appropriate for externally occurring tumors but also is used to great benefit for patients with metastases to the chest and in some patients with brain cancer. Neoplasms for which the author has seen consistent and obvious therapeutic benefit of Xue Fu Zhu Yu Tang include ***mast cell tumors, thyroid adenocarcinoma, pulmonary metastases of a variety of different tumors, and superficial hemangiomas and hemangiosarcomas***. The practitioner should continue use of the formula until pulse, tongue, physical, and historical findings of Blood deficiency and Blood stasis abate. A *suggested starting dose* of granular concentrate is ¼ tsp per 10 to 15 lb of body weight, or 60 to 75 mg/kg of body weight, at least once daily.
- **Ge Xia Zhu Yu Tang** (Drive Out Blood Stasis from Below the Diaphragm Decoction) is indicated especially for ***hepatomegaly and splenomegaly from neoplasia***. Ge Xia Zhu Yu Tang appears to help extend survival times for patients with hepatic neoplasms especially. Guiding signs for the use of this formula are a purple tongue, a wiry or choppy pulse, and abdominal pain in the cranial or mid-abdomen and along the costal arch. A *suggested starting dose* of granular concentrate is ¼ tsp per 10 to 15 lb of body weight, or 60 to 75 mg/kg of body weight, at least once daily.

- **Shao Fu Zhu Yu Tang** (Drive Out Blood Stasis from the Lower Abdomen Decoction) is indicated for Blood stasis tumors of the lower abdomen. Specific examples include ***bladder tumors, prostatic tumors, tumors of the ovaries or uterus, and even liver tumors or cirrhosis***. Hallmarks of a patient that may benefit include evidence of Yang deficiency, such as the seeking of heat, hind limb weakness, and incontinence. The patient may also have a pale, lavender, or purple tongue and a wiry or choppy pulse. The formula may have exceptional benefit in the treatment of bladder neoplasia when the bladder is firm and painful and when there is a pronounced history of hematuria. The practitioner can add 20 g of Hua Shi (Talc) to 100 g of the base formula to augment the benefits of the formula in bladder neoplasia. **Shao Fu Zhu Yu Tang,** like **Ge Xia Zhu Yu Tang,** has good ability to relieve pain. A *suggested starting dose* of granular concentrate is ¼ tsp per 10 to 15 lb of body weight, or 60 to 75 mg/kg of body weight, at least once daily.
- **Yunnan Bai Yao** is a formula that appears to offer some relief of bleeding and pain in inoperable ***abdominal hemangiosarcomas***. Without the use of an antineoplastic formula in addition to Yunnan Bai Yao, survival is likely to be prolonged a few months at most. A *suggested starting dose* of granular concentrate is ¼ tsp per 10 to 15 lb of body weight, or 60 to 75 mg/kg of body weight, at least once daily.
- When Blood stasis appears to arise chiefly because of Qi stagnation, Qi-moving formulas may be considered. **Chai Hu Shu Gan San** (Bupleurum Ease the Liver Powder) contains **Si Ni San** (Four Cold Extremities Powder) with Xiang Fu and Chuan Xiong added to relieve pain in the upper abdomen and around the costal arch. It is thus especially appropriate for upper abdominal tumors, such as ***hepatic and gastric tumors.*** Guiding signs to its use are mental depression, moodiness, hypochodriac distention and pain, chest fullness, belching, indigestion, abdominal distention, a lavender tongue, and a wiry or taut pulse. It should be combined with **Xuan Fu Dai Zhe Tang** for gastric cancer. A *suggested starting dose* of granular concentrate

is ¼ tsp per 10 to 15 lb of body weight, or 60 to 75 mg/kg of body weight, at least once daily.

- **Xi Jiao Di Huang Tang** (Decoction of Rhinoceros Horn and Rehmannia) is a formula that cools and moves Blood. Guiding signs include high fever, delirium, dark red tongue, a thready and rapid pulse, epistaxis, bloody stool, hematuria, purple-black ecchymoses, and melena. Modern versions of the formula replace Xi Jiao (Rhinoceros Horn) with Shui Niu Jiao (Water Buffalo Horn), which is from a domesticated species, or Bai Mao Gen (Imperata). A *suggested starting dose* of granular concentrate is ¼ tsp per 10 to 15 lb of body weight, or 60 to 75 mg/kg of body weight, at least once daily.
- Acupuncture points useful in Blood deficiency, Qi stagnation, and Blood stasis include ST 37, ST 39, BL 17, BL 20, BL 18, BL 21, CV 12, SP 10, LI 4, BL 40, LI 11, and ST 36. Specific point indications can be found in Appendix E. In general, the points that feel most turgid, swollen, thickened, or warm should figure prominently in the prescription.

Supportive formulas

- Some formulas can be of tremendous benefit in palliative care and improvement in the quality of life of the patient even though they may not reliably reduce tumor mass. This approach may be especially important in advanced or chronic cases of neoplasia. These formulas may be used alone or to help counter the side effects of conventional treatments. The formulas may also possess some direct effect against tumors, depending on the case.
- For Liver Blood deficiency, **Bu Gan Tang** (Nourish the Liver Decoction) can be considered. This formula is a Blood tonic and a mild Yin tonic. Guiding signs to its use include eye dryness, fear aggression, irritability, a dull or dry coat, a tendency to muscle spasms and cramping pains, a pale tongue, and a thin and slightly wiry pulse. A *suggested starting dose* of granular concentrate is ¼ tsp per 10 to 15 lb of body weight, or 60 to 75 mg/kg of body weight, at least once daily. The formula should not be used in Damp cases.

- For Spleen Qi deficiency, **Si Jun Zi Tang** (Four Gentlemen Decoction) can be used. Guiding signs include pallor, soft voice, weakness of the arms and legs, abdominal distention, loss of appetite, vomiting, borborygmi, diarrhea, a pale tongue, and a weak pulse. A *suggested starting dose* of granular concentrate is ¼ tsp per 10 to 15 lb of body weight, or 60 to 75 mg/kg of body weight, at least once daily.
- For Qi and Yin deficiency, **Sheng Mai San** (Generate the Pulse Decoction) can be considered. This formula contains just three herbs, Ren Shen, Mai Men Dong, and Wu Wei Zi, which serve to replenish Qi and body fluids. Signs that a patient may need this formula include a pale or red tongue, a feeble or weak pulse, fatigue, shortness of breath, thirst, a chronic cough, and mouth dryness. A *suggested starting dose* of granular concentrate is ¼ tsp per 10 to 15 lb of body weight, or 60 to 75 mg/kg of body weight, at least once daily.
- **Da Bu Yuan Jian** (Great Tonify the Source Decoction) is used to nourish Yin and Blood. It also mildly tonifies Spleen Qi to increase strength and appetite, and is used to relieve low back pain and stiffness. This formula can be used when the patient also has dry eyes or hair, a lusterless coat, a pale or red tongue, and a frail pulse. A *suggested starting dose* of granular concentrate is ¼ tsp per 10 to 15 lb of body weight, or 60 to 75 mg/kg of body weight, at least once daily.
- For Qi and Blood deficiency, **Ba Zhen Tang** (Eight Treasures Decoction) should be considered. This formula acts to tonify the Spleen Qi and nourish Blood. Guiding signs include a pale tongue, a thready pulse or a gigantic and weak pulse, pallor, fatigue, shortness of breath, palpitations, loss of appetite, and anemia. A *suggested starting dose* of granular concentrate is ¼ tsp per 10 to 15 lb of body weight, or 60 to 75 mg/kg of body weight, at least once daily.
- **Ren Shen Yang Ying Tang** (Ginseng Support the Nutritive Qi Decoction) is used when the patient exhibits emaciation, pallor, inappetance, insomnia, cognitive deficiencies, chilliness, incontinence, and anemia. The patient generally has a pale tongue and a

weak, thready pulse. A *suggested starting dose* of granular concentrate is ¼ tsp per 10 to 15 lb of body weight, or 60 to 75 mg/kg of body weight, at least once daily.

- For Yin deficiency with Empty Heat, **Zhi Bai Di Huang Wan** (Anemarrhena, Phellodendron, and Rehmannia Pill) can be considered. Guiding signs for this formula include coat dryness, heat intolerance, thirst, low back stiffness and hind limb weakness, colitis, weight loss, dehydration, a red, dry tongue, and a thin, rapid, or floating pulse. A *suggested starting dose* of granular concentrate is ¼ tsp per 10 to 15 lb of body weight, or 60 to 75 mg/kg of body weight, at least once daily.
- For Stomach Yin deficiency, **Yi Wei Tang** (Benefit the Stomach Decoction) can be considered. This formula acts to replenish Lung and Stomach Yin. Such Yin deficiencies manifest as thirst, hunger, dry cough, retching, upper abdominal pain, hiccough, fever, dry and hard stools, a red, dry tongue, and a thready, rapid pulse. This formula may be of particular benefit in gastric or lung cancer. A *suggested starting dose* of granular concentrate is ¼ tsp per 10 to 15 lb of body weight, or 60 to 75 mg/kg of body weight, at least once daily.
- For the older gastric cancer patient, the practitioner should consider using a combination of **Li Zhong Tang** (Cultivate the Center Decoction) and **Liu Jun Zi Tang** (Six Gentlemen Decoction). Li Zhong Tang acts to dispel cold from the Spleen and Stomach, and Liu Jun Zi Tang acts to replenish Spleen Qi. Patients that benefit from this combination have a pale, swollen, or moist tongue, a weak, slow, or soft pulse, lack of thirst, decreased appetite, watery diarrhea, productive cough, vomiting, shortness of breath, eructations, and abdominal pain that is ameliorated by pressure. A *suggested starting dose* of granular concentrate is ¼ tsp per 10 to 15 lb of body weight, or 60 to 75 mg/kg of body weight, at least once daily.
- For Kidney Yang deficiency, **You Gui Wan** (Restore the Right Pill) should be considered because it is a vigorous Kidney Yang tonic. It is used for patients that exhibit

pallor, chilliness, urinary incontinence, stiff and weak low back and knees, a pale, swollen, wet tongue, and a deep, slow, weak pulse. A *suggested starting dose* of granular concentrate is ¼ tsp per 10 to 15 lb of body weight, or 60 to 75 mg/kg of body weight, at least once daily.

Herb/Biopharmaceutical Interactions

- Berberine may upregulate cellular multidrug resistance pumps and result in decreased retention of chemotherapeutic agents (Lin, 1999).
- Controversy exists about the use of antioxidant approaches during radiation or chemotherapy, since conventional therapies may rely on the infliction of oxidative damage on neoplastic cells for some of their antineoplastic effect. Several antioxidant agents may actually enhance chemotherapy and radiation effectiveness, however, including Milk Thistle *(Silybum marianum)*, which has the additional benefit of protecting hepatocytes from any hepatotoxic effects of chemotherapeutic drugs (Invernizzi, 1993; Scambia, 1996). A generalized edict against the use of antioxidants in patients receiving chemotherapy may therefore be detrimental because it may potentially delay the discovery of synergistic relationships between alternative therapies and chemotherapeutic approaches. More research is needed to identify which antioxidant agents may benefit chemotherapeutic protocols, and which may hinder them.

ADENOCARCINOMA, NASAL

Paradigmatic Options

- When clinical presentation agrees, the protocol outlined previously for tumors arising from Damp or Toxic Heat should be considered.

AUTHORS' CHOICES:

SM: Toxic Heat protocol.
SW: Diet; antioxidants; high doses of Vitamin A; Fish Oil; Garlic; Turmeric; mixed flavonoids; IP6; Chinese herbs; chemotherapy when appropriate.

LIPOMA AND OTHER FATTY LUMPS

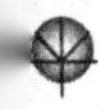

Paradigmatic Options

- Historically, the physical appearance of an abnormality was taken fairly literally in Chinese medicine. Lipomas appear similar to phlegm in texture and color and so were considered accumulations of congealed Dampness and Phlegm. A readily achievable goal in the management of lipomas is to halt further development of the tumors by addressing constitutional tendencies to Dampness and Phlegm through the use of generally appropriate diets and herbs. Herbal formulas used include Dampness-draining formulas such as **San Ren Tang** (Three Seeds Decoction), **Wei Ling Tang** (Decoction to Dispel Dampness in the Spleen and Stomach), and **Si Miao San** (Four Marvels Powder). These formulas are discussed at length elsewhere in the text. Dietary strategies to consider include avoiding food allergens, reducing carbohydrate content, and providing food preparations that ensure completeness of digestion.
- Specific approaches have also been advocated for the treatment of existing tumors. A barrier to tumor absorption and dissemination would seem to be their relatively low vascularity. Some of the formulas listed contain Blood-moving herbs to attempt to increase local circulation to the area of the tumor.
- For Spleen Qi deficiency that results in Phlegm accumulation, one approach that has been advocated is the combination of **Gui Pi Wan** (Restore the Spleen Pill), **Er Chen Tang** (Two Cured Herbs Decoction), and **Xiao Jing Pian.** The latter is a proprietary formula with considerable toxic potential owing to its content of scorpion and seeds of the *Nux vomica* plant, which is a natural source of strychnine. These two toxic ingredients are used in some formulas to help break down masses and unblock the channels. Two ingredients that assist them in this formula are Ban Xia and Di Long. The rest of the herbs are used to invigorate the Blood and warm the channels. The *recommended dose* for **Xiao Jing Pian** is 0.3 g or 3 capsules two to three times daily.

- Xiao Jing Pian employs a dynamic used in **Xiao Huo Luo Dan** (Minor Invigorate the Collaterals Pill), which is considerably less toxic. Practitioners concerned about the toxic potential of Xiao Jing Pian may wish to substitute Xiao Huo Luo Dan. **Er Chen Tang** is a simple general formula to transform Phlegm. **Gui Pi Wan** completes the dynamic by tonifying Spleen Qi and tonifying Blood deficiency to reduce Blood stasis. A *suggested starting dose* of granular concentrate of the Gui Pi Wan, Xiao Huo Luo Dan, and Er Chen Tang combination is ¼ tsp per 10 to 15 lb of body weight, or 60 to 75 mg/kg of body weight, at least once daily.

Nontoxic Formulas Advocated for Lipomas in the Human Literature *(Fruehauf, 1995)*

- For Phlegm coagulation with Qi deficiency that manifests in patients as multiple lipomas, shortness of breath, weak voice, poor appetite, low body weight, a pale tongue, and a fine or weak pulse, the practitioner can consider **Liu Jun Zi Tang** (Six Gentlemen Decoction) with Ban Xia added. A *suggested starting dose* of granular concentrate is ¼ tsp per 10 to 15 lb of body weight, or 60 to 75 mg/kg of body weight, at least once daily.
- For Phlegm coagulation associated with Blood stagnation that perhaps manifests as multiple, firm, and poorly circumscribed lipomas, blue discoloration of the skin, a purple tongue, and a wiry pulse, a combination of Hu Po, Chen Xiang, Tao Ren, Hong Hua, San Leng, E Zhu, Dang Gui, Ban Xia, Zhe Bei Mu, and Zhu Li can be considered to transform Phlegm and strongly move Blood. A *suggested starting dose* of granular concentrate is ¼ tsp per 10 to 15 lb of body weight, or 60 to 75 mg/kg of body weight, at least once daily.
- For Phlegm coagulation with Yang deficiency that manifests as multiple lipomas, cold extremities, an aversion to cold, pallor, abdominal pain, a fat, pale tongue, and sunken slow pulses, **Yang He Tang** (Yang Activating Decoction) with Zhe Bei Mu and Xi Xin can be considered. A *suggested starting dose* of granular

concentrate is ¼ tsp per 10 to 15 lb of body weight, or 60 to 75 mg/kg of body weight, at least once daily.

AUTHORS' CHOICES:

SM: Address constitutional tendencies to Dampness and Phlegm through diet and basic herbal formulas.
SW: Correct diet according to patient needs; Chinese herbal formulas.

LIVER (HEPATIC ADENOCARCINOMA, HEPATOMA)

Alternative Options with Conventional Bases

- S-Adenosylmethionine (SAMe) to augment hepatic glutathione stores.

Herbs

- **Curcumin** (Turmeric, *Curcuma longa*): prevents carcinogenesis and induces apoptosis in human hepatic adenocarcinoma cell lines in vitro (Jiang, 1996; Lin, 1998). This spice is fairly well tolerated when added to homemade diets for dogs and cats.
- **Sho-saiko-to:** prevented development of hepatocellular carcinoma in humans with cirrhosis (Shimizu, 2000). An important herb contained in this formula is Chinese Skullcap *(Scutellaria baicalensis)*, which contains baicalin, baicalein, and saikosaponin-a, all of which have been shown to have antitumor activity in vitro (Motoo, 1994).
- **Chai Hu Gui Zhi Tang:** suppressed liver lesion development, inhibited cell proliferation, and induced apoptosis in an induced model of hepatic carcinogenesis (Tatsuta, 2000).

Paradigmatic Options

- The practitioner should use the most appropriate formulas discussed in the general section on cancer treatment to address liver cancer. For all of the following formulas, a *suggested starting dose* of granular concentrate is ¼ tsp per 10 to 15 lb of body weight, or 60 to 75 mg/kg of body weight, at least once daily. Some leading candidates for consideration include the following:

- **Chai Hu Su Gan San** (Bupleurum Ease the Liver Powder) for patients with Liver Qi stagnation that manifests as cranial abdominal pain, bloating, decreased appetite, depression, a lavender tongue, and a taut pulse.
- For Qi and Blood stagnation that manifests as sharp pain in the cranial abdomen, firm palpable masses, a purple tongue, and a choppy and perhaps deep and thready pulse, **Ge Xia Zhu Yu Tang** (Drive Out Stasis from Below the Diaphragm Decoction) can be used. When icterus accompanies evidence of Blood stasis, about 15 g of Yin Chen Hao is added to 100 g of Ge Xia Zhu Yu Tang.
- When Spleen Qi deficiency results in the accumulation of Dampness, the practitioner should consider combining **Si Jun Zi Tang** and **Er Chen Tang.** Patients that may benefit reportedly have evidence of dull cranial abdominal pain, fatigue, nausea, poor appetite, a distended abdomen, a pale tongue, and a deep, thin, weak pulse.
- For patients that exhibit evidence of Yin deficiency with internal Heat, **Er Zhi Wan** (Two Ultimates Pill) combined with **Qing Hao Bie Jia Tang** (Decoction of Sweet Wormwood and Tortoise Shell) should be considered. Er Zhi Wan is a moderately strong formula that clears Empty Heat and stops bleeding in Yin-deficient patients without dampening them. Qing Hao Bie Jia Tang nourishes Yin and dispels Heat. Patients that benefit may have insomnia and night-time restlessness, weakness in the low back and knees, dull cranial abdominal pain, a poor appetite, fatigue, low fever, night panting, heat in paws, a dry mouth, bleeding gums, a red, dry tongue, and a thin, rapid pulse. Some authors find this formula to be especially useful for patients that are undergoing chemotherapy.
- **Chai Hu Gui Zhi Tang** (Bupleurum and Cinnamon Twigs Decoction) is a combination of **Gui Zhi Tang** and **Xiao Chai Hu Tang.** Patients that may benefit

from this formula may exhibit alternating chills and fever, digestive signs reminiscent of the Liver overacting on the Spleen, abdominal fullness, belching, muscle aches and stiffness, a floating pulse, and a pale or red tongue.

AUTHORS' CHOICES:

SM: Appropriate Chinese herbal formula and supportive diet therapy.
SW: Diet; antioxidants; Fish Oil; Garlic; Turmeric; mixed flavonoids; Chinese herbs.

LUNG (PRIMARY OR METASTATIC)

Alternative Options with Conventional Bases

- **Shi Quan Da Bu Tang combined with interferon A/D:** had a better antimetastatic effect than either interferon or the herbal formula alone in a mouse model of metastatic renal cell carcinoma (Muraishi, 2000).
- **Keishi-ka-kei-to:** inhibited metastasis of melanoma in a mouse model (Suzuki, 1997).

Paradigmatic Options

- As previously mentioned, **Xue Fu Zhu Ye Tang** (Drive Out Stasis in the Mansion of Blood Decoction) is perhaps the single most useful formula for metastatic lung tumors. Realistic expectations are an obvious improvement in quality of life, with reductions in dyspnea and coughing. However, tumor mass reduction may not be seen despite these clinical improvements. A *suggested starting dose* of granular concentrate is ¼ tsp per 10 to 15 lb of body weight, or 60 to 75 mg/kg of body weight, at least once daily. The formula should not be discontinued as long as improvements are maintained.
- Formulas advocated for human primary lung cancer that may be applicable to animals include the following:
  - **Dao Tan Tang** (Phlegm-Resolving Decoction) for accumulations of Dampness, Phlegm, and Toxic Heat. This

is an antitussive formula that resolves Phlegm. Guiding signs include a white, frothy coating on the tongue, a slippery pulse, dyspnea, a productive cough, vomiting, fullness and oppression of the chest, restlessness, and loss of appetite. **Ting Li Da Zao Xie Fei Tang** (Purge the Lung with Lepidium and Jujube Decoction) can also be considered when the patient has asthma, facial edema, cough with profuse sputum, chest distention, dysuria, insomnia, a wet or frothy tongue, and a slippery pulse. A *suggested starting dose* of granular concentrate is ¼ tsp per 10 to 15 lb of body weight, or 60 to 75 mg/kg of body weight, at least once daily.

- For primary lung cancer associated with Empty Fire, **Sha Shen Mai Men Dong Tang** (Glehnia and Ophiopogon Decoction) can be considered. This formula nourishes the Lung and Stomach Yin to promote the secretion of body fluids. It is used when there is evidence of a dry throat, thirst, a dry cough, tenacious sputum, a red tongue, and a weak, rapid pulse. A *suggested starting dose* of granular concentrate is ¼ tsp per 10 to 15 lb of body weight, or 60 to 75 mg/kg of body weight, at least once daily.
- For cases of Qi and Yin Deficiency, **Sheng Mai San** (Generate the Pulse Powder) can be used. For Qi, Blood, and Yang deficiency, **Shi Quan Da Bu Tang** (Ten Ingredients for Complete Tonification Decoction) can be considered. This formula consists of **Ba Zhen Tang** with Huang Qi and Rou Gui added to address further Spleen Qi and Kidney Yang deficiency. A *suggested starting dose* of granular concentrate is ¼ tsp per 10 to 15 lb of body weight, or 60 to 75 mg/kg of body weight, at least once daily.

AUTHORS' CHOICES:

SM: Supportive therapy with diet and appropriate Chinese herbal formula.

SW: Diet; antioxidants; Fish Oil; Garlic; Turmeric; mixed flavonoids; IP6; Chinese herbs.

LYMPHOMA

Alternative Options with Conventional Bases

Nutrition

- **A specific combination of Arginine and Fish Oil:** was found to enhance disease-free intervals and survival times in dogs with lymphoma (Ogilvie, 2000). Arginine may inhibit tumor growth and metastasis, and it enhances immune function. Fish Oil decreases inflammation and may inhibit metastasis as well. These supplements are available in the proportions and doses tested in the commercial diet, N/D.

Paradigmatic Options

- Various formulas have been suggested for acute leukemic varieties of lymphoma. Some of these clinical presentations are probably more common in humans than in animals, but the formulas may be of assistance when animals exhibit the same signs. Most of these formulas have been discussed in the general section on the role of Blood stasis in tumor formation.
- For Excess Heat in the Blood that is manifested as high fever, bleeding, anemia, involvement of a variable array of organs, a dark-red tongue, and a rapid pulse, **Xi Jiao Di Huang Tang** (Rhinoceros and Remhannia Decoction) can be considered. A *suggested starting dose* of granular concentrate is ¼ tsp per 10 to 15 lb of body weight, or 60 to 75 mg/kg of body weight, at least once daily. See the General section at the beginning of this chapter for information on how this formula is modified to eliminate the need for Xi Jiao as an ingredient.
- For Blood stasis that manifests as palpable abdominal masses, low-grade fever, dry mouth, a purple tongue, and deep, thin, choppy pulses, **Ge Xia Zhu Yu Tang** (Drive Out Stasis from Below the Diaphragm Decoction) can be used. A *suggested starting dose* of granular concentrate is ¼ tsp per 10 to 15 lb of body weight, or 60 to 75 mg/kg of body weight, at least once daily.
- For Qi and Yin deficiency that is manifested as lower fever, fatigue, sweating during the day or night, heat in the paws and chest, lower lumbar weakness and pain, a

pale tongue, and deep and thready pulses, **Sheng Mai San** (Generate the Pulse Powder) should be considered. A *suggested starting dose* is ¼ tsp per 10 to 15 lb of body weight, or 60 to 75 mg/kg of body weight, at least once daily.

In Cases of Chronic Leukemic Disorders

- For Liver Yin and Blood deficiency that manifests as low-grade fever, irritability, dry mouth, nighttime restlessness and panting, low body weight, bruising, epistaxis, a tender tongue, and a thready and rapid pulse, **Bu Gan Tang** (Nourish the Liver Decoction) can be considered. A *suggested starting dose* of granular concentrate is ¼ tsp per 10 to 15 lb of body weight, or 60 to 75 mg/kg of body weight, at least once daily.
- **Ba Zhen Tang** (Eight Precious Ingredients Decoction) can be considered for Qi and Blood deficiency. Signs for use include pallor, shortness of breath, fatigue, dizziness, panting, a pale tongue, and a thready and weak pulse. A *suggested starting dose* of granular concentrate is ¼ tsp per 10 to 15 lb of body weight, or 60 to 75 mg/kg of body weight, at least once daily.
- For chronic Blood stasis tumors that are manifested as a hard mass in the cranial abdomen, upper abdominal bloating, bruising, bone pain, epistaxis, or hematochezia, **Ge Xia Zhu Yu Tang** should be considered. A *suggested starting dose* of granular concentrate is ¼ tsp per 10 to 15 lb of body weight, or 60 to 75 mg/kg of body weight, at least once daily.
- For bleeding related to leukemia, **Yun Nan Bai Yao** can be considered. See Chapter 9 for herb forms and doses.
- For lymphoma that is manifested as lymphadenopathy, an approach based on the Damp and Toxic Heat protocol described in the first section of this chapter frequently yields some benefit in my (SM) practice. This may be particularly true for animals receiving concurrent chemotherapy, in that responsiveness of the tumor to chemotherapy seems to be significantly enhanced relative to animals not receiving alternative therapies. Animals that respond often have several of the clinical traits associated with accumulation of Dampness and

Phlegm. Coinciding lameness caused by deformities from degenerative joint disease may also improve with use of this approach. Lymphoma is the tumor type for which the cell differentiation effects of Vitamin A have been researched the most in humans. Ginger can be added to the Hoxsey-like formula to reduce the possibility of any gastrointestinal side effects for animals without marked Heat signs. The treatment rationale for the Damp and Toxic Heat protocol section provides basic advice on how to alter the Hoxsey-like formula.

- If signs of Spleen Qi deficiency or any other abnormalities appear, the Hoxsey-like formula can be used simultaneously with the appropriate Chinese herbal formula. Use of formulas containing the Qi tonic Ren Shen (Ginseng) provide the patient with Ginseng's potential benefit of promoting lymphoblast differentiation.
- A Chinese herbal formula that may be considered for lymphoma manifested as peripheral lymphadenopathy is **Tao Hong Er Chen Tang** (Two Cured Herbs Decoction with Carthamus and Persica). The formula is made by combining approximately 15 g of Tao Ren and 12 g of Hong Hua with approximately 35 g of Er Chen Tang. This formula is indicated for cases that appear to have elements of both Blood stasis and Phlegm accumulation arising from Spleen Qi deficiency. Specific signs for its use include weight loss, poor appetite, enlarged lymph nodes, a pale or lavender tongue, and soft to tight pulses. The formula is probably insufficient by itself to control tumor development but may yield good results when combined with conventional chemotherapeutics, even when these are administered at lower than normal doses or intervals. This strategy may be useful in animals that seem relatively intolerant of chemotherapy alone. A *suggested starting dose* of granular concentrate is ¼ tsp per 10 to 15 lb of body weight, or 60 to 75 mg/kg of body weight, at least once daily.
- Alcohol extracts of the following Western herbs can be combined in the indicated ratios to successfully support the action of **Xue Fu Zhu Yu Tang** and

abbreviated or mild chemotherapy protocols in the treatment of thoracic lymphoma: 3 parts Red Clover, 3 parts Red Root *(Ceanothus americanus)*, 1 part Pokeroot, and 3 parts Gumweed *(Grindelia* spp.). Animals that benefit the most exhibit signs of Blood stasis and Phlegm accumulation such as a lavender tongue, a chronic productive cough, thin, wiry pulses, and perhaps splenomegaly. A *suggested starting dose* is 0.2 ml per 5 lb of body weight, at least once daily.

- For all these approaches the institution of the appropriate dietary measures discussed in the general section on the treatment of cancer appears to enhance results.

AUTHORS' CHOICES:

SM: Diet; appropriate formula.
SW: Chemotherapy; diet; antioxidants; Fish Oil; Garlic; Turmeric; mixed flavonoids; IP6.

MAMMARY CANCER

Alternative Options with Conventional Bases

- A case control study of European dogs that developed mammary cancer indicated that obesity and homemade diets are risk factors. Serum retinol concentrations were lower in patients with mammary cancer. A high intake of beef was particularly associated with development of cancer, although low chicken intake was also a risk (Alenza, 1998). If a homemade diet is recommended for mammary cancer patients, it may be best to avoid beef and concentrate on poultry or fish.
- **Rosemary** *(Rosmarinus officinalis)*: has been suggested as one herbal treatment for mammary cancer. One constituent of Rosemary, carnosol, suppressed tumorigenesis in a rat model of induced mammary cancer (Singletary, 1996). Rosemary extract also increased intracellular levels of the chemotherapeutic agents doxorubicin and vinblastine by overcoming a

multidrug resistance pump in a mammary cancer cell line (Plouzek, 1999). These studies suggest that Rosemary may be added to homemade diets to aid in prevention of breast cancer and may be a useful adjunct in chemotherapy for mammary adenocarcinoma.

- **Conjugated linoleic acid** (CLA): is cytotoxic to mammary cancer cells in vitro (O'Shea, 2000) and inhibits growth and metastasis of implanted mammary tumors in vitro and in mice at 0.1% to 1% of the diet (Hubbard, 2000). CLA is thought to increase sensitivity of cancer cells to normal levels of oxidative stress (Devery, 2001). CLA is contained in meat and dairy products, especially milk fat.
- **Phytoestrogens:** have been recommended as an adjunctive treatment for mammary cancer in dogs, undoubtedly because they appear to be useful in humans. However, their greatest use in humans is for prevention and for management of menopausal signs after chemotherapy. Since dogs do not tend to have estrogen-responsive tumors, the value of phytoestrogens as treatment is suspect.

Paradigmatic Options

- When the tumor appears to arise from Liver Qi stagnation and is manifested as apparent distention and pain in the mammary glands, depression, abdominal discomfort on palpation, a lavender tongue with a thin white or yellow coating, and a wiry pulse, **Chai Hu Su Gan San** (Bupleurum Ease the Liver Powder) can be considered. A *suggested starting dose* of granular concentrate is ¼ tsp per 10 to 15 lb of body weight, or 60 to 75 mg/kg of body weight, at least once daily.
- When an apparent imbalance of the Chong and Ren Mai extraordinary vessels is manifested as a painful mass in the mammary gland, abnormal heat cycles, dry mouth, a red, dry tongue, and a wiry or thready pulse, a combination of **Er Xian Tang** (Decoction of Curculigo and Epimedium) and **Xiang Bei Yang Yong Tang** (Cyperus and Fritillaria Decoction to Nourish the Nutritive Qi) can be given. A *suggested starting dose* of granular concentrate is ¼ tsp per 10 to 15 lb of body

weight, or 60 to 75 mg/kg of body weight, at least once daily. Acupuncture points to address this imbalance are KI 6, LU 7, SP 4, and PC 6.

- **Xiang Bei Yang Ying Tang** appears to have clinical potential in the management of human breast cancer. It addresses Qi and Blood deficiency with Qi, Blood, and Phlegm stagnation that causes masses on the neck, breasts, and axillae. Patients that benefit may have a pale or purple tongue and a weak or choppy pulse. A *suggested starting dose* of granular concentrate is ¼ tsp per 10 to 15 lb of body weight, or 60 to 75 mg/kg of body weight, at least once daily. Potentially useful acupuncture points to support the action of this formula include ST 39, ST 37, PC 6, ST 14, SI 1, GB 41, and Tai Yang.
- **Er Xian Tang** is used to address Kidney Yin and Yang deficiency accompanied by excess Liver fire that leads to menopausal hot flashes and urinary frequency.
- **Yi Qi Yang Yong Tang** is closely related to Xiang Bei Yang Ying Tang. They share many of the same ingredients, but a much greater proportion of the former's ingredients are Qi tonics. The main purpose of this formula is to tonify Qi and Blood, and it has some Blood-moving properties. It is best indicated for patients that have a thin body, pallor, shortness of breath, panting at night, poor appetite, loose stool, a pale, white-coated tongue, and a deep, weak, and thready pulse. Its ingredients are as follows:

Dang Shen	30 g
Huang Qi	30 g
Bai Zhu	10 g
Fu Ling	12 g
Dang Gui	15 g
Chuan Xiong	9 g
Shu Di Huang	15 g
Bai Shao	15 g
Dan Shen	15 g
Xiang Fu	10 g
Bei Mu	10 g

A *suggested starting dose* of granular concentrate is ¼ tsp per 10 to 15 lb of body weight, or 60 to 75 mg/kg of body weight, at least once daily.

AUTHORS' CHOICES:

SM: Surgical removal; chicken- or fish-based diet; appropriate herbal formula.
SW: Surgery; diet; CLA; IP6; antioxidants; Fish Oil; Garlic; Turmeric; mixed flavonoids.

MAST CELL TUMOR

Alternative Options with Conventional Bases

- **Vitamin C:** has been suggested as an inhibitor of mast cell degranulation in allergy models, but the evidence has not been convincing. Some veterinarians claim that Vitamin C is toxic to mast cells, and use for mast cell tumors is recommended at up to 50 mg/kg of body weight per day, qid. Aside from reversible diarrhea at high doses this vitamin is nontoxic and has other benefits, so it may be worth using, but because of Vitamin C's prooxidant effects, other antioxidants should also be provided.

Paradigmatic Options

- **Xue Fu Zhu Yu Tang** with added San Leng and E Zhu seems to be an extremely effective formula for preventing recurrence after surgical excision. The formula is best suited to superficially occurring mast cell tumors arising from Liver Blood deficiency that leads to Blood stasis. Even some animals with tumors metastatic to a single lymph node have entered apparent remission. Repeated aspirates of the lymph nodes after several months' use of the formula have shown no presence of mast cells. A *suggested starting dose* of granular concentrate is ¼ tsp per 10 to 15 lb of body weight, or 60 to 75 mg/kg of body weight, at least once daily.

AUTHORS' CHOICES:

SM: Xue Fu Zhu Yu Tang with San Leng and E Zhu; diet.
SW: Diet; antioxidants; Fish Oil; Garlic; Turmeric; mixed flavonoids.

MELANOMA

Alternative Options with Conventional Bases

Nutrition

- **Melatonin:** slows melanoma proliferation in vitro (Cos, 2001). A case series in human melanoma patients suggested improved outcomes (Gonzalez, 1991). The general section earlier in the chapter discusses other effects of Melatonin. The *dose* recommended by Boik is equivalent to approximately 0.2 mg/lb of body weight.

Herbs

- **Cordyceps** *(Cordyceps sinensis)*: given to mice at 100 to 200 mg/kg of body weight inhibited metastasis in mice implanted with an immortalized melanoma cell line (Nakamura, 1999).
- **Juzen-taiho-to, Sho-saiko-to,** and **Keishi-ka-kei-to:** decreased metastasis of melanoma in a variety of mouse models (Kato, 1998; Utsuyama, 2000).

Paradigmatic Options

- The appropriate herbal formula and dietary strategy should be used for the case based on the information given in the initial section in this chapter. Melanoma may manifest itself either as Blood stasis or as Toxic Heat.

AUTHORS' CHOICES:

SM: Appropriate diet and herbal formula.
SW: Diet; antioxidants; Melatonin; Fish Oil; Garlic; Turmeric; mixed flavonoids; Chinese herbal formulas.

MYCOSIS FUNGOIDES

Alternative Options with Conventional Bases

Nutrition

- **Fatty acids:** anecdotal reports suggest that γ-linolenic acid (GLA) from Evening Primrose Oil given at 30 mg/kg of body weight daily improves outcomes.

Linoleic acid (LA) was reported to lead to remission in a small group of dogs (Peterson, 1999). It is supplied by Safflower Oil that is *not* genetically altered and is administered at 3 ml/kg of body weight twice weekly. The brand used in the original report is Hollywood and is available from health food stores. Supporting data are lacking; in fact, the preponderance of evidence suggests that ω-6 fatty acids enhance tumorigenesis in most situations. It may be advisable to reserve this therapy for patients that are not responding well to chemotherapy and ω-3 fatty acids.

Paradigmatic Options

- The appropriate herbal formula and dietary strategy should be used based on the information given in the initial section in this chapter and in the section on Lymphoma. Damp Heat strategies are more likely to yield results than Blood stasis approaches.

AUTHORS' CHOICES:

SM: Appropriate diet and herbal formula.
SW: Chemotherapy; diet; antioxidants; Fish Oil; Garlic; Turmeric; mixed flavonoids.

OSTEOSARCOMA

Alternative Options with Conventional Bases

- **Retinoic acid:** induced differentiation and cell death in canine osteosarcoma cells in vitro, and when given orally to athymic mice implanted with canine osteosarcoma cells, it reduced pulmonary metastases (Barroga, 2000; Hong, Kadosawa, 2000; Hong, Mochizuki, 2000; Hong, Ohashi, 2000). There are case reports of human osteosarcoma patients who achieved partial and total remission after receiving all-trans retinoic acid, with or without concurrent treatment with interferon. The dose used in one study was 90 mg/m^2 3 days per week (Todesco, 2000). In dogs we have used 5000 IU/lb of body weight by injection every 3 weeks. Oral treatment also may be possible.

- **Vitamin D_3**: induces differentiation of canine osteosarcoma cells in vitro (Barroga, 2000) and reduces growth and metastasis of osteosarcoma in mice (Hara, 2001). The dose I (SM) use for Vitamin D is 750 IU per lb of body weight, given by subcutaneous injection every 3 to 4 weeks.
- Spontaneous remission of osteosarcoma in dogs has been reported, making evaluation of alternative and conventional treatments difficult.

Paradigmatic Options

- The Damp and Toxic Heat protocol may benefit dogs with osteosarcoma for which owners decline surgical amputation. Boneset is typically added to the formula to relieve bone pain. Degrees of response to the protocol vary from complete apparent remission, to improved 1- and 2-year survival rates, to no benefit whatsoever, and the formula may not be effective in suppressing metastases in dogs that have had the affected limb amputated. In dogs that respond well, a crucial element to their success has been the absolute avoidance of trauma until significant tumor shrinkage or reossification has occurred. Trauma to the weakened bone seems to reactivate the tumor, at which point any improvements reverse and the treatment fails. Trauma can be inflicted by any heavy exercise.

AUTHORS' CHOICES:

SM: Damp and Toxic Heat protocol.
SW: Vitamin A; diet; antioxidants; Fish Oil; Garlic; Turmeric; mixed flavonoids.

PARANEOPLASTIC SYNDROMES

Paradigmatic Options

- Anemia is often associated with Blood deficiency. When Blood deficiency arises from Spleen deficiency and leads to signs of cognitive dysfunction or ulcerations on the tip of the tongue, **Gui Pi Wan** (Restore the Spleen Pill) can be considered. When elements of Qi, Blood, and Yang deficiency are present, **Shi Quan Da Bu Wan** (Ten Ingredients for Complete and Great Tonification Pill) should be used. When pale, watery hemorrhage, urinary incontinence, abdominal bloating, poor appetite, watery stool, exhaustion, a pale tongue, and a feeble or weak but gigantic pulse are present, **Bu Zhong Yi Qi Wan** (Tonify the Center and Boost the Qi Pill) can be considered. A *suggested starting dose* of granular concentrate for all formulas is ¼ tsp per 10 to 15 lb of body weight, or 60 to 75 mg/kg of body weight, at least once daily.

- For intermittent fevers, a formula containing **Chai Hu** should be given. The formula should be appropriate for other signs exhibited by the patient. Candidate formulas include **Si Ni San, Xiao Yao San, Chai Hu Shu Gan San,** and **Xiao Chai Hu Tang** (Minor Bupleurum Decoction). A *suggested starting dose* of granular concentrate for all formulas is ¼ tsp per 10 to 15 lb of body weight, or 60 to 75 mg/kg of body weight, at least once daily.
- For acute management of bleeding tendencies, **Yun Nan Bai Yao,** also known as San Qi, can be considered. A list of doses and dose forms for this herb can be found in Chapter 9, as can other formulas for long-term control of hemorrhage.
- For painful Blood stasis, Dan Shen, Yu Jin, or Chuan Xiong can be used either alone or added to an herbal formula matched to the presentation of the patient.

AUTHORS' CHOICES:

SM: Use the appropriate Chinese herbal formula.
SW: Diet; antioxidants; Fish Oil; Garlic; Turmeric; mixed flavonoids.

PERIANAL ADENOCARCINOMA

Paradigmatic Options

Traditional Chinese Medicine

- The appropriate herbal formula and dietary strategy should be used based on the information given in the initial section in this chapter. Perianal tumors are more likely to be manifestations of Dampness and Toxic Heat.

AUTHORS' CHOICES:

SM: Damp Heat protocol; other formulas as indicated.
SW: Diet; antioxidants; Fish Oil; Garlic; Turmeric; mixed flavonoids.

SQUAMOUS CELL CARCINOMA

Paradigmatic Options

Traditional Chinese Medicine

- The appropriate herbal formula and dietary strategy should be used based on the information given in the initial section in this chapter. Squamous cell carcinoma is usually a manifestation of Dampness and Toxic Heat.

AUTHORS' CHOICES:

SM: Appropriate diet and herbal formula.
SW: Diet; piroxicam where appropriate; antioxidants; IP6; Fish Oil; Garlic; Turmeric; mixed flavonoids.

TRANSITIONAL CELL CARCINOMA

Alternative Options with Conventional Bases

- **Garlic:** in a controlled trial using mice that were implanted with bladder carcinoma cells, those receiving Garlic in their water (50 mg/100 ml) had reductions in tumor volume (Riggs, 1997).

- **Astragalus** *(Astragalus membranaceous)*: was shown to protect mice from development of bladder tumors when they had been given a chemical bladder cancer inducer (Kurashige, 1999).

Paradigmatic Options

- **Shao Fu Zhu Yu Tang** is possibly the most important Chinese herbal formula to address bladder tumors. The practitioner can add 20 g of Hua Shi to 100 g of the base formula to "guide" its action to the bladder and soften the bladder mass. Patients that respond best have evidence of Yang deficiency. For patients that exhibit Heat signs, the Damp and Toxic Heat protocol may be used.

AUTHORS' CHOICES:

SM: Shao Fu Zhu Yu Tang with added Hua Shi.
SW: Diet; piroxicam; IP6; Garlic.

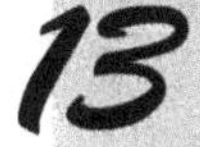

CASE REPORT

Squamous Cell Carcinoma in a German Shepherd

HISTORY

Duke, a 7-year-old, male, neutered German shepherd, was brought with a chief complaint of squamous cell carcinoma of the tongue of approximately 3 months' duration. The tumor began as a small, red nodule on the right edge of the tongue. Within a few months the normal tongue tissue had been replaced by a large, raised, irregularly shaped mass with indistinct borders 3 inches in length. A complete blood count and chemistry panel showed no irregularities. Biopsy of the mass showed it to be a squamous cell carcinoma. Histologic features and tumor behavior led the pathologist to anticipate both locally aggressive behavior and distant metastasis. No treatment could be advised for the squamous cell carcinoma, and a poor prognosis was given. The owner consulted me (SM) to see if any alternative therapies could be offered and shifted Duke to a diet of chicken breast, carrots, broccoli, and cauliflower supplemented by a small amount of canned dog food.

Further questioning revealed that Duke had had hind limb stiffness ever since bilateral cranial cruciate ruptures were repaired within 2 years of each other. The last surgery had been approximately 2 years earlier. Ongoing signs included stiffness on rising and initiating movement that disappeared with continued movement. Weather had no apparent impact on the degree of Duke's stiffness.

Duke also had pemphigus foliaceus that had been diagnosed from biopsies of an extensive crusting nasal lesion that was worse over the nasal alae. Current therapy consisted of 25 mg of prednisone given orally every other day, but the nasal lesions persisted despite this therapy.

Duke also had recurrent skin problems distinct from the pemphigus lesions. These were erythematous lesions with brown crusts, focused in the inguinal and axillary regions. Various ointments and shampoos had been used in the past to palliate these lesions. Duke also had a history of eye and ear discharge without excessive inflammation.

In general, Duke preferred cool conditions. He had a strong appetite but low thirst. He would snap and growl at small dogs but was otherwise somewhat withdrawn.

PHYSICAL EXAMINATION

Physical examination revealed that Duke was drooling copious tenacious saliva and there was a large tumor along the right side of his tongue. The tumor was red, irregularly shaped, and denuded of epithelium, and had a necrotic focus midway along its 3- to 4-inch length. The tumor was accompanied by marked halitosis. No lymphadenopathy was present.

Duke's pulses were broad and wiry. He had large yellow flakes of dander disseminated throughout his coat and adherent to the skin. He appeared to be in pain when his knees were touched. He also had vertebral fixations throughout his lumbar spine, was overweight, and was panting and restless. His agitation precluded any attempt at chiropractic treatment.

ASSESSMENT

From a conventional medical perspective, the diagnoses of pemphigus foliaceus and squamous cell carcinoma were well substantiated. In Chinese medicine, lesions along the edge of the tongue correspond to problems with the Liver. Involvement of the Liver was also suggested by Duke's irritability, the weakness of his ligaments, and the distribution of lesions in areas associated with the Liver channel, such as the inguinal region.

The Liver is prone to accumulating Damp Heat, which was signified in Duke's case by the abundant Heat signs (heat intolerance, red lesions, panting, restlessness, and agitation) and Dampness symptoms (elevated appetite with depressed thirst, yellow flakes of dander, tenacious, ropy saliva, halitosis, and wiry pulses). In cancer, Damp Heat is considered to have congealed into a type of Toxic Heat that results in severely destructive lesions such as squamous cell carcinoma of the tongue.

TREATMENT

The two separate conditions that affected Duke, pemphigus foliaceus and squamous cell carcinoma, are often amenable to the same treatment, namely the Hoxsey-like formula discussed previously. This formula was prescribed at a dose of 3 ml twice daily, and the formula was augmented by adding 10 ml of Yellow Dock and 15 ml of Agrimony to 75 ml of base formula to address mucosal ulceration. Whole herb alcohol extracts of all herbs were used. The Hoxsey-like formula was anticipated to assist in cell differentiation through its content of genistein or other constituents, and to help resolve the pemphigus lesions by enhancing liver function (Chapter 9 gives further information on the treatment of pemphigus foliaceus).

Duke was given an injection of 750,000 IU of Vitamin A coupled with 112,500 IU of Vitamin D to promote cell differentiation. These injections were repeated monthly throughout his treatment. Duke's diet was modified with additions of liver and leafy greens so that it contained higher amounts of Vitamin A.

Duke was prescribed an EFA supplement (3-V Caps; DVM Pharmaceuticals Inc.). This supplement contains EPA, DHA, and Vitamins A, D, and E. Of particular interest was DHA, which acts synergistically to enhance Vitamin A–mediated differentiation of tumor cells. Duke was prescribed enough 3-V Caps to provide 167 mg of DHA three times daily.

OUTCOME

Duke received his first follow-up examination 9 days after he was first seen. Some mild signs of improvement were seen, in that drooling was reduced and the necrotic center of the tongue appeared to have resolved. The Hoxsey-like formula dosage was increased to four times daily to speed improvements, and the prednisone dosage was reduced to 12.5 mg every other day to reduce any associated immune depression that might interfere with tumor resolution.

Three weeks later, improvements in Duke's condition were more obvious and included an absence of salivation and obvious healing of the tongue. The tongue was much less red and swollen along its right side. There was still an irregular, roughened surface at the tumor site, but it was considerably paler. Duke was also becoming more playful, and his appetite was more normal or even a little depressed. These improvements were slightly offset by an increase in dandruff, eye discharge, conjunctival reddening, and pruritus. Prednisone therapy had been discontinued, however, which suggested that these signs had been present before, but masked by steroid use. The pemphigus lesions had resolved. Treatment was continued, and homeopathic Sulfur (30C given once daily for 1 week) was prescribed to address the dermatitis.

One month later, Duke's tongue was healing over a defect formerly occupied by the tumor. Epithelium extended from the upper surface of the tongue over the irregular tongue edge. The nose remained healed, but the Sulfur had had no appreciable impact on Duke's general skin complaints. Given Duke's improvements, the dose of the Hoxsey-like formula was reduced to twice daily from four times daily. A 50:50 combination of whole herb alcohol extracts of Goldenseal and Alfalfa was administered both to moisten the skin and to help reduce his mild superficial pyoderma. Duke's treatment was otherwise unchanged.

Over the next 3 months, Duke remained stable with continuing mild pyoderma. Various other formulas had been tried after the failure of the Alfalfa-Goldenseal combination, including Long Dan Xie Gan Tang and Si Miao San, but none of these had produced lasting benefit to his skin condition. In contrast, his tongue now appeared grossly normal except for the defect left behind as the tumor disappeared. The pemphigus lesions had now recently reappeared on the nasal alae, however, despite continued use of the Hoxsey-like formula. The Hoxsey-like tincture was also modified with Agrimony being replaced by 15 ml of Sarsaparilla *(Smilax officinalis)*, an herb popular in the 19th century for "humid" flaking skin lesions such as psoriasis in humans. No other changes were made in Duke's treatment.

At the last check, approximately 2 months later, and 7 months after his initial presentation, all of Duke's problems were lessened. The pemphigus was once again in remission as was, apparently, the tumor. The skin lesions were also now largely resolved, although subsequent outbreaks also proved highly responsive to various antibiotic protocols. Duke's therapy with the essential fatty acid supplement, the new version of the Hoxsey-like tincture, monthly injections of Vitamins A and D, and his homemade diet continued.

COMMENTS

Duke's case illustrates the general usefulness of the Hoxsey-like formula in some of veterinary medicine's most serious small animal disorders. This case also underscores the synergistic approach to neoplasia discussed in this chapter. Multiple modalities that alone may prove only partially effective may be combined to much greater advantage if they share a common general goal. Cell differentiation was thus promoted here by the Hoxsey-like formula's content of berberine, genistein, and possibly other constituents, as well as the use of supplemental Vitamin A, a diet high in Vitamin A, and Vitamin A synergists such as DHA. Even the Hoxsey-like formula's lipotropic effect of enhancing liver metabolism may be of benefit to the treatment of cancer, for example, by increasing the liver's reductive capacity so that oxidative damage to DNA might be minimized.

Treatment of cancer with alternative therapies produces a spectrum of results. For a significant number of patients, natural therapies are palliative or even ineffective. A significant population of cancer patients seem to be capable of enduring remission when tumors, which otherwise typically recur, are debulked or excised. When tumors cannot be excised, they may still become static and exhibit an absence of growth or metastasis, which results in survival rates that seem to compete with or even exceed those expected with conventional management. Duke's case represents the best of what alternative approaches to cancer can accomplish, with a large aggressive tumor that apparently entered remission. Whether the remission will endure is not yet known at the time of writing, but the exceptional results of this case and others like it occur frequently enough to suggest that alternative therapies should receive much more attention in cancer research.

SM

REFERENCES

Alenza DP, Rutteman GR, Pena L, Beynen AC, Cuesta P. Relation between habitual diet and canine mammary tumors in a case-control study. *J Vet Intern Med* 12(3):132-139, 1998.

Austin S, Dale EB, DeKadt S. Long term follow-up of cancer patients using Contreras, Hoxsey and Gerson therapies. *J Naturopathic Medicine* 5:74-76, 1994.

Barroga EF, Kadosawa T, Okumura M, Fujinaga T. Influence of vitamin D and retinoids on the induction of functional differentiation in vitro of canine osteosarcoma clonal cells. *Vet J* 159(2):186-193, 2000.

Barroga EF, Kadosawa T, Okumura M, Fujinaga T. Inhibitory effects of 22-oxa-calcitriol and all-trans retinoic acid on the growth of a canine osteosarcoma derived cell-line in vivo and its pulmonary metastasis in vivo. *Res Vet Sci* 68(1):79-87, 2000.

Bensky D, Gamble A. *Chinese Herbal Medicine Materia Medica,* revised ed. Seattle, 1993, Eastland Press.

Boik, John. *Natural Compounds in Cancer Therapy.* Princeton, Minn, 2001, Oregon Medical Press.

Cos S, Garcia-Bolado A, Sanchez-Barcelo EJ. Direct antiproliferative effects of melatonin on two metastatic cell sublines of mouse melanoma (B16BL6 and PG19). *Melanoma Res* 11(2):197-201, 2001.

Devery R, Miller A, Stanton C. Conjugated linoleic acid and oxidative behavior in cancer cells. *Biochem Soc Trans* 29(Pt 2):341-344, 2001.

Ehling D. *The Chinese Herbalist's Handbook,* revised ed. Santa Fe, NM, 1996, Inword Press.

Fruehauf H. *The Treatment of Difficult and Recalcitrant Diseases with Chinese Herbs: A Collection of Case Studies.* Portland, Ore, 1995, ITM.

Gonzalez R, Sanchez A, Ferguson JA, Balmer C, Daniel C, Cohn A, Robinson WA. Melatonin therapy of advanced human malignant melanoma. *Melanoma Res* 1(4):237-243, 1991.

Hara K, Kusuzaki K, Takeshita H, Kuzuhara A, Tsuji Y, Ashihara T, Hirasawa Y. Oral administration of 1 alpha hydroxyvitamin D_3 inhibits tumor growth and metastasis of a murine osteosarcoma model. *Anticancer Res* 21(1A):321-324, 2001.

Hong SH, Kadosawa T, Mochizuki M, Matsunaga S, Nishimura R, Sasaki N. Effect of all-trans and 9-cis retinoic acid on growth and metastasis of xeno-transplanted canine osteosarcoma cells in athymic mice. *Am J Vet Res* 61(10):1241-1244, 2000.

Hong SH, Mochizuki M, Nishimura R, Sasaki N, Kadosawa T, Matsunaga S. Differentiation induction of canine osteosarcoma cell lines by retinoids. *Res Vet Sci* 68(1):57-62, 2000.

Hong SH, Ohashi E, Kadosawa T, Mochizuki M, Matsunaga S, Nishimura R, Sasaki N. Retinoid receptors and the induction of apoptosis in canine osteosarcoma cells. *J Vet Med Sci* 62(4):469-472, 2000.

Hubbard NE, Lim D, Summers L, Erickson KL. Reduction of murine mammary tumor metastasis by conjugated linoleic acid. *Cancer Lett* 150(1):93-100, 2000.

Invernizzi R, Bernuzzi S, Ciani D, Ascari E. Silymarine during maintenance treatment of acute promyelocytic leukemia. *Hematologia* 78:340-341, 1993.

Jiang MC, Yang-Yen HF, Yen JJ, Lin JK. Curcumin induces apoptosis in immortalized NIH 3T3 and malignant cancer cell lines. *Nutr Cancer* 26(1):111-120, 1996.

Kaegi E. Unconventional therapies for cancer. 4. Hydrazine sulfate. *Can Med Assoc J* 158:1327-1330, 1998.

Kaegi E. Unconventional therapies for cancer. 6. 714-X. *Can Med Assoc J* 158:1621-1624, 1998.

Kato M, Liu W, Yi H, Asai N, Hayakawa A, Kozaki K, Takahashi M, Nakashima I. The herbal medicine Sho-saiko-to inhibits growth and metastasis of malignant melanoma primarily developed in ret-transgenic mice. *J Invest Dermatol* 111(4):640-644, 1998.

Kurashige S, Akuzawa Y, Endo F. Effects of astragali radix extract on carcinogenesis, cytokine production, and cytotoxicity in mice treated with a carcinogen, *N*-butyl-*N'*-butanolnitrosoamine. *Cancer Invest* 17(1):30-35, 1999.

Lin LI, Ke YF, Ko YC, Lin JK. Curcumin inhibits SK-Hep-1 hepatocellular carcinoma cell invasion in vitro and suppresses matrix metalloproteinase-9 secretion. *Oncology* 55(4):349-353, 1998.

Lin HL, Liu TY, Lui WY, Chi CW. Up-regulation of multidrug resistance transporter expression by berberine in human and murine hepatoma cells. *Cancer* 85(9):1937-1942, 1999.

Motoo Y, Sawabu N. Antitumor effects of saikosaponins, baicalin and baicalein on human hepatoma cell lines. *Cancer Lett* 86(1):91-95, 1994.

Muraishi Y, Mitani N, Yamaura T, Fuse H, Saiki I. Effect of interferon-alpha A/D in combination with the Japanese and Chinese traditional herbal medicine juzen-taiho-to on lung metastasis of murine renal cell carcinoma. *Anticancer Res* 20(5A):2931-2937, 2000.

Naiman I. *Cancer Salves: A Botanical Approach to Treatment.* Poulsbo, Wash, 2000, Seventh Ray Press.

Nakamura K, Yamaguchi Y, Kagota S, Kwon YM, Shinozuka K, Kunitomo M. Inhibitory effect of *Cordyceps sinensis* on spontaneous liver metastasis of Lewis lung carcinoma and B16 melanoma cells in syngeneic mice. *Jpn J Pharmacol* 79(3):335-341, 1999.

Ogilvie GK. Interventional nutrition for the cancer patient. *Clin Tech Small Anim Pract* 13(4):224-231, 1998.

Ogilvie GK, Fettman MJ, Mallinckrodt CH, Walton JA, Hansen RA, Davenport DJ, Gross KL, Richardson KL, Rogers Q, Hand MS. Effect of Fish Oil, arginine, and doxorubicin chemotherapy on remission and survival time for dogs with lymphoma: a double-blind, randomized placebo-controlled study. *Cancer* 88(8):1916-1928, 2000.

O'Shea M, Devery R, Lawless F, Murphy J, Stanton C. Milk fat conjugated linoleic acid (CLA) inhibits growth of human mammary MCF-7 cancer cells. *Anticancer Res* 20(5B):3591-3601, 2000.

Riggs DR, DeHaven JI, Lamm DL. *Allium sativum* (garlic) treatment for murine transitional cell carcinoma. *Cancer* 79(10):1987-1994, 1997.

Plouzek CA, Ciolino HP, Clarke R, Yeh GC. Inhibition of P-glycoprotein activity and reversal of multidrug resistance in vitro by rosemary extract. *Eur J Cancer* 35(10):1541-1545, 1999.

Scambia G, De Vincenzo R, Ranelletti FO, Panici PB, Ferrandina G, D'Agostino G, Fattorossi A, Bombardelli E, Mancuso S. Antiproliferative effect of silybin on gynaecological malignancies: Synergism with cisplatin and doxyrubicin. *Eur J Cancer* 32A:877-882, 1996.

Shamsuddin AM. Metabolism and cellular functions of IP6: a review. *Anticancer Res* 19(5A):3733-3736S, 1999.

Shimizu I. Sho-saiko-to: Japanese herbal medicine for protection against hepatic fibrosis and carcinoma. *J Gastroenterol Hepatol* (15 suppl): D84-D90, 2000.

Singletary K, MacDonald C, Wallig M. Inhibition by rosemary and carnosol of 7,12-dimethylbenz[a]anthracene (DMBA)-induced rat mammary tumorigenesis and in vivo DMBA-DNA adduct formation. *Cancer Lett* 104(1):43-48, 1996.

Suzuki F, Kobayashi M, Komatsu Y, Kato A, Pollard RB. Keishi-ka-kei-to, a traditional Chinese herbal medicine, inhibits pulmonary metastasis of B16 melanoma. *Anticancer Res* 17(2A):873-878, 1997.

Tatsuta M, Iishi H, Baba M, Narahara H, Yano H, Sakai N. Suppression by Chai-hu-gui-zhi-tang of the development of liver lesions induced by *N*-nitrosomorpholine in Sprague-Dawley rats. *Cancer Lett* 152(1):31-36, 2000.

Todesco A, Carli M, Iacona I, Frascella E, Ninfo V, Rosolen A. All-trans retinoic acid and interferon-alpha in the treatment of a patient with resistant metastatic osteosarcoma. *Cancer* 89(12):2661-2666, 2000.

Utsuyama M, Seidlar H, Kitagawa M, Hirokawa K. Immunological restoration and anti-tumor effect by Japanese herbal medicine in aged mice. *Mech Ageing Dev* 122(3):341-352, 2001.

Yeung H. *Handbook of Chinese Herbal Formulas.* Los Angeles, 1995, Self-published.

Yeung H. *Handbook of Chinese Herbs.* Los Angeles, 1996, Self-published.

14

Therapies for Neurologic Disorders

CERVICAL SPONDYLOMYELOPATHY (WOBBLER SYNDROME)

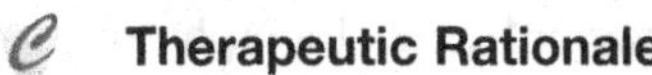

Therapeutic Rationale

- Identify specific pathologic causes, which may include vertebral canal stenosis, vertebral instability, disk protrusion, compression from synovial cysts, or hypertrophy of the ligamentum flavum.
- Reduce risk of trauma.
- Stabilize.
- Reduce pain.

Alternative Options with Conventional Bases

- **Diet:** cervical vertebral malformation may have a developmental component similar to hip dysplasia. Some practitioners have successfully used caloric restriction in "at risk" dogs (diagnosed early).
- **Robert Jones–type cervical collar:** can be made with towels and a wide Velcro strip (Durkes, personal communication). This collar has been used very successfully in my (SW) practice when owners were unwilling or unable to go forward with diagnostics or corrective surgery. The collar can be used for 2 to 8 weeks at a time as needed.
- **Methylsulfonylmethane** (MSM): has been used as an antiinflammatory for various painful musculoskeletal disorders and appears to be safe for long-term use. One *suggested dose* is 20 mg/lb of body weight daily.
- **Glycosaminoglycans:** abnormal compressive forces in spinal disease have been shown to change proteoglycan content of intervertebral disks in dogs (Hutton, 1998).

Supplementation with glycosaminoglycans for intervertebral disk disease has not been examined but may be administered to dogs with unstable spinal segments when supporting disk integrity and vertebral endplate structure may improve function and decrease pain.

Paradigmatic Options

Chiropractic

- Wobbler syndrome encompasses a variety of potential underlying disorders. In some cases the compression is independent of the position of the neck, whereas in others it varies with neck position. Detailed imaging studies using plain film radiographs, myelography, and MRI can differentiate the cause of Wobbler syndrome and the degree of its persistence. These studies are highly advisable when the practitioner has access to referral for them. Compression from disk protrusion and vertebral instability should be ruled out before hand manipulation methods of chiropractic adjustment are used (Halderman, 1991). Cases for which surgery promises complete rapid resolution, or in which neurologic deficits are worsening, should be approached surgically. When any doubt regarding the usefulness of surgery exists and when risks of chiropractic treatment have been completely evaluated, conservative management using chiropractic may be attempted to see if an acceptable degree of clinical improvement can be attained. Such improvement is often seen after the first adjustment. Careful application of low-force adjustment techniques using spring-loaded devices may lessen but not eliminate the risk of complications in patients with Wobbler syndrome treated with chiropractic.
- That chiropractic can cause deterioration in Wobbler syndrome is well known, which prompts well-intentioned practitioners to counsel complete avoidance of these techniques. However, prudent chiropractic treatment by qualified veterinary chiropractors using low-force techniques can be of significant benefit in some cases of Wobbler syndrome.

- The reason that chiropractors can greatly relieve the ataxia of a "wobbler," on occasion within minutes, is that they appear to be able to quickly relieve shear stresses on unstable joints. Patients that benefit the most from chiropractic often have multiple vertebral fixations throughout the spine, even in areas not immediately adjacent to the site of cord compression. These fixations result in large blocks of several vertebrae becoming functionally immobile so that they can only move as a single unit. Excursions of movement at facet joints between two adjacent blocks of vertebrae then become abnormally large to compensate for the loss of movement at the facets within the "fused" block. Wobbler syndrome can conceivably result from spinal cord impingement by such hypermobile vertebrae. Fusions between vertebrae that promote this hypermobility are often not osseous, even in cases in which advanced spondylosis deformans has been identified. Responsiveness to chiropractic adjustment suggests that the fusions are more functional and are possibly maintained by muscle spasms and microcalcification of ligaments.
- The release of fixations and the restoration of palpable mobility within the fused blocks seem to immediately relieve the hypermobile tendencies of joints that have had to provide the otherwise rigid spine with some flexibility. These improvements are seen even when the hypermobile joint that is producing the signs of Wobbler syndrome is not manipulated or adjusted. Such improvement may be manifested clinically as a reduction of ataxia within the first 24 to 48 hours, if not sooner.
- After the initial treatment repeated chiropractic examinations are necessary for a few weeks to ensure that motion of the individual vertebrae is being maintained. Treatment of any underlying factors predisposing to vertebral fixation will replace the need for ongoing chiropractic treatment, and acupuncture and herbal medicine can play a significant role in such treatment. In addition, supplements to enhance the health and suppleness of cartilage and connective tissue are often prescribed.

- A final cautionary note should be made regarding the use of chiropractic in Wobbler syndrome by inexperienced practitioners. As mentioned previously, skilled practitioners avoid manipulating hypermobile joints. An unskilled practitioner may, however, inadvertently manipulate an unstable joint and exacerbate the problem. Only prudent chiropractic treatment by an experienced practitioner should be applied to animals with cervical instability.

Acupuncture

- Acupuncture treatment of meridians coursing through the cervical and paraspinal regions may reduce the recurrence of generalized vertebral fixations. Generally useful points that are thought to have a powerful influence over these regions include BL 40, BL 60, BL 58, TH 5, GB 41, SI 3, GB 39, LI 4, LU 7, BL 25, GB 20, and GB 21. In addition, the acupuncturist should evaluate the patient from a traditional Chinese medical perspective, using pulse and tongue diagnosis and a thorough review of the history. The goal of such an evaluation is to identify and differentiate any underlying deficiencies, excesses, and Zang-Fu patterns that may be contributing to Dampness accumulation, Qi stagnation, Blood stasis, and inflexibility.

Chinese Herbs

- For all of the following formulas, a *recommended starting dose* of granular concentrate is ¼ tsp per 10 to 15 lb of body weight, or 60 to 75 mg/kg of body weight, divided into two daily doses.
- When Blood deficiency leads to an increased tendency to Qi stagnation and muscle spasm, **Xue Fu Zhu Yu Tang** (Eliminate Stasis in the Mansion of Blood Decoction) can be very useful.
- **Qiang Huo Sheng Shi Tang** (Decoction of Notopterygium to Dispel Dampness) may also be used, with or without the modifications suggested in the section on meningitis later in the chapter. This formula is used for patients that have pronounced rigidity and

pain of the back of the neck, a normal or pale tongue, and a taut and floating pulse.

- **Du Huo Ji Sheng Tang** (Decoction of Pubescent Angelica and Loranthus) can be considered for older, chilly animals with multiple deficiencies and for patients with a suggestion of lingering hind limb weakness and low back stiffness even when the ataxia has otherwise improved. To 100 g of base formula is added 12 g Qiang Huo (Notopterygium) to better address neck stiffness and pain and 9 g Chuan Wu Tou (Aconite) to relieve generalized pain. Prolonged use of Aconite is potentially toxic.
- **Xiao Huo Luo Dan** (Minor Activate the Collateral Pills) and **Da Huo Luo Dan** (Major Activate the Circulation Pills) have been advocated in the treatment of Wobbler syndrome. These pills contain Chuan Wu Tou (Aconite) and are therefore also potentially toxic long term.
- Some older chilly dogs seem to respond well to a more nonspecific Kidney-tonifying formula than Du Huo Ji Sheng Tang, such as **Shen Qi Wan** (Kidney Qi Pills). This formula is available from some herb distributors as **Rehmannia 8**, or **Ba Wei Di Huang Wan.** When ordering Ba Wei Di Huang Wan to administer to a patient with Wobbler syndrome, practitioners should ensure that they are ordering the version that contains Ginger and Aconite (a nontoxic form), rather than the version that contains Astragalus and Schisandra.
- Many other formulas have been developed in Chinese medicine to treat pain, stiffness, and impeded circulation. Although the formulas mentioned have been highly effective for Wobbler syndrome, the practitioner may identify others that are more appropriate to a particular case. The practitioner is always encouraged to make a precise diagnosis from a Chinese medical perspective and to choose a formula appropriate to that diagnosis and the clinical presentation of the patient.

AUTHORS' CHOICES:

SM: Chiropractic; acupuncture; herbs to address underlying disorders.
SW: Cervical collar; acupuncture.

DEGENERATIVE MYELOPATHY

Therapeutic Rationale

- Since the cause of degenerative myelopathy (DM) is unknown, different therapeutic regimens have been suggested based on the possibility of autoimmune disorder, vitamin E deficiency, vitamin B deficiency, or simple degenerative disorder.
- Maintain neurologic integrity and muscular function through acupuncture.

Alternative Options with Conventional Bases

- Most of the information in this section is derived from the experience and recommendations of Roger Clemmons DVM, PhD (University of Florida) who advocates the theory that DM is a canine version of multiple sclerosis (MS).

Antioxidants

- **Antioxidants:** reduce fat peroxidation and may modulate inflammatory cytokines; therefore antioxidants are used as antiinflammatories.
- **Vitamin E:** is fat soluble and is considered especially important in the treatment of DM. It may be administered at 400 to 2000 IU daily. Antioxidant vitamins and minerals may be most effective when administered in combination, and Vitamin C, Selenium, and Beta-carotene may also have beneficial effects on oxidative damage of the nervous system.
- **N-Acetylcysteine** (NAC): has been shown to inhibit apoptosis associated with neurodegenerative conditions (Deigner, 2000). A *suggested dose* for NAC is 25 mg/kg of body weight three times a day for 2 weeks, then tid every other day.
- **Vitamin D:** may be deficient in patients with MS (Hayes, 2000), and Vitamin D supplementation has been suggested. Vitamin D is potentially toxic in high doses given long term. One *suggested dose* is 750 IU per lb of body weight monthly by subcutaneous injection.

- **B vitamins:** folate and B_{12} deficiencies have been found in some patients with MS and deficiency can cause demyelination disorders (Bottiglieri, 1996). Clemmons suggests a B complex that provides 50 to 100 mg of most of the B vitamins daily for a German shepherd or dogs of similar weight.

Antiinflammatories

- **Bromelain:** Clemmons has found circulating immune complexes in the serum of dogs that have DM and believes that they contribute to the disease. Bromelain has antiinflammatory properties and may degrade immune complexes. When Bromelain is given in high doses, some is absorbed intact (Castell, 1997) and it may be a useful adjunct treatment.

Immunotherapy

- Based on the theory that immunotherapy with organ- or disease-specific proteins can be used to induce immune tolerance in immune-mediated disease, some recent work showed that administering specific nervous system protein epitopes may reduce pathologic conditions in a model of multiple sclerosis (McFarland, 2001). Some dog owners have purchased bovine or ovine brain as a dietary supplement for their pets that have DM. Alternatively, companies that manufacture glandulars may be able to supply "spinal cord" glandular products. The risk of spongiform encephalopathy transferred to dogs from animals used for these supplements is unknown.

Paradigmatic Options

Chinese Medicine

- Degenerative myelopathy and hind limb proprioceptive deficits in dogs, like feline hyperesthesia syndrome, may be best understood from the Chinese medical perspective as an example of an excessive external pathogen clogging an Extraordinary Vessel. True DM and idiopathic hind limb proprioceptive deficit disorders are discussed here together because their clinical presentation is similar and, in most cases, a final differentiation between the two via histopathologic examination of the myelin sheath is not made.

- Many veterinary acupuncturists assume the affected channel in both these disorders is the Du Mai because DM affects the central nervous system, which the path of the Du Mai closely approximates. Other acupuncturists target the Bladder channel and its adjacent Hua Tuo Jia Ji, lured by the intimate association between the path of the Bladder channel and the sciatic nerve.
- Although these approaches are popular, the results of their application in treating DM and hind end proprioceptive deficits are typically poor. The reason for the poor outcomes is at least in part that veterinary acupuncturists are at times too easily swayed by their knowledge of neuroanatomy in the selection of acupuncture points. The end result is a point prescription that seems sensible from a neurologic perspective but is contrary to Chinese medical theory. For example, the typical clinical presentation of a Du Mai disorder more closely resembles feline hyperesthesia, in which too much energy is ascending to the head, than it does DM, in which energy fails to descend to the feet. Similarly, although the Bladder channel is important in the acupuncture treatment of DM, it is not considered in Chinese medicine to be the main channel that confers mobility to the hind limbs.
- A syndrome that fits the presentation of DM very well is obstruction of the Extraordinary Vessel known as the Dai Mai. Like the other Extraordinary Vessels, the Dai Mai has its own unique set of symptoms that arise when it becomes clogged by pathogenic excess and these symptoms represent an extreme form of the Vessel's normal function. The excess accumulation affecting the Dai Mai in DM appears to be Phlegm.
- The Dai Mai runs around the body like a girdle, which accounts for its translation as the Girdling Vessel or the Belt Vessel. It thus traverses all the other meridians that connect the upper and lower body. Its function is to gather in the waist to the spine, thus giving support to the entire upper body. When it is filled with pathogenic excess, the Dai Mai cinches the Yang channels that cross

beneath it too tightly, which results in a broad-scale failure of Yang Qi to descend to the legs.

- Ancient descriptions of symptoms of obstruction of the Dai Mai closely parallel what we witness in dogs with DM, namely, the appearance of lower limb paralysis. In addition, the Dai Mai is treated through needling of the Gall Bladder channel, which is the channel considered by Chinese medicine as most important in conferring the ability to move the legs.
- The net result of having all the Yang energy in the upper body is profound weakness or paralysis of the lower limbs and signs of Heat and agitation in the upper body. Veterinarians commonly attempt to treat the problem by strengthening Kidney Yang, but usually to no avail. The real problem may be a trapping of Yang energy above Yin, with consistent benefits of acupuncture therapy seen only when the Dai Mai is "opened" and the Yang channels are released to resume their normal pattern of flow downward into the leg.
- One other pathway may cause DM and hind end proprioceptive deficits. This mechanism is almost the opposite of the mechanism just discussed; instead of being "hot above and cold below," the patient is "hot below." This is known as Damp Heat accumulation in the lower jiao and is one manifestation of Wei Syndrome, an atonic and paralytic condition of the hind limbs that has been proposed as a means of interpreting and treating DM. Less advanced cases of Damp Heat accumulation in the lower burner are common problems in dogs and cats and result in tendencies to colitis, vulvar inflammation, and cystitis. In severe cases, Damp Heat accumulation can cause the weakening and withering of the lower limbs and pain in the lower back. The disorder can still be treated by opening the Dai Mai, however, so that circulation is improved between the upper and lower halves of the body. Additional acupuncture points are used to drain Damp Heat from the lower jiao.
- Differentiation of the two presentations of DM can be difficult. In general, though, obstruction of the Dai Mai by pathologic excesses of Phlegm so that Yang Qi is unable to descend is attended by a lavender, coated

tongue and slippery pulses. Entrapment of Damp Heat in the lower jiao is attended by a red, moist tongue and slippery, wiry pulses.

Acupuncture

- In treating both types of disorders, the most important goal is to open the Dai Mai to promote the normal descent of Yang Qi down the Stomach, Gall Bladder, and Bladder channels into the leg. Points used to open the Dai Mai are GB 41 and TH 5. In addition, a painful point can usually be found on affected animals ventromedial to the ileum. This point is analogous to GB 26 in humans and should be needled.
- Additional points that trace the approximate path of the Dai Mai can be selected to treat other aspects of the case, such as the tendency for deficient Yang in the lower body and the tendency toward the accumulation of Dampness and Phlegm in the channels. BL 22, 40, and 28 help drain obstructing Dampness and Phlegm and also allow stimulation of the Bladder channel, the second most important channel carrying Yang Qi to the lower leg. Needling CV 12 helps reduce the formation of Dampness and Phlegm by the middle burner, and GB 25 tonifies the Kidney Yang.
- BL 25, 26, or 27 may be of benefit because of their strong influence on the sciatic nerve root, as well as the flow of Qi down the Bladder channel.
- Administration of electroacupuncture seems to enhance treatment efficacy, since increased limb tone and muscle strength often become evident immediately following the acupuncture treatment. Current is passed from BL 22 or 25 to BL 40, using intensities just below those required to produce muscular contraction. Dispersing current may also be focused on distal active points such as GB 41, BL 60, and BL 40.
- Reasonable expectations are for further deterioration to halt in over half of affected patients, although weekly treatment is often necessary to maintain this level of improvement. Dogs that respond usually also regain limb strength and some measure of conscious proprioception. Possibly one third of treated dogs fail to

respond. Clinical experience with this protocol suggests that respondents typically remain stable or continue to slowly improve over extended periods despite the frequent tendency of this disorder to wax and wane.

Chinese Herbs

- Chinese herbal treatment seems to augment the successes seen with acupuncture treatment of DM and hind limb proprioceptive deficits. For dogs that are "hot above and cold below," **Xiao Huo Luo Dan** (Minor Invigorate the Collaterals Pill) can be used. For dogs that have Damp Heat accumulation in the lower burner, **Si Miao San** (Four Miracles Powder) can be considered. Si Miao San can be adapted as a treatment for Wei Syndrome (Wu, 1997), but it appears effective for dogs with DM in its original form as well. Some older animals that appear truly Kidney Qi deficient do well on **Du Huo Ji Sheng Tang** (Pubescent Angelica and Loranthus Decoction). A *recommended starting dose* of granular concentrate for all these formulas is ¼ tsp per 10 to 15 lb of body weight, or 60 to 75 mg/kg of body weight, divided into two daily doses.
- Another formula that has been advocated for treatment of DM is **Tan Hua Fang,** which is available from Jing Tang Herbal. The formula is potentially toxic because of its content of Aconite and *Nux vomica. Nux vomica* is a natural source of strychnine, which stimulates the spinal cord. It is indicated for paralysis and paresis caused by stagnation that is manifested as a purple tongue, rapid pulse, and sensitivity on palpation of the spine. The ingredients of the patent formula include Dang Gui, Chuan Xiong, Chi Shao Yao, Hong Hua, Mo Yao, Xue Jie, and Ru Xiang to move Blood; various insects including Quan Xie or Tu Bie Chong and Wu Gong to "tunnel through obstructions"; Du Zhong, Xu Duan, Gu Sui Bu, Ba Ji Tian, Gou Ji, Niu Xi, and Bu Gu Zhi to strengthen the lower back and limbs and tonify Kidney Qi and Yang; Fu Zi and Wu Yao to warm Kidney Yang; Huang Qi to tonify Qi; Ma Qian Zi *(Nux vomica)* to break up obstructions to circulation; and

Tian San Qi and Gan Cao to harmonize the action of the ingredients and reduce toxic potential. This herbal formula should be given strictly as recommended by the manufacturer, for no longer than 2 weeks.

AUTHORS' CHOICES:

SM: Electroacupuncture; Chinese herbs.
SW: Acupuncture; Chinese herbs; antioxidants and enzymes.

EPILEPSY

See the general section on Seizures later in the chapter.

FACIAL PARALYSIS

Therapeutic Rationale

- Identify treatable causes, which include otitis media or interna, hypothyroidism, neoplasia, encephalitis, polyneuropathy, and facial neuritis.

Paradigmatic Options

- Facial paralysis has many causes, but paradigmatic treatments are largely chosen symptomatically based on clinical presentation.

Homeopathy

- **Causticum 30C** sid prn: used especially for right-sided facial paralysis accompanied by general tendencies to hind limb weakness, separation anxiety at night, and urinary incontinence. The remedy may also be used for left-sided facial paralysis when signs otherwise agree, but cases of right-sided paralysis seem to benefit more in my (SM) experience.

Chinese Medicine

- When unilateral occurrence of facial paralysis appears to follow exposure to a cold wind, it is said to arise from an

invasion of Wind-Cold. As a peripheral neurologic disorder, it may be especially amenable to acupuncture.
- Local points to consider: SI 18, ST 6, ST 8, TH 17.
- Regional points to consider: GB 20.
- Distant points to consider: LI 4, LU 7, TH 5, any of ST 41 through 44, SI 3.

- **Qian Zheng San** (Restore the Normal Position Powder) has been advocated for facial paralysis caused by invasions of Wind and Wind-Phlegm, but it is potentially toxic. Addition of 9 g Jing Jie (Schizonepeta), 12 g Fang Feng (Ledebouriella), and 6 g Bai Zhi (Angelica) to 30 g of base formula may dilute its toxicity and increase the formula's Wind-dispersing properties. A *recommended starting dose* of granular concentrate is ¼ tsp per 10 to 15 lb of body weight, or 60 to 75 mg/kg of body weight, divided into two daily doses.

AUTHORS' CHOICES:

SM: Acupuncture; Causticum when symptoms agree.
SW: Acupuncture if idiopathic.

FELINE HYPERESTHESIA SYNDROME

Therapeutic Rationale
- Control seizures.
- Reduce skin irritation and panniculitis.
- Rule out other musculoskeletal and central nervous system (CNS) disorders and abscessation of the tail head.

Alternative Options with Conventional Bases
Nutrition
- **Rule out food allergies** as a cause of dermatitis.
- **Antioxidants:** some practitioners have claimed that antioxidants are useful and may ameliorate unidentified steatitis or other inflammatory disorder.
- **Carnitine:** Shelton has suggested that some of these cats have a vacuolar myopathy and that Carnitine, in

addition to coenzyme Q_{10}, Riboflavin, and Vitamin E, may be worth trying (March, 1999).

Herbs

- **St. John's Wort** *(Hypericum perfoliatum;* SJW): selective serotonin reuptake inhibitors (SSRIs) such as fluoxetine have been recommended for feline hyperesthesia, based on the theory that this condition represents dopaminergic hyperinnervation. SJW has SSRI properties. An interesting note is that SJW traditionally was used in herbal and homeopathic form for peripheral nerve irritation, which makes this herb intriguing as a potential treatment for hyperesthesia syndrome.

Paradigmatic Options

Homeopathy

- **Arsenicum album 30C** sid prn: patients that benefit are fearful, anxious, and ravenous, have a past medical history of colitis, crave their owner's attention, and are cold, thirsty, and intensely pruritic in areas where lesions cannot be identified.
- **Zincum metallicum 30C** sid prn: should be considered in cases arising promptly following conventional medical treatment of dermatologic disorders.

Chinese Medicine

- In Chinese medicine, not all neurologic problems are internal medical disorders. Whereas idiopathic epilepsy and vestibular syndromes are caused by energy rebelling upward inside the body, the convulsions of feline hyperesthesia seem to be caused by energy rising up on the outside of the body and are elicited when particular areas, usually on the dorsum, of the body are touched.
- The pathway of rising energy in feline hyperesthesia syndrome is up the Bladder, Du Mai, and Yang Qiao Mai channels. The latter two are Extraordinary Vessels, and a commonly forgotten function of the Extraordinary Vessels is to absorb superficial pathogens

and prevent them from entering the body. Indeed, this is the only function of the Extraordinary Vessels acknowledged by the *Nei Jing*. The Extraordinary Vessels can be considered a means by which excess pathogenic energy can be absorbed and stored by the body so that it does not mix with the usable Qi in the rest of the body.

- In feline hyperesthesia syndrome, pathologic excesses appear to accumulate in the downward-flowing Bladder channel and its associated Luo-connecting vessel and spill over into adjacent channels anytime a cat with feline hyperesthesia syndrome is touched on its back. The nearest channels to the Bladder channel are the Extraordinary Vessels known as the Yang Qiao Mai and the Du Mai. When an animal is healthy, they function to help deliver energy to the brain, thus maintaining consciousness. When pathogenic Qi suddenly spills from the Bladder channel into these two Extraordinary Vessels, pathologic levels of Qi reach the brain, which culminates in seizures.
- The Bladder channel is a Tai Yang channel, which means it is typically attacked by Cold. In feline hyperesthesia syndrome, however, the offending pathogen is Damp Heat and Phlegm. It is nonetheless logical for this Heat or Yang pathogen to accumulate in the Tai Yang channels, since they are located in the most Yang regions of the body.
- Patients that are susceptible to invasions of Damp Heat and Phlegm are those in which a certain amount of Damp Heat is already being internally generated. The invasion of exterior Damp Heat thus simply represents the straw that breaks the proverbial camel's back, which has already been weakened by internal Damp Heat accumulation. The goals of acupuncture treatment of feline hyperesthesia are thus not only to disperse the channel pathogen, but also to strengthen the Spleen function, clear Heat, and drain Dampness. The role of Damp Heat and Phlegm in feline hyperesthesia is confirmed in affected cats having a swollen, red tongue with tenacious saliva and yellow coating, and a rapid pulse.

- Despite the esoteric nature of the Chinese medical perspective, the Western medical perspective on feline hyperesthesia syndrome is not all that different. Even from the Western perspective, it appears the seizures are peripherally mediated, possibly through a process called "kindling," and are aggravated by increased cutaneous inflammation. Flea control measures and hypoallergenic diets may thus aid greatly in the control of this condition when allergic dermatitis is thought to coexist. Interestingly, Phlegm pathogens arising in Spleen-deficient animals often correlate in conventional medicine to symptoms arising from food sensitivities.
- Since feline hyperesthesia syndrome is an external type of seizure disorder, acupuncture is extremely well suited to its treatment and favorable outcomes may be even more complete and more likely than in the treatment of idiopathic epilepsy. The goals in the acupuncture treatment of feline hyperesthesia are to open the Bladder channel, regulate the Du Mai and Yang Qiao Mai, clear Heat, and drain Dampness. Local points in areas of heightened sensitivity are used to open the Bladder channel, but *only* after distal points have already been inserted. If distal points have not been inserted to regulate the Du Mai and Yang Qiao Mai, needling local points may simply spill more Qi into the Extraordinary Vessels and create more seizures.
- Points to regulate the Du Mai and Yang Qiao Mai include SI 3 and BL 62. Points to clear Heat include LI 11, SP 10, LI 4, and BL 40. BL 40 is especially important here because it is the "command point" for the entire back and it also relieves itch by having a strong Blood-cooling effect. SP 9, BL 28, and BL 22 are used to further regulate the Bladder channel and drain Dampness.
- For extremely agitated and painful cats, initial physical treatment might simply be chiropractic to relieve the vertebral fixations that are often present in these cases. Often, the lower lumbar and sacral vertebrae are rigid and unyielding, particularly adjacent to the areas of greatest pain. Chiropractic treatment can be considered

a crude method of initiating the movement of Qi when it has become stagnant.

- A Chinese herbal formula that shows promise for use in feline hyperesthesia syndrome is one that is used in the treatment of tetanus, also a peripherally mediated CNS disorder, in humans. The formula is based on **San Ren Tang** (Three Seeds Decoction). To 75 g of base formula, the practitioner adds 9 g Di Long (Earthworm), 9 g Qin Jiao (Large Gentian Root), and 9 g Si Gua Luo (Loofah). The practitioner may also consider adding 6 g Du Huo (Angelica Root), 9 g Fang Feng (Ledebouriella), and 6 g Man Jing Zi (Vitex fruit) to enhance the formula's pain-relieving properties and to obtain more rapid control of seizures. A *recommended starting dose* of granular concentrate is ¼ tsp per 10 to 15 lb of body weight, or 60 to 75 mg/kg of body weight, divided into two daily doses.

Western Herbal Medicine

- **A combination of** 2 parts Red Clover *(Trifolium pratense)*, 2 parts Skullcap *(Scutellaria laterifolia)*, 3 parts Passion Flower *(Passiflora incarnata)*, and 3 parts Stinging Nettles *(Urtica dioica)* seems effective for some cases of feline hyperesthesia syndrome. The usefulness of Passion Flower and Skullcap in seizures is discussed in the general section on Seizures. Nettles is a cooling herb specific for cases in which pruritus is associated with extreme excitability. Red Clover has a reputation for efficacy in childhood eczema and can transform accumulations of Dampness and Phlegm. In summary, this formula addresses many of the treatment objectives identified for feline hyperesthesia syndrome from a Chinese medical perspective. Johnny-Jump-Up *(Viola tricolor)* may be added to the formula to further relieve nervous irritability, especially when the animal has moist skin eruptions. Linden Flowers *(Tilia europea* and *T. americana)* have been combined with Nettles by some practitioners to reduce irritability and itch. A *suggested starting dose* is 0.2 ml of the combined formula per 5 lb of body weight, divided into two daily doses.

AUTHORS' CHOICES:

SM: Acupuncture; herbal medicine; avoid food allergies; control fleas.
SW: Evaluate for allergic skin disorders and fleas; Chinese herbs; acupuncture; chiropractic.

FLY BITING SEIZURES

See the general section on Seizures later in the chapter.

IDIOPATHIC VESTIBULAR SYNDROME

Therapeutic Rationale

- Support patient while problem resolves, usually within 2 to 3 weeks.

Alternative Options with Conventional Bases

- **Ginger** *(Zingiber officinale)*: appears to be effective for motion sickness and seasickness in people (Ernst, 2000) and may be worth trying for nausea caused by vestibular disturbances in dogs.

Paradigmatic Options

Chinese Medicine

- From a Chinese medical point of view, idiopathic vestibular syndrome in dogs shares an almost identical pathogenesis with idiopathic epilepsy. The general section on Seizures can be consulted for additional information. The main cause of idiopathic vestibular disorder in dogs is Upward Disturbance of Wind Phlegm, which is treated with **Ban Xia Bai Zhu Tian Ma Tang** (Pinellia, Atractylodes, and Gastrodia Decoction). The addition of 15 to 20 g of Jiang Can (Silkworm Casing) to 100 g of base formula seems to help the patient return to equilibrium more rapidly than without treatment. Interestingly, Jiang Can seems to produce this effect even in recovered patients that have a lingering head tilt, when the conventional medical assumption might be that permanent neuronal damage has occurred. The improvements seen in animals receiving Ban Xia Bai Zhu Tian Ma Tang with added Jiang Can suggest that at least some of this damage may not be irreversible. In patients that are treated with Chinese herbal therapy, lingering head tilts are rarely seen. A *recommended starting dose* of granular concentrate is ¼ tsp per 10 to 15 lb of body weight, or 60 to 75 mg/kg of body weight, divided into two daily doses.

- Although older canines are more commonly affected with idiopathic vestibular syndrome, a similar condition appears to occasionally arise in cats of any age. When Spleen Qi deficiency leading to the production of Phlegm is in evidence, **Ban Xia Bai Zhu Tian Ma Tang** with added Jiang Can seems to be effective. The success of this digestion-improving formula in so many cases of vestibular syndrome in canines and felines implies that the disorder, like idiopathic epilepsy, may be at least partly due to underlying food sensitivity. The prohibitions against unprocessed raw food diets mentioned for epilepsy seem also to apply to cats suffering from vestibular syndrome, since dramatic worsening of symptoms immediately after institution of these diets has been observed in Spleen-deficient animals.
- An additional cause of idiopathic vestibular syndrome in dogs is, as in epilepsy, Yin deficiency leading to Empty Fire and the generation of an Internal Wind. **Zhi Bai Di Huang Wan** (Anemarrhena, Phellodendron, and Rehmannia Pill) is the treatment of choice in these usually agitated patients, and they typically have a floating, forceful pulse and a red tongue. A *recommended starting dose* of granular concentrate is ¼ tsp per 10 to 15 lb of body weight, or 60 to 75 mg/kg of body weight, divided into two daily doses.
- Acupuncture points used to treat idiopathic vestibular syndrome are essentially the same as those used in epilepsy. A list of recommended points and their rationale can be found in the general section on Seizures.

AUTHORS' CHOICES:

SM: Ban Xia Bai Zhu Tian Ma Tang or Zhi Bai Di Huang Wan, depending on case details.
SW: Supportive care while condition resolves on its own; Ginger for nausea or discomfort.

INTERVERTEBRAL DISK DISEASE

For cervical disk disease, see the Cervical Spondylomyelopathy section.

Therapeutic Rationale

- Minimize spinal movement in acute stages.
- Reduce pain and inflammation.
- Maintain muscular strength throughout recovery.
- Give bladder care.

Alternative Options with Conventional Bases

- **Glycosaminoglycans:** abnormal compressive forces in spinal disease have been shown to change proteoglycan content of intervertebral disks in dogs (Hutton, 1998). Supplementation with glycosaminoglycans for intervertebral disk disease (IVD) has not been examined but may be administered to dogs with unstable spinal segments when supporting disk integrity and vertebral endplate structure may improve function and decrease pain.
- **Prolotherapy:** consists of injections of a mild irritant into or around an unstable joint to achieve stabilization through fibrosis. Irritants that produce the sclerosing effect include 50% dextrose, lidocaine, sodium morrhuate, and a zinc-phenol solution. An interesting discussion and case series may be found on the website http://www.prolotherapy.com/articles/myers.htm. Prolotherapy is not widely used in veterinary medicine at this time.
- **Hyperbaric oxygen:** has been suggested as an adjunct treatment to reduce free radicals formed after severe spinal trauma.

- **Dimethyl sulfoxide** (DMSO): may reduce pain and inflammation. Some veterinarians apply it topically over the affected area of the spine (whether this concentrates DMSO in that area before it is absorbed systemically is unknown). Care is necessary in handling DMSO.
- **MSM:** a DMSO derivative that is used clinically as an antiinflammatory agent.

Paradigmatic Options

Homeopathy

- Animals in acute pain may benefit from **Hypericum perfoliatum 30C** given up to three times daily.

Chiropractic

- Studies are needed to evaluate the efficacy of chiropractic in the management of IVD. In human patients, chiropractic is usually recommended for patients with disk protrusion that causes spinal pain and no neurologic deficits. However, many animal patients have nuclear extrusion that causes spinal cord compression, which is normally a contraindication to chiropractic adjustment. It is in these cases that surgical intervention is typically advised.
- Chiropractic appears beneficial in subacute and chronic cases of IVD, possibly for the same reasons it is useful in Wobbler syndrome. Adjustment of fixations away from the site of disk calcification or extrusion may reduce any joint strain or hypermobility at the site of the damaged disk, lessening progression of the lesion and allowing the disk to heal in place more quickly. For this reason, extended periods of strict rest in dogs with IVD are potentially deleterious in that they promote gradually increasing areas of vertebral fixation. Only in acute cases of IVD is cage rest appropriate, from the chiropractic perspective.

Acupuncture

- Unlike DM, hind limb weakness after disk prolapse or rupture seems to chiefly involve the Bladder channel. The Gall Bladder and Stomach channels appear secondarily involved. Therapeutic goals are to restore normal Qi flow down the Bladder channel into the leg by use of chiropractic and acupuncture. Points that are frequently useful include BL 40, BL 60, BL 28, BL 54, GB 30, LV 3, GB 34, GB 29, ST 38, and GB 39, as well as points above and below the site of obstruction. Rather than using radiographs to establish the level of channel obstruction, the practitioner is advised to place needles above and below any line transecting the spine where, on moving distally from this point, a decline in radiant heat as measured by a hand held above the skin is present. Electroacupuncture may prove beneficial in management of these cases, with dispersing treatments applied above any identified "thermocline" and distally at BL 40 or 60.

Chinese Herbs

- For each of the following formulas, a *recommended starting dose* of granular concentrate is ¼ tsp per 10 to 15 lb of body weight, or 60 to 75 mg/kg of body weight, divided into two daily doses.
- Various formulas have been advocated for pain relief in cases of IVD, including **Xiao Huo Luo Dan** and **Da Huo Luo Dan** (respectively, Minor and Major Invigorate the Collaterals Pills). Phlegm, Qi stagnation, and Blood stasis should be prominent in cases in which these formulas are applied. The tongue would be purple, and the pulse wiry and perhaps fast. The formulas should not be used over a long term because of their toxic potential.
- Kidney-deficient animals may benefit from **Du Huo Ji Sheng Tang** (Pubescent Angelica and Loranthus Decoction). In such a case the dog would have a pale tongue, caudal spinal pain or weakness, aggravation in cold weather, weakness in the rear, and pulses that are forceful and wiry.
- **Bu Yang Huan Wu Tang** (Tonify Yang and Normalize the Five Viscera Decoction) has been proposed for use in IVD. This formula was developed specifically to treat Qi-deficient presentations of intracranial hemorrhage in humans. Its usefulness may extend to Qi-deficient presentations of IVD in dogs.

- **Sang Ji Sheng San** is primarily a Yang tonic formula for Bony Bi Syndrome, and it may be useful in dogs with chronic IVD, spondylosis, and osteoarthritis.
- If none of the above formulas suits the clinical presentation of the patient, the reader should consult Chapter 12. Formulas that are generally effective in the treatment of arthropathies are often also effective for disorders involving facet joints and intervertebral disks.
- Once animals have become ambulatory, an evaluation of the patient using traditional Chinese medicine (TCM) to identify underlying disease patterns is recommended, with the view that treatment of these underlying tendencies will decrease the risk of further injury.

AUTHORS' CHOICES:

SM: Hypericum in acute cases; acupuncture and chiropractic in subacute cases; glycosaminoglycans to reduce frequency of episodes in the long term; appropriate Chinese herbal formula.

SW: Very short-term exercise restriction according to animal's comfort level; electroacupuncture; chondroitin supplementation to reduce frequency of episodes long term.

MENINGITIS AND ENCEPHALITIS

Therapeutic Rationale

- Identify predisposing or associated injury, infection, or immune compromise.
- Control seizures.

Alternative Options with Conventional Bases

Nutrition

- **Antioxidants,** including *N*-acetylcysteine (Auer, 2000), Vitamins E, C, and A, Selenium, and Beta-carotene, may reduce tissue damage. One *suggested dose* for *N*-acetylcysteine is 25 mg/kg of body weight tid for 14 days, then tid qod.

- **Bromelain** has established systemic antiinflammatory effects and has been suggested in treatment of CNS inflammatory disorders.

Paradigmatic Options

- Septic meningitis should be treated with antibiotics, but aseptic meningitis may be amenable to adjunct therapies. Treatment is multipronged and aimed at restoring normal mobility and circulation through the neck region, as well as controlling febrile tendencies.
- A differential diagnosis of suspected meningitis is simple atlantooccipital joint fixation. This syndrome is a common chiropractic syndrome and is not accompanied by fever. Affected animals frequently yelp at night during sleep, presumably because inadvertent movements during sleep elicit compression of the greater occipital nerve where it emerges between the atlas and the occiput. Affected animals become able to eat or drink only from raised surfaces and are unable to lower the head to the floor level. Displacement of the atlas is frequently palpable and demonstrable on plain film radiographs but is usually overlooked by practitioners not familiar with chiropractic medicine. Symptoms are immediately relieved by chiropractic adjustment of the atlas, and normal motion is restored.
- When meningitis has been confirmed clinically, several modalities are combined to reduce fever and promote normal neck movement and circulation. Treatment sessions should be at least daily, and preferably several times daily, until the condition is resolved. A useful protocol is the following.

Chiropractic

- Gentle chiropractic adjustment of all fixations should be attempted first to restore as much movement as possible. If some degree of stiffness lingers after adjustment, it signals the presence of a more serious disorder than simple atlantooccipital fixation.

Acupuncture

- Acupuncture treatment should be initiated next. Aseptic meningitis can be considered in its initial stages an invasion of the Tai Yang layer (Bladder and Small Intestine channels) by Wind and Dampness. This pathogenic invasion may spill over into the adjacent Du Mai and the Shao Yang (Triple Burner and Gall Bladder) regions. Acupuncture points are chosen to do the following:
    - Release the Tai Yang meridians: LI 4, LU 7, BL 40, BL 60, SI 3, BL 10.
    - Regulate the Du Mai: SI 3 and BL 62 (or BL 60), GV 14.
    - Open the Shao Yang meridians: TH 5, GB 20, GB 21.
    - Clear Heat: TH 5, LI 4, GV 14.
    - Reduce fever: LI 4, GV 14, BL 40, LI 11, GV 4, Er Jian.
- Some of these points are also useful to treat neck and occipital pain, as noted above.
- Drops in the body temperature of febrile animals can be impressively rapid, by as much as 1° to 2° Fahrenheit within 20 to 30 minutes. Some of this loss of body heat appears to be mediated by increased rate and depth of respiration during treatment.
- In addition, any focal areas of spasm or pain should be needled. Needles should be retained with the dog lying quietly for as long as possible.

Chinese Herbs

- For high fever with severe pain, **Chai Ge Jie Ji Tang** (Decoction of Bupleurum and Pueraria to Relieve the Muscles) can be considered. This is arguably the best formula for sterile or aseptic meningitis in dogs. The tongue is red, and the pulse may be slippery, rapid, and full. Facial features are often red and congested. This formula should be used for patients for which homeopathic Belladonna would seem applicable (for more information on Belladonna indications, refer to the section on homeopathy below). A *recommended starting dose* of granular concentrate is ¼ tsp per 10 to 15 lb of body weight, or 60 to 75 mg/kg of body weight, divided into two daily doses.

- **Qiang Huo Sheng Shi Tang** (Decoction of Notopterygium to Dispel Dampness) with 6 g Fang Ji (Stephania Root), 4 g Fu Zi (Aconite), or 4 g Chuan Wu Tou (Sichuan Aconite) added to about 40 g of the base formula. This formula is more effective for a patient with modest fever, but severe pain and nuchal rigidity. The pulse is floating and tight, and the tongue may appear normal. Long-term use of this enhanced formula presents a risk of toxicity because of its content of aconite, and Fang Ji is under scrutiny as being potentially toxic. The base formula is nontoxic. A *recommended starting dose* of granular concentrate is ¼ tsp per 10 to 15 lb of body weight, or 60 to 75 mg/kg of body weight, divided into two daily doses.
- **Xue Fu Zhu Yu Tang** (Drive Out Stasis in the Mansion of Blood) may be used in Blood stasis cases. The pulse is wiry, and the tongue is lavender or purple. Other signs of Blood deficiency may also be present in the medical history or on physical examination. These include tendencies to frequent dreaming, fear aggression, fine dander, itch, mild, dry papular dermatitis lesions, poor hair regrowth, recurrent mast cell tumors, and muscle spasm or tightness. A *recommended starting dose* of granular concentrate is ¼ tsp per 10 to 15 lb of body weight, or 60 to 75 mg/kg of body weight, divided into two daily doses.

Western Herbs

- A **Western herbal formula** that may help relax the neck muscles and relieve pain is made from 4 parts Passion Flower, 1 part Lobelia *(Lobelia inflata)*, 2 parts Hops *(Humulus lupulus)*, 2 parts Prickly Ash Bark *(Xanthoxylum clava-herculis)*, and 1 part Comfrey *(Symphytum officinale)*. Lobelia comprises no more than 10% of the formula because of its toxic potential. Lobelia is considered quite possibly the most powerful Qi mover in all of Western herbal medicine. Prickly Ash is considered a Blood mover. Passion Flower is considered a strong antispasmodic, and Hops and Comfrey together mobilize Phlegm accumulations obstructing the channels. There are no herbs in this formula to reduce fever, so consideration might be given to adding Willow Bark *(Salix alba)* for its salicylate content. A *suggested starting dose* is 0.2 ml of the combined formula per 5 lb of body weight, divided into two daily doses.

- **Comfrey:** has recently been generally abandoned for internal use because of concern over the hepatotoxicity of its pyrrolizidine alkaloids. Practitioners may thus wish to exclude it from the above formula. Unfortunately, clinical experience with the formula without Comfrey has not been obtained, but benefit can probably still be expected.
- **Yellow Jasmine** *(Gelsemium sempervirens):* seems to have a particular relaxing effect on the muscles in the occipital region and also seems to clear Heat from the head from a Chinese medical perspective. It should be considered for Western herbal formulas to address neck pain and aseptic meningitis. Like Lobelia, it is potentially toxic and should compose only perhaps 10% of a larger formula, such as the Western herbal formula described in this section.
- From a Chinese medicine point of view, it is crucial to rule out Blood stasis in the brain for animals that have cortical symptoms and are suspected of having meningoencephalitis. This differentiation is especially important to make if a history of head trauma cannot absolutely be ruled out. Blood stasis is ruled out by response to therapy, particularly homeopathic Arnica montana, as described below.

Homeopathy

- **Belladonna 30C:** up to three times daily and then tapering to once daily or as needed. It should be used for acutely painful dogs that are sensitive to the slightest touch and have marked reddening of the sclera, muzzle, and oral mucosa.
- **Arnica montana 30C:** given up to three times daily and then tapering as needed. Clinical experience with Arnica suggests that patients often demonstrate improved neurologic function within 1 hour in cases of Blood stasis, regardless of the duration of the illness. The benefits of Arnica are not restricted to cerebral hemorrhage and

edema after trauma but seem to extend even to cases of cerebrovascular accident in both humans and dogs. Improvements can be seen with the use of Arnica weeks or even years after the initial onset of symptoms.

AUTHORS' CHOICES:

SM: Sterile meningitis—acupuncture; Chai Ge Jie Ji Tang. Cortical lesions—Arnica montana to rule out Blood stasis and cerebral edema.

SW: Sterile meningitis—steroids; acupuncture; Chinese herbs.

PAIN, GENERAL

Alternative Options with Conventional Bases

- **DL-Phenylalanine** (DLPA): may inhibit decarboxylation of endogenous opioids or work by other mechanisms through the endogenous analgesia system.

Herbs

- Many of the herbs discussed in the section on pain in Chapter 12 may also be appropriate here. These may include Willow, Devil's Claw *(Harpagophytum procumbens)*, Ginger, and others.
- **Corydalis** *(Corydalis yanhusuo* and other species): inhibits the reticular activating system (RAS) of the brain stem, and chronic use may result in tolerance and cross-tolerance with morphine (Huang, 2000). This herb, along with two others (Du Huo [Pubescent Angelica] and Bai Jiang Cao [Patrinia]), was shown to reduce pain from inflammation in a rat model (Wei, 1999).

Paradigmatic Options

- From a Chinese medical perspective, all pain is a manifestation of obstructed circulation of Qi and Blood. Therefore some very general recommendations may be made concerning the relief of pain using alternative treatment methods. The paramount consideration in relieving pain, however, is the identification of the underlying disorder so that specific therapy, whether alternative or conventional, may be rendered. Only some general approaches will be listed here.

Acupuncture

- Practitioners should be aware of some of the most important acupuncture points for addressing various regions of the body:
  - LI 4 addresses head and facial pain.
  - ST 36 can be used for any kind of abdominal pain.
  - GB 34 can be used for any muscular pain, as well as pain in the costal region and the lateral flanks.
  - BL 40 relieves pain along the entire back.
  - LU 7 addresses pain of the posterior (i.e., dorsal) head and neck.
  - LI 4 and LIV 3 are paired to address pain caused by Qi stagnation anywhere in the body.
  - BL 17 is indicated in all cases of Blood stasis; BL 11, ST 37, and ST 39 are also useful in this regard.
  - BL 60 addresses both low back pain and pain of the head and neck when the Bladder channel is involved.
  - BL 10 relieves pain in the occiput.
  - PC 6 can relieve chest pain.
  - GB 20 and 21 govern the flow of Qi through the shoulders, occiput, and lateral neck.
  - TH 5 governs Qi flow throughout the lateral head and neck.
  - BL 25 is important in pain referable to the sciatic nerve.
  - GB 29 and 30 help hip pain.
  - GB 41 helps temporal and eye pain.
  - ST 8 helps frontal pain.
- Various "alarm points" may prove useful to address pain in particular organs:
  - CV 3 for uterine and bladder pain.
  - CV 12 for stomach and upper abdominal pain.
  - LIV 14 for gastric pain and inflammation (although LIV 14 is the Liver alarm point).
- In addition, areas of heightened sensitivity and muscle spasm should always be needled in pain cases, even if they do not correspond to known acupuncture points.

A useful general strategy for pain relief is to first identify the channel with which locally painful points are associated. Insert a needle into a distal point that seems sensitive, swollen, warm, or "sticky" on the same channel. Then insert a needle into the locally painful point. Repeat for as many channels as are affected, usually three or fewer.

Acupressure and Shiatsu

- Acupressure or massage can be extremely effective for relieving pain and for enhancing the results of an ensuing acupuncture treatment. Qi and Blood stagnation secondary to Blood deficiency are especially amenable to massage. Muscle spasms and tightness are often present. These patients also may have solicited manual contact by the owners at home and may prefer to lie on the sore limb on a hard surface. The tongue is often pale or lavender, and the pulse thin and wiry.
- Acute Blood stasis, such as by severe local trauma, may be aggravated by massage. The tongue in these patients is often purple, the pulse wiry, and the animal may have a history of avoiding any kind of pressure or contact on the painful area.
- The practitioner should not use point pressure at first in massaging painful areas, since it can elicit further muscle spasm. Instead, the practitioner should use a broad application of moderate pressure, such as with the thenar and hypothenar eminences of the hand, and massage in a slow circular motion. As the practitioner feels the muscles begin to relax, pressure can be applied using a circular motion more specifically to areas of local pain. Direct pressure over bony prominences should be avoided. As the muscles relax more, the area of massage can be expanded to regions above and below the painful area on the channel that runs through the area of pain. The practitioner should work from upstream to downstream, following the flow of Qi along the particular channel, crossing over and working the painful area as he or she does so.

Chiropractic

- Chiropractic is effective at promptly relieving pain attributable to vertebral body fixations with resultant nerve root compression. Clinical experience shows that relief commonly occurs within minutes of treatment.
- Chiropractic, acupuncture, and acupressure have a synergistic relationship. Acupuncture and massage can soften muscles that are in spasm, making fixations easier to release. Chiropractic can be thought of as a crude but effective method of suddenly relieving obstructions to Qi flow through the area to which it is applied.

Chinese Herbs

- **Bu Gan Tang** (Boost the Liver Decoction) can be considered for dogs with muscle spasms. These dogs should have thin, wiry pulses, pale or lavender tongues, and not even a hint of Dampness or Phlegm in their presentations.
- For Qi stagnation secondary to Blood deficiency that is progressing to Blood stasis, **Xue Fu Zhu Yu Tang** (Drive Stasis from the Mansion of Blood Decoction) can be considered. Muscle spasms are not prominent in affected patients, but case presentation is otherwise similar to patients receiving **Bu Gan Tang** (Boost the Liver Decoction).
- **Shao Fu Zhu Yu Tang** (Drive Stasis from the Lower Abdomen Decoction) should be used for Blood stasis in the lower abdomen. This formula contains Corydalis, the pain-relieving herb described in further detail in the following paragraphs.
- **Wu Yao Tang** (Lindera Decoction) can be used for animals with lower abdominal and bladder pain and an irritable temperament.
- The following herbs may be added to formulas to help address pain:
  - Xiang Fu (Cyperus) for pain in the lower abdomen and along the costal arch; Mu Xiang (Saussurea) for pain in the upper abdomen; Wu Yao (Lindera) for pain in the lower abdomen caused by Qi stagnation from Cold; Yan Hu Suo (Corydalis) for both Qi and Blood stasis—this herb has a special affinity for the lower abdomen

but may be used for pain anywhere; Hui Xiang (Fennel) is surprisingly effective at relieving abdominal pain and cramping, especially in older animals.
- **Herbs that relieve superficial pain:** Ru Xiang (Boswellia or Frankincense)—a species of Boswellia used in Ayurvedic medicine has been extensively adopted in over-the-counter preparations for joint inflammation and pain. The Chinese medical use of Ru Xiang is similar; Mo Yao (Commiphora) is extensively used for superficial pain.
- **Herbs that relieve pain by warming:** Fu Zi (prepared Aconite); Gan Jiang (Ginger); Rou Gui (Cinnamon); Wu Zhu Yu (Evodia)—specific for when Liver and Stomach are affected by cold; Wu Yao for pain in the lower abdomen; Chuan Wu Tou (Sichuan Aconite—potentially toxic) and Cao Wu Tou (Aconite) for superficial pain and pain in the extremities.

- A number of modern formulas are based on Yan Hu Suo (Corydalis). These are largely combinations of Shao Yao Gan Cao Tang with added Corydalis. The formulas include **Corydalis 5, Great Corydalis, Corydalis Formula,** and **Corydalin** and are available from a variety of Chinese herb manufacturers. These empirical formulas have broad applications in the treatment of pain, and practitioners who do not have the detailed knowledge necessary to make a TCM diagnosis may want to consider using them.

Western Herbs

- **Black Cohosh** *(Actea racemosa):* for uterine cramping in particular; early Western herbalists used this herb for all kinds of pain, and it was often combined with Prickly Ash Bark.
- **Devil's Claw:** an antiinflammatory herb popular for joint pain relief.
- **Mint** *(Mentha piperita)***Oil:** can be used topically as a local anesthetic.
- **Prickly Ash Bark:** for Blood stasis.
- **Valerian** *(Valeriana officinalis):* has antispasmodic activity in both skeletal and smooth muscle; may be especially useful in Blood-deficient dogs prone to spasm.

- **Wild Yam** *(Dioscorea villosa):* for smooth muscle spasm.
- **Willow:** a natural source of nonsteroidal antiinflammatory salicylates.
- **Yucca** *(Yucca schidigera):* contains steroidal saponins that may have antiinflammatory activity. Yucca can be combined with Prickly Ash Bark to avoid occasional gastrointestinal (GI) upset.

Homeopathy

- **Arnica montana** 30C sid to tid: for any acute trauma, especially if attended by bruising and pain that steadily worsens with motion.
- **Colocynthis** 30C sid to tid: for abdominal pain that causes the patient to adopt a hunched position.
- **Dioscorea villosa** 30C sid to tid: for abdominal pain that is relieved by stretching out the abdomen.
- **Hypericum perforatum** 30C sid to tid: for "road rash" and shooting pain, especially if the pain is related to nerve compression or damage.
- **Rhus toxicodendron** 30C sid to tid: for tendinomuscular injuries that are worse with initial movement but improve with sustained gentle movement; patients are often Blood deficient from a Chinese medical perspective and have a history of overexertion leading to chronic lameness with no structural cause. Patients that respond to this remedy may also benefit from **Lycopodium clavatum 30C** if the pain is chronic or if the dog is also fear aggressive.
- **Ruta graveolens** 30C sid to tid: for pain that is worse with extended immobility, but also with even the slightest exertion—no rest for this patient! The patient's injury often involves a ligament or bone or is otherwise more structural; a good example is a healing fracture or a partial cruciate tear.
- **Symphytum officinalis** 30C sid: for pain relating to healing fractures. Clinical impressions of Symphytum are consistent with folklore, which maintains that this herb speeds the rate of fracture healing. It also may promote fusion of nonunion fractures, even when repeated attempts at surgical repair have failed.

AUTHORS' CHOICES:

SM: Address underlying cause; use herbs and homeopathics appropriate to the presentation; acupuncture and chiropractic often afford immediate relief.

SW: Acupuncture; chiropractic; DLPA; Corydalis formulas.

PERIPHERAL NEUROPATHY

Therapeutic Rationale

- Identify etiology if possible.
- Control immune-mediated damage if present.
- Use physical therapy.

Alternative Options with Conventional Bases

- **Alpha-lipoic acid** (thioctic acid): has been shown to improve signs of diabetic polyneuropathy in human clinical trials. In humans these improvements were associated with large doses of approximately 600 mg daily. However, toxicity has been seen in dogs and cats with administration of large doses. The *recommended dose* for cats is no more than 25 mg daily; the *recommended dose* for dogs is up to 200 mg daily for large dogs.
- **St. John's Wort:** a traditional remedy for painful neuropathy. It can be used as the herb or in homeopathic form.
- **Gosha-jinki-gan,** a Kampo formula: was shown to possess antinociceptive activity in diabetic mice and was inhibited by administration of dynorphin antiserum and kappa-opioid receptor antagonists. The principal herb at work in this study was shown to be processed aconite tuber (Suzuki, 1999).

Chinese Medicine

- Acupuncture points noted for the ability to relieve paresthesias in the extremities that are associated with neuropathy are the extra points known as the Ba Xie ("eight evils") and Ba Feng ("eight winds") points. The Ba Xie points are between the digits of the forelimbs at the metacarpophalangeal joints. The practitioner can access these points by angling the needles toward the spaces between the metacarpals from the toe webs. The Ba Feng are in the corresponding positions on the hind limbs.

AUTHORS' CHOICES:

SM: Ba Xie and Ba Feng points.
SW: Alpha-lipoic acid; acupuncture.

SEIZURES, GENERAL

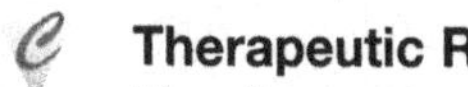

Therapeutic Rationale

- The diagnosis of "epilepsy" is oversimplified, since a number of syndromes may cause recurrent seizures. The alternative therapies described below may help in a percentage of cases depending on the cause, but at this point mechanisms are largely unknown and treatment must be trial and error.
- The practitioner should attempt to control seizures, since they usually become more frequent if untreated. Potassium bromide is emerging as a first choice over phenobarbital. Newer anticonvulsants may be necessary—felbamate, gabapentin, chlorazepate, valproic acid, and possibly other drugs from human medicine.

Alternative Options with Conventional Bases

Nutrition

- **Hypoallergenic diet:** a correlation between food, neurotransmitter production, and behavior is increasingly recognized, and there are numerous case reports of allergy and its relationship to epilepsy (Ballarini, 1990; Campbell, 1970, 1974; Collins, 1994; Crayton, 1981). Dogs with signs of allergies tend to respond more readily to hypoallergenic diets, which mirrors a study in humans in which only patients with other symptoms (headache, abdominal disorders, or hyperkinetic behavior) responded to elimination diets (Egger, 1989). Certain breeds fit this profile, including Labrador retrievers, golden retrievers, German shepherds, and some terriers.

- **Ketogenic diets** (Thomas, 2000): these diets were introduced in 1921 and are regaining a place in treatment of humans with epilepsy. A high-fat, low-carbohydrate, low-protein diet induces ketosis, which may have some effect on vagal function. The diet, a liquid emulsion, is composed of a 3:1 to 4:1 ratio of fats to proteins and carbohydrates. Solid food is gradually introduced provided seizures are controlled and ketosis is adequate. Ketogenic diets are potentially dangerous, however, and direct medical supervision is required in humans, usually by hospitalization. The diets are considered unhealthy for actively growing children and possibly for animals as well. These diets are unpalatable for people, and compliance has been a problem, but the most serious problem with these diets in dogs is that dogs are more resistant to ketosis. The diets have not been in popular use in canine epilepsy by alternative practitioners and cannot be highly recommended at this time. Potential side effects include hyperlipidemia, hypoglycemia, protein deficiency, urolithiasis, vomiting, diarrhea, and abdominal pain. A clear contraindication would be a history of pancreatitis.
- ***N,N*-Dimethylglycine** (DMG): a glycine receptor agonist that is thought to have anticonvulsant activity in gamma-aminobutyric acid (GABA)-deficient seizure models. Although DMG is in popular clinical use, controlled trials to date show little anticonvulsant activity.
- **Antioxidant vitamins:** in some studies human epileptic patients have been shown to have lower plasma vitamin A and C levels (Sudha, 2001). One reviewer suggests that astrocytes in particular have a role in reducing vitamin C and releasing this active form to aid in scavenging reactive oxygen species generated during seizures (Wilson, 1997). The role of antioxidant nutrients has not been studied in seizuring dogs, nor has the effect of supplementing antioxidants to

epileptic patients. Many clinicians use antioxidant preparations safely for epileptic patients with variable results, and supplementation appears worth trying.

- **Taurine:** in humans central nervous system amino acid imbalance is receiving increasing attention. Taurine is an inhibitory amino acid that appears to be released from the hippocampus during seizure activity (Wilson, 1996). In vitro studies suggest that Taurine released during seizure activity may have a protective effect (Saransaari, 2000). Whether these elevated Taurine levels represent a protective effect or are causally related to seizure activity is a matter of debate. Clinically, Taurine supplementation to prevent seizures has not been uniformly successful. Taurine-deficient diets have been shown to decrease seizure activity in some models (Eppler, 1999), but if seizures are a problem in animals eating diets low in taurine, supplementation may be attempted. Doses range from 250 to 1000 mg bid.
- **Magnesium:** low magnesium levels lead to neuromuscular hyperexcitability and reduce seizure threshold in epileptic models. Supplementation has occasionally reduced seizure frequency in canine epileptic patients. Magnesium supplementation is contraindicated in animals with renal failure. The *recommended dose* is 10 mg and up qd (1 to 2 mEq/kg/day) (about 5 mg/lb of body weight).
- **Manganese:** low manganese levels have been associated with epilepsy in humans and rats.
- **Cholodin:** a vitamin and mineral supplement that contains choline and phosphatidylcholine, which are acetylcholine precursors. The role of acetylcholine in kindling seizures is poorly understood, but anecdotal reports have suggested that cholodin helps reduce seizure frequency.
- **Melatonin:** has been recognized as an anticonvulsant in many models and may interact with GABA, benzodiazepine, or other receptors or contribute to dopaminergic activity (Stewart, 2001). Many dogs with epilepsy have most seizures at night when melatonin levels are highest, but one study suggested that melatonin has a proconvulsant effect (Sandyk, 1992).

- In contrast, some studies suggest that circadian rhythm is disrupted in some human patients with epilepsy. Although dosage is uncertain, the practitioner should consider a dose of 0.3 to 5 mg, once in the evening or bid.
- **Chai Hu Long Gu Mu Li Tang:** was shown in several in vitro seizure models to inhibit sodium and calcium channels, stabilize neuronal membrane excitability, and inhibit glutamate release (Wu, 2000).
- **Tian Ma Gou Teng Yin:** a very common prescription for seizures. It showed anticonvulsant and antioxidant activity in an induced seizure rat model of epilepsy (Hsieh, 1999).
- **Saiko-keishi-to-ka-shakuyaku** (TJ-960): a Kampo herbal formula that is often used for seizures. In one study it appeared to reduce seizure frequency and improve cognition (Nagakubo, 1993). Anecdotal reports of use in dogs have not been encouraging.

Other Therapies

- Acupuncturists often note that epileptic seizures seem better controlled with sustained, frequent treatments. Gold bead or suture implants are often used to this end (Durkes, 2001).
- Client education for home management of long seizures: The owner should apply intermittent digital pressure (10 to 60 seconds per compression at intervals of 2 to 15 minutes) to the superior eyelid of one or both eyes to compress the globe into the orbit (Speciale, 1999).

Paradigmatic Options

Bach Flower Remedies

- **Rescue Remedy:** is popular for animals with epilepsy and seizures. Despite its popularity and low toxicity, we believe it is too weak and nonspecific a treatment to be relied on for effective control of seizures.

Homeopathy

- **Cicuta virosa 30C:** may be given initially up to three times daily and then tapered to the minimum effective dose, to animals with seizures manifested as pronounced opisthotonos and extensor rigidity. Some of these patients are considered to be Liver Blood deficient from the Chinese medical perspective.

- **Belladonna 1M:** administered as a single dose to attempt to abort the development of seizures in animals with obvious prodromes.
- **Nux vomica 30C:** should be considered for epilepsy, particularly in aggressive chilly cats with a history of low-back tightness and hind limb weakness. Patients that benefit may be thirsty, suffer seizures early in the morning, and be affected with mild tics and spasms between seizures. A *recommended starting dose* is one dose daily for 1 to 2 weeks, tapering to the lowest effective dose.
- **Strychninum 30C:** may be effective in preventing violent sudden convulsions that throw an animal off its feet. The minimum effective dose should be given up to three times daily to start.

Chinese Medicine

- Chinese medical treatments for seizures evolved without practitioners having knowledge of the various causes of the condition from a conventional perspective. Therefore the different therapeutic approaches outlined in this section are applied based solely on Chinese medical evaluations, and not conventional medical evaluations. As our understanding of alternative strategies progresses in the coming years, we may find that a Chinese medical cause of epilepsy can be superimposed perfectly over a particular cause identified by conventional medicine. However, we are not at that point and Chinese medicine must be considered a medical system unto itself.
- The most common cause of seizures in dogs in Chinese medicine appears to be an Upward Disturbance of Wind Phlegm. Upward Disturbance of Wind Phlegm is also a common cause of idiopathic vestibular syndrome in dogs and vestibular disorders in cats.
- The Chinese pathophysiology behind this disorder is somewhat elaborate. In Upward Disturbance of Wind Phlegm, Spleen Qi deficiency causes the formation of Dampness and Phlegm, which accumulate in and

obstruct the middle jiao. Accumulations are eventually sufficient to cause "Qi counterflow," and the Qi rebels upward and carries Dampness and Phlegm with it. The counterflowing Qi produces the restlessness and convulsions of the patient, and the accumulation of Phlegm in the upper reaches of the body "obstructs the sensory orifices" and causes an unconscious state during seizures.

- Upward Disturbance of Wind Phlegm is suspected when other signs of Dampness and Spleen or Stomach disharmony are present in a patient. These signs include poor appetite, weight gain, chronic vomiting, lack of energy, and a tendency to sleep deeply or appear stuporous.
- Another cause of idiopathic epilepsy in dogs is Yin deficiency with Empty Fire. The Empty Heat or Fire stirs up an internal Wind, and the rising gusts of this Wind produce convulsions or sudden vertigo.
- The two disorders are not difficult to differentiate. Patients with Phlegm accumulations appear stuporous, whereas Yin-deficient patients appear highly agitated. Both disorders may be attended by Heat, since Dampness and Phlegm accumulations become hot in the body as they "compost." Wind-Phlegm patients appear to be considerably more damp and encumbered, however, than do Yin-deficient patients. The encumbrance is often manifested as a long-term tendency to weight gain. Patients affected by Yin deficiency with Empty Fire exhibit obvious signs of Dryness such as weight loss.
- Final definitive differentiation between the two syndromes is made with pulse and tongue diagnosis. A pale or red tongue with a peeled or absent coating and a thin, rapid, wiry, and floating pulse signify the loss of Yin, resultant Empty Heat, and rising energy. A soft or slippery pulse and a pale, swollen, or wet tongue point to a Spleen Qi deficiency that has caused a Dampness accumulation.
- Acupuncture treatment protocols for idiopathic epilepsy with an Upward Disturbance of Wind Phlegm include descending the Qi with PC 6, ST 8, GB 6, GB 9, Er Jian, and ear Shen Men; removing Phlegm obstructions of

the Heart and Shen with BL 15, CV 14, or PC 6; and transforming Phlegm accumulations with ST 40 and PC 6. When substantial Damp Heat has accumulated, the practitioner should consider GB 43 and LIV 2.

- Acupuncture protocols for Yin deficiency leading to Empty Fire and Yang rising may include the points KI 2 and KI 3 to nourish Yin and clear Empty Fire; LIV 3 and LI 4 to move Qi, nourish Liver Yin, and clear Heat from the Head; CV 4 to tonify Essence and descend Qi; GV 20 to descend Qi; GB 20 to extinguish Wind; and BL 18 and BL 23 to nourish Liver and Kidney Yin.
- Chinese herbal protocols exist for management of both causes of idiopathic epilepsy. Upward Disturbance of Wind Phlegm is treated with the rather benign formula known as **Ban Xia Bai Zhu Tian Ma Tang** (Pinellia, Atractylodes, and Gastrodia Decoction). The anticonvulsant effect of this formula may be made even more powerful by the addition of 20 g of Jiang Can (Silkworm Casing) to 100 g of the base formula. A *recommended starting dose* of granular concentrate is ¼ tsp per 10 to 15 lb of body weight, or 60 to 75 mg/kg of body weight, divided into two daily doses.
- Despite its gentle action, clinical experiences with the formula have been impressive. A limited number of dogs may become seizure free; the majority have generally reduced frequency and intensity of seizure episodes even with eventual substantial reductions or even gradual cessation of anticonvulsant medication. From a Chinese medical perspective anticonvulsant medications seem to aggravate the underlying Damp Heat condition that causes idiopathic epilepsy, which perhaps explains why some patients remain refractory to treatment or even worsen despite increasing doses of conventional medications.
- In extremely hot, Damp cases, **Long Dan Xie Gan Tang** (Gentian Purge the Liver Decoction) may be used to gain initial control of seizures. A *recommended starting dose* of granular concentrate is ¼ tsp per 10 to 15 lb of body weight, or 60 to 75 mg/kg of body weight, divided into two daily doses. This formula will have to be discontinued eventually in favor of a milder formula such as **Ban Xia**

Bai Zhu Tian Ma Tang, which is more suited to long-term use. Long Dan Xie Gan Tang should absolutely be avoided unless the patient's pulses are strong. The practitioner should discontinue its use if the patient exhibits any loss of appetite or decline in energy. **Di Tan Tang** (Scour Phlegm Decoction) may be added to, or may be used simultaneously with, Long Dan Xie Gan Tang to extend the application of the latter to more Spleen Qi–deficient cases. When two formulas are being used simultaneously, the *recommended starting dose* of granular concentrate is ⅛ tsp per 10 to 15 lb of body weight, or 60 to 75 mg/kg of body weight, given once daily.

- The perceived success of **Ban Xia Bai Zhu Tian Ma Tang** in many cases of epilepsy suggests that epilepsy may well be a type of food sensitivity reaction, since the formula is heavily directed toward enhancing completeness of digestion from a Chinese medical perspective. There is not yet recognition in conventional medicine that food sensitivities may play a role in the generation of idiopathic epilepsy in animals, although the link has been established between food sensitivities and epilepsy in humans (Werbach, 1996). Frequent responses of epileptic patients to Chinese herbal formulas that focus on Spleen Qi deficiency, Dampness, and Phlegm strongly suggest that such a link may eventually be identified in animals.
- The link between diet and epilepsy remains a strong clinical impression on the part of alternative veterinary medical practitioners. One alarming observation thus far is that dairy products used to disguise medications may actually promote seizure tendencies in some animals. "Overnutrition" appears to be a concern in other patients. This association has been recorded in the human literature as well, with children being observed to be predisposed to seizures after the consumption of very large meals (Werbach, 1996). Factors that may promote completeness of digestion in animals include highly processed diets and high-carbohydrate diets. Ketogenic diets are discussed earlier in this section. Some animal owners and veterinarians speculate that these diets may provide some benefit in the control of

seizures in animals, and from the Chinese perspective such diets may be especially beneficial in cases arising from an accumulation of Dampness and Phlegm.

- Another type of diet widely recommended in the lay literature and by some holistic veterinary practitioners is one comprising raw foods. Clinical experience with these diets has shown them to be harmful to some animals, but beneficial for others. These foods are harder to digest from a Chinese medical perspective, producing a greater burden on the Spleen Qi with the resultant elaboration of Dampness. They may, however, slow digestion and absorption, reducing tendencies to "overnutrition." Spleen deficiency and Dampness arising from overnutrition are seen in animals with strong pulses, and raw foods may be considered for these patients. Raw foods should probably be used only with caution in genuinely Spleen Qi–deficient animals with feeble pulses. If in doubt, test the tolerance of an epileptic animal to raw foods by feeding only small amounts mixed in with the normal diet.
- The main formula for cases of idiopathic epilepsy that are perceived to arise from Yin deficiency leading to Empty Fire and the generation of an internal Wind is **Zhi Bai Di Huang Wan** (Anemarrhena, Phellodendron, and Rehmannia Pill). Patients that benefit from this formula have a red and dry tongue and a floating, forceful pulse. The animal's seizures may be notable for an absence of drooling and for the patient's remaining conscious throughout the seizure. A *recommended starting dose* of granular concentrate is ¼ tsp per 10 to 15 lb of body weight, or 60 to 75 mg/kg of body weight, divided into two daily doses.
- Many other herbal formulas have been advocated for use in epilepsy in both humans and animals. They are summarized in the following paragraphs. For all these formulas a *recommended starting dose* of granular concentrate is ¼ tsp per 10 to 15 lb of body weight, or 60 to 75 mg/kg of body weight, divided into two daily doses.
- **Di Tan Tang** (Scour Phlegm Decoction) for Upward Disturbance of Wind Phlegm. This formula is similar to **Ban Xia Bai Zhu Tian Ma Tang.** The practitioner may

add 15 g of Jiang Can to 100 g of the base formula to make it a more powerful anticonvulsant.

- **Ding Xian Wan** (Arrest Seizures Pill) for initial control of seizures only. This formula is potentially toxic and should not be used over the long term. Patients that respond to Ding Xian Wan may also respond to Ban Xia Bai Zhu Tian Ma Tang and Di Tan Tang, making the use of this potentially toxic formula sometimes unnecessary.
- **Tian Ma Gou Teng Yin** (Gastrodia and Uncaria Decoction) is the single most important formula for epilepsy arising from Liver Blood deficiency that has generated internal Wind. This formula may be overused at present, but it will benefit a significant proportion of epileptic dogs simply because the canine species appears highly prone to Blood deficiency. Signs of Blood deficiency in dogs include thin, wiry pulses and pale to lavender tongues. Fear aggression and anxiety are common. **Zhen Gan Xi Feng Tang** (Sedate the Liver and Extinguish Wind Decoction) can be used for Blood-deficient patients that fail to respond to Tian Ma Gou Teng Yin.
- **Cang Pu Yu Jin Tang, Yang Yin Xi Feng San,** and **Bu Xue Xi Feng San** are other formulas that have been recommended for idiopathic epilepsy. Cang Pu Yu Jin Tang is used primarily for obstruction of the Heart orifices; it removes Phlegm and opens the orifices. Yang Yin Xi Feng San nourishes Yin and extinguishes Wind. Bu Xue Xi Feng San tonifies Blood and Qi and extinguishes Wind. It is used for Qi and Blood deficiency and Liver Blood deficiency seizures.
- Other formulas of lesser importance for dogs include **Jian Ling Tang** (Construct Roof Tiles Decoction) and **Qi Ju Di Huang Wan** (Lycium, Chrysanthemum, and Rehmannia Pill). In patients benefiting from these two formulas both Yin deficiency and Blood deficiency are in evidence.

Western Herbal Medicine

- **Skullcap** *(Scutellaria laterifolia)*: is a Western herbal nervine, and *S. baicalensis* is commonly found in TCM formulas for a number of different disorders. Skullcap was used in the United States by the Eclectics and other early naturopaths as a specific for seizures. It is best used in tincture or as a fresh plant. One additional herb that enjoyed an even greater reputation for addressing neurologic and hyperexcitability disorders in early Western herbalism is Passion Flower. It can be combined with Skullcap to create a small herbal formula for use in epilepsy. The addition of Hops appears to make the formula more powerful still. This triad seems to embody the dynamic required of a successful treatment approach from a Chinese medical perspective, which is to cool the upper body, descend Qi, and transform Phlegm. Suggested ratios of the three herbs are 4 parts Passion Flower, 3 parts Skullcap, and 3 parts Hops. A *suggested starting dose* is 0.2 ml of the combined formula per 5 lb of body weight, divided into two daily doses. Larger amounts may be used if results are encouraging but incomplete.

Cautions

- The interactions between herbs and anticonvulsant drugs are uncertain, and the practitioner should carefully monitor patients with intractable seizures that are being treated with both.

AUTHORS' CHOICES:

SM: Long Dan Xie Gan Tang; Ban Xia Bai Zhu Tian Ma Tang; hypoallergenic or elimination diet.
SW: Hypoallergenic diets; acupuncture; Chinese herbal formulas as appropriate.

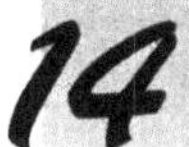

CASE REPORT
Suspected Feline Hyperesthesia Syndrome

HISTORY

Teddy, an 11-pound stray male cat, was brought for treatment by a client in whose yard he had lived for a few months. The chief complaint was acute hind limb paralysis. The client had observed several apparent seizures in Teddy, elicited when he turned around to lick his back. Teddy's hind limbs became paralyzed after a particularly strong seizure 1 week earlier during which the client saw a series of violent spasms pass through Teddy's flanks.

The client sought veterinary care once Teddy lost hind limb control. A local veterinarian presumptively diagnosed acute thromboembolism of the external iliac arteries and gave a poor prognosis. The practitioner declined to offer treatment, which prompted the client to seek alternative veterinary medical treatment a few days later.

On Teddy's arrival at my (SM) clinic, I immediately palpated the cat's femoral arteries and found a clear pulse present on both sides. The presence of both paresis and seizures suggested a possible multifocal lesion in the central nervous system, and consultation with a nearby board-certified veterinary neurologist was advised. The client said he would consider this advice but requested that we proceed with an evaluation.

PHYSICAL EXAMINATION

Teddy had a normal body temperature of 102.3° F and a normal heart rate of 180 beats per minute. His femoral pulses were easily palpated bilaterally but were thin and wiry from a Chinese medical perspective. His tongue was wet and swollen and had a thick yellow coating. At the start of the examination, Teddy's bladder was very full and could not be expressed.

Teddy exhibited marked pruritus and thick accumulations of flea dirt over the lower lumbar region. During the examination, Teddy showed sudden urges to lick his hind limbs and feet. His attempts to do so produced seizure-like activity with the sudden onset of generalized extensor rigidity, tremors, and urinary and fecal incontinence. The urine and feces appeared grossly normal.

Palpation of Teddy's limbs revealed no evidence of pain or fractures. The hind limb musculature was poorly developed, however, and the lumbar region was rigid. Heat radiated palpably from the region of the fourth lumbar vertebra, where Teddy was markedly sensitive to touch.

A cranial nerve examination revealed apparently normal audition, deglutition, and tongue movements. Withdrawal reflexes and crossed extensor reflexes were detected in both limbs. Both hind limbs exhibited extensor rigidity, making it difficult to evaluate patellar deep tendon reflexes. Teddy's pupils were equal and reactive to light. Fundic examination revealed no evidence of retinal pathologic change. Ocular movements were normal.

No laboratory evaluations were possible because of the financial constraints of the client.

ASSESSMENT

Thromboembolism of the external iliac arteries was ruled out by the presence of clear and distinct bilateral femoral pulses. Differential diagnoses that could have been ruled out with further diagnostic testing included feline infectious peritonitis, cryptococcosis, toxoplasmosis, feline leukemia virus infection, and feline immunodeficiency virus infection. A diagnosis of feline hyperesthesia syndrome was strongly suspected, however, on the basis of the extreme pruritus and the immediate development of seizures when Teddy responded to the skin irritation by licking or grooming himself.

From a Chinese medical perspective, the wiry pulses, heat over the region of L4, and thickly coated, wet tongue implied that there was an obstruction to Qi flow in the lumbar area caused by the accumulation of Damp Heat and Phlegm. In feline hyperesthesia syndrome a latent accumulation of Dampness and Phlegm in the channels caused by an underlying Spleen deficiency is viewed as being aggravated by an external invasion of Wind-Phlegm and Wind-Damp. In the lumbar region the Bladder channel carries Qi downward to the legs and the adjacent Yang Qiao Mai and Du Mai channels carry energy up to the brain. In feline hyperesthesia syndrome the obstruction to Qi flow is in the Bladder channel and touching the cat in the region of the obstruction spills stagnant Qi into the adjacent Du Mai and Yang Qiao Mai. The rush of Qi into the brain produces the sudden onset of epilepsy. Teddy's inability to move his hind legs, and that his bladder could not be expressed, signified the obstruction of Qi flow in the Bladder channel.

TREATMENT

It is my opinion (SM) that involvement of the cerebral cortex in feline hyperesthesia syndrome is functional, with the true lesion located peripherally. I think seizures are induced through "kindling," when repetitive afferent impulses produced by skin inflammation bring cerebral cortical activity close to the seizure threshold. Any added tactile stimulation results in the production of afferent impulses that exceed this threshold, producing a seizure. Given Teddy's hind limb paresis, a lumbar spinal cord lesion may have compounded the hyperesthesia. Fortunately, the same acupuncture prescription could be used to treat both problems.

A priority in treatment from a conventional medical perspective was to reduce peripheral nerve irritation. In Teddy's case this especially included measures to control fleas. Imidacloprid (Advantage) was applied according to manufacturer's directions.

From a Chinese medical perspective a major priority was the restoration of Qi flow down the Bladder channel. Chiropractic is an effective way of crudely moving Qi on a regional basis through the spinal region. This is demonstrated by the conversion of wiry pulses to moderate pulses in animals and humans receiving chiropractic treatment. Chiropractic also serves to potentially reduce afferent impulses by relieving paresthesias arising from nerve root compression. For all these reasons, chiropractic manipulation was the chief treatment performed on Teddy's first visit.

On Teddy's second visit 3 days later acupuncture was used to help promote normal Qi movement through the Bladder channel. Acupuncture was not used on the first visit for fear of eliciting further afferent impulses and subsequent seizures. Now that chiropractic had initiated the normal movement of Qi and had reduced any afferent impulses caused by paresthesias from nerve root compression, acupuncture treatment was deemed safe to use.

In addition to moving Qi down the Bladder channel, the acupuncture was used to help regulate Qi flow up the Du Mai and Yang Qiao Mai. The points selected were BL 21, 25, 26, 40, and 62; SI 3; PC 6; ST 40; LIV 2; and GV 2 and 20. Distal points were placed first to begin regulating the three channels. Only then were local points inserted to disperse local accumulations. The needles were vigorously reduced.

A hypoallergenic diet was prescribed on the second visit in case some of Teddy's skin inflammation and resultant afferent impulses were due to food allergies. No herbal medicines or pharmaceuticals were prescribed.

Teddy was treated with acupuncture on two additional visits 18 and 22 days after his first visit.

OUTCOME

After chiropractic adjustment on Teddy's first visit his bladder could be easily expressed and his paresis was slightly lessened. When Teddy arrived for his second treatment 3 days later his seizures had already stopped. He was able to flex his limbs slightly with sufficient motivation. Conscious proprioceptive deficits in both hind limbs were now evident. His tongue was unchanged, and his pulses were now rapid and wiry. Immediately after the acupuncture treatment on the second visit, Teddy's paresis was noticeably reduced and he exhibited increased normal movements of the hind limbs and coordinated attempts to walk.

After his third visit, Teddy was able to walk a few steps on his own. Teddy had another seizure a few days later and again became partly paretic. Acupuncture was administered the same day, and Teddy regained his ability to walk a few steps immediately afterward. The benefits of acupuncture to Teddy were clear, given the obvious "dose-response" relationship to acupuncture Teddy exhibited on his second and fourth visits.

Six weeks after his initial examination, Teddy was weak but could walk with only occasional knuckling of the right hind limb. At his last follow-up 4 months later, Teddy had regained his ability to walk normally and had had no further seizures. He was being fed a home-cooked, turkey-based hypoallergenic diet.

SM

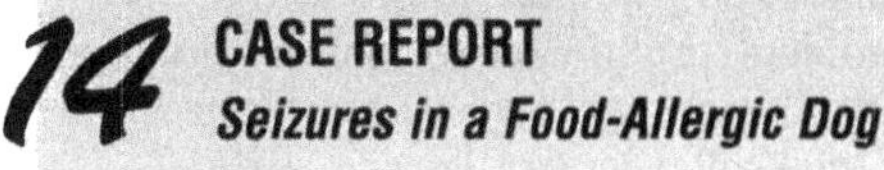

14 CASE REPORT
Seizures in a Food-Allergic Dog

HISTORY

Prior, a 6-year-old, male, neutered Labrador retriever presented with a history of seizures; he had had approximately five to six in the previous 6 months. The owner also reported a history of pedal pruritus and recurrent otitis. Prior's regular veterinarian had initiated phenobarbital therapy 1 month before (60 mg bid) after a routine biochemical profile and complete blood cell count proved normal. The owner sought natural medicine as an alternative because of Prior's increased appetite and mild personality changes and her own research suggesting that phenobarbital has the potential to cause liver toxicity. Prior's diet was a premium dry dog food, and he was receiving no supplements at that time.

PHYSICAL EXAMINATION

On examination, Prior was noted to have mild yeast otitis and to be mildly overweight, but no other abnormalities were found.

ASSESSMENT

Rule-outs for seizures in a 6-year-old Labrador include immune-mediated disease, space-occupying lesions, meningitis, other primary brain lesions, and "idiopathic" epilepsy. Because Prior had signs of allergies—pedal pruritus and otitis—allergy was considered a possible cause of his seizures.

TREATMENT

A commercial elimination diet of venison and potato was recommended, and his owner was given thorough counseling about other sources of food. The client was given the option to try additional nutraceuticals such as magnesium supplements and dimethylglycine, but she decided not to use them. Marine Fish Oil as a source of eicosapentanoic acid and docosahexanoic acid was recommended to help control signs of allergic dermatitis. The client was advised to reduce the phenobarbital dosage over the next 2 weeks, then to discontinue it completely and to call if Prior's seizures resumed.

OUTCOME

At the time of latest follow-up 2 years later, Prior had had no additional seizures and was not being given phenobarbital. His owner was very compliant regarding his diet, rotating between commercial venison, duck, and fish diets. Prior's allergies continued to cause skin problems, but the owner had stopped giving him Fish Oil. His owner was advised to begin food challenges to broaden Prior's diet choices.

COMMENTS

Learning to use herbs and nutraceuticals may seem complicated, but diet can be a very powerful treatment and is a simple first step in treatment of many disorders. In my practice (SW), certain breeds of dogs that have a high prevalence of allergies and develop "epilepsy" appear to have diet-responsive seizure disorders. These breeds include Labrador retrievers, golden retrievers, and German shepherds.

SW

REFERENCES

Auer M, Pfister LA, Leppert D, Tauber MG, Leib SL. Effects of clinically used antioxidants in experimental pneumococcal meningitis. *J Infect Dis* 182(1):347-350, 2000.

Ballarini G. Animal psychodietetics. *J Small Anim Pract* 3:523-532, 1990.

Bottiglieri T. Folate, vitamin B_{12}, and neuropsychiatric disorders. *Nutr Rev* 54(12):382-390, 1996.

Campbell MB. Allergy and epilepsy. In Speer F, editor. *Allergy of the Nervous System*. Springfield, Ill, 1970, Charles C Thomas.

Campbell MB. Neurological and psychiatric aspects of allergy. *Otolaryngol Clin North Am* 7:805, 1974.

Castell JV, Friedrich G, Kuhn CS, Poppe GE. Intestinal absorption of undegraded proteins in men: presence of bromelain in plasma after oral intake. *Am J Physiol* 273(1 Pt 1):G139-146, 1997.

Collins JR. Seizures and other neurologic manifestations of allergy. *Vet Clin North Am Small Anim Pract* 24(4):735, 1994.

Crayton JW. Epilepsy precipitated by food sensitivity: report of a case with double-blind placebo controlled assessment. *Clin Electroencephalogr* 12(4):192-198, 1981.

Deigner HP, Haberkorn U, Kinscherf R. Apoptosis modulators in the therapy of neurodegenerative diseases. *Expert Opin Investig Drugs* 9(4):747-764, 2000.

Durkes TE. Gold bead implants. In Schoen AM, editor. *Veterinary Acupuncture: Ancient Art to Modern Medicine,* ed 2. St. Louis, Mo, 2001, Mosby.

Egger J, Carter CM, Soothill JF, Wilson J. Oligoantigenic diet treatment of children with epilepsy and migraine. *J Pediatr* 114(1):51-58, 1989.

Eppler B, Patterson TA, Zhou W, Millard WJ, Dawson R Jr. Kainic acid (KA)-induced seizures in Sprague-Dawley rats and the effect of dietary taurine (TAU) supplementation or deficiency. *Amino Acids* 16(2): 133-147, 1999.

Ernst E, Pittler MH. Efficacy of ginger for nausea and vomiting: a systematic review of randomized clinical trials. *Br J Anaesth* 84(3):367-371, 2000.

Gascon G, Patterson B, Yearwood K, Slotnick H. *N,N*-Dimethylglycine and epilepsy. *Epilepsia* 30(1):90-93, 1989.

Halderman S. *Principles and Practice of Chiropractic,* ed 2. Norwalk, Conn, 1991, Appleton & Lange.

Hayes CE. Vitamin D: a natural inhibitor of multiple sclerosis. *Proc Nutr Soc* 59(4):531-535, 2000.

Hsieh CL, Tang NY, Chiang SY, Hsieh CT, Lin JG. Anticonvulsive and free radical scavenging actions of two herbs, *Uncaria rhynchophylla* (MIQ) Jack and *Gastrodia elata* Bl., in kainic acid-treated rats. *Life Sci* 65(20):2071-2082, 1999.

Huang KC. *The Pharmacology of Chinese Herbs.* Boca Raton, Fla, 2000, CRC Press.

Hutton WC, Toribatake Y, Elmer WA, Ganey TM, Tomita K, Whitesides TE. The effect of compressive force applied to the intervertebral disc in vivo: a study of proteoglycans and collagen. *Spine* 23(23):2524-2537, 1998.

March PA et al. Electromyographic and histological abnormalities in epaxial muscles of cats with feline hyperesthesia syndrome. In the Proceedings of the ACVIM Forum 704, 1999 (abstr).

McFarland HI, Lobito AA, Johnson MM, Palardy GR, Yee CS, Jordan EK, Frank JA, Tresser N, Genain CP, Mueller JP, Matis LA, Lenardo MJ. Effective antigen-specific immunotherapy in the marmoset model of multiple sclerosis. *J Immunol* 166(3):2116-2121, 2001.

Nagakubo S, Niwa S, Kumagai N, Fukuda M, Anzai N, Yamauchi T, Aikawa H, Toyoshima R, Kojima T, Matsuura M, et al. Effects of TJ-960 on Sternberg's paradigm results in epileptic patients. *Jpn J Psychiatry Neurol* 47(3):609-620, 1993.

Pirog JE. *The Practical Application of Meridian Style Acupuncture.* Berkeley, Calif, 1996, Pacific View Press.

Sandyk R, Tsagas N, Anninos PA. Melatonin as a proconvulsive hormone in humans. *Int J Neurosci* 63(1-2):125-135, 1992.

Saransaari P, Oja SS. Taurine and neural cell damage. *Amino Acids* 19 (3-4):509-526, 2000.

Seiler N, Sarhan S. Synergistic anticonvulsant effects of GABA-T inhibitors and glycine. *Naunyn Schmiedebergs Arch Pharmacol* 326(1):49-57, 1984.

Speciale J, Stahlbrodt JE. Use of ocular compression to induce vagal stimulation and aid in controlling seizures in seven dogs. *J Am Vet Med Assoc* 214(5):663-665, 1999.

Stewart LS. Endogenous melatonin and epileptogenesis: facts and hypothesis. *Int J Neurosci* 107(1-2):77-85, 2001.

Sudha K, Rao AV, Rao A. Oxidative stress and antioxidants in epilepsy. *Clin Chim Acta* 303(1-2):19-24, 2001.

Suzuki Y, Goto K, Ishige A, Komatsu Y, Kamei J. Antinociceptive effect of Gosha-jinki-gan, a Kampo medicine, in streptozotocin-induced diabetic mice. *Jpn J Pharmacol* 79(2):169-175, 1999.

Thomas W. Idiopathic epilepsy in dogs. *Vet Clin North Am* 30(1):183-206, 2000.

Wei F, Zou S, Young A, Dubner R, Ren K. Effects of four herbal extracts on adjuvant-induced inflammation and hyperalgesia in rats. *J Altern Complement Med* 5(5):429-436, 1999.

Werbach M. *Nutritional Influences on Illness,* ed 2. Tarzana, Calif, 1996, Third Line Press.

Wilson CL, Maidment NT, Shomer MH, Behnke EJ, Ackerson L, Fried I, Engel J Jr. Comparison of seizure-related amino acid release in human epileptic hippocampus versus a chronic, kainate rat model of hippocampal epilepsy. *Epilepsy Res* 26(1):245-254, 1996.

Wilson JX. Antioxidant defense of the brain: a role for astrocytes. *Can J Physiol Pharmacol* 75(10-11):1149-1163, 1997.

Wu HM, Huang CC, Li LH, Tsai JJ, Hsu KS. The Chinese herbal medicine Chai-Hu-Long-Ku-Mu-Li-Tan (TW-001) exerts anticonvulsant effects against different experimental models of seizure in rats. *Jpn J Pharmacol* 82(3):247-260, 2000.

Wu Y, Fischer W. *Practical Therapeutics of Traditional Chinese Medicine.* Brookline, Mass, 1997, Paradigm Publications.

Yeung H. *Handbook of Chinese Herbs.* Los Angeles, 1996, Self-published.

Yeung H. *Handbook of Chinese Herbal Formulas.* Los Angeles, 1996, Self-published.

Ziegler D, Reljanovic M, Mehnert H, Gries FA. Alpha-lipoic acid in the treatment of diabetic polyneuropathy in Germany: current evidence from clinical trials. *Exp Clin Endocrinol Diabetes* 107(7):421-430, 1999.

15

Therapies for Ophthalmologic Disorders

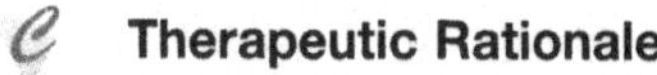

CATARACTS

Therapeutic Rationale

- Manage blood sugar if the patient has diabetic cataracts.

Alternative Options with Conventional Bases

Systemic Herbs

- **Bilberry** *(Vaccinium myrtillus):* contains anthocyanins that may have beneficial effects on microcirculation. It is often recommended for cataracts but is probably more appropriate for retinal diseases.
- **Butterfly Bush** *(Buddleia officinalis):* common in Chinese herbal formulas for eye problems. It contains flavonoids (apigenin, luteolin) and retards cataractogenesis in vitro (Matsuda, 1995).
- **Pa Wei Di Huan Wan** and **Zhang Yan Ming:** were effective in inhibiting lens sorbitol formation in vitro (Chiou, 1992).

Topical Herbs

- **Cineraria, Dusty Miller,** or **Silver Ragwort** *(Senecio cineraria):* has been used in dogs for management of cataracts of various types, based on data from the 1950s. Anecdotally, use of this herb has resulted in improvements. The extract is irritating and must be diluted by at least 50% unless the practitioner uses a preparation that is specifically prepared for use in dogs. It is usually administered for at least 6 months to achieve full benefits. Cataract clearing may be incomplete in advanced cases, and clearing typically begins around the circumference of the lens.

Nutrition

- Carotenoid deficiencies may cause cataracts. The practitioner should ask about the animal's diet and, if it is homemade, ensure that sufficient balance and supplementation are being given.
- **Vitamin C:** has been shown in human epidemiologic studies to be protective against cataract formation (Mares-Perlman, 2000). In the only randomized controlled trial in people the evidence for Vitamin C alone was not as strong but multiple antioxidant vitamin and mineral supplements reduced the incidence of cataracts (Seddon, 1994).
- **Vitamin E:** Vitamin E levels appear to be inversely correlated with cataract incidence in people, and supplementation may reduce incidence and progression in humans and rats (Lyle, 1999; Seth, 1999). More recent work suggests that Vitamin E applied topically (either as a phospholipid liposome vehicle or as 1% Vitamin E acetate) is effective in slowing the progression of cataracts.
- **Alpha-lipoic acid** (or thioctic acid): has been shown to be protective in a number of in vitro models of lens damage.
- **Zinc:** although lens zinc concentrations may decrease with age, no support for supplementing Zinc alone to arrest the progression of cataracts is evident. In a study of dogs, zinc acetate had no positive effect and may have increased lens opacity when it was applied topically (MacMillan, 1989).
- **Taurine:** has a protective effect in in vitro models of diabetic cataractogenesis.

Paradigmatic Options

Traditional Chinese Medicine

- Interpretations of physical findings in Chinese medicine are often very literal. For example, a purple mass would be labeled as denoting Blood stasis. According to this line of thinking a murkiness located where there is normally crystal clarity, such as in cataracts, would suggest an underlying accumulation of "turbidity" in the body.

- Turbidity is considered unwanted material and is equated to pollution. Treatment of cataracts requires not just attention to the lens, but also an overall improvement of the body's economy. Particular treatment objectives for cataracts would include the transformation of Phlegm and the draining of Dampness, since Dampness and Phlegm are the two most common labels assigned to internal pollutants. In addition, treatment goals would involve addressing either the content of the patient's diet or the ability of the patient to adequately digest and assimilate, since all Dampness and Phlegm are considered to come from the Spleen, which is somewhat arbitrarily assigned the role of digestion in the body.
- Therapies that show special promise of fitting this blueprint for the treatment of cataracts include the following.

Homeopathy

- **Calcarea carbonica 30C**: once daily for 3 to 4 weeks, then as needed after a reexamination of the eye for improvements in opacity or vision. Patients most likely to respond to Calcarea manifest many other symptoms that are considered responsive to the remedy, including intractable weight gain, timidity, aggravation from damp weather, a "nursemaid" mentality toward other animals, and teeth that are easily worn down.

Chinese Medicine

- Any formula that is appropriate for the signs in the patient's other organ systems, supports the Spleen, drains Dampness, and transforms Phlegm may be suitable as internal support for animals with cataracts. When these formulas appear to be of benefit, the practitioner should consider reviewing the patient's diet to identify possible allergens or ingredients to which the patient may be sensitive. Raw and low-carbohydrate diets might be considered for hot and excessive patients; bland, low-residue, and easy-to-digest diets might be considered for frail, weak, thin patients.

- Two formulas that address the Spleen and that have shown great potential in the treatment of ophthalmic disease in humans are **Wu Ling San** (Hoelen Five Herb Formula) and **Fu Ling Gui Zhi Bai Zhu Gan Cao Tang** (Atractylodes and Hoelen Combination). Both have similar ingredients and indications except that Wu Ling San has added herbs to promote urination, drain Damp, and clear Heat. It has been noted that diabetes mellitus in dogs, with its attendant cataracts, also often presents as a Spleen Qi–deficient Damp Heat case. Dogs with diabetes that are given these formulas may theoretically manifest both an improvement in glucose tolerance and an improvement in vision. Wu Ling San should be considered for patients that have a floating pulse, coated tongue, and signs of Dampness in the upper reaches of the body (e.g., vomiting of water, dizziness, cough, foamy saliva). Fu Ling Gui Zhi Bai Zhu Gan Cao Tang can be used for patients that have a soft and slippery pulse, a scalloped and wet tongue, and signs of Dampness and Phlegm in the upper body (e.g., cough, dizziness, tiredness, and sluggishness). A *suggested starting dose* of granular concentrate for both formulas is ¼ tsp per 10 to 15 lb of body weight, or 60 to 75 mg/kg of body weight, given at least once daily.
- When the patient appears to be dried out rather than Damp from a Chinese medical perspective, Yin- and Blood-tonifying formulas such as **Qi Ju Di Huang Wan** and **Si Wu Tang** should be considered. These formulas are contraindicated in cases in which the animal is considered to be primarily Spleen Qi deficient. In practice, these formulas seem to have a more important role in the treatment of corneal disease than of cataracts. A *suggested starting dose* of granular concentrate for both formulas is ¼ tsp per 10 to 15 lb of body weight, or 60 to 75 mg/kg of body weight, given at least once daily.

Western Herbal Medicine

- **Cineraria, Dusty Miller,** or **Silver Ragwort:** in light of the role Phlegm and Dampness play in the generation of cataracts and in the disruption of circulation to the eye the counterirritant effect of Cineraria gains new appropriateness. By attracting circulation to the eye Cineraria may be metaphorically said to aid in flushing turbidity from the eye. Counterirritants also have a reputation for decongesting internal structures directly below the region to which they are applied.

- Cineraria is typically advocated for cataracts that are in the early stage of development, which almost precludes its use in dogs or cats except for those belonging to the most vigilant owners. Nevertheless, clinical experience with the herb as a dilute eyedrop suggests that some improvement in vision can be expected beginning from the periphery inward, even in advanced cataracts. In cases of juvenile cataracts, early use of the herb seems to reliably halt further cataract development. Unfortunately, Cineraria is becoming increasingly difficult to find commercially because of liability concerns. Practitioners may soon have to manufacture their own eyedrops from the tincture and assume the responsibility for making sure the drops are sterile, filtered, and diluted by a minimum of 50% in normal saline.

Cautions

- St. John's Wort: caution is advised if animals are exposed to large amounts of sunlight. Hypericin strongly reacts with sunlight and can damage the lens if it is contained in lens proteins (Schey, 2000).
- Vitamin C: it has been suggested that high doses of Vitamin C may have a prooxidant effect that would accelerate oxidative damage at relevant (and unknown) doses (Davies, 1995). The balance of the evidence, however, points to the value of supplementing antioxidants in preventing cataracts.

AUTHORS' CHOICES:

SM: Dilute Cineraria tincture topically in tandem with oral administration of Dampness-draining and Spleen-tonifying formulas.
SW: Antioxidant combination orally; Cineraria tincture topically.

CONJUNCTIVITIS

Therapeutic Rationale

- Manage primary causes (e.g., infection, allergy, keratoconjunctivitis sicca [KCS], environmental, immune-mediated, glaucoma, uveitis).
- Manage inflammation.

Alternative Options with Conventional Bases

Topical Herbs

- **Eyebright** *(Euphrasia officinalis):* traditionally used for conjunctivitis; it contains tannins (similar to Tea *[Camellia sinensis]*) that may have antiinflammatory activity. Eyebright also contains Quercetin, a bioflavinoid, the usefulness of which is described below.
- **Tea:** contains tannins and flavonoids; diluted tea is used tid prn as an antiinflammatory. It should be made daily to prevent contamination.

Nutrition

- **Quercetin and other flavonoids:** may inhibit mast cell degranulation (Kimata, 2000), but clinical effects in patients have not been investigated. Anecdotal reports are occasionally positive. These therapies should be used at a dose proportional to the human recommended doses—approximately 50 to 400 mg tid.
- **L-Lysine:** administration resulted in less severe conjunctivitis in cats inoculated with feline herpesvirus in the conjunctival sac compared with cats that received placebo. The dose used was 500 mg bid, and cats receiving this dose had higher plasma lysine levels (Stiles, 2002).

Paradigmatic Options

Chinese Medicine

- From a Chinese medical perspective, chronic conjunctivitis seems most often to be a by-product of an internal imbalance. The excessive discharge from the eyes can be taken quite literally as a sign of internal Dampness accumulation in channels of the body, most often the Gall Bladder channel. Internal treatment with herbal formulas to stop the manufacture of Dampness by the Spleen will greatly reduce the amount of eye discharge.

- The Gall Bladder is the Yang counterpart of the Liver, and Liver disorders in the body often eventually involve the Gall Bladder channel. Thus the other main cause of conjunctivitis in small animals is a Liver disorder.
- Direct treatment of the Gall Bladder may be attempted through acupuncture. For example, the Chinese name for GB 41 on the foot is translated as "Foot Overlooking Tears." GB 41 seems to be especially effective for acute epiphora when a direct ocular irritant cannot be found.
- Chinese herbal treatment is the most common method used in Chinese medicine to treat conjunctivitis. The focus in Chinese herbal treatment is on treatment of the underlying disorder and not just the conjunctivitis. Most often, this disorder also affects the skin, and Chapter 5 gives more information about which herbal formula may be most appropriate.
- When a Liver condition caused by a Yin or Blood deficiency or by dryness from upflaring Liver or Gall Bladder Fire is perceived to be the underlying cause of conjunctivitis, two herbs that are frequently added to formulas to improve conjunctivitis are Gou Qi Zi (Lycium Fruit) and Ju Hua (Chrysanthemum). Improvements in mucoid conjunctivitis in KCS can be quite dramatic in Liver Blood– or Yin-deficiency cases when these two herbs are added to the formula. A measurable improvement in tear production is not unusual in such cases.
- For Liver Yin and Blood deficiency, **Qi Ju Di Huang Wan** (Lycium, Chrysanthemum, and Rehmannia Pill) and **Ming Mu Di Huang Wan** (Improve Vision Pill with Rehmannia) can be used. Signs of deficiency include as dry coat, failure of hair to regrow after clipping, powdery dander, KCS, fear aggression, thin pulses, and a pale or lavender tongue. For Upflaring Liver Fire manifested as dominance aggression, irritability, weeping or exudative skin lesions, severe itch, a red tongue, and forceful wiry pulses, **Long Dan Xie Gan Tang** (Gentian Purge the Liver Decoction) can be considered. Gou Qi Zi and Ju Hua should be added

to the latter two formulas to enhance their ability to address conjunctivitis. The herbs should be present in as high a percentage of the formula as any other ingredients. A *suggested starting dose* of granular concentrate for all three formulas is ¼ tsp per 10 to 15 lb of body weight, or 60 to 75 mg/kg of body weight, given at least once daily.

- When conjunctivitis alone is the focus of treatment, the following formulas may be of benefit:
  - For Liver Qi stagnation resulting in early-stage Liver Wind Rising or Liver Heat, **Fang Feng San** (Ledebouriella Powder) has been recommended by some authors (Xie, 2000). Signs include rubbing at the eyes, redness, serous or mucoid discharge, red tongue, and superficial and wiry or taut, rapid, or surging pulse. Fang Feng San contains Fang Feng (12%), Jing Jie (12%), Chan Tui (8%), Huang Lian (8%), Huang Qin (8%), Long Dan Cao (8%), Shi Jue Ming (10%), Qing Xiang Zi (8%), Jue Ming Zi (10%), Mo Yao (8%), and Gan Cao (8%).
  - For Liver Heat and stagnation, **Jue Ming San** (Haliotis Powder) has been recommended by some authors (Xie, 2000). Signs include swollen lids, ocular discharge, photophobia and miosis, corneal opacity, possible history of trauma, history of stress (indicating Liver Yang rising into eyes), a red or pale tongue, and a surging fast, or deep and weak pulse. Jue Ming San is composed of Shi Jue Ming (15%), Jue Ming Zi (15%), Gu Jing Cao (8%), Mi Meng Hua (8%), Huang Lian (7%), Zhi Zi (10%), Huang Qin (8%), Mo Yao (7%), Huang Qi (8%), Huang Yao Zi (7%), and Bai Yao Zi (7%).

Western Herbal Medicine

- **Eyebright:** especially suited to patients that appear Damp or Spleen Qi deficient from a Chinese medical perspective. It is arguably the single most important treatment in conjunctivitis caused by Dampness accumulation in the head. Eyebright can be taken as part of a larger herbal formula containing equal parts of Peppermint *(Mentha piperita)* and Elder Flowers *(Sambucus nigra)*. In Chinese medicine Mint has the reputation of clearing Heat and redness from the eyes and Elder Flowers, like Eyebright, contain substantial amounts of Quercetin. A *suggested starting dose* of the oral formula is 0.2 ml per 5 lb of body weight given at least once daily.

- Eyebright is also available commercially as eyedrops, either alone or in combination with other herbs. Homeopathic preparations of Euphrasia appear to have similar efficacy in conjunctivitis as the crude herb but are more restricted in their use in the sense that the patient must match the symptoms calling for the use of Euphrasia in the homeopathic literature.
- **Chamomile Flowers** (*Matricaria* spp.): often advocated for use topically as an eyewash, either alone or in combination with equal amounts of Eyebright and Fennel (*Foeniculum vulgare*). Chamomile enjoys a reputation as an antiinflammatory herb when applied topically, but it may be more beneficial in cases in which the underlying dynamic seems to involve the Liver from a Chinese medical perspective. This Chamomile, Eyebright, and Fennel combination may also be taken internally, thus eliminating the need for preparation of sterile eyewashes from aqueous herbal extracts. The oral version of the formula is thought to effect decongestion of the sinuses, possibly improving drainage when it is impeded by inflammation around the lacrimal duct. Nasal decongestion may be enhanced by the addition of Pleurisy Root (*Asclepias tuberosa*) to oral formulas. The resultant formula should contain approximately equal amounts of all constituents. This formula may also decongest the conjunctiva itself. A *suggested starting dose* of the oral formula is 0.2 ml per lb of body weight given at least once daily.

AUTHORS' CHOICES:

SM: Treatment of the underlying disorder, usually an allergy problem, with the appropriate herbal formula (see Chapter 5). For Dampness conditions confined to the eye or head alone, Eyebright (topically, orally) either alone or in combination with other Western herbs.

SW: Tea, topically; Fish Oil, diet changes, and Quercetin systemically to address allergies if present; Chinese herbal formulas.

FELINE HERPES KERATITIS

Therapeutic Rationale

- Suppress viral replication and prevent recrudescence.
- Manage ocular inflammation.

Alternative Options with Conventional Bases

Topical Treatments

- **Autologous serum:** the patient's serum, spun down and given to the client in a red top tube as a topical treatment, qid. Serum contains alpha$_2$-macroglobulins that have anticollagenase activity as well as growth factors that may enhance corneal healing. It may also contain antiherpesvirus antibodies. The serum must be refrigerated.
- **Zinc—25% ocular wash:** Zinc suppresses herpesvirus replication (Arens, 2000) and may inhibit certain metalloproteinases that contribute to ulcer formation (Smith, 1999).
- ***Melia azedarach:*** meliacine, an extract of this herb, was shown to suppress clinical signs of ocular herpes in mice treated topically tid for 4 days (Alche, 2000).
- **Herbal eyewashes** containing Eyebright (a source of tannins that may coagulate proteins to form a sort of collyrium of the ulcer), Calendula *(Calendula officinalis)*, and other herbs have been used by some practitioners.

Systemic Treatments

- **Lemon Balm** *(Melissa officinalis):* a controlled trial using a topical form of Lemon Balm for people with recurrent herpes indicated that the extract was effective in reducing symptoms (Koytchev, 1999). In vitro studies suggest that Lemon Balm extract inactivates herpes simplex virus 1 (HSV-1) (Dimitrova, 1993). Based on anecdotal reports, success is greatest when the herb is mixed in food at 500 mg to 1 g daily.
- **Lysine:** believed to suppress blood arginine levels, inhibiting herpesvirus replication (Collins, 1995). In a study that examined the effect of L-lysine on the development of conjunctivitis in cats inoculated with herpesvirus, lysine administration resulted in less severe

clinical signs and higher plasma lysine levels, but plasma arginine levels were not different from the placebo group (Stiles, 2002). In naturopathic medicine, increased lysine:arganine ratios are considered more important in supporting herpesviral activity than the absolute plasma level of either amino acid. Dosage is 500 mg bid.

- **Propolis:** has efficacy against human herpesvirus and has been shown to increase healing in corneal lesions (Ozturk, 2000; Vynograd, 2000).
- **Stephania** *(Stephania tetranda):* an extract of Stephania, tetrandine, inhibited development of keratitis in mice infected with HSV-1 by modulating the immune and inflammatory response (Hu, 1997). Stephania is not usually used alone but as a component of Chinese herbal formulas.

Paradigmatic Options

Chinese Medicine

- From a Chinese medical perspective Liver disorders are much less common in cats than in dogs. Accordingly the formulas used to treat corneal conditions in dogs are seldom indicated in cats. In felines the main source of pathologic conditions is not the Liver but the Spleen. Specifically, herpetic keratitis in cats often occurs in patients that have a Spleen Qi deficiency with secondary Dampness accumulation.
- An interesting herbal formula that may show promise in the treatment of herpetic ulcerations in cats is **Dang Gui Nian Tong Tang** (Angelica Squeeze Out the Pain Decoction). This formula is rarely used in China but is widely used in Japan. It dries Damp, clears Heat, and dispels Wind, but protects the Spleen Qi in a variety of acute painful superficial disorders of the limbs and skin. It has been advocated for use in humans for herpetic eruptions of the head. A *suggested starting dose* of granular concentrate is ¼ tsp per 10 to 15 lb of body weight, or 60 to 75 mg/kg of body weight, divided into two daily doses.

Western Herbal Medicine

- **Eyebright:** can be considered to dry Dampness from a Chinese medical perspective, and early 20th-century use of the herb in American Eclectic herbalism was in patients with pulses that corresponded to Spleen Qi deficiency from a Chinese medical perspective. Accordingly Eyebright, whether in crude or homeopathic form, is frequently successful in the alleviation of herpes keratitis in cats. It can be combined synergistically with Lemon Balm orally for an even greater clinical effect. Eyebright may be used orally, topically, or in homeopathic form.

AUTHORS' CHOICES:

SM: Eyebright topically, orally, or homeopathically.
SW: Lysine orally; Lemon Balm orally; Eyebright topically.

GLAUCOMA

Therapeutic Rationale

- Reduce intraocular pressure to prevent permanent blindness.

Alternative Options with Conventional Bases

- **Coleus** *(Coleus foskolii)*: forskolin, an extract of Coleus, is a protein kinase A activator that reduces aqueous humor production, but it is also an alpha-adrenergic agonist and should probably be used in clinical experiment only as a topical drug. We have no experience with this herb.
- **Jaborandi** *(Pilocarpus jaborandi)*: pilocarpine, an extract of Jaborandi, is a parasympathomimetic drug used in glaucoma cases.
- **Glycine:** dogs with primary glaucoma have high intraocular glutamate and low intraocular glycine concentrations (Brooks, 1997). Some practitioners have suggested that supplementation with Glycine may be helpful (Fox, 1972).
- **Alpha-lipoic acid:** studies (mostly in Russian) have suggested that alpha-lipoic acid may be useful in

management of glaucoma. The dosage for cats is up to 25 mg daily; dosage for dogs is approximately 1 to 5 mg/kg of body weight, up to a maximum of 200 mg daily.

Chinese Medicine

- An excess of energy in the head is considered to underlie acute glaucoma according to Chinese medicine. The source of the excess energy is Liver Yang Rising. Signs include irritability, vomiting, severe ocular pain, a deep-red tongue, and a wiry pulse. **Long Dan Xie Gan Tang** (Gentian Purge the Liver Decoction) can be used to treat patients with acute glaucoma.
- A formula advocated for glaucoma caused by rising Liver Yang is **Zhen Gan Xi Feng Tang** (Decoction to Subdue the Endogenous Wind in the Liver). Indications for its use are similar to those for Long Dan Xie Gan Tang, but this formula is less drying and possibly less debilitating to the patient in the event of a misdiagnosis.
- When the rising of Liver Yang into the eyes is caused by a Liver Yin deficiency, **Ming Mu Di Huang Wan** (Vision Improving Six Herbs Rehmannia Tea) should be considered. Patients that benefit from this formula may not be as acutely affected, have a floating or thin and rapid pulse and a red but dry tongue, may be elderly, and may have a history of KCS and low-grade allergic dermatitis.
- A *suggested starting dose* of granular concentrate for all three formulas is ¼ tsp per 10 to 15 lb of body weight, or 60 to 75 mg/kg of body weight, divided into two daily doses.
- Acupuncture points used for glaucoma include GB 37, LIV 3, LIV 2, KI 3 (especially in Yin-deficient cases), LI 4, GB 20, Tai Yang, and BL 2. The latter two are local points, and the first three address hyperactivity in the Liver and Gall Bladder channels. GB 20 is a regional point. LI 4 clears Heat from the head.

Cautions

- Diuretic herbs may potentiate the action and side effects of carbonic anhydrase inhibitor diuretics.

AUTHORS' CHOICES:

SM: Conventional treatment or appropriate Chinese herbal formula.
SW: Conventional treatment; alpha-lipoic acid.

INDOLENT ULCERS

Therapeutic Rationale

- Address infection.
- Control protease activity.
- Protect defect.

Alternative Options with Conventional Bases

- **L-Lysine:** 250 to 500 mg bid for herpetic ulcers. See Feline Herpes Keratitis section.
- **Vitamin A:** severe long-term deficiency of Vitamin A is associated with retinal problems and xerophthalmia in humans. True deficiencies are unlikely in dogs and cats that eat balanced diets, although *optimal* Vitamin A doses in the diet may yet have to be established. Topical administration of Vitamin A palmitate in oil has nevertheles been recommended by some practitioners.
- **Autologous serum:** serum may act as an anticollagenase and antiprotease in melting ulcers and may contain growth factors as well. The serum should be separated and filtered through a sterile 0.22-µm filter into a sterile injection vial. After drawing off 0.4-ml portions, the practitioner dispenses drops from that syringe without the needle (Maggs, 1997; Tsubota, 1999).

Paradigmatic Options

- The prominent cause of indolent ulcers from a holistic medical perspective is a Yin or Blood deficiency syndrome causing reduced tear production. Although plasma drops would be prescribed according to a different rationale, their application to the indolent ulcer would thus seem exceedingly appropriate from the holistic perspective.

Chinese Medicine

- A *suggested starting dose* of granular concentrate for the following formulas is ¼ tsp per 10 to 15 lb of body weight, or 60 to 75 mg/kg of body weight, divided into two daily doses.
- **Long Dan Xie Gan Tang** (Gentian Purge the Liver Decoction) is advocated for patients suffering pain and inflammation. Shi Jue Ming (Haliotis Shell) may be added, as may Gou Qi Zi (Lycium Fruit) and Ju Hua (Chrysanthemum) to enhance clinical efficacy. This formula is contraindicated in cases in which digestive weakness is present and in debilitated animals. It should also not be used for patients that have advanced dryness with powdery dander, poor hair growth, weight loss, a thin and dry tongue, and a thin, floating pulse. Use should be stopped immediately if loss of appetite, lethargy, or watery diarrhea occurs. Clinical indications for the use of this formula include swollen lids, ocular discharge, photophobia and miosis, corneal opacity, heat intolerance, excessive appetite and thirst, aggression, a red or pale tongue, and a surging, fast pulse.
- For Yin deficiency syndrome, **Qi Ju Di Huang Wan** should be considered. Guiding symptoms include late-stage or chronic ulcers, thick, mucoid ocular discharge, pupil atrophy and dilation indicating some blindness, corneal opacity or general clouding, and a thin, rapid, or floating pulse. The tongue may be delicate, pale, and peeled, dry and red.
- Mi Meng Hua *(Buddleia officinalis)* may be useful for indolent ulcers because of its reputation in Chinese medicine for preserving blood supply to the superficial eye tissues. It may be added to any of the formulas listed, given that it is appropriate in both excess and deficient types of cases.
- Topical use of Eyebright eyedrops may support the action of the Chinese herbs listed by helping reduce the progression of lesions.
- Useful acupuncture points for congestive cases include ST 8, GB 20, LI 4, BL 10, CV 12, and ST 43. ST 8 decongests the head and treats the eye. It is a major intersection point for the Gall Bladder and Stomach meridians, both

of which are important in eye disorders. GB 20 is a regional point important in treating eye disorders. LI 4 clears Heat from the entire facial region. BL 10 is a regional point to treat eye disorders by decongesting the Bladder channel where it originates at the medial canthus. CV 12 is an important point to stop the formation of congesting Dampness in dogs and cats. ST 43 is a distal point with secondary indications of clearing Heat and redness from the eye and face.

AUTHORS' CHOICES:

SM: Qi Ju Di Huang Wan for Yin deficiency; autologous serum; apply Eyebright topically.

SW: Conventional treatments including acetylcysteine; autologous serum; Qi Ju Di Huang Wan.

KERATOCONJUNCTIVITIS SICCA

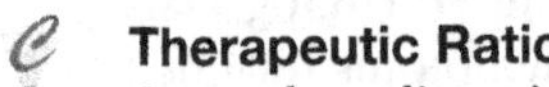

Therapeutic Rationale

- Control predisposing and secondary disorders.
- Keep eyes clean.
- Provide lubrication.

Paradigmatic Options

Chinese Medicine

- Keratoconjunctivitis sicca (KCS) is almost invariably associated with Blood deficiency in dogs. Blood deficiency seems to underlie over half of all cases of allergic dermatitis in dogs, and allergic dermatitis and KCS are often found to coexist in the same patient.
- KCS seldom has to be treated primarily and seems highly responsive to herbal formulas appropriate to the manifestation of Blood deficiency in the patient. Other common clinical syndromes arising from Blood deficiency include recurrent mast cell tumors; superficial neoplasms such as hemangiomas,

hemangiosarcomas, and thyroid adenocarcinomas; masticatory myositis; and fear aggression.

- To address KCS in patients with other Blood deficiency–related complaints, the practitioner should use the formula appropriate to the underlying problem and, if desired, add additional herbs to address KCS. Additional herbs that are of benefit include Gou Qi Zi (Lycium Fruit), Ju Hua (Chrysanthemum), and Mi Meng Hua (Buddleia Flower).
- For all of the following formulas, a *suggested starting dose* of granular concentrate is ¼ tsp per 10 to 15 lb of body weight, or 60 to 75 mg/kg of body weight, given at least once daily.
- The basic herbal formula for Blood deficiency is **Si Wu Tang** (Four Materials Decoction). The main herbal formula for Blood deficiency that causes allergic dermatitis is **Si Wu Xiao Feng Yin** (Four Materials Eliminate the Wind Decoction). For superficial neoplasms arising from Blood deficiency, **Xue Fu Zhu Ye Tang** (Drive Out Stasis in the Mansion of Blood Decoction) can be used. Guiding symptoms for all of these formulas include thin, wiry pulses, a pale or lavender tongue, fear aggression, fine dander, excessive dreaming, and slow hair regrowth.
- When Blood deficiency has progressed to Yin deficiency, **Qi Ju Di Huang Wan** (Lycium, Chrysanthemum, and Rehmannia Pill) can be considered. The section on indolent ulcers includes further discussion of this formula.
- Acupuncture point prescriptions are aimed at enhancing Blood production in the body. They include BL 18, SP 6, CV 12, ST 36, and LIV 3. GB 41 may be needled to influence tear production. GB 20 can indirectly affect the eyes. LI 4 influences the entire face and aids in the tonification of Qi and Blood.

AUTHORS' CHOICES:

SM: Si Wu Xiao Feng Yin; Xue Fu Zhu Ye Tang.
SW: Cyclosporin topically.

RETINAL DISEASE, INCLUDING PROGRESSIVE RETINAL ATROPHY

Therapeutic Rationale

- Reduce inflammation when present.
- Address nutritional deficiency.
- Address underlying disorders.

Alternative Options with Conventional Bases

Systemic Herbs

- **Bilberry:** older studies done in Italy suggest that Bilberry improves retinal function. This effect is believed referable to its content of bioflavonoids. Over-the-counter products for human use in retinal disorders frequently include bioflavonoid extracts from other plants, most notably Rutin. These bioflavonoid extracts show some evidence of being able to preserve the vascular integrity of the retina. The *suggested dose* is 60 to 240 mg bid.

Nutrition

- **Zinc:** thought to be related to the development of human macular degeneration. The dosage in dogs and cats is approximately 4 mg/kg of body weight daily po for Zinc methionine; 10 mg/kg of body weight daily po for Zinc sulfate; and 5 mg/kg of body weight daily po for Zinc gluconate.
- **Taurine:** Taurine deficiency retinopathy is recognized in cats. Although it is unlikely to occur if the cat is eating a balanced diet, homemade diets may be deficient in Taurine. Taurine is safe and worth supplementing as a trial to any cat with retinal blindness.
- **Antioxidants:** Vitamin E deficiency can damage retinal photoreceptors, and retinal lesions are observed in dogs with Vitamin E deficiency (Davidson, 1998). Vitamin A may be helpful in preventing human retinal diseases.
- **Fish Oil:** docosahexanoic acid (DHA) deficiency has been implicated in retinal degeneration (Waldron, 1998), and DHA has been suggested as helpful in arresting the progress of the disease.

Paradigmatic Options

- Progressive retinal atrophy seems to be consistently associated with relatively severe Damp Heat accumulations in the head from a Chinese medical perspective. This Damp Heat may be metaphorically construed to dry out and sear the blood supply to the retina. The patient with progressive retinal atrophy (PRA) is thus significantly hotter than the damp patient with cataracts when their symptoms and clinical findings are interpreted from the Chinese medical perspective. More aggressive Damp Heat–clearing herbs are usually called for in patients with PRA to halt further deterioration.
- Sight is seldom restored when it has been completely lost in chronic cases. The best chance for sight preservation is in early cases and when an animal is acutely affected.
- Success in halting vision deterioration with the formulas listed in the following section suggests that the animal's diet should be reviewed for possible allergens or compounds to which the animal is sensitive.
- Dietary recommendations cited for cataracts may be followed.

Chinese Medicine

- **Long Dan Xie Gan Tang** (Gentian Purge the Liver Decoction) is an exceptional formula for clearing Damp Heat from the Liver, Gall Bladder, and head, especially in cases of acute onset. However, the formula may cause severe lethargy and loss of appetite if it is used inappropriately. It should be used only when the patient's tongue is red and the pulse is excessive (wiry, forceful, or rapid). Once the patient's condition is stabilized, long-term use of **Si Miao San** can be considered.
- For cases in which some Spleen Qi deficiency is evident, precluding the use of Long Dan Xie Gan Tang, **Si Miao San** (Four Miracles Powder) can be considered. Although not as specific for eye disorders as Long Dan Xie Gan Tang, Si Miao San does stop the further creation of Dampness by the Spleen, possibly preventing additional vision loss.

- A *suggested starting dose* of granular concentrate for both formulas is ¼ tsp per 10 to 15 lb of body weight, or 60 to 75 mg/kg of body weight, divided into two daily doses.
- Acupuncture treatment of PRA should make liberal use of distal points, including LI 4, GB 41, LIV 2 and 3, TH 4 and 5, and GB 37. A useful local point is Tai Yang. All of these points are powerful in their effect of clearing Heat from the head and eyes.

Chiropractic

- Cervical and upper thoracic vertebral fixations are common in dogs with PRA. Their presence might be construed from a chiropractic point of view as promoting congestion in the head and neck. From a Chinese medical point of view, this congestion would aggravate the body's tendency to accumulate Heat pathogens in the head. Adjustment of vertebral fixations when it is otherwise deemed safe to do so is recommended in the treatment of PRA.

AUTHORS' CHOICES:

SM: Bilberry and other bioflavonoid compounds; chiropractic adjustment; Damp Heat–clearing herbal formulas appropriate to the case supplemented by acupuncture.

SW: Antioxidants; Bilberry; appropriate Chinese herbal formula in acute cases.

15 CASE REPORT
Ulcerative Conjunctivitis in a Dog

HISTORY

Taz, a 4-month-old, male Bichon Frise, had a history of pannus of acute onset. Taz had received the final in his series of multivalent puppy vaccinations less than 1 month earlier and had become "sick, hot, and listless" 10 days later. His veterinarian at the time tentatively diagnosed an acute bacterial infection, hospitalized the dog, and initiated treatment with parenteral fluids and antibiotics. While Taz was hospitalized, he had severe conjunctival swelling. This swelling continued even as Taz generally improved in response to treatment. The veterinarian prescribed a 10-day course of oral corticosteroids followed by a 10-day course of antihistamines. Taz did not respond to either drug.

Shortly after the drugs were discontinued, Taz's conjunctivitis worsened and the conjunctiva became severely ulcerated. In addition, copious epiphora developed. Taz was taken to the veterinary emergency clinic, and after physical examination autoimmune conjunctivitis was presumptively diagnosed. Lifelong treatment with corticosteroids was prescribed along with an eye ointment containing topical hydrocortisone that ameliorated the swelling slightly. Dissatisfied with Taz's response to treatment and concerned about the possible side effects of giving her dog corticosteroids for life, the owner discontinued use of the corticosteroids, and consulted a veterinarian with a special interest in alternative medicine.

Further questioning revealed that Taz had a history of eye discharge ranging from green-yellow to black. He was a nervous dog, and his appetite had recently become reduced by about 50% for unknown reasons. His diet consisted of a well-known brand of dry puppy food. Taz was described as extremely thirsty and somewhat polyuric.

PHYSICAL EXAMINATION

On physical examination, Taz's conjunctivae were severely ulcerated and bleeding, with the right eye particularly affected. Fluorescein dye tests ruled out any accompanying corneal pathologic problems. Taz's tongue was pale, lavender, and dry. His pulses were thin, rapid, and wiry.

ASSESSMENT

In Chinese medicine, severe destructive lesions of any type or at any location are described as caused by Toxic Heat. Toxic Heat is also the term applied to illnesses that sweep through a community accompanied by especially severe symptoms. Toxic Heat thus equates with epidemics in conventional medicine. The tendency for the body to occasionally manifest toxic Heat signs in response to vaccinations is thus not unexpected, given that they are modified live forms of organisms that spread in epidemic fashion.

Besides ulcerative conjunctivitis, signs of Heat exhibited by Taz included yellow discharges, rapid, wiry pulses, extreme thirst, high fever, and bright red hemorrhage. Extreme Heat may "injure the Qi," which results in a loss of appetite and extreme listlessness.

The external structures of the eyes are considered to fall under the influence of the Chinese medical concept of the Liver. Taz's Chinese medical diagnosis was thus considered to be Toxic Heat accumulation in the Liver. **Long Dan Xie Gan Tang** (Gentian Purge the Liver Decoction) was prescribed, given its ability to drain severe Heat accumulations from the Liver channel. It is also commonly considered for any severe acute pathologic condition of the eye, including conjunctivitis. Even though Taz did not have the typical tongue appearance calling for use of this formula in dogs, the history and physical findings otherwise provided a compelling case for its use. Two grams each of granular concentrates of Ju Hua *(Chrysanthemum)*, Bo He *(Mentha)*, and Man Jing Zi *(Vitex)* were added to 25 g of base formula to improve Long Dan Xie Gan Tang's ability to clear redness, inflammation, and Heat from the eyes. Taz was prescribed ¼ tsp twice daily.

OUTCOME

Within 4 days Taz's eye condition appeared improved. His water consumption had decreased dramatically, although his appetite remained low and he had even vomited yellow fluid twice one morning. His energy level had improved, however. Physical examination revealed his conjunctival swelling and inflammation to be approximately 50% resolved. Taz's pulses remained rapid but were less wiry, and his tongue remained slightly pale pink to lavender. Because of concern that the vomiting may have represented an injury of the Spleen Qi by the aggressive cooling action of the formula, Taz's dose of Long Dan Xie Gan Tang was reduced by half.

Ten days later, Taz's conjunctival inflammation had largely resolved. His appetite had returned, and there had been no further incidences of vomiting. His thirst and pulses were now normal. Shortly afterward the formula was discontinued, and the condition did not recur.

SM

REFERENCES

Alche LE, Berra A, Veloso MJ, Coto CE. Treatment with meliacine, a plant derived antiviral, prevents the development of herpetic stromal keratitis in mice. *J Med Virol* 61(4):474-480, 2000.

Arens M, Travis S. Zinc salts inactivate clinical isolates of herpes simplex virus in vitro. *J Clin Microbiol* 38(5):1758-1762, 2000.

Bensky D, Gamble A. *Chinese Herbal Materia Medica*, revised ed. Seattle, 1993, Eastland Press.

Biswas NR, Beri S, Das GK, Mongre PK. Comparative double blind multicentric randomised placebo controlled clinical trial of a herbal preparation of eye drops in some ocular ailments. *J Indian Med Assoc* 94(3):101-102, 1996.

Brooks DE, Garcia GA, Dreyer EB, Zurakowski D, Franco-Bourland RE. Vitreous body glutamate concentration in dogs with glaucoma. *Am J Vet Res* 58(8):864-867, 1997.

Chiou GC, Stolowich NJ, Zheng YQ, Shen ZF, Zhu M, Min ZD. Effects of some natural products on sugar cataract studied with nuclear magnetic resonance spectroscopy. *J Ocul Pharmacol* 8(2):115-120, 1992.

Collins K, Nasisse M, Moore C. In vitro efficacy of L-lysine against feline herpesvirus type-1. *Proceedings of the American College of Veterinary Ophthalmology*, p.141, 1995.

Das GK, Pandey RM, Biswas NR. Comparative double masked randomised placebo controlled clinical trial of a herbal eye drop preparation in trachoma and conjunctivitis. *J Indian Med Assoc* (10):383-384, 1995.

Davidson MG, Geoly FJ, Gilger BC, McLellan GJ, Whitley W. Retinal degeneration associated with vitamin E deficiency in hunting dogs. *J Am Vet Med Assoc* 213:645-651, 1998.

Davies KJ. Oxidative stress: the paradox of aerobic life. *Biochem Soc Symp* 61:1-31, 1995.

Dimitrova Z, Dimov B, Manolova N, Pancheva S, Ilieva D, Shishkov S. Antiherpes effect of *Melissa officinalis* L. extracts. *Acta Microbiol Bulg* 29:65-72, 1993.

Fox SL. The use of glycine in the reduction of intraocular pressure. *Eye, Ear, Nose Throat Mon* 51:35, 1972.

Fruehauf H, Dharmananda S. *Pearls from the Golden Cabinet: The Practitioner's Guide to the Use of Chinese Herbs and Traditional Formulas*. Portland, Ore, 1994, Institute for Traditional Medicine.

Hu S, Dutt J, Zhao T, Foster CS. Tetrandrine potently inhibits herpes simplex virus type-1-induced keratitis in BALB/c mice. *Ocul Immunol Inflamm* 5(3):173-180, 1997.

Kilic F, Bhardwaj R, Caulfeild J, Trevithick JR. Modelling cortical cataractogenesis. 22. Is in vitro reduction of damage in model diabetic rat cataract by taurine due to its antioxidant activity? *Exp Eye Res* 69(3):291-300, 1999.

Kimata M, Shichijo M, Miura T, Serizawa I, Inagaki N, Nagai H. Effects of luteolin, quercetin and baicalein on immunoglobulin E–mediated mediator release from human cultured mast cells. *Clin Exp Allergy* 30(4):501-508, 2000.

Koytchev R, Alken RG, Dundarov S. Balm mint extract (Lo-701) for topical treatment of recurring herpes labialis. *Phytomedicine* 6(4):225-230, 1999.

Lyle BJ, Mares-Perlman JA, Klein BE, Klein R, Palta M, Bowen PE, Greger JL. Serum carotenoids and tocopherols and incidence of age-related nuclear cataract. *Am J Clin Nutr* 69(2):272-277, 1999.

MacMillan AD, Nelson DL, Munger RJ, Wolf ED, Scagliotti RH, Bellhorn RW, Shaw D, Schmidt G, Dice PF. Efficacy of zinc citrate ascorbate for treatment of canine cataracts. *J Am Vet Med Assoc* 194(11):1581-1582, 1989.

Maggs DJ, Nasisse MP. Effects of oral L-lysine supplementation on the ocular shedding rate of feline herpesvirus (FHV-1) in cats. Proceedings of 28th

Annual Meeting of the American College of Veterinary Ophthalmology, Santa Fe, NM, 1997.

Mares-Perlman JA, Lyle BJ, Klein R, Fisher AI, Brady WE, VandenLangenberg GM, Trabulsi JN, Palta M. Vitamin supplement use and incident cataracts in a population-based study, *Arch Ophthalmol* 118(11):1556-1563, 2000.

Matsuda H, Cai H, Kubo M, Tosa H, Iinuma M. Study on anti-cataract drugs from natural sources. II. Effects of buddlejae flos on in vitro aldose reductase activity. *Biol Pharm Bull* 18(3):463-466, 1995.

Mills S, Bone K. *Principles and Practice of Phytotherapy*. New York, 2000, Churchill Livingstone.

Ozturk F, Kurt E, Cerci M, Emiroglu L, Inan U, Turker M, Ilker S. The effect of propolis extract in experimental chemical corneal injury. *Ophthalmic Res* 32(1):13, 2000.

Schey KL, Patat S, Chignell CF, Datillo M, Wang RH, Roberts JE. Photooxidation of lens alpha-crystallin by hypericin (active ingredient in St. John's Wort). *Photochem Photobiol* 72(2):200-203, 2000.

Seddon JM, Christen WG, Manson JE, LaMotte FS, Glynn RJ, Buring JE, Hennekens CH. The use of vitamin supplements and the risk of cataract among US male physicians. *Am J Public Health* 84(5):788-792, 1994.

Seth RK, Kharb S. Protective function of alpha-tocopherol against the process of cataractogenesis in humans. *Ann Nutr Metab* 43(5):286-289, 1999.

Smith VA, Hoh HB, Easty DL. Role of ocular matrix metalloproteinases in peripheral ulcerative keratitis. *Br J Ophthalmol* 83(12):1376-1383, 1999.

Stiles J, Townsend WM, Rogers QR, Krohne SG. Effect of oral administration of L-lysine on conjunctivitis caused by feline herpesvirus in cats. *Am J Vet Res* 63(1):99-103, 2002.

Tsubota K, Goto E, Shimmura S, Shimazaki J. Treatment of persistent corneal epithelial defect by autologous serum application. *Ophthalmology* 106(10):1984-1989, 1999.

Vynograd N, Vynograd I, Sosnowski Z. A comparative multi-centre study of the efficacy of propolis, acyclovir, and placebo in the treatment of genital herpes (HSV). *Phytomedicine* 7(1):1-6, 2000.

Waldron MK, Spencer AL, Bauer JE. Role of long-chain polyunsaturated n-3 fatty acids in the development of the nervous system of dogs and cats. *J Am Vet Med Assoc* 213:619-621, 1998.

Weiss RF, Fintelmann V. *Herbal Medicine*, ed 2. New York, 2000, Thieme.

Xie H, Veterinary Herbal Medicine Training Program (class notes). Chi Institute of Chinese Medicine, Reddick, Fla, pp 37-38, 2000.

16

Therapies for Respiratory Disorders

ASTHMA, FELINE

Therapeutic Rationale

- Manage underlying disorders, including lung parasites.
- Manage inflammation.
- Control bronchoconstriction.

Alternative Options with Conventional Bases

- Some practitioners have noted that asthmatic cats often have acute exacerbations of their disease shortly after being vaccinated. A thorough consideration of the risk versus the need for protection against feline viral diseases is advisable.

Nutritional Therapies

- Food allergens are increasingly recognized as a factor in human allergic respiratory disease (Baker, 2000). An elimination diet trial occasionally improves signs in asthmatic cats.
- **Fish Oil:** in a study of asthmatic children a small dose of Fish Oil decreased symptom scores (Nagakura, 2000). Fish is a common food allergen in cats, so Fish Oil should be considered in the context of investigating the role of food allergy. Fish Oil as a supplement should be given to cats as ½ to 1 capsule daily (containing approximately 200 mg of docosahexanoic acid [DHA] and 300 mg of eicosapentaenoic acid [EPA]).
- **Antioxidants:** their role in asthma has been the focus of much asthma research. Antioxidant "defense" mechanisms appear to be compromised in human asthma patients, and low dietary intake of antioxidant

vitamins may or may not be related to the severity of the disease (Picado, 2001; Soutar, 1997). In one animal model, Vitamin E reduced ovalbumin-induced bronchospasm by 51% (Stetinova, 2000). Large clinical intervention trials are not available. Antioxidant supplementation is safe and may have benefit. We recommend a mixed supplement containing at least Vitamin E, Vitamin C, and Selenium.

- **Magnesium:** used in human medicine as an emergency intravenous bronchodilator in acute asthma attacks. Hypomagnesemia appears to be common in humans with asthma (Alamoudi, 2000). How this finding relates to cats that eat complete and balanced diets is unknown, although low serum magnesium is a common finding in hospitalized cats and is associated with lower survival (Toll, 2002). In the single trial in which Magnesium supplements were given to stable, chronic asthmatic patients, Magnesium was given intravenously only once and there was no effect. If asthmatic patients have some metabolic defect interfering with Magnesium availability, it is possible that long-term supplementation would be of greater benefit.
- **Pyridoxine:** has been suggested to benefit asthmatic patients. Pyridoxine corrects a metabolic abnormality in some human patients, but in a controlled trial 300 mg daily of Pyridoxine was not effective in improving measurements of respiratory compromise.

Herbs

- **Herbs that have been used traditionally** but for which no support can be found include Khella *(Ammi visnaga)*, Licorice *(Glycyrrhiza uralensis)*, and Lobelia *(Lobelia inflata)*. The latter is a very powerful herb that should be used cautiously.
- **Butterbur** *(Petasites formosanus):* has spasmolytic and antimuscarinic activity that supports its traditional use in asthma (Ko, 2001). It contains hepatotoxic pyrrolizidine alkaloids.
- ***Tylophora indica asthmatica:*** a traditional Ayurvedic herb that may have antiallergic activity but is associated with adverse effects when given alone.

- **Coleus** *(Coleus forskolii):* a traditional Ayurvedic herb that has mild bronchodilating activity.
- **Coltsfoot** *(Tussilago farfara):* has been used in Western herbal medicine and traditional Chinese medicine (TCM). It contains a mucilage and inhibits platelet-activating factor (PAF). The Coltsfoot constituent tussilagone was also shown to have a pressor effect in cats and dogs when given intravenously (IV) and stimulated respiration. Although Coltsfoot may be effective (no animal or clinical studies to evaluate it are available), it contains pyrrolizidine alkaloids, which have been associated with hepatic venoocclusive disease.
- **Ginkgo** *(Ginkgo biloba):* also contains factors that inhibit PAF, which is thought to play a role in the inflammatory cascade in asthma. Ginkgo extract has been shown to inhibit bronchoconstriction in a guinea pig model (Touvay, 1986).
- **Saiboku-To:** has been found effective in humans and laboratory animal models but has not been tested in dogs or cats. In a study of human subjects (Nakajima, 1993), Saiboku-To downregulated $beta_2$ receptors and $beta_2$ agonist activity. Two in vitro studies on dog respiratory epithelium suggest that the formula generates nitric oxide (Tamaoki, 1995) and potentiates beta-adrenergic function (Tamaoki, 1993). Saiboku-To has been associated with the development of inflammatory pneumonitis in humans after long-term use. It should be used only to lower the dose of conventional drugs and not as a long-term or a single agent.
- **Xiao Qing Long Tang** (Minor Blue-Green Dragon Decoction): has shown an ability to suppress bronchial inflammation in allergic mice (Kao, 2000). Its use has not been investigated in dogs, cats, or people but we have used it with success in cats in clinical practice.
- **Ja Wai San Zi Tang:** a modern formula. Li and others developed a version of it (MSSM-002) containing Perilla (Zi Su Zi), Descurainia (Ting Li Zi), Apricot (Xing Ren), Scutellaria (Huang Qin), Sophora (Ku Shen), Angelica (Dang Gui), Peony (Bai Shao), Kudzu (Ge Gen), Platycodon (Jei Gen), Licorice (Gan Cao),

Jujube (Da Zao), Ginger (Sheng Jiang), Pteria (Zhen Zhu Mu), and Reishi (Ling Zhi). In this study MSSM-002 not only suppressed the airway pressure-time index to a degree equivalent to dexamethasone, but also resulted in different cytokine profiles than dexamethasone. MSSM-002 shifted a TH2 pattern to a TH1 pattern, which suggests a different mechanism than that of dexamethasone.

Paradigmatic Options

Homeopathy

- **Silica 30C:** should be considered for asthma in cats that have an apparent vulnerability to respiratory infections that settle in the chest. Patients that benefit have a persistent cough, often with profuse mucoid sputum. Abundant rattling in the chest may be heard. The animals may be timid, noise sensitive, chilly, constipated, small in stature, and prone to chronic abscesses and weight loss. A *recommended dosage* is three pellets one to three times daily as needed.

Chinese Herbs

- In Chinese medicine asthma arises from a failure of Lung Qi to descend from its accumulation in the chest. Lung Qi obstruction by Phlegm accumulation is the most common cause of asthma in felines. A main cause of Phlegm accumulation in humans is consumption of foods to which the person is allergic, especially carbohydrates such as wheat and wheat-containing foods. A similar carbohydrate intolerance may be a cause of feline asthma.
- There are several herbal formulas to address Phlegm Obstruction of the Lungs as a cause of asthma. When Phlegm accumulations have slowly become heated by their prolonged presence in the body, the usual prescription is **Ding Chuan Tang** (Arrest Wheezing Powder). Suggestive signs that this formula may be of benefit include cough with yellow sputum, dyspnea, wheezing, increased thirst, possible fever, possible thick nasal discharge, a rapid, slippery pulse, and a red, moist, swollen tongue. A *suggested starting dose* is ¼ tsp

per 10 to 15 lb of body weight, or 60 to 75 mg/kg of body weight, divided into two daily doses.

- **Ding Chuan Tang** contains moderate amounts of Ephedra (Ma Huang), the natural source of the bronchodilator ephedrine, which accounts for some of its antiasthma activity. Other formulas containing small to moderate amounts of Ma Huang are also prescribed for asthma in cats if signs seem to warrant their use. These formulas contain only small amounts of ephedrine and thus are not associated with ephedrine toxicity. A further safeguard against side effects is to use the formulas only for appropriate patients. Two of these formulas are **Ma Xing Shi Gan Tang** (Ephedra, Apricot Kernel, Gypsum, and Licorice Decoction) and **Xiao Qing Long Tang** (Minor Blue-Green Dragon Decoction).
- In Chinese mythology the Blue-Green Dragon is the symbol for Yang energy, and its ascent into the sky epitomizes the triumph in the springtime of warm and dry Yang over cold and wet Yin. This legend inspired the name of the Chinese herbal formula for asthma that uses warming and drying herbs to help patients overcome attacks of coughing caused by copious bronchial fluid secretions. Patients that benefit from **Xiao Qing Long Tang** may be febrile but exhibit cold intolerance and dyspnea. They may also have accumulations of edema and a tendency to lassitude. The pulse is typically floating, and the tongue is pale, slimy, and wet. A *suggested starting dose* is ¼ tsp per 10 to 15 lb of body weight, or 60 to 75 mg/kg of body weight, divided into two daily doses.
- **Ma Xing Shi Gan Tang** (Ephedra, Apricot Kernel, Gypsum, and Licorice Decoction) is another formula to consider for chilly asthmatic cats that have a dry cough with minimal evidence of Phlegm. The animals are still short of breath, but exhibit an excess of internal heat despite their chills with elevated thirst, floating, rapid, or slippery pulses, and a red tongue. This presentation is seen mainly in acute cases.
- Not all formulas effective for asthmatic cats contain ephedrine. **Su Zi Jiang Qi Tang** (Perilla Descend the Qi Decoction) is frequently effective in relieving asthma in

older cats, manifesting as a recurrent or persistent moist cough. Patients may show early evidence of renal azotemia on laboratory tests, a swollen, lavender tongue, tenacious saliva, and a slippery or wiry pulse. Other signs include hind limb weakness and low back stiffness. A *suggested starting dose* is ¼ tsp per 10 to 15 lb of body weight, or 60 to 75 mg/kg of body weight, divided into two daily doses.

- When the animal shows less evidence of intolerance to cold and merely exhibits signs indicating an accumulation of Phlegm, a combination of **Er Chen Tang** (Two Cured Decoction) and **San Zi Yang Qin Tang** (Three Seeds Nursing the Parents Decoction) can be considered. The patient tends to have a recurrent cough that is worse on rising in the morning with expectoration of abundant white phlegm. Nausea, vomiting, fatigue, a poor appetite, loose stools, a wet and pale tongue, and a slippery pulse may also be present. A *suggested starting dose* is ¼ tsp per 10 to 15 lb of body weight, or 60 to 75 mg/kg of body weight, divided into two daily doses.
- Other causes of feline asthma seem to be rare in our practices, but some authors believe that they occur. One such cause is Lung Yin deficiency. A variety of herbal formulas have been developed to address coughing caused by Lung dryness. **Sha Shen Mai Dong Tang** (Glehnia and Ophiopogon Decoction) is a predominantly nourishing and moistening formula that is used to treat animals that have Lung Yin deficiency manifested as a low, dry cough, no nasal discharge, increased thirst, heat intolerance, a red, dry tongue, and a thready, weak pulse. A *suggested starting dose* is ¼ tsp per 10 to 15 lb of body weight, or 60 to 75 mg/kg of body weight, divided into two daily doses.
- When sputum accumulations are thicker, more yellow, and even purulent, **Qing Fei Zhi Suo Fang** can be considered. It contains 12 g Bei Sha Shen, 12 g Tian Men Dong, 12 g Mai Men Dong, 6.5 g Ren Shen, and 11.5 g each Bai He, Bei Mu, Xing Ren, Gua Lou Pi, and Dong Gua Ren. Patients that benefit may cough more at night, be thirsty, and have a red, dry tongue and a rapid and thin pulse. When the cough is frequent, dry,

and exhausting in a Yin-deficient patient, **Mai Wei Di Huang Wan** (Ophiopogon, Schizandra, and Rehmannia Pill) should be considered. Animals that benefit are often older and exhibit signs of Kidney Yin deficiency, including weight loss, weakness, a red, dry tongue, and a floating, thin, and perhaps rapid pulse. A *suggested starting dose* for both formulas is ¼ tsp per 10 to 15 lb of body weight, or 60 to 75 mg/kg of body weight, divided into two daily doses.

- As chronic coughing continues, injury to Lung Qi may arise as well as injury to Lung Yin. The classic formula for this disorder in humans is **Mai Men Dong Tang** (Ophiopogon Decoction). Feline patients that benefit have mild Phlegm accumulations and depletion of Lung Qi and Yin. Signs include weakness and shortness of breath from a chronic, dry cough with tenacious phlegm. Patients are thirsty and have a red, dry tongue tip and a weak, rapid pulse. A *suggested starting dose* is ¼ tsp per 10 to 15 lb of body weight, or 60 to 75 mg/kg of body weight, divided into two daily doses.
- **Bu Fei Tang** (Tonify the Lung Decoction) may also be considered for the Qi- and Yin-deficient patient. Signs include a chronic asthmatic cough with thin and scanty sputum, low energy, a weak voice, cold intolerance, pallor, and weakness. The practitioner should consider Bu Fei Tang over Mai Men Dong Tang when the patient has slight evidence of a lingering Phlegm-Heat condition. The tongue is typically pale in this patient, and the pulse is often soft. A *suggested starting dose* is ¼ tsp per 10 to 15 lb of body weight, or 60 to 75 mg/kg of body weight, divided into two daily doses.
- Bu Fei Tang contains some components of a small formula known as **Sheng Mai San** (Generate the Pulse Powder). This is the classic formula for strongly tonifying Qi, nourishing Yin, and stopping coughing. Unlike Bu Fei Tang, it has no Heat-clearing or Phlegm-transforming action. A *suggested starting dose* is ¼ tsp per 10 to 15 lb of body weight, or 60 to 75 mg/kg of body weight, divided into two daily doses.
- As Qi deficiency becomes more severe, it progresses from simple Lung Qi deficiency to Lung and Kidney Qi

deficiency. The patient has a chronic asthmatic cough, feeble respiration, shortness of breath, aversion to cold, exercise intolerance, and a pale, wet tongue. A formula to address this problem is **Ren Shen Ge Jie San** (Ginseng and Gecko Powder). It acts to tonify Lung and Spleen Qi and to enable the Kidneys to grasp descending Lung Qi. This formula contains a smaller formula, **Shen Jie San,** which contains only Ren Shen (Ginseng) and Ge Jie (Gecko). These two "herbs" act to tonify Lung and Kidney Qi, respectively. Included with them in the larger formula are herbs that allow the formula to address complications of Spleen and Lung Qi deficiency, including Phlegm and Dampness accumulations that have resulted in wheezing, yellow sputum, and Heat in the chest. This formula may be useful for the management of asthma in aged cats. A *suggested starting dose* is ¼ tsp per 10 to 15 lb of body weight, or 60 to 75 mg/kg of body weight, divided into two daily doses.

- As in Western herbalism mustard poultices are used in Chinese medicine to relieve chest congestion. Advocates of this technique apply mustard, known in Chinese medicine as Bai Jie Zi Tu Fa, to the skin over BL 13, 20, 43, and 44. The mustard should be washed off the skin after approximately 10 minutes of exposure, and it should be used only to supplement the effects of oral formulas by being applied as needed up to twice daily.
- Acupuncture can augment the action of Chinese herbal formulas. For Yin deficiency the practitioner should consider BL 13, LU 5, LU 7, and KI 6. For Phlegm accumulations, BL 13, BL 20, LU 9, SP 3, ST 40, LI 4, PC 6, and SP 4 should be considered. Asthmatic cats often have upper thoracic fixations that should be relieved through chiropractic manipulation. Not surprisingly, many acupuncture points in the upper thoracic area can be used to address asthma, including the extra point Ding Chuan, BL 12, and BL 13.

Hydrotherapy

- **"Hot Fomentations"** are a traditional hydrotherapy technique used by naturopathic physicians to rapidly relieve pulmonary congestion. They appear to also be effective in cats with acute pulmonary congestion and mild to moderate dyspnea. A small hand towel is soaked in water, wrung out, and microwaved until steaming hot but not too hot to hold. When the towel is at the right temperature, it is wrapped around the cat's chest and left in place for 3 minutes. Then a cold cloth wrung out tightly after being soaked in ice water is vigorously rubbed over the cat's chest for 1 minute. The entire process is repeated two more times. After just this simple procedure, an obvious and immediate improvement often occurs in the cat's level of dyspnea. The efficacy of this technique uses the same hemodynamic reflexes as a mustard poultice to relieve pulmonary congestion. Increased perfusion of superficial vessels and capillaries is believed to produce a reflexive vasoconstriction in visceral structures located immediately beneath.

Cautions

- Herbs said to contain sympathomimetic amines (Aniseed, Capsicum, Parsley, Vervain) or hypertensive activity (Bayberry, Broom, Blue Cohosh, Licorice) may interact with or increase the activity of common bronchodilators.

AUTHORS' CHOICES:

SM: Appropriate Chinese herbal formula; Su Zi Jiang Qi Tang; Ren Shen Ge Jie San; hypoallergenic and low-carbohydrate diet.
SW: Hypoallergenic or homemade diet; Fish Oil; Xiao Qing Long Tang or other Chinese herbal formulas.

BRONCHITIS, CANINE

Therapeutic Rationale

- Suppress cough.
- Reduce bronchoconstriction and reactivity.
- Reduce chronic inflammation, which leads to bronchoconstriction and excess mucus production.
- Improve partial arterial oxygen tension.
- Treat infections, if present.

Alternative Options with Conventional Bases

Nutritional Therapies

- Food allergens are increasingly recognized as a factor in human allergic respiratory disease (Baker, 2000). An attempt to improve the quality of the animal's diet, and perhaps institute an elimination program, occasionally proves helpful.
- **Fish Oil:** in a study of asthmatic children a small dose of Fish Oil decreased symptom scores (Nagakura, 2000). Fish Oil supplements should be given as one capsule daily (containing approximately 120 mg of DHA and 180 mg of EPA) per 10 to 15 lb of body weight.
- **Antioxidants:** their role in asthma have been the focus of much asthma research. Antioxidant "defense" mechanisms appear to be compromised in human patients with asthma, and low dietary intake of antioxidant vitamins may or may not be related to the severity of the disease (Picado, 2001; Soutar, 1997). In one animal model Vitamin E reduced ovalbumin-induced bronchospasm by 51% (Stetinova, 2000). Larger clinical intervention trials are not available. Antioxidant supplementation is safe and may have benefit. We recommend a broad-spectrum antioxidant supplement.
- ***N*-Acetylcysteine** (NAC): has been suggested for treatment of asthma. Studies in laboratory animals have been encouraging, but clinical studies in humans have yielded less encouraging results (Grandjean, 2000; Stey, 2000). A case series in German reports that six dogs treated with NAC improved (Staudacher, 1989).
- **Pyridoxine:** has been suggested to benefit asthmatic patients. Pyridoxine corrects a metabolic abnormality in some human patients, but in a controlled trial 300 mg daily of Pyridoxine was not effective in improving measurements of respiratory compromise.

Herbs

- **Herbs that have been used traditionally** but for which no support can be found include Khella, Licorice, and Lobelia. The latter is a powerful herb that should be used cautiously.

- **Butterbur** *(Petasites formosanus):* has spasmolytic and antimuscarinic activity that supports its traditional use in human allergic respiratory disease (Ko, 2001). It contains hepatotoxic pyrrolizidine alkaloids.
- ***Tylophora indica asthmatica:*** a traditional Ayurvedic herb that may have antiallergic activity but is associated with adverse effects when given alone.
- **Coleus:** a traditional Ayurvedic herb that has mild bronchodilating activity.
- **Coltsfoot:** has been used in Western herbal medicine and TCM. It contains a mucilage and inhibits platelet activating factor (PAF). Although Coltsfoot may be effective (no animal or clinical studies to evaluate it are available), it contains pyrrolizidine alkaloids, which have been associated with hepatic venoocclusive disease. The Coltsfoot constituent tussilagone was also shown to have a pressor effect in cats and dogs when given IV, and it stimulated respiration.
- **Ginkgo:** also contains ginkgolides that inhibit PAF, which is thought to play a role in the inflammatory cascade in asthma. Ginkgo extract has been shown to inhibit bronchoconstriction in a guinea pig model (Touvay, 1986).
- **Ren Shen Ge Jie San:** a traditional formula for long-standing Lung Qi deficiency that has been clinically helpful in managing canine allergic bronchitis. It has not been examined experimentally. Nonetheless, *Panax ginseng,* one of its components, has shown an ability to relax human bronchial smooth muscle by generating nitric oxide (Tamaoki, 2000).
- **Mai Men Dong Tang** (Ophiopogon Formula): appears to increase tracheal mucociliary transport velocity and decrease airway fluid protein content (Tai, 1999).
- **Saiboku-To:** has been found effective in humans and laboratory animal models but has not been tested in dogs or cats. In a study of human subjects (Nakajima, 1993), Saiboku-To downregulated beta$_2$ receptors and beta$_2$ agonist activity. Two in vitro studies on dog respiratory epithelium suggest that the formula generates nitric oxide (Tamaoki, 1995) and potentiates beta-adrenergic function (Tamaoki, 1993). Saiboku-To has

been associated with the development of inflammatory pneumonitis in humans after long-term use. It should be used only to lower the dose of conventional drugs and not as a long-term or a single agent.

- **Xiao Qing Long Tang** (Minor Bupleurum Decoction): has shown an ability to suppress bronchial inflammation in allergic mice (Kao, 2000). Its use for dogs, cats, or people has not been investigated, but we have used it with success in asthmatic cats in clinical practice.
- **Ja Wai San Zi Tang:** a modern formula. Li and others developed a version of it (MSSM-002) containing Perilla (Zi Su Zi), Descurainia (Ting Li Zi), Apricot (Xing Ren), Scutellaria (Huang Qin), Sophora (Ku Shen), Angelica (Dang Gui), Peony (Bai Shao), Kudzu (Ge Gen), Platycodon (Jei Gen), Licorice (Gan Cao), Jujube (Da Zao), Ginger (Sheng Jiang), Pteria (Zhen Zhu Mu), and Reishi (Ling Zhi). In this study MSSM-002 not only suppressed airway pressure-time index to a degree equivalent to dexamethasone, but also resulted in different cytokine profiles than dexamethasone. MSSM-002 shifted a TH2 pattern to a TH1 pattern, which suggests a different mechanism than that of dexamethasone.

Paradigmatic Options

Homeopathy

- Many remedies are listed for chronic cough. A few of the most effective or most commonly called for in my practice (SM) are discussed in this section. Although it is contrary to the tenets of classic homeopathy, different remedies can be used simultaneously as sort of a "homeopathic herbal formula" to achieve better effect.
- **Antimonium tartaricum 30C:** should be considered for cough with copious mucus that is aggravated when the animal is lying down, in warm rooms, and in cold, damp weather. The rattling of mucus in the chest may be audible. The *recommended dosage* is one to three times daily.
- **Bryonia alba 30C:** should be considered for a dry, hacking cough that is worse with exercise or even the slightest motion and better when the animal lies still,

especially with the head elevated. The *recommended dosage* is up to three times daily as needed.

- **Dulcamara 30C:** may prove effective for productive coughs that are aggravated by damp weather. Coughs may be spasmodic with excessive mucous secretions. There may be vomiting of white tenacious mucus and coughing of mucus after physical exertion. The *recommended dosage* is one to three times daily.
- **Phosphorus 30C:** can be considered for coughing and vomiting in very affectionate animals, especially when a loss of voice has occurred.

Chinese Herbs

- In my (SM) experience the cause of chronic cough in the majority of canine patients is Blood stasis. Indeed, in both Chinese and Western herbal traditions herbs that addressed chronic cough are invariably Blood movers. Centuries before it achieved prominence in the treatment of menstrual irregularities and bleeding disorders in humans, the original use of the famous Blood mover Dang Gui *(Angelica sinensis)* was for the treatment of chronic cough. It is an underlying predisposition to Blood deficiency that makes the dog predisposed to Blood stasis, just as a river with a low water level is more prone to breaking up into stagnant pools and oxbows.
- **Xue Fu Zhu Yu Tang** (Drive Out Stasis in the Mansion of Blood Decoction) is extremely well adapted to the treatment of chronic cough in dogs. Its numerous ingredients fulfill all the actions on a large scale that **Si Wu Tang** (Four Materials Decoction, which is part of Xue Fu Zhu Yu Tang) uses on a small scale to make Xue Fu Zhu Yu Tang one of the premier formulas to nourish Blood. That is, the formula recognizes through its ingredients the interdependence of Blood volume and ease of Blood circulation and the interdependence of Qi flow on Blood flow. All the herbs in the formula focus their efforts on moving Qi, moving Blood, or nourishing Blood, except Jie Geng, which guides the formula to the upper jiao and the lungs. The practitioner should consider this formula for dogs with thin, wiry pulses and a pale-pink or lavender tongue.

Guiding symptoms also include hacking, spasmodic, dry coughs, powdery fine dander, poor hair regrowth, a dry coat, fear aggression, dry eyes, mild intermittent lameness without apparent structural cause, a tendency to muscle spasms, dry forms of otitis externa, and allergic dermatitis with mild dry lesions and persistent itch. A *suggested starting dose* is ¼ tsp per 10 to 15 lb of body weight, or 60 to 75 mg/kg of body weight, divided into two daily doses.

- Although Xue Fu Zhu Yu Tang deserves the reputation of being the main formula to consider in tracheobronchitis caused by Blood deficiency and Blood stasis, another Blood formula that is more specific to lung complaints may be useful. This formula is **Bai He Gu Jin Tang** (Lily Bulb Preserve the Metal Decoction). Specifically, Bai He Gu Jin Tang moistens Lung Yin, moves Blood to stop cough, clears Empty Heat, and cools Blood to stop bleeding. The cooling and hemostatic actions of the formula make it especially worth considering for cases of hemoptysis resulting from Empty Fire, which is its traditional use. Its content of Blood tonics may also make it applicable for Blood-deficient dogs with dry, chronic cough, a tender tongue (pale to pink with thin edges and a lavender center), and a thin pulse. A *suggested starting dose* is ¼ tsp per 10 to 15 lb of body weight, or 60 to 75 mg/kg of body weight, divided into two daily doses.
- Acupuncture points that may potentiate the action of the two formulas in stopping chronic spasmodic coughs include BL 17, BL 11, ST 37, ST 39, and SP 10 to move and regulate the Blood; BL 13 and CV 17 to disperse the Lung Qi and move Blood in the chest; and LIV 3 to move Liver Qi and nourish Liver Blood.
- Other formulas that have been suggested for tracheobronchitis include the combination of **Er Chen Tang** (Two Cured Decoction) and **San Zi Yang Qin Tang** (Three Seeds Nursing the Parents Decoction). The patients that respond best reportedly have Phlegm-Cold manifested as a loud, wet cough, possible nasal discharge, lack of thirst, a wet, pale tongue, and a tight, slow pulse. They may have a recurring cough that is worse on rising in the morning with expectoration of

abundant white phlegm. There may also be nausea, vomiting, fatigue, a poor appetite, and loose stools. A *suggested starting dose* is ¼ tsp per 10 to 15 lb of body weight, or 60 to 75 mg/kg of body weight, divided into two daily doses. Acupuncture points to support the use of this formula include SP 4, PC 6, CV 12, and ST 40 to descend Qi and stop Phlegm formation.

- For Lung Qi and Yin deficiency leading to chronic dry cough, **Ren Shen Wu Wei Zi Tang** (Ginseng and Schizandra Decoction) should be considered. This formula is used to stop coughing in animals when no suggestion of Phlegm is present and the cough appears to be nonproductive. Huang Qi and Fang Feng can be added to the formula to reduce the patient's vulnerability to infectious tracheobronchitis. This formula may also be a consideration for use in some cases of thymic lymphoma when symptoms agree. Specific guiding symptoms to the use of this formula also include chronic forceless coughing, shortness of breath, fatigue, loss of appetite, weight loss, a pale tongue, and a soft pulse. A *suggested starting dose* is ¼ tsp per 10 to 15 lb of body weight, or 60 to 75 mg/kg of body weight, divided into two daily doses. Acupuncture points to treat Lung Yin deficiency include BL 13, LU 9, ST 36, and KI 3. Acupuncture points to address Qi deficiency include BL 13, BL 20, LU 9, ST 36, CV 12, CV 6, and CV 4.
- A formula that may be considered for older animals when the practitioner suspects that chronic cough has led to Kidney Qi deficiency is **Shen Qi Wan** (Kidney Qi Pill). Guiding signs and symptoms include shortness of breath, aversion to cold, exercise intolerance, and a pale, wet tongue. A *suggested starting dose* is ¼ tsp per 10 to 15 lb of body weight, or 60 to 75 mg/kg of body weight, divided into two daily doses.
- **Shen Qi Wan** might be especially useful for general support after **Su Zi Jiang Qi Tang** (Perilla Descend the Qi Decoction) has stabilized the patient's condition by resolving any tendency toward asthmatic cough with profuse saliva and sputum. Other signs indicating the potential usefulness of Shen Qi Wan and Su Zi Jiang Qi

Tang include low back pain or stiffness and hind limb weakness. Su Zi Jiang Qi Tang should be considered when the tongue is pale and lavender with tenacious saliva and the pulses are taut or slippery or weak. A *suggested starting dose* is ¼ tsp per 10 to 15 lb of body weight, or 60 to 75 mg/kg of body weight, divided into two daily doses. Acupuncture points to support the action of these two formulas are PC 6, ST 40, CV 12, KI 3, BL 23, and CV 4.

- Consideration can also be given to **Xiao Qing Long Tang** (Minor Blue-Green Dragon Decoction), **Bai He Gu Jin Tang** (Lily Bulb Preserve the Metal Decoction), and **Ren Shen Ge Jie San** (Ginseng and Gecko Powder). These formulas are discussed more fully in the section on Feline Asthma.

Western Herbs

- Western herbs, as prescribed by early "energetic" traditions, were extremely effective at dealing with chronic coughs, and were often superior to many Chinese formulas developed to address pulmonary complaints. Western herbal formulas that were used in the 1800s frequently fulfilled four principal objectives through their ingredients: improve pulmonary circulation, relax airway spasm, moisten airway linings, and dry up excess secretions. The herbs that fulfill these goals are discussed briefly below.
- Chronic coughing is considered in Chinese medicine to be caused by stagnant Blood in the chest. These coughs are distinguished by their "barking" or resonant nature. Interestingly, early Western herbal traditions held the same view, and herbs used to stop chronic coughing were also used to increase circulation in general. Examples of Blood-moving Western herbs to stop chronic coughs include **Red Root** *(Ceanothus americanus)*, **Gumweed** *(Grindelia squarrosa, G. camporum,* and other species), and even **Red Clover** *(Trifolium pratense)*. Some Blood-moving herbs that were used for congestive heart failure were used to treat chronic cough of respiratory origin, including **Bugleweed** *(Lycopus virginicus)*, **Motherwort** *(Leonurus cardiaca)*, and **Lily**

of the Valley *(Convallaria majalis)*. Herbs that warmed and invigorated the circulation were used to augment the action of Blood-moving herbs, especially **Lobelia** *(Lobelia inflata)*, **Cayenne** *(Capsicum)*, and **Pleurisy Root** *(Asclepias tuberosa)*.

- Demulcent herbs were used to moisten the airways to relieve dry tickling coughs and emolliate viscid airway secretions. These included **Marshmallow** *(Althea officinalis)*, **Slippery Elm** *(Ulmus fulva)*, and **Comfrey** *(Symphytum officinale)*. Comfrey has fallen into disfavor because of its toxic potential, but it was used frequently until the last decade because of its additional antitussive properties.
- Excessive airway secretions were also treated with Western herbs. Useful herbs included **Elecampane** *(Inula helenium)*, **Lobelia** *(Lobelia inflata)*, and **White Horehound** *(Marrubium vulgare)*.
- Antispasmodic herbs were employed to reduce resonant types of coughs. Antispasmodic herbs included **Licorice** *(Glycyrrhiza glabra)* and **Cherry Bark** *(Prunus* spp.). **Cherry bark** is an extremely effective antitussive but is potentially toxic in large doses because it contains small amounts of cyanide-containing compounds. Cherry Bark is still considered safe enough to be sold over the counter for human use. Licorice also acted to moisten airways.
- A shotgun formula for chronic pulmonary complaints popular in the 19th century contained herbs from all of these categories. Its ingredients were **Pleurisy Root, Comfrey Root, Licorice, Elecampane, Lobelia, Horehound,** and **Red Clover.** Although specific ratios for the different herbs were not listed, equal parts of each herb would produce an effective formula for a wide variety of etiologies. Note the effectiveness of these formulas even in the absence of strong antimicrobial constituents.

Cautions

- Herbs said to contain sympathomimetic amines (Aniseed, Capsicum, Parsley, Vervain) or hypertensive activity (Bayberry, Broom, Blue Cohosh, Licorice) may interact with or increase the activity of common bronchodilators.

AUTHORS' CHOICES:

SM: Xue Fu Zhu Yu Tang; homeopathic remedies.
SW: Diet improvement; Fish Oil; Chinese and Western herbs.

FELINE VIRAL UPPER RESPIRATORY DISEASE, ESPECIALLY HERPESVIRUS

Therapeutic Rationale

- Provide nutritional and fluid support.
- Control secondary bacterial infections.

Alternative Options with Conventional Bases

Nutritional Therapies

- **L-Lysine:** has been shown to reduce herpesvirus replication in cell cultures containing low arginine levels, but the effectiveness of simply adding L-lysine to an affected animal's normal diet is still in doubt. A recent controlled trial of eight cats showed that supplementation of 500 mg bid reduced clinical signs of conjunctivitis when cats were inoculated with FHV-1 (Stiles, 2002). Long-term use of L-lysine is often necessary, but the safety of high levels of L-lysine administered over a long term is unknown.
- **Vitamin C:** as ascorbate it inactivated herpes simplex virus in vitro, both alone and in combination with copper (Sagripanti, 1997). Vitamin C is one of the most popular alternative treatments for herpesvirus infection in cats, but it has not been investigated in clinical trials. Cats usually tolerate a dose of 250 mg daily well; overdose may lead to diarrhea.

Herbs

- **Echinacea** *(Echinacea purpurea, E. angustifolia):* has been examined extensively in the prevention and treatment of acute viral upper respiratory disease in humans. Echinacea probably acts on the innate immune system to activate mononuclear cells.
- Studies reporting on a total of 910 human subjects, all published in German, appear to suggest that Echinacea

significantly shortens the severity and duration of upper respiratory symptoms (the common cold). If used preventively it may enhance immunopathologic processes that account for some of the symptoms of viral upper respiratory infection (Percival, 2000). Echinacea use has not been examined in cats but is popular among cat owners. The literature on Echinacea warns consistently against use of the herb longer than 2 weeks. This is less a warning about toxicity than it is a guideline for effective use. Echinacea probably exerts its full effect on mononuclear cell production of cytokines within 2 weeks. Longer use will probably not have additional benefit and has been suggested to result in induction of tolerance by the animal's system. This is one reason that Echinacea is not recommended for long-term maintenance of cats infected with feline leukemia virus, feline immunodeficiency virus, or other chronic viral disease but is recommended to be used symptomatically for acute infections instead.

- **Lemon Balm** *(Melissa officinalis)*: has shown activity against HSV-1 in vitro. For cats, it is mixed in food at 500 mg to 1 g divided daily.

Paradigmatic Options

- See Chapter 9.

Homeopathy

- Homeopathy can be a profoundly useful way of managing acute viral upper respiratory infections in cats. Large populations can be treated easily, prophylactically, and inexpensively, thus making homeopathy the treatment of choice for clinics and kennels in which these infections tend to occur on a regular basis. Informal surveys of cat populations treated by homeopathic medicine have shown them to generally recover more quickly than cats treated with conventional medicine.
- **Allium cepa 30C:** useful for profuse, irritating serous nasal discharge that causes sneezing. The animal may also have lacrimation, burning, and photophobia of the eyes. The *recommended dosage* is one to three times daily as needed.

- **Belladonna 30C:** for cats with high fever, deep-red tongue, irritability and sensitivity to touch, nasal excoriations, inappetence, and dehydration. The *recommended dosage* is one to three times daily as needed.
- **Euphrasia officinalis 30C:** should be considered for cats with serous ocular discharge that may irritate the skin, swelling of the cheeks and lower lids, and possibly a profuse, bland nasal discharge. It is also helpful for persistent ophthalmia manifested as marked photophobia, blepharospasm, and blisters or ulcers of the cornea. The *recommended dosage* is one to three times daily as needed.
- **Ferrum phosphoricum 30C:** to rapidly reduce high fevers associated with initial viral infection. There are minimal symptoms that indicate its use beyond the fever and redness of the mouth, nose, and tongue. The *recommended dosage* is one to three times daily.

AUTHORS' CHOICES:

SM: Homeopathy.
SW: L-Lysine; Lemon Balm; Echinacea.

RHINITIS AND SINUSITIS

Therapeutic Rationale

- Depends on cause, which may be infectious, neoplastic, allergic, trauma, or foreign body.

Alternative Options with Conventional Bases

Nutritional Therapies

- Although food allergy is not a common cause of chronic rhinitis and sinusitis, its possibility as a cause to be ruled out is recognized in human medicine. Elimination diets should be considered in dogs and cats with chronic rhinitis.
- **Antioxidants:** may be clinically tested in the treatment of chronic rhinitis. In one study decreased antioxidants

were measured in the nasal mucosa of affected human patients (Westerveld, 1997). Considering the probable immune-enhancing capacity of antioxidants their effects may be multiple. A broad-spectrum antioxidant supplement is recommended.

Herbs

- **Nettles** *(Urtica dioica):* has been recommended as a single herb effective in the treatment of many allergic symptoms. In a double-blind, randomized trial of human patients, Nettles was effective in reducing symptoms (Mittman, 1990).
- **Butterbur** *(Petasites hybridus):* as effective as the antihistamine cetirizine in a controlled trial of 125 human patients with seasonal allergic rhinitis. The herb was supplied as extract ZE 339° standardized to 8 mg of total petasine per tablet; one tablet, four times daily (Schapowal, 2002). This herb may be difficult to find because suppliers are concerned about its pyrrolizidine alkaloid content, but this trial found no adverse effects. The extract can be given in doses proportional to that used in humans in this trial.
- **Sho-seiryu-to** (Minor Blue Green Dragon, Xiao Qing Long Tang): effective modulating inflammation of the nasal mucosa (Ikeda, 1994; Kao, 2000; Tanaka, 1998).

Paradigmatic Options

Homeopathy

- **Pulsatilla 30C:** may be helpful for bland or cream-colored nasal discharges in clingy, sensitive animals. The appetite of patients that benefit may be poor or sporadic, with the animal often eating only as long as the owner remains by the food dish. The *recommended dosage* is one to three times daily.

Chinese Herbs

- The most popular Chinese herbal formula among veterinarians for the management of rhinitis and sinusitis is **Cang Er Zi San** (Xanthium Powder). It has reportedly been very effective when used orally or as a steam treatment, although the exact method by which the formula is aerosolized as a vapor is not discussed. A single herb with similar Phlegm-dispelling effects that has been administered by steam inhalation in chronic sinusitis is Shi Chang Pu.

- Human patients that benefit from Cang Er Zi San have purulent nasal discharges, frontal and temporal headaches, and floating pulses. It is my (SM) impression that the popularity of this formula is undeserved given the infrequency with which it produces results. Some practitioners attempt to enhance its efficacy with the addition of 6 g Huang Qin, 9 g Ju Hua, 9 g Ge Gen, and 9 g Lian Qiao per 30 g of base formula for patients that appear to suffer from Wind-Heat. Their symptoms include increased thirst, yellow or green discharges, and a rapid, floating pulse. Acupuncture points that may reinforce the action of Cang Er Zi San include LU 7, LI 4, Bi Tong, LI 20, Yin Tang, and GB 20. The needle in Tai Yang should be retained as long as possible and even removed later at home by the owner.
- Another formula combination for use in Wind-Heat leading to sinusitis is **Huang Qin Hua Shi Tang** (Scutellaria and Talcum Decoction) with **Cang Er Zi San.** Animals that may benefit from this combination are described as having a turbid, yellow discharge, nasal congestion, loss of sense of smell, redness of the nasal cavity, nasal pain, headache, fatigue, loss of appetite, and perhaps even diarrhea. The tongue is red and the pulse is rapid, slippery, or soft. These symptoms describe not only a Wind-Heat invasion but also a coinciding Damp Heat of the Spleen and Stomach. A *suggested starting dose* is ¼ tsp per 10 to 15 lb of body weight, or 60 to 75 mg/kg of body weight, divided into two daily doses. Acupuncture points to support treatment include LI 20, Bi Tong, GV 23, SP 9, SP 6, ST 36, LI 4, and Yin Tang.
- When the patient has Spleen Qi deficiency leading to Phlegm accumulation, some authors advocate the use of **Bu Zhong Yi Qi Tang** (Tonify the Center to Boost the Qi Decoction) combined with **Cang Er Zi San** and given topically by inhalation. Patients that benefit

manifest chronic fatigue, nasal congestion, or clear discharge after overexertion. The tongue is pale and the pulse is soft. Bu Zhong Yi Qi Tang is apparently chosen to boost Spleen and Lung Qi in order to bolster Wei Qi, the superficial layer of protective Qi that prevents invasion of Pathogenic Winds. A *suggested starting dose* is ¼ tsp per 10 to 15 lb of body weight, or 60 to 75 mg/kg of body weight, divided into two daily doses.

- A more traditional formula used to strengthen Wei Qi is **Yu Ping Feng San** (Jade Wind Screen Powder). This formula is to be used between bouts of sinusitis. It should not be used in patients in which Qi deficiency is not present. A *suggested starting dose* is ¼ tsp per 10 to 15 lb of body weight, or 60 to 75 mg/kg of body weight, divided into two daily doses.
- A formula some herbalists advocate for sinusitis is **Xiao Qing Long Tong** (Minor Blue-Green Dragon Decoction). This formula was previously discussed in the section on Feline Asthma. It is recommended for use in animals with sinusitis when secretions are copious and the patient is cold intolerant. Other possible symptoms include a wet cough, dyspnea, accumulations of edema, and a tendency to lassitude. The pulse is typically floating and the tongue pale, slimy, and wet. A *suggested starting dose* is ¼ tsp per 10 to 15 lb of body weight, or 60 to 75 mg/kg of body weight, divided into two daily doses.

Western Herbs

- Acute, chronic, or recurrent sinusitis may be disorders for which traditional Western herbal approaches are more successful than Chinese herbal and modern botanical approaches. Both Chinese and modern medical herbal approaches to sinusitis seem, when analyzed pharmacologically, to emphasize the use of herbs with antimicrobial and immune-enhancing activity. Early Western herbalism seemed to view sinusitis as arising from chronically poor circulation through the sinuses, thereby reducing access of the immune system to the mucosal surfaces. Thus, although traditional Western herbal formulas contained herbs that would probably be categorized as drying Damp and dispersing Wind Heat by Chinese medical standards, they also contained herbs that would be classified as Qi movers. Even the Dampness-drying herbs, such as Eyebright *(Euphrasia officinalis)* and Elderberry Flower *(Sambucus nigra)*, seem to act by reducing sinus swelling via inhibiting mast cell degranulation. In contrast, most popular Chinese herbal formulas to address sinusitis are noticeably lacking in Qi movers, or herbs to improve general circulation.

- A deceptively simple formula that I (SM) have observed repeatedly to improve sinus circulation in sinusitis in dogs, cats, and humans is a combination of 15 ml Elderberry Flower, 10 ml Chamomile *(Matricaria recutita)*, 10 ml Pleurisy Root *(Asclepias tuberosa)*, and 15 ml Eyebright. Alcohol extracts are used. A *suggested starting dose* is 0.2 ml per 5 lb of body weight given twice daily. This is a safe and reasonably palatable formula that can be given for extended periods. Its lack of antimicrobial herbs does not seem to interfere with its potential for efficacy in bacterial sinusitis. It should be considered for use in any case of chronic sinus inflammation.

AUTHORS' CHOICES:

SM: Elderberry Flower and Pleurisy Root combination (see Western Herbs).
SW: Elimination diet; Fish Oil; Chinese herbs.

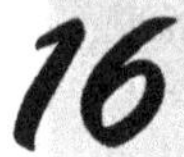

CASE REPORT
Chronic Cough and Collapsing Trachea in a Dog

HISTORY

Holly, an 11-year-old, female, spayed Yorkshire Terrier, was brought for treatment of a chronic cough secondary to a collapsing trachea. The collapsing trachea had been observed several years earlier, when the coughing first began, on survey lateral radiographs of the chest. No cardiac abnormalities had been observed, and no treatment had been prescribed. Over the succeeding years Holly's cough had become steadily worse.

At the time of presentation Holly's cough seemed worse at night and during periods of agitation. Since she was prone to anxiety, including fear of loud or unusual noises and of being left alone, it seemed to the owners that Holly was coughing all the time. The cough was described as "honking," and the owners often woke during the night to find Holly gasping for air. Holly also no longer seemed able to bark.

Holly had a tendency to abdominal bloating and gas. She also had chronic halitosis caused by severe periodontal disease. Because of concerns about anesthetic, risk dental scaling and polishing had not been performed.

Holly had had episodes of what were described as possible absence seizures in the past, characterized by episodic stiffness, trembling, and leaning against a wall for support. During these episodes Holly would not respond if her owners called to her and would bump into things as she staggered, which suggested a possible loss of sight. The episodes ceased after treatment with the Chinese herbal formula Tian Ma Gou Teng Yin.

Other problems noted in Holly's medical history included a chronic left eye discharge and a tendency to occasionally vomit bile around 8 AM if she had not had a bowel movement or was exceptionally anxious.

A complete blood count and chemistry examination 3 months before the consultation for the collapsing trachea had disclosed no significant abnormalities, except for a slightly low thyroxine level with normal TSH levels, which was assessed as secondary to chronic illness. After the blood draw Holly displayed enduring and significant bruising around the venipuncture site. The owners had been told that if any other bleeding or bruising episodes were observed, a blood clotting panel would be required to rule out any hemorrhagic diatheses.

Regarding her general physical tendencies, Holly preferred to be warm. She had a good appetite and a normal level of thirst.

PHYSICAL EXAMINATION

On physical examination Holly was noted to have fetid breath accompanying dental tartar accumulation. The conjunctiva of the left eye was slightly red, although no discharge was in evidence. An inspiratory crackle was heard bilaterally during auscultation of the lungs, even when Holly was panting. No heart murmur was heard on auscultation. Her pulses were thin, wiry, and regular, and her tongue was a deep red-purple color. No precordial thrill was palpable. Holly paced restlessly and exhibited a deep hacking cough when she was not being examined.

ASSESSMENT

Holly was assessed as having a collapsing trachea given the previous radiographic findings and the "barking" cough that was aggravated by excitement and agitation. Pulmonary edema secondary to congestive heart failure was considered a possibility because of the dyspnea and coughing episodes at night and the crackling heard on physical examination. In the absence of any signs of cardiac disease, chronic bronchitis could not be ruled out. The owners agreed to obtain further radiographs to rule out cardiac complaints if initial treatment attempts were unsuccessful.

From a Chinese medical perspective, Blood stasis was considered to be present in Holly's chest. Evidence for Blood stasis included the chronic loud cough, the bruising previously noted at the venipuncture site, and the purple discoloration to the tongue. Qi stagnation frequently accompanies Blood stasis and was suggested by the wiry pulses, abdominal bloating, and Holly's chronic state of agitation. Liver Blood deficiency may even have aggravated tendencies to Blood and Qi stasis, and was suggested by the apparent responsiveness of Holly's seizures to Tian Ma Gou Teng Yin and by her tendency to fearfulness.

TREATMENT PLAN

Treatment goals were to move Qi and move Blood. As mentioned in Chapter 4, these are common objectives in the holistic management of congestive heart failure. The same herbs were frequently used to address both conditions in early herbal traditions, so definitively ruling out cardiac disease was not strictly necessary before treatment could begin. Blood tonification was avoided in case it aggravated any pulmonary edema. Because of the cardiac overtones of Holly's case, herbs that improved cardiovascular function and relieved coughing were initially selected.

A Western herbal formula containing alcohol extracts of the following herbs was prepared: 10 ml of Lobelia, 25 ml of Dandelion, 10 ml of Licorice, 15 ml of Grindelia, 15 ml of Elecampane, and 25 ml of Lily of the Valley. Holly was prescribed a heavy dose of the formula of 2 ml twice daily. Lobelia was prescribed to relieve the coughing and also help reduce pulmonary edema, Dandelion was prescribed as a potassium-sparing diuretic, Licorice was prescribed to relax airway spasms and reduce coughing, Grindelia is an important herb to relieve asthma in humans, Elecampane was prescribed to dry airway secretions and reduce coughing, and Lily of the Valley was prescribed for its cardiac glycoside content.

OUTCOME

Holly was reassessed after 2 weeks. The owners had noted increased urination, suggesting that the Dandelion was effective as a diuretic. Coughing and shortness of breath were mildly improved, although the owners still woke to find her dyspneic in the middle of the night. Her dyspnea was described as a "hunger for air." Mucus was seen in the stool, and Holly was avoiding the warm places she had previously sought such as under the bedclothes. Her abdomen continued to be distended. In addition, the owners felt that Holly's eyes appeared to bulge after the tincture was administered.

On physical examination, the crackling sounds in the lungs were reduced but still present. Holly appeared to be coughing less during her physical examination, but her cough was still harsh and honking. Palpation of the abdomen revealed no evidence of organomegaly or ascites. Holly's pulses were still thin, and her tongue was still purple and red. She was also passing extremely malodorous flatus. The owners had not noted this phenomenon at home.

Holly was assessed as being modestly improved, and the tincture was continued at a dose of 1 ml daily. Homeopathic Carbo vegetabilis 30C was also prescribed, beginning at a dose of 2 pellets in the evening, and then to be reduced to the minimum effective frequency as her signs improved. Carbo vegetabilis was prescribed because of the hallmark symptoms of an aversion to being covered up, pronounced abdominal bloating and flatulence, dyspnea at night while sleeping, cyanotic discoloration of the tongue, and "air hunger."

When Holly was reevaluated 3 weeks later, some further improvements were noted. When she was given Carbo vegetabilis 30C twice daily by mistake, Holly's shortness of breath was greatly alleviated and she had also begun barking again. However, these effects were lost when she was given the originally prescribed dose of Carbo vegetabilis once daily. Coughing was still noted when Holly was excited or in dry air. She continued to be anxious and restless, and her eyes still seemed to be bulging to the owner. On physical examination, inspiratory crackles were auscultable over the left thorax only when Holly's mouth was closed. The tongue was still red-purple, and her heart sounds continued to be normal. Her pulses remained thin but were less wiry. The malodorous flatus had resolved.

In early Western herbalism, bulging eyes were considered to be a hallmark indication for the use of Passion Flower, an anxiolytic nervine discussed in Chapter 3. A new tincture was prepared that contained 10 ml of alcohol extracts each of Motherwort, Passion Flower, Bugleweed, Comfrey, and Licorice to be given at a dosage of 1 ml twice daily. Motherwort and Bugleweed would relieve Blood stasis in the chest, simultaneously addressing both the chronic cough and the possible cardiac complaints. Comfrey was used to moisten the airways and relieve coughing triggered by dryness. Passion Flower was provided as an anxiolytic. Licorice was used to relieve bronchospasm and associated coughing. In addition to the herbal formula, Carbo vegetabilis 30C was continued at a dose of three pellets once daily.

Two months after beginning treatment, Holly was reevaluated. She was coughing much less often and had regained her ability to bark even though she had had no tincture for 3 days before the examination. The owner no longer felt that Holly's eyes were bulging. Holly also appeared considerably more relaxed. The last episode of "air hunger" could not be recalled. Halitosis, flatulence, and abdominal bloat were all similarly resolved. Physical examination revealed that inspiratory crackles were no longer present. Holly was relaxed during her appointment, and her tongue was a deep pink color. No coughing was heard. Holly's treatment with the revised tincture and homeopathic remedy was continued, although future visits were planned to determine if a single herbal formula or homeopathic could be devised that would address all outstanding signs Holly might have. In the event that Holly's signs worsened again, plans were made for survey radiographs of the thorax.

DISCUSSION

Conventional medical research is designed to identify treatments that improve the greatest number of patients with a particular problem. In so doing depth of effect is sacrificed for breadth of effect to a certain extent. In complementary medicine the opposite situation exists: breadth of effect is often sacrificed for depth of effect. This reflects the general observation many have made regarding natural medicine, that some patients seem to benefit dramatically and others not at all. Indeed, optimum results are thought more likely in natural medicine when a treatment is exactly matched to a patient, and a large portion of this text is devoted to helping a practitioner choose which of the many alternative therapies discussed for a given disorder will best suit the particular patient. Over the past several centuries, guiding symptoms have been of key importance in most herbal traditions in helping choose the right treatment. Often these symptoms are the very ones that would be dismissed as incomprehensible or irrelevant, such as the bulging eyes or extreme flatulence in Holly's case.

Holly's case illustrates how early medical systems were able to provide considerable depth of effect even in the absence of modern diagnostic methods. When conclusive diagnoses are not available because of technical or funding constraints, metaphoric means of evaluating patients frequently become the key to effective treatment. In the case of cardiac and chronic respiratory disorders, the same general problem of Blood stasis in the chest frequently pervades both.

Practitioners should note the use of Comfrey for Holly. Use of this herb is actively discouraged because of possible hepatic side effects. It was selected because it fulfilled two major objectives of moistening airways and stopping coughing. Other demulcent herbs could probably have been used to moisten the airways, including Slippery Elm and Marshmallow, and other antitussive herbs could have been used to stop coughing.

It is important to note how homeopathy was used in Holly's case to address some features of her condition and an herbal formula was designed to address the remaining concerns. Use of the two produced an effect that possibly neither could have produced alone.

SM

REFERENCES

Alamoudi OS. Hypomagnesaemia in chronic, stable asthmatics: prevalence, correlation with severity and hospitalization. *Eur Respir J* 16(3):427-431, 2000.

Baker JC, Ayres JG. Diet and asthma. *Respir Med* 94(10):925-934, 2000.

Bensky D, Gamble A. *Chinese Herbal Medicine Materia Medica,* revised ed. Seattle, 1993, Eastland Press.

Boericke W. *Materia Medica with Repertory,* ed 9. Santa Rosa, Calif, 1927, Boericke & Tafel.

Day C. *The Homeopathic Treatment of Small Animals: Principles and Practice.* Saffron Walden, UK, 1990, CW Daniel.

Dimitrova Z, Dimov B, Manolova N, Pancheva S, Ilieva D, Shishkov S. Antiherpes effect of *Melissa officinalis* L. extracts. *Acta Microbiol Bulg* 29:65-72, 1993.

Grandjean EM, Berthet P, Ruffmann R, Leuenberger P. Efficacy of oral long-term *N*-acetylcysteine in chronic bronchopulmonary disease: a meta-analysis of published double-blind, placebo-controlled clinical trials. *Clin Ther* 22(2):209-221, 2000.

Ikeda K, Wu DZ, Ishigaki M, Sunose H, Takasaka T. Inhibitory effects of sho-seiryu-to on acetylcholine-induced responses in nasal gland acinar cells. *Am J Chin Med* 22(2):191-196, 1994.

Kao ST, Wang SD, Wang JY, Yu CK, Lei HY. The effect of Chinese herbal medicine, xiao-qing-long-tang (XQLT), on allergen-induced bronchial inflammation in mite-sensitized mice. *Allergy* 55:1127-1133, 2000.

Ko WC, Lei CB, Lin YL, Chen CF. Mechanisms of relaxant action of *S*-petasin and *S*-isopetasin, sesquiterpenes of *Petasites formosanus*, in isolated guinea pig trachea. *Planta Med* 67(3):224-229, 2001.

Li XM, Huang CK, Zhang TF, Teper AA, Srivastava K, Schofield BH, Sampson HA. The Chinese herbal medicine formula MSSM-002 suppresses allergic airway hyperreactivity and modulates TH1/TH2 responses in a murine model of allergic asthma. *J Allergy Clin Immunol* 106(4):660-668, 2000.

Maggs DJ, Collins BK, Thorne JG, Nasisse MP. Effects of L-lysine and L-arginine on in vitro replication of feline herpesvirus type. *Am J Vet Res* 61(12):1474-1478, 2000.

Mittman P. Randomized, double-blind study of freeze-dried *Urtica dioica* in the treatment of allergic rhinitis. *Planta Med* 56:44-47, 1990.

Nagakura T, Matsuda S, Shichijyo K, Sugimoto H, Hata K. Dietary supplementation with fish oil rich in omega-3 polyunsaturated fatty acids in children with bronchial asthma. *Eur Respir J* 16(5):861-865, 2000.

Murphy R. *Lotus Materia Medica.* Pagosa Springs, Colo, 1995, Lotus Star Press.

Naeser MA. *Outline Guide to Chinese Herbal Patent Medicines in Pill Form.* Boston, Mass, 1990, Boston Chinese Medicine.

Nakajima S, Tohda Y, Ohkawa K, Chihara J, Nagasak Y. Effect of Saiboku-to (TJ-96) on bronchial asthma. *Ann NY Acad Sci* 685:549-560, 1993.

Percival SS. Use of echinacea in medicine. *Biochem Pharmacol* 60:155-158, 2000.

Picado C, Deulofeu R, Lleonart R, Agusti M, Mullol J, Quinto L, Torra M. Dietary micronutrients/antioxidants and their relationship with bronchial asthma severity. *Allergy* 56(1):43-49, 2001.

Sagripanti JL, Routson LB, Bonifacino AC, Lytle CD. Mechanism of copper-mediated inactivation of herpes simplex virus. *Antimicrob Agents Chemother* 41(4):812-817, 1997.

Schapowal A. Randomised controlled trial of butterbur and cetirizine for treating seasonal allergic rhinitis. *BMJ* 324:144-146, 2002.

Soutar A, Seaton A, Brown K. Bronchial reactivity and dietary antioxidants. *Thorax* 52(2):166-170, 1997.

Staudacher G, Staudacher M. New approaches to the secretolytic therapy of chronic bronchitis in dogs. *Berl Munch Tierarztl Wochenschr* 102(3):95-99, 1989.

Stetinova V, Grossmann V. Effects of known and potential antioxidants on animal models of pathological processes (diabetes, gastric lesions, allergic bronchospasm). *Exp Toxicol Pathol* 52(5):473-479, 2000.

Stey C, Steurer J, Bachmann S, Medici TC, Tramer MR. The effect of oral *N*-acetylcysteine in chronic bronchitis: a quantitative systematic review. *Eur Respir J* 16(2):253-262, 2000.

Stiles J, Townsend WM, Rogers QR, Krohne SG. Effect of oral administration of L-lysine on conjunctivitis caused by feline herpesvirus in cats. *Am J Vet Res* 63(1):99-103, 2002.

Stiles J, Townsend W, Rogers Q, Krohne S. The effect of oral LN-lysine on the course of feline herpesvirus conjunctivitis. In proceedings of the 31st Annual Meeting American College of Veterinary Ophthalmologists, Montreal, Quebec, Canada, 2000.

Tai S, Kai H, Isohama Y, Moriuchi H, Hagino N, Miyata T. The effect of maimendongtang on airway clearance and secretion. *Phytother Res* 13(2):124-127, 1999.

Tamaoki J, Chiyotani A, Takeyama K, Kanemura T, Sakai N, Konno K. Potentiation of beta-adrenergic function by saiboku-to and bakumondo-to in canine bronchial smooth muscle. *Jpn J Pharmacol* 62(2):155-159, 1993.

Tamaoki J, Kondo M, Chiyotani A, Takemura H, Konno K. Effect of saiboku-to, an antiasthmatic herbal medicine, on nitric oxide generation from cultured canine airway epithelial cells. *Jpn J Pharmacol* 69(1):29-35, 1995.

Tamaoki J, Nakata J, Kawatani K, Tagaya E, Nagai A. Ginsenoside-induced relaxation of human bronchial smooth muscle via release of nitric oxide. *Br J Pharmacology* 130:1859-1864, 2000.

Tanaka A, Ohashi Y, Kakinoki Y, Washio Y, Yamada K, Nakai Y, Nakano T, Nakai Y, Ohmoto Y. The herbal medicine shoseiryu-to inhibits allergen-induced synthesis of tumour necrosis factor alpha by peripheral blood mononuclear cells in patients with perennial allergic rhinitis. *Acta Otolaryngol Suppl* 538:118-125, 1998.

Toll J, Erb H, Birnbaum N, Schermerhorn T. Prevalence and incidence of serum magnesium abnormalities in hospitalized cats. *J Vet Intern Med* 16(3):217-221, 2002.

Touvay C, Etienne A, Braquet P. Inhibition of antigen-induced lung anaphylaxis in the guinea-pig by BN 52021 a new specific paf-acether receptor antagonist isolated from *Ginkgo biloba. Agents Actions* 17(3-4):371-372, 1986.

Westerveld GJ, Dekker I, Voss HP, Bast A, Scheeren RA. Antioxidant levels in the nasal mucosa of patients with chronic sinusitis and healthy controls. *Arch Otolaryngol Head Neck Surg* 123(2):201-204, 1997.

Yan W. *Practical Therapeutics of Traditional Chinese Medicine.* Brookline, Mass, 1997, Paradigm Publications.

Yeung H. *Handbook of Chinese Herbal Formulas.* Los Angeles, 1995, Self-published.

Yeung H. *Handbook of Chinese Herbs.* Los Angeles, 1996, Self-published.

17

Therapies For Reproductive Disorders

METRITIS

Therapeutic Rationale

- Identify and treat infection.

Paradigmatic Options

Chinese Medicine

- Dia Xia, or "vaginal discharge," is a common disorder in humans. It includes discharge from any source, including endometritis, metritis, open pyometra, and vaginitis. Various formulas have been developed to treat the disorder in women, and they are listed here for consideration for use in animals with vulvar discharge. As with most disorders in Chinese medicine, Dai Xia can be broadly classified into excess and deficiency types. Excess types of Dai Xia include Downpour of Damp Heat and Heat Toxin. Deficiency types include Spleen Qi deficiency, Kidney Yin deficiency, and Kidney Yang deficiency.

Heat Toxin vulvar discharge

- Heat Toxin vulvar discharge is characterized by a sudden onset of foul, purulent discharge that would be considered septic in conventional medicine. Other signs of Heat that may be present include fever and heat intolerance, irritability, severe malaise, excessive thirst with poor appetite, abdominal pain, and perhaps dark, scanty urine. The tongue is typically red to purple, may have a yellow coating, and may be dry, depending on the severity of the heat. The pulse is rapid and forceful and easily palpated. The Chinese herbal formula advocated for this condition is **Huang Lian Jie**

Du Tang (Antiphlogistic Decoction of Coptis). This formula is extremely bitter and must be given in capsules. It must never be given to a deficient animal because it may cause diarrhea and loss of appetite. Other uses of this strong antimicrobial preparation include septicemia, dysentery, pneumonia, acute urinary tract infections, and abscessation.
A *recommended starting dose* is ¼ tsp per 15 lb of body weight, or approximately 60 to 75 mg/lb of body weight, divided into two daily doses.

Damp Heat vulvar discharge

- Damp Heat vulvar discharge is similar to Heat Toxin vaginal discharge but may be more chronic and established in nature. There is usually a heavy, foul, and thick discharge. However, the patient may not appear as severely or acutely ill as in cases of Heat Toxin discharge. Other symptoms may include local itching, dark, scanty urine, heat intolerance, loss of appetite and increased thirst, loss of thirst and increased appetite, thick tan flakes of dander, and other complaints consistent with Damp Heat in the past medical history. The tongue is red or purple and is usually wet. The pulse is slippery and wiry and may be rapid. Formulas to consider for this disorder include **Zhi Dai Fang** (Discharge Checking Formula) and **Long Dan Xie Gan Tang** (Gentian Drain the Liver Decoction). The practitioner should choose Zhi Dai Fang for animals that are not too irritable and have signs of Dampness prevailing over signs of Heat. The discharge may be blood streaked. Long Dan Xie Gan Tang should be used for hotter animals with more forceful pulses, irritability or aggression, and heat intolerance. A *recommended starting dose* for either formula is ¼ tsp per 15 lb of body weight, or approximately 60 to 75 mg/lb of body weight, divided into two daily doses.
- Useful acupuncture points to use with these formulas include CV 3, SP 9, SP 6, LI 11, SP 10, and LIV 2. CV 3 is a local point that addresses the uterus and lower jiao. SP 9 stops the Spleen from manufacturing obstructing Dampness. SP 6 moves the Qi of the lower jiao to expel

the discharge. LI 11 clears Damp Heat, and SP 10 and LIV 2 cool the Blood and the Liver meridians in the lower jiao, respectively.

Spleen Qi deficiency vulvar discharge

- Spleen Qi deficiency has a completely different presentation from the previous two categories. The patient may be fatigued or listless and have a copious, thin discharge with minimal odor, a tendency to loose stools, and a poor appetite. Blood may be present in the discharge. There may even be edema in the hind paws. The tongue is usually pale and may have a slimy coating. The pulse feels weak or even choppy. The formula for this condition is **Wan Dai Tang** (Discharge Ceasing Decoction). This formula tonifies and even literally lifts the Spleen Qi at the same time it drains Damp and stops mild bleeding.
- When Heat signs are slightly more prominent in a weaker animal with deficient pulses, **Yi Huang Tang** (Transforming Yellow Decoction) should be considered. This formula focuses less on tonifying the Spleen and more on having an astringent effect on the copious and perhaps yellow discharge. It also clears more Heat than Wan Dai Tang. A *recommended starting dose* for either formula is ¼ tsp per 15 lb of body weight, or approximately 60 to 75 mg/lb of body weight, divided into two daily doses.
- Acupuncture points to consider in treating Spleen Qi deficiency types of vulvar discharge include ST 36, SP 6, ST 40, BL 20, SP 9, and CV 4.

Kidney Yang deficiency vulvar discharge

- As deficiency signs and Coldness signs become more prominent, the disease progresses from simple Qi deficiency to a more severe Kidney Yang deficiency. At this point there may be a continuous discharge of a thin white or clear mucus, cold intolerance, frequent need to urinate, even in the middle of the night, pale urine, loose stools, anestrus or delayed estrus, difficulty in getting pregnant, low back pain with weak and cold extremities, a pale tongue, and a deep, slow, or weak pulse. The formula used for this disorder is usually **Nei Bu Wan** (Internal Supplementation Pill). A *recommended starting dose* is ¼ tsp per 15 lb of body weight, or approximately 60 to 75 mg/lb of body weight, divided into two daily doses.

- Useful acupuncture points for Kidney Yang deficiency leading to vaginal discharge include CV 4, BL 23, and KI 3 to tonify the Kidneys.

Kidney Yin deficiency vulvar discharge

- The other deficiency that may be recognized is Kidney Yin deficiency. In these cases there is a sticky, odorless, blood-tinged, and perhaps excoriating discharge. The patient usually has a light build, may be restless especially at night, may be constipated with dry feces, and may experience vaginal irritation. There may also be elevated thirst and a tendency to dream frequently. The pulse is usually rapid and thin. The tongue appears red and somewhat dry. For these patients, **Zhi Bai Di Huang Wan** (Anemarrhena, Phellodendron, and Rehmannia Pill) should be considered. A *recommended starting dose* is ¼ tsp per 15 lb of body weight, or approximately 60 to 75 mg/lb of body weight, divided into two daily doses.
- Useful acupuncture points for Kidney Yin deficiency leading to vaginal discharge include CV 3, SP 6, KI 6, and BL 23.

Blood stasis vulvar discharge

- Bloody types of discharges may be more amenable to Blood-moving formulas. Some case reports have suggested that a Blood-moving formula composed of Pu Huang, Dang Gui, and Wu Ling Zhi was effective for metritis in sheep. It should be considered for use in Blood stasis when the animal exhibits dark, bloody discharges, wiry or irregular pulses, and a purple tongue. In dogs with pale or lavender tongues, choppy or wiry pulses, and postpartum metritis or retained lochia, **Sheng Hua Tang** (Generation and Transformation Decoction) can be considered. A *recommended starting dose* for either formula in companion animals is ¼ tsp per 15 lb of body weight, or approximately 60 to 75 mg/lb of body weight, divided into two daily doses.

- Another Blood-moving formula has similarly been used in Blood stasis cases of canine metritis in which there is some suggestion of Damp Heat (Xie, 2000). A *recommended starting dose* for the formula is ¼ tsp per 15 lb of body weight, or approximately 60 to 75 mg/lb of body weight, divided into two daily doses. The ingredients of this formula are the following:

Yi Mu Cao	20%
Huang Bai	20%
Hong Hua	10%
Dang Gui	19%
Xiang Fu	11%
Cang Zhu	9%
Lai Fu Zi	11%

Western Herbal Medicine

- A basic Western herbal formula with a long history of use in cases of vaginal discharge is a mixture of equal parts of liquid extracts of Cranesbill *(Geranium maculatum)*, Bethroot *(Trillium erectum)*, Marshmallow *(Althea officinalis)*, and Agrimony *(Agrimonia eupatoria)*. It can be used to treat Damp Heat discharge (see Chinese Medicine section). A *recommended starting dose* is 0.1 ml per 2½ lb of body weight, given up to three times daily.

AUTHORS' CHOICES:

SM: Appropriate Chinese herbal formula, with rigorous follow-up in very ill animals to ensure compliance and efficacy.

SW: Luteolysis when appropriate; antibiotics when positive culture and signs agree; Chinese herbs; acupuncture.

PYOMETRA

- See section on Metritis. We recommend surgery or luteolytic drugs for frank closed pyometra. As with any potentially life-threatening condition, open pyometra should be managed with extreme caution and diligent follow-up if using unproven alternative medical treatments.

VAGINITIS

Therapeutic Rationale

- Address underlying causes (anatomic abnormalities, subclinical urinary incontinence, obesity-induced fat folds over vulva, etc.).
- Identify and suppress pathogenic bacteria.
- Reduce inflammation.

Alternative Options with Conventional Bases

- **Change the animal's diet**, since food allergy may be associated with inflammation of many mucosal surfaces.
- **Probiotics:** long used in treatment of women with vaginitis. A recent study indicates that oral lactobacillus supplementation improves the clinical course and results in lactobacillus deposition in the vagina (Reid, 2001). Probiotics are live organisms, and commercial products are frequently labeled inaccurately because of shifts in bacterial populations in the production facilities and reduction in viable organisms on store shelves. In general, only very fresh, refrigerated, or freeze dried products should be used, and even for small dogs we use high doses of one to three times the labeled dose for humans, unless gastrointestinal upset occurs, in which case lower doses are then used.

Paradigmatic Options

Chinese Herbs

- Two Chinese herbal formulas that have been advocated for use in vaginitis are **Er Miao San** (Two Marvels Powder) and **Yu Dai Wan** (Cure Discharge Pill). Yu Dai Wan is specifically for vaginal discharge caused by Damp Heat when the discharge is thick, and perhaps red tinged. Er Miao San, when combined with Huai Niu Xi and Cang Zhu to make **Si Miao San** (Four Marvels Powder), is an extremely important formula in alternative veterinary medicine with application to many disorders. Si Miao San should be used when the animal seems to have marked Heat signs (e.g., a red tongue, slippery and wiry pulses, heat intolerance, elevated appetite or thirst, but usually not both) and a history of Damp Heat accumulation resulting from Spleen Qi deficiency indicated by cystitis, colitis, weeping rashes, an oily coat, and hind limb weakness. A *recommended starting dose* for either formula is ¼ tsp per 15 lb of body weight, or approximately 60 to 75 mg/lb of body weight, divided into two daily doses.

AUTHORS' CHOICES:

SM: Appropriate Chinese herbal formula; probiotics.
SW: Diet changes; probiotics; Chinese herbs.

17 CASE REPORT
Chronic Vaginitis in a Bernese Mountain Dog

HISTORY

Gayla, a 6-year-old, female, spayed Bernese mountain dog, was brought for treatment of chronic vaginitis and lameness. The vaginitis was of 1 year's duration and was marked by a redness and swelling of the vulva and a profuse mucoid discharge. The problem was originally diagnosed by a different veterinarian as a recurrent urinary tract infection when urinalysis revealed increased numbers of white blood cells and a culture of the urine was positive for *Escherichia coli*. Whether the sample was obtained by cystocentesis or free-catch is unknown. No signs of dysuria or stranguria had been observed.

Gayla's past medical history included gingivitis, halitosis, and "arthritis." The owner recalled that homeopathic Baptisia may have helped the gingivitis and halitosis, although she could not remember the potency or dosage regimen used. Gayla tended to have excess saliva production even when halitosis and gingivitis were absent.

Lameness caused by congenital hip dysplasia was an ongoing concern, and the referring veterinarian advised the owner that the left anterior cruciate ligament was also probably deteriorating. This assumption was made because of Gayla's chronic tendency to lameness of the left hind leg accompanied by a tendency for the left knee to rotate outward during walking. No radiographs or cranial drawer tests were performed to substantiate this diagnosis. Gayla's hind limb lameness resulted in her having difficulty standing up after sitting or lying down, and she had little interest in exercise. The owner had tried various physical interventions to aid Gayla's hind limb discomfort. She felt that magnet therapy, Tellington Touch, and massage had all been of some benefit.

Forelimb lameness had recently become a problem. Acute painful swelling of the elbows and knees developed after Gayla was given an oral antibiotic for the vaginitis. Use of oral antibiotics was discontinued, but a topical antibiotic preparation (Panalog) had no effect on reducing the vaginal discharge. Elbow and knee swelling was also triggered by damp weather, as well as by the most recent annual vaccination, although the owner could not recall the type of vaccine used. The lameness was aggravated by Gayla's overall tendency to gain weight.

Minor health complaints included development of warts on her elbows, loose stools, and snoring while sleeping.

Gayla's ravenous appetite was currently being assuaged with a homemade diet consisting of raw poultry organs and meat, ground bones, and grated vegetables. Although it had no effect on her lameness and vaginitis, the raw food did cause Gayla to have more formed stools. Halitosis developed, however, when her diet was supplemented with an additive containing kelp, alfalfa, vitamin E, vitamin C, and apple cider vinegar, so the dietary supplement was discontinued. Bovine colostrum had been administered in the past as a nutritional supplement and, although amounts given could not be recalled, the owner felt that it increased the Gayla's overall energy.

Numerous medicinal supplements were being given, including methylsulfonylmethane (MSM), Willow Bark, and Deer Antler. None of these therapies had any apparent effect on the vaginitis or lameness.

Gayla exhibited low thirst. She enjoyed both warm and cool temperatures but generally preferred warm, soft surfaces. She had recently and inexplicably developed a fear of thunderstorms. She interacted well with other animals and people but had a tendency to be protective of her food and to shy away from rambunctious animals. The owner felt that this evasiveness was an effort by Gayla to protect her hips from trauma.

PHYSICAL EXAMINATION

A copious murky white vulvar discharge was found during the physical examination of Gayla. Her vaginal area seemed quite painful to the touch, although no vulvar swelling or redness was seen. There was also no evidence of pain overlying the kidneys at the thoracolumbar junction, lessening the likelihood of pyelonephritis. Gayla's pulses were thin, forceless, and superficial (i.e., soft), and her tongue varied from pink to red. Her hair and skin were normal except for greasiness of the fur around the ears. Active acupuncture points included SP 6, SP 9, LI 11, BL 26, and BL 24. LI 11 was centered over the region of greatest elbow swelling and was warm to the touch. Gayla's body temperature was 101.8° F. Findings of abdominal palpation were normal. Drawer tests were not performed.

LABORATORY EVALUATION

Urinalysis of a midstream urine sample provided findings consistent with previous results. That is, rod-shaped bacteria and white blood cells were present in abundance. No culture and sensitivity test was performed. No other laboratory test was performed.

ASSESSMENT

Since Gayla exhibited no signs of abnormal urination, her history of pyuria was interpreted as probably secondary to a chronic bacterial vaginosis given the copious thick exudates from the vulva. Her joint complaints may have reflected polyarthritis, but further testing was not performed at the time of the initial assessment.

From a Chinese medical perspective, Gayla had Dampness accumulations in the joints and vagina. Dampness in the joints was signaled by the swelling that was aggravated in damp weather. The mucous discharge from the vagina was similarly viewed as reflecting Dampness. General body-wide tendencies to Dampness accumulation are reflected by a tendency to snore, weight gains, coat greasiness, and warts. The tendency of this Dampness to become Damp Heat, in spite of Gayla's temperature preferences, was signaled by the occasional red tongue, the warmth and swelling around SP 9 and LI 11, halitosis, and increased appetite coinciding with decreased thirst.

In Chinese medicine the original source of Dampness and Damp Heat accumulations in the body is always deficient

Spleen function. Multiple signs of Spleen deficiency were present, including soft pulses and the swelling noted at Spleen Qi tonification points such as BL 24, BL 26, and SP 6. Administration of antibiotics, which are energetically cold, tends to further damage Spleen Qi. In Gayla's case, antibiotics seemed to aggravate the development of Dampness in the joints.

The Spleen deficiency may have been leading to a secondary Blood deficiency in Gayla as evidenced by the possible weakening of the cruciate ligaments, although cruciate ligament disease remained unconfirmed. Other Blood deficiency signs included increased anxiety around other animals and during thunderstorms.

Treatment goals from a Chinese medical perspective were to drain Dampness, gently clear Heat, and tonify the Spleen.

TREATMENT

Si Miao San (Four Marvels Powder), consisting of only four herbs, satisfied the treatment goals and was prescribed for Gayla. Phellodendron, one of the four ingredients, contains a phytochemical known as berberine that has antimicrobial properties. Subsequent aggravation of the elbow swelling was prevented by two of the other ingredients in the formula that act to support the Spleen. As mentioned in the text, the formula is used for hind end weakness secondary to Damp Heat accumulations as well as for vaginitis. Gayla was given approximately 1 tsp of the granular concentrate form of Si Miao San in her food twice daily.

Gayla's diet was not changed, and no additional supplements and medications were used.

OUTCOME

Gayla was brought for a follow-up evaluation 3 weeks later. The vaginal discharge had apparently ceased, although the owner felt that some mucosal reddening was present. Gayla was able to rise more easily. She was now more willing to go on walks, and lameness was pronounced only in the mornings when she began to move. Painful areas seemed restricted to the left knee and elbow.

Physical examination revealed the vulva and vagina to be pain free with no apparent reddening. Vaginal fluid was scanty to absent. Cytology of an impression smear of the vaginal wall revealed occasional mononuclear cells, well-differentiated polymorphonuclear cells, and a minimal presence of bacteria. No phagocytosis or toxic change was noted.

Since Damp Heat signs had largely disappeared from Gayla's lower body, the formula was discontinued and **Tao Hong Yin** (Persica and Carthamus Beverage) with added **Di Long** was prescribed to address Gayla's forelimb lameness and to disperse further Dampness from the channels. Within a couple of weeks of starting the Tao Hong Yin, Gayla became more playful and active. After an additional 5 weeks, some vulvar discharge was noted and the owner refilled the Si Miao San prescription for intermittent use on an as-needed basis. Twelve months after her initial presentation, Gayla remained free of vaginal discharge despite the discontinuation of Si Miao San 2 months earlier. The formula was discontinued completely.

DISCUSSION

The original goals of antibiotic therapy were fulfilled in Gayla using Si Miao San. Unlike antibiotics, however, Si Miao San did not aggravate Gayla's lameness complaints.

Gayla's response to Si Miao San helped guide the choice of Tao Hong Yin as the herbal formula to use for her lameness. Tao Hong Yin has significant Dampness-dispersing properties because of its content of Wei Ling Xian (Clematis).

As in other cases in this text, Gayla's case demonstrates how improvements in the chief complaint are often attended by improvements in the other signs that supported the metaphoric diagnosis. Until conventional research can validate the efficacy of the Chinese herbal formulas proposed in this text, a pervasive improvement in an animal's condition is a strong indication to a holistic practitioner that the chosen treatment has been beneficial.

SM

REFERENCES

Ehling D. *The Chinese Herbalist's Handbook,* revised ed. Santa Fe, NM, 1996, Inword Press.

Reid G, Bruce AW, Fraser N, Heinemann C, Owen J, Henning B. Oral probiotics can resolve urogenital infections. *FEMS Immunol Med Microbiol* 30(1):49-52, 2001.

Xie H. Veterinary Herbal Medicine Training Program, class notes, Session V, p 135, Reddick, Fla, 2000.

Yan W. *Practical Therapeutics of Traditional Chinese Medicine.* Brookline, Mass, 1997, Paradigm Publications.

Yeung H. *Handbook of Chinese Herbs.* Los Angeles, 1996, Self-published.

18

Therapies for Urologic Disorders

BENIGN PROSTATIC HYPERTROPHY/ HYPERPLASIA

Therapeutic Rationale

- Reduce hormonal stimulation for prostatic tissue.

Alternative Options with Conventional Bases

Nutritional Therapies

- **Plant sterols**: β-Sitosterol appears to improve clinical parameters in men with benign prostatic hypertrophy/ hyperplasia (BPH) (Wilt, 2000). Sterols are contained in many plants, but the commercial product Moducare is probably a more concentrated source.

Herbs

- **Saw Palmetto** *(Serenoa repens):* acts as a 5-alpha reductase inhibitor, and is effective in reducing symptoms in human BPH. It has been tested in dogs and was not effective in correcting measurements of BPH; however, these dogs were asymptomatic (Barsanti, 2000), so a true parallel to the demonstrated efficacy in human BPH has not yet been investigated.
- **Nettles** *(Urtica dioica):* may be mildly effective in human males with BPH. Nettles are commonly used in combination with other herbs. Only the root is considered to have activity in BPH.
- **Pygeum** *(Pygeum africanus):* has been shown in clinical trials to reduce symptoms associated with BPH in men (Ishani, 2000). The mechanism by which it works is unknown, and Pygeum use has not been popular in dogs to date.

Chinese Medicine

- For all of the formulas listed below, a *suggested starting dose* of granular concentrate is ¼ tsp per 10 to 15 lb of body weight, or 60 to 75 mg/kg of body weight, given in divided doses twice daily.
- The Chinese herbal formulas advocated for use in prostate disease are usually those that clear Damp Heat in the lower body, including **Ba Zheng San** (Eight Corrections Powder) and **Long Dan Xie Gan Tang** (Gentian Purge the Liver Decoction). These formulas are for use in "excessive" cases only, such as a dog with a dark-red tongue, forceful, tense, rapid pulses, and dysuria. Ba Zheng San acts specifically on the genitourinary tract and has ingredients that promote proper urethral sphincter function and completeness of voiding. Long Dan Xie Gan Tang has a broader effect on the body and might be considered when the animal has a tendency toward dominance aggression, nighttime restlessness and pacing, and a past medical history of other syndromes amenable to Long Dan Xie Gan Tang, including epilepsy, hyperadrenocorticism, and moist pyoderma.
- For older, weaker, chilly dogs, **Bei Xie Fen Qing Yin** (Decoction of Hypoglauca Yam to Separate the Clear) can be considered. The original version of this formula had four herbs that acted to warm the Kidney and aid in the "separation of the clear and the turbid," which is supposed to occur in the Bladder, powered by the Kidney. A later version of the formula, known as **Bei Xie Fen Qin Yin II**, is less warming, more cooling, and more Dampness draining. Practitioners should be sure to double-check which version of the formula they have before using it for a patient.
- Patients that appear to have Blood stasis (signs include a pale or purple tongue, wiry pulses, lower abdominal pain, firm palpable mass, and chilliness) should be treated with **Shao Fu Zhu Yu Tang** (Drive Out Stasis from the Lower Abdomen Decoction).

- **Si Miao San** (Four Marvels Powder) can be considered as a treatment to prevent recurrence in susceptible animals. This formula is also to be used in animals with chronic tendencies to Damp Heat, manifesting as recurrent colitis, cystitis, low back tightness, hind limb weakness, and heat intolerance.

Western Herbs

- Other Western herbs of potential benefit in the treatment of prostate disorders in the dog are listed below. They can be used alone or in combination and include the following:
  - **Hydrangea** *(Hydrangea arborescens):* for painful and inflamed prostates.
  - **Horsetail** *(Equisetum arvense)* and **Cleavers** *(Galium aparine):* used to soften hypertrophic and fibrotic lesions.
- These are herbs that address "excess" prostate conditions, whereas Saw Palmetto is an herb more appropriate to "deficiency" types of disorders. Since canine prostate disorders seem to be primarily of the "excess" type, more attention should probably be paid to the potential of these lesser-known herbs. A *suggested starting dose* of the above herbs, whether alone or combined in a formula (3 parts Hydrangea, 2 parts Cleavers, and 3 parts Horsetail), is 0.2 ml per 5 lb of body weight, divided into two daily doses.

AUTHORS' CHOICES:

SM: Appropriate Chinese herbs.
SW: Saw Palmetto Berry; Nettles root; plant sterols.

CALCULI, GENERAL

Therapeutic Rationale

- Cystotomy when necessary.
- Decrease urine concentration.
- Decrease calculus precursors.

Alternative Options with Conventional Bases

Herbs

- **Diuretic herbs:** in combination with increased fluid intake diuresis may theoretically reduce crystallization and stone formation by diluting urinary solutes. Diuretic herbs that have been recommended include Corn Silk *(Zea mays)*, Dandelion *(Taraxacum officinale)*, Horsetail *(Equisetum arvense)*, and Parsley *(Petroselinum crispum)*. Corn Silk was not shown to have diuretic activity in one study (Doan, 1992). Dandelion may have diuretic properties (Racz-Kotilla, 1974). Four species of Horsetail were shown to have diuretic activity in one study (Perez Gutierrez, 1985).
- **Demulcent herbs:** thought to reduce inflammation by coating tissues with a mucilaginous substance; how this occurs in the urinary tract after oral ingestion is unclear. Demulcent herbs recommended for urinary tract inflammation include Marshmallow Root *(Althea officinalis)*, Corn Silk, Parsley, and others.
- **Antimicrobial herbs:** have been used when stones have formed as a result of chronic urinary tract infection. See the section on Urinary Tract Infection for information on Uva-Ursi *(Arctostaphylos uva-ursi)*, Buchu *(Barosma betulina* or *Agathosma betulina)*, and Cranberry *(Vaccinium macrocarpon)*.
- **pH-modifying herbs:** Uva-Ursi and Horsetail *(E. arvense)* have a reputation for increasing urinary pH (Grases, 1994), but documentation is slim. If these herbs decrease urinary acidity (or raise urinary pH), they may be contraindicated in cases of struvite urolithiasis.

Other herbs for urinary calculi

- **Gravel Root** *(Eupatorium purpureum)*: a traditional antilithic. It contains toxic pyrrolizidine alkaloids and so should be used cautiously if at all. **Hydrangea** *(Hydrangea arborescens)* also carries the common name Gravel Root.
- **Horsetail:** high in silicon and contains thiaminase. In addition to its diuretic activity (Perez Gutierrez, 1985), Horsetail is thought to have antimicrobial actions possibly related to saponins (Grases, 1994).

- **Couch Grass** or **Dog Grass** *(Elymus repens)*, **Stone Root** *(Collinsonia canadensis)*, and **Hydrangea:** said to have diuretic effects, but no studies are available on these herbs.

Nutritional Therapies

- **Taurine** and **Carnitine:** A report on dogs with cystinuria indicated that three of five dogs observed had carnitinuria. Cystinuric dogs excreted less taurine in their urine than healthy dogs. The authors in this study suggest that cystinuria may be a risk factor for taurine and carnitine deficiency (Sanderson, 2001). Supplementing dogs that have cysteine crystals or calculi with Carnitine and Taurine is low risk and may have some utility.

Paradigmatic Options

Chinese Medicine

- Crystals and calculi represent a more severe form of Damp Heat accumulation in the Bladder than that discussed in the Chinese medical section on urinary tract infections. Dampness is present in such abundance in these patients that it is congealing into uroliths.
- The Chinese herbal formula typically advocated in Chinese medicine for urolithiasis in humans is **Shi Wei San** (Pyrrosia Leaf Powder). This formula drains Dampness, clears Heat, and expels stones. Its antilithic properties are reportedly enhanced with the addition of Jin Qian Cao (Lysimachia), Hai Hin Sha (Lygodium Spores), and Ji Nei Jin (Chicken Gizzard Lining). Hematuria can be reduced with the addition of Xiao Ji (Small Thistle), Pu Huang (Bulrush Pollen), and Mu Dan Pi (Moutan Bark) to the base formula. A *suggested starting dose* of granular concentrate is ¼ tsp per 10 to 15 lb of body weight, or 60 to 75 mg/kg of body weight, divided into two daily doses.

Western Herbs

- Clinical experience with the combination of Hydrangea, Stone Root, Gravel Root, and Corn Silk discussed in the section on Western herbal treatment of urinary tract infections suggests that this formula is an effective urinary acidifier. Clinical experience in my (SM) practice demonstrates that it is effective in acidifying the urine pH and dissolving uroliths in dogs. This benefit exists even when acidifying diets are not used. However, uroliths in successfully treated cases were not chemically analyzed. Extended use of this formula over several months yielded no toxic effects. A *suggested starting dose* is 0.2 ml per 5 lb of body weight of the combined herbal formula, given twice daily.

- In Chinese medicine Dampness is considered a type of unusable body fluid that is manufactured by faulty digestion. This underscores the recognized link between diet and uroliths. Dietary control of struvite uroliths seems to be more than a matter of including urinary acidifiers and controlling magnesium levels, however. Excess levels of congealed Dampness and Phlegm commonly correlate with food allergies or sensitivities and incomplete digestion. It is noteworthy that one of the Chinese "herbs" used specifically for urinary calculi is the lining of chicken gizzard. Metabolites of its content of ventriculin are credited with producing a delayed increase in secretion of gastric juices, which in turn promotes increased gastric acidity and completeness of digestion. This increased acid secretion may play an indirect role in urinary tract acidification.
- The herbal formula containing Hydrangea, Stone Root, and Gravel Root may also help acidify urine by regulating circulation through the bladder wall so that tendencies to hematuria are lessened. Blood and transudates seem to have an alkalinizing effect on urine, and the apparent benefit of herbs that regulate microcirculation suggests that chronic low-grade cystitis is an antecedent event to many cases of urethral obstruction.

AUTHORS' CHOICES:

SM: Hydrangea, Stone Root, Corn Silk, and Gravel Root combined.
SW: Increase water in the diet; herbal diuretics in combination.

CHRONIC RENAL DISEASE OR FAILURE

Therapeutic Rationale

- Treat inciting causes when possible.
- Monitor and maintain hydration.
- Monitor and correct mineral and electrolyte disturbances.
- Control secondary effects of uremia.

Alternative Options with Conventional Bases

Nutritional Therapies

- **ω-3 fatty acids:** in one clinical trial dogs receiving ω-3 polyunsaturated fatty acids (PUFA) from marine Fish Oil were shown to have slowed glomerular changes and preserved renal architecture compared with dogs receiving ω-6 PUFA from safflower oil or tallow (Brown, 1998). The *recommended dose* for Fish Oil is 500 mg PUFA or one double-strength capsule per 5 to 10 lb of body weight.
- **B vitamins:** administration of cyanocobalamin and folate has been associated with beneficial changes in plasma homocysteine and blood lipid levels in humans, and increased intracellular thiamine protects against some effects of uremia. The doses given are higher than dietary requirements. Although it is not known whether B vitamin administration has the same benefit to dogs and cats, patients with chronic renal disease appear to feel and eat better when given B vitamin complex or a vitamin-mineral complex recommended for dogs or cats. This may be due to increased losses of B vitamins caused by chronic polyuria.
- **Bromelain:** has been shown to reduce inflammation and disease progression in cases of glomerulonephritis or immune-mediated glomerular disease in rats (Sebekova, 1999).

Herbs (Box 18-1)

- **Chinese Rhubarb** *(Rheum officinale,* Niao Du Jing in traditional Chinese medicine [TCM], or *Rheum palmatum,* Da Huang in TCM): a component of some

BOX 18-1 Herbs for the Urinary Tract

Diuretics
Corn Silk
Parsley
Dandelion
Horsetail
Bearberry
Buchu

Demulcents
Corn Silk
Marshmallow
Slippery Elm

Antimicrobials
Bearberry

pH-modifying
Bearberry
Horsetail

Others (antiinflammatory?)
Rhubarb
Asparagus
Gravel Root (Eupatorium)
Gravel Root (Hydrangea)
Stone Root (Collinsonia)

TCM combinations for renal disease and has been extensively investigated in China and Japan for its effects on failing kidneys. Various mechanisms have been posited, including alterations in nitrogen metabolism (rhubarb is a laxative) changes in arachidonic acid metabolism and cytokine modulation, or decreases in fibronectin levels. In one study (Zhang, 1996) administration of *R. officinale* reduced proteinuria and glomerular damage in rats. In another study in which human patients with renal failure were treated in one of three different ways—rhubarb *(R. officinale)* alone, rhubarb plus captopril, or captopril alone—end-stage renal failure within 25 to 40 months of treatment occurred at the lowest rate (13.1%) in the group receiving both captopril and rhubarb, next lowest (25.9%) in the rhubarb group, and highest (54.3%) in the group receiving only captopril (Leishi, 1996). Rhubarb is sometimes administered as an enema in China. Chronic use of rhubarb as a laxative will dehydrate the patient. If this occurs, lower doses may have to be used, together with other supportive treatments.

- **Asparagus** *(Asparagus officinalis;* Tian Men Dong in TCM): a traditional treatment for Kidney Yin deficiency.

Some herbalists believe that Tian Men Dong can "cleanse" the kidneys and act as a mild diuretic, although the Chinese herbal literature does not document these effects. Nephrologists warn that Asparagus is high in oxalates and is a contraindicated food for patients with a history of oxalate urinary calculi.

- **Liu Wei Di Huang Tang** (Six Flavor Tea, Rehmannia 6): a combination of six herbs *(Rehmannia glutinosa* Root, *Cornus officinalis* Fruit, *Dioscorea batatas* Root, *Paeonia suffruticosa* Root Bark, *Alisma plantago-aquatica* Tuber, and *Poria cocos)*. In a study of rats with one kidney or partially ligated kidneys resulting in sharply elevated blood pressure and renal function deterioration, subjects treated with Liu Wei Di Huang Tang had reduced hypertension and mortality compared with rats receiving no treatment. The authors of this study theorize that Liu Wei Di Huang actually enhances renal blood flow (Li, 1974).
- **Astragalus** *(Astragalus membranaceus)* and **Rehmannia** *(Rehmannia glutinosa):* Chinese studies on a combination of these two herbs indicated that the combination resulted in significant improvements in humans and laboratory animals with nephritis compared with control animals (Su, 1993).
- **Wen Pi Tang** (Onpi-to): has been investigated in Japan and in one series of eight cases was thought to slow progression of renal failure (Mitsuma, 1999).
- ***Clerodendron trichotomum:*** the single herb was shown to cause renal vasodilation and increased urinary output when given intravenously to dogs (Lu, 1994). This herb is used only in Chinese herbal formulas.

Other Considerations

- **Overvaccination**: Recent work (Lappin, 2002) suggests that subcutaneous panleukopenia, rhinotracheitis, and calicivirus (FVRCP) vaccination of cats may play a role in the development of chronic kidney disease. These vaccines are produced on and contain feline kidney cell tissue. When cats were given feline kidney cell tissue or these vaccines subcutaneously, they developed antibodies to kidney tissue. Intranasal FVRCP vaccinated cats did not develop these antibodies. This emerging data may provide one more reason to vaccinate more cautiously than we have in the past.

Paradigmatic Options

Chinese Medicine

- The treatment of chronic renal failure, particularly in cats, is one of the best ways for a conventional veterinary practitioner to witness firsthand the expanded therapeutic possibilities and outcomes offered by alternative medicine. This is because chronic renal failure, unlike many other conditions in which alternative medicine is applied, benefits from the same approach in almost every case. It seems reasonable to predict that, even if no other alternative medicines are used, every veterinary practice in North America will have herbal formulas to treat chronic renal failure on its shelves within the next decade. The Chinese metaphoric understanding of the Kidneys and their relationship to the Spleen accounts beautifully for the constellation of signs usually associated with chronic renal failure in cats.
- One of the best ways to understand the Chinese medical perspective of the role of the Kidney in the body is to imagine a cooking pot over a fire. The Kidney is the fire itself, the ultimate provider of vital energy in the body. The flame of this fire is like an oil lamp dependent on a certain amount of precious fluid to maintain it. In the body that fluid is known as Yin and the spark that ignites it into a flame is Yang. This Yang is, in part, handed down from the upper reaches of the body the way a hand reaches down to light a candle on a table.
- One of the first jobs of the Kidney is to use some of its flame to evaporate a small amount of Yin so that it rises as a cloud of mist to cool and moisten the Yang in the upper reaches of the body. An axis of balance is thus established when the hot Yang of the upper body lights the flame that serves, indirectly, to cool it. Without this balance the upper body has an innate tendency to become overheated and the lower body

tends to become cool. A prominent sign of Excess Heat in the upper body is thirst, whereas the fading fire of the Kidney is reflected, as we might expect, in a failure to concentrate urine so that valuable water is lost.

- Over the flame of life in the Kidney sits the cooking pot, which is equated with digestion in Chinese medicine. The organs assigned this role of digestion in Chinese medicine are the Spleen and Stomach. When the flame is adequate, cooking is adequate and digestion and assimilation are complete. When the flame is too low, cooking is inadequate and scum forms on the surface of the pot's contents, similar to what happens to hot soup as it cools.
- The pot itself is primarily considered to be the Stomach, and the movement of the contents of the pot into general circulation is considered the province of the Spleen. When this metaphoric scum (known in Chinese medicine as Phlegm) accumulates as a result of a failing fire in the Kidney, the first organ it affects is the Stomach. As the Phlegm accumulates, it begins to disrupt the normal downward flow of energy in the digestive tract and vomiting results.
- All of the signs of chronic renal failure as it is typically seen in veterinary practice, including polyuria, polydipsia, chronic vomiting, the seeking of heat, and weight loss (representing a failure to assimilate by the Spleen), are explained by this elaborate model of fading Kidney fire. The explanation might seem contrived to fit the signs of chronic renal failure, except for the apparent effectiveness of the Chinese herbal formulas it suggests as a treatment.
- One of the most popular Chinese herbal formulas for the treatment of Kidney failure in cats is **Shen Qi Wan** (Kidney Qi Pill), which is also known as **Ba Wei Di Huang Wan** or **Rehmannia 8.** Another formula occasionally is sold under the name Ba Wei Di Huang Wan, but it has different ingredients. The practitioner treating chronic renal failure needs to use the formula containing Fu Zi (prepared Aconite, which is nontoxic) and Rou Gui (Cinnamon). These two herbs provide the spark that will reignite the flame of the Kidneys when

the connection between the upper and lower parts of the body has been lost. The other herbs contained in Rehmannia 8 make up the smaller formula known as **Liu Wei Di Huang Wan** (Rehmannia 6). These herbs metaphorically replenish the oil or fuel that allows the Kidney flame to burn.

- **Rehmannia 8** is applied to all cases of chronic renal failure in small animals presenting with polyuria, polydipsia, seeking of heat, vomiting, poor appetite, and weight loss. Despite the research supporting the benefits of **Rehmannia 6** to renal perfusion in rats, the use of Rehmannia 6 alone is contraindicated in chilly patients because increased vomiting and loss of appetite are potential outcomes. Aconite and Cinnamon should be present for typical improvements to be seen, which are reductions in blood urea nitrogen (BUN) and creatinine to normal or high-normal levels; reduction or cessation of vomiting; improved appetite and weight gain; increased urinary specific gravity, sometimes to levels exceeding minimal concentrating ability; reduced thirst; and reduced urine volume. Some cats that respond to Rehmannia 8 live for years when it is consistently used. Improvements may be seen even before low-protein diets and fluid therapy have been instituted.
- The perceived enhanced effectiveness of Rehmannia 8 over Rehmannia 6 may be explained by the invigorating effects Cinnamon and Aconite typically are thought to have on circulation. This increased circulation may increase renal clearance more than Rehmannia 6 (the base formula) alone can. Rehmannia 6 is only for use in cats with chronic renal failure that have heat intolerance, a red, dry, small tongue, and rapid, floating pulses. Rehmannia 8 is indicated for the majority of cats that are affected by uncomplicated chronic renal failure that have pale, wet, swollen tongues and a strong desire to seek heat. A *suggested starting dose* of granular concentrate of both of these formulas is ¼ tsp per 10 to 15 lb of body weight, or 60 to 75 mg/kg of body weight, given at least once daily.

- Despite the studies previously noted indicating the efficacy of Rhubarb in humans with renal failure, the positive response of cats to "warming" formulas suggests that veterinary practitioners should proceed with caution in the use of "cooling" herbs such as Rhubarb in chronic renal failure cases. Cooling herbs may be much more applicable in animals with "hot" and "excessive" presentations, such as acute renal failure, active renal inflammation, and glomerulonephritis. Only very small doses of Rhubarb as part of an overall warming formula such as **Wen Pi Tang** (Warm the Spleen Decoction) should be contemplated for use in chilly cats with chronic renal failure.
- If improvements in renal perfusion and clearance are truly the mechanism by which Rehmannia 6 and Rehmannia 8 work, new light begins to be shed on the pathophysiology of chronic renal failure. Even though 60% to 75% of the original kidney mass may no longer be functioning, a significant portion of nephrons may not yet have degenerated to the point of ischemic necrosis. Some of these nephrons may still be able to function well enough if reperfused, resulting in the restoration of minimal concentrating ability and adequate renal function. This might especially be true in patients treated early in the disease process, since clinical experience with Rehmannia 8 suggests that animals with renal insufficiency respond the best. However, improvements have also been seen in animals in much more advanced states of renal failure.
- The use of **Jin Suo Gu Jing Wan** has also been advocated for use in chronic renal failure. This formula may be more appropriate if urinary incontinence, soft stools, pale or white vaginal discharge, and perhaps seminal emission are part of the clinical presentation. **Zhen Wu Tang** (Water-Controlling God Decoction) is an intensely warming formula, mainly used for edema but advocated by some for treating chronic renal failure. Limited clinical experience with this formula in cats with chronic renal failure has not been rewarding. A *suggested starting dose* of granular concentrate for both

of these formulas is ¼ tsp per 10 to 15 lb of body weight, or 60 to 75 mg/kg of body weight, divided into two daily doses.

- Special considerations exist for treatment of chronic renal failure in cats that are also clinically hyperthyroid. Formulas that should be considered for use in these patients include **Er Xian Tang** (Decoction of Curculigo and Epimedium) and **Zhi Bai Di Huang Wan** (Anemarrhena, Phellodendron, and Rehmannia Pill). Consult Chapter 8 for further information on treating these patients.
- Some patients brought for treatment of chronic renal failure have serum BUN and creatinine levels that are only occasionally inappropriate relative to urine specific gravity. At other times, they may appear to have adequate urine concentrating ability. From a Chinese medical point of view these patients often demonstrate signs of Spleen Qi deficiency only (e.g., poor appetite, fatigue, soft pulses, pale tongue). Signs of Dampness caused by Yang deficiency (e.g., craving heat, vomiting, wet tongue, slippery pulses) may not yet be in evidence. Tonification of Spleen Qi using formulas such as **Wei Ling Tang** (Decoction to Dispel Dampness in the Spleen and Stomach) and perhaps **Si Miao San** (Four Miracles Powder) may be effective in forestalling consistent signs of renal insufficiency. **Shi Pi Yin** (Spleen Tonic for Edema) may be especially helpful in patients with Spleen Qi deficiency accompanied by edema and poor appetite.
- Spleen Qi formulas may be used in tandem with **Shen Qi Wan** for patients in which both Spleen and Kidney tonification is desired. Spleen tonification may help forestall Kidney Qi deficiency, since the Spleen is the source of all postnatal Essence. This Essence is stored in the Kidney and is converted into Yin and Yang from which the body's flame of life (i.e., Qi) is generated.

Acupuncture and Moxibustion

- An appropriate herbal formula can be considered the most important aspect of Chinese medical treatment of chronic renal failure. Acupuncture and moxibustion may be used to enhance the effectiveness of the herbal approach, and may be applied to KI 3, BL 23, GV 4, and CV 4 (if accessible), regardless of whether the case is of the "hot" or "cold" variety. Acupuncture and moxibustion may reflexively increase renal blood flow. Local heat from other sources also appears to have been effective in stimulating renal blood flow. Direct moxibustion should be used only with the utmost caution in animals because the risk of burning is greater than that of indirect moxa.

Western Herbs

- Few Western herbs have the reputation for efficacy that Rehmannia 8 seems to have. Goldenrod *(Solidago canadensis)* is reputed to have the ability to promote urine production and lower BUN levels. Limited clinical experience with this herb in chronic renal failure in cats has not been encouraging.
- Other herbs with rational bases but little support include Dandelion, Horsetail, and Marshmallow *(Althea officinalis)*. Dandelion Leaf is a diuretic and has been used traditionally for kidney failure, presumably in advanced oliguric, acute, or end-stage renal failure. Horsetail is sometimes recommended for kidney failure. Since it is a mild diuretic, this use is presumably only for oliguric, acute, or end-stage renal failure. Althea Root is a traditional demulcent and mild diuretic. It is sometimes recommended for chronic renal failure but is probably more appropriate for inflammatory conditions of the urinary tract because of its mucilage content.
- Western herbs may have more application in the management of acute renal failure manifesting as anuria and oliguria. For example, Juniper *(Juniperus communis)* appears to have a powerful stimulatory effect on glomerular filtration and Juniper Oil has been used successfully to stimulate urine flow in older dogs affected with anuria. This ability of Juniper to increase urine production has been attributed to its content of terpenes. Terpenes have a reputation for increasing renal blood flow by causing inflammation of the

glomerulus, although this claim has not been substantiated. Many modern Western herbalists therefore avoid Juniper in renal failure cases. It should be noted, however, that Western herbalism is almost alone in its use of single herbs. Most advanced herbal traditions did not use single herbs but combined herbs in formulas to provide a balanced effect without undue side effects. The use of Juniper in smaller amounts, either alone or in combination with other herbs, may significantly reduce the risk of renal "exhaustion" relative to when Juniper is used alone.

- The following are some guidelines for the use of Juniper. It should be used only in oliguric and anuric animals. Use should be minimized or avoided in inflammatory conditions of the glomeruli. A *recommended starting dose* might be one drop of alcohol extract per 4 lb of body weight in divided doses daily. If the effect is inadequate, dosage should be increased to a maximum of one drop per lb of body weight daily in divided doses. Use should be discontinued once urine production has been reestablished or if there is no clinical benefit after 3 to 4 days.

Chiropractic

- Hind limb weakness is a common complaint in animals with renal insufficiency and is characteristic of declining Kidney Qi. It is also common, however, for some of this hind limb weakness to be caused by reduced mobility and abnormal positioning of the lower lumbar vertebrae and the sacrum. Adjustment of such fixations can produce improvements in hind limb strength that seem to be immediate. Examination of the spine should also extend to the thoracic and cervical regions, since vertebral fixations tend to amass where there are other fixations.

Cautions

- Chinese herbal combinations containing aristolochic acid have been associated with kidney failure and urothelial cancer. In some products the herbs *Aristolochia westlandi* (Guang Fang Ji) and *Aristolochia manshuriensis* (Guan Mu Tong) are incorrectly substituted for the nontoxic herbs

Stephania tetrandra (Han Fang Ji), *Clematis armandii* (Chuan Mu Tong), *Akebia* (Mu Tong), and others. Reputable companies will provide assurance that their products are free of aristolochic acid.

- Diuretic herbs may increase toxicity of some antiinflammatory drugs.
- Diuretic herbs may increase potential for hypokalemia if administered with diuretic drugs or with corticosteroids (Poppenga, 2002). Dandelion is reported to be a potassium-sparing diuretic.
- Marshmallow may decrease absorption of other drugs.
- Chromium has been associated with kidney damage in human patients taking 600 μg or more daily (Cerulli, 1998; Wasser, 1997). There has been some suggestion that the damage was actually caused by contaminants, but this has not been confirmed.
- Licorice *(Glycyrrhiza glabra)* used on a long-term basis leads to hyperaldosteronism, accompanied by hypokalemia, sodium retention, and hypertension. Licorice should be used with great care in renal failure patients. The deglycyrrhizinated forms of licorice do not possess this toxic potential.

AUTHORS' CHOICES:

SM: Rehmannia 8; conventional care as needed; chiropractic when needed.
SW: Fish Oil; Rehmannia 6 or Rehmannia 8; home fluid therapy.

FELINE LOWER URINARY TRACT DISEASE

Therapeutic Rationale

- Reduce crystalluria.
- Reduce stress.
- Prevent and treat obstructions.

Alternative Options with Conventional Bases

Nutritional Therapies

- **Ascorbic acid:** may acidify urine, but most studies have shown equivocal or negative results (Castellow, 1996;

Hetey, 1980). Interestingly, one study in horses suggested that Vitamin C is effective in reducing urine pH (Wood, 1990). If a cat has persistently alkaline urine, a trial of Vitamin C at 125 to 250 mg bid will probably be risk free.

Herbs

- **Cranberry:** widely believed to acidify urine, but the few studies analyzing this effect do not support this effect (Habash, 1999; Kinney, 1979; Tsukada, 1994).
- **Choreito** (Zhu Ling San or available commercially as Polyporus combination): has been shown to decrease struvite crystalluria and hematuria in cats with feline lower urinary tract disease (FLUTD) (Buffington, 1994, 1997a, 1997b).

Chinese Herbs

- The crystals of FLUTD represent a more severe form of the Damp Heat accumulation in the Bladder than that discussed in the Chinese medical section on urinary tract infections. Dampness is present in such abundance in these cases that it is congealing into mucus, crystals, and urethral plugs.
- The Chinese herbal formula typically advocated in Chinese medicine for urolithiasis in humans is **Shi Wei San** (Pyrrosia Leaf Powder). This formula drains Dampness, clears Heat, and expels stones. Its antilithic properties are reportedly enhanced with the addition of Jin Qian Cao (Lysimachia), Hai Hin Sha (Lygodium Spores), and Ji Nei Jin (Chicken Gizzard Lining). Hematuria can be reduced with the addition of Xiao Ji (Small Thistle), Pu Huang (Bulrush Pollen), and Mu Dan Pi (Moutan Bark) to the base formula. A *suggested starting dose* of granular concentrate is ¼ tsp per 10 to 15 lb of body weight, or 60 to 75 mg/kg of body weight, divided into two daily doses.

Western Herbs

- Clinical experience with the combination of Hydrangea, Stone Root, Gravel Root, and Corn Silk discussed in the section on Western herbal treatment of urinary tract infections suggests that this formula is an effective urinary acidifier. This benefit exists even when acidifying diets are not used. It has been used successfully to prevent recurrences of urolithiasis in cats and to abort the development of urinary tract obstruction in early cases. Despite Eupatorium's content of pyrrolizidine alkaloids, long-term toxic effects on the liver of small animals receiving this formula for several months have not been identified.

- In Chinese medicine Dampness is considered a type of unusable body fluid that is manufactured by faulty digestion, underscoring the recognized link between diet and urethral obstruction. Dietary control of FLUTD might seem to be more than a matter of including urinary acidifiers and controlling magnesium levels. Excess levels of congealed Dampness and Phlegm commonly correlate with food allergies or sensitivities and incomplete digestion. It is noteworthy that one of the Chinese "herbs" used specifically for urolithiasis in humans is Chicken Gizzard Lining. Metabolites of its content of ventriculin are credited with causing an increase in the secretion of gastric juices, which in turn promotes increased gastric acidity and completeness of digestion. This increased acid secretion may also play an indirect role in urinary tract acidification. In general, however, the mechanism by which Chinese herbal formulas reduce or dissolve stones is unclear.
- The herbal formula containing Hydrangea, Stone Root, Corn Silk, and Gravel Root may also help acidify urine by regulating circulation through the bladder wall so that tendencies to hematuria are lessened. Blood and transudates seem to have an alkalinizing effect on urine, and the apparent benefit of herbs that regulate microcirculation suggests that chronic low-grade cystitis is an antecedent event to many cases of urethral obstruction.
- **Saw Palmetto:** traditionally used for dysuria. Most studies demonstrating the efficacy of Saw Palmetto in BPH (discussed previously) focus on improvements in urination dynamics as evidence of its effects and assume these are attributable to a reduction in prostate

size. Liposterolic extracts of Saw Palmetto have been shown, however, to contain a compound with calcium channel–blocking activity that confers a spasmolytic effect on rat uterus, bladder, and aorta. Saw Palmetto appears to be clinically effective in FLUTD only in substantial doses. A *recommended starting dose* is one capsule of dried herb, or 30 drops of alcohol extract three to six times daily, tapering as signs of dysuria abate. Practitioners are advised to use whole herb in alcohol tincture form until the active ingredient is identified and emphasized in standardized extracts.

Cautions

- Uva-Ursi, used in urinary tract infections, may reduce the effectiveness of urinary acidifiers (Poppenga, 2002).

AUTHORS' CHOICES:

SM: Saw Palmetto for postobstruction urethral spasm; Hydrangea, Corn Silk, Stone Root, and Gravel Root to prevent recurrences and abort pending obstruction.

SW: Canned or fresh food; Choreito based on symptoms and long term if necessary.

INCONTINENCE

Therapeutic Rationale

- Identify cause (e.g., urinary tract infection, calculi, tumors, estrogen deficiency).

Alternative Options with Conventional Bases

Nutritional Therapies

- Food allergy has been implicated in some cases of incontinence, and elimination diets may be worth investigating for some dogs' diets (Guilford, 1999).

Herbs

- **Soy isoflavones:** these are phytoestrogens, compounds that bind to certain types of estrogen receptors. There are anecdotal reports of occasional success when soy isoflavones were used for treatment of estrogen-responsive incontinence in spayed female dogs. A provisional dose is approximately 0.5 to 2 mg/lb of body weight daily.

- **Wild Yam** *(Dioscorea* spp.): has also been used for estrogen-responsive incontinence, but probably inappropriately. This use is based on a misconception that Wild Yam contains progesterone, when in reality it contains diosgenin, a precursor used in steroid synthesis that is probably not converted to progesterone in the body.

Paradigmatic Options

- The maintenance of urinary continence is a complex process. It is the by-product of a metaphoric upward pull within the body. In Chinese medicine Qi or energy propels the movement of all fluid, so the first requirement of continence is adequate energy. Adequate pulling force, the second requirement, comes from the upper body and includes being conscious of the bladder. The third requirement is a minimum of "downward drag" or "accumulations" that serve to inspire the urge to urinate. Incontinence with fear is considered to be a type of downward drag in which retreat of the organism is so forcibly downward as to expel urine. Each of these three avenues (strength or Qi, conscious state, and downward accumulations) is discussed in further detail below.

Inadequate Energy Levels

- In Chinese medicine the Kidneys are the storage area of the body's Qi, or energy reserves. Kidney Qi or Yang deficiency is thus considered to be an important cause of incontinence. The Kidney is also responsible for the integrity of the lower orifices and for ensuring that urine is adequately concentrated. Declining Kidney Qi thus easily leads to urinary incontinence because of its association with general lack of strength, poor sphincter integrity, and the tendency to produce dilute urine that further challenges maintenance of sphincter tone.

- Several formulas have potential application for this form of incontinence. **Suo Quan Wan** (Shut the Sluice Pill) is a small formula to warm the Kidney Yang and Bladder and astringe urine leakage. For extra power, 40 g of it is combined with about 75 g of **Bu Zhong Yi Qi Tang** (Tonify the Center and Augment the Qi Decoction). Signs calling for this combined formula might include digestive weakness, fatigue, previous hemorrhagic tendencies, a soft pulse, a pale tongue, abdominal bloating, and the tendency to prolapse. In addition, some practitioners have found the addition of about 15 g of Sang Piao Xiao (Mantis Egg Casing) to 40 g of Suo Quan Wan to treat urinary incontinence to be effective. For all of these formulas, a *suggested starting dose* of granular concentrate is ¼ tsp per 10 to 15 lb of body weight, or 60 to 75 mg/kg of body weight, divided into two daily doses.
- A general formula for Kidney Qi deficiency and all its attendant problems is **Shen Qi Wan** (Kidney Qi Pill), also known as **Rehmannia 8** (Ba Wei Di Huang Wan). This formula is discussed in the section on chronic renal failure, and practitioners are reminded to obtain the version of the formula that contains Cinnamon and Aconite. For long-term use, some practitioners recommend using 50 g **Rehmannia 6** (Liu Wei Di Huang Wan) and adding 6 g Cinnamon and 12 g Schizandra (Wu Wei Zi). Schizandra is credited with an astringent action that stops fluid leakages of many types. For all these formulas, a *suggested starting dose* of granular concentrate is ¼ tsp per 10 to 15 lb of body weight, or 60 to 75 mg/kg of body weight, divided into two daily doses.
- **Jin Suo Gu Jin Wan** (Metal Lock Pill to Stabilize the Essence) has been advocated for use in Kidney-deficient types of incontinence in animals. This formula is somewhat "neutral" and has a consolidating stabilizing action that is used to treat spermatorrhea in fatigued patients with Lung or Spleen Qi deficiency. Its use has been expanded to include urinary incontinence. A *suggested starting dose* of granular concentrate is ¼ tsp per 10 to 15 lb of body weight, or 60 to 75 mg/kg of

body weight, divided into two daily doses. A more vigorously tonifying formula that still consolidates or acts as an astringent is **Wu Bi Shan Yao Wan** (Dioscorea Pill). This formula is used in cases of Kidney deficiency as opposed to Lung or Spleen deficiency. A *suggested starting dose* of granular concentrate is ¼ tsp per 10 to 15 lb of body weight, or 60 to 75 mg/kg of body weight, divided into two daily doses.

- Acupuncture treatment of this type of incontinence uses points that strengthen the Qi of the body, including KI 3, KI 7, GV 4, BL 23, BL 20, CV 4, CV 6, ST 36, and LI 4.

Reduced Conscious Control

- The effect of the upper regions of the body, including consciousness, in the maintenance of continence has been likened to the ability to hold water in a straw by placing a finger on the top end. One extremely important formula that maintains continence in this fashion is **Sang Piao Xiao San** (Mantis Egg Casing Powder). Sang Piao Xiao San is a somewhat rich tonifying formula that acts to gather, descend, and penetrate the Shen (i.e., consciousness) so that the Heart and Kidneys are reconnected and the mind becomes aware of the bladder. A *suggested starting dose* of granular concentrate is ¼ tsp per 10 to 15 lb of body weight, or 60 to 75 mg/kg of body weight, divided into two daily doses.
- As briefly mentioned in the section on Chronic Renal Failure, a connection between the Heart and Kidney is necessary for life. Descent of Heart Yang provides the spark that helps keep the flame of life in the Kidneys alive. In return, the Kidney fire "steams" some of the Kidney Yin so that it rises to keep the Heart Yang cool and the spirit calm. Hormones in Chinese medicine are known as "celestial water" and are considered a precious component of Kidney Yin; it is not surprising to find them playing a role in the maintenance of continence.
- Hormone-responsive urinary incontinence is a type of Kidney Yin deficiency that results in a failed connection

between the Heart and Kidney. It is typically worse at night, as are all Yin deficiency syndromes. Hormone supplementation effectively equates to supplying the body with a form of Yin that can be used to cool the Heart Yang, calm the Shen, redirect the Heart Yang downward to restore consciousness of urination, and restore the normal axis of control between the Heart and the Kidney.

- Plants containing phytoestrogens are understood to reconnect the Heart and the Kidney in Chinese medicine. Dan Dou Chi (Prepared Soy Bean) is thus used for both Yin deficiency and mental restlessness and irritability. It is not surprising to learn that its isoflavones may be useful in the management of hormone-responsive urinary incontinence. Other plants that contain phytoestrogen, such as Alfalfa *(Medicago sativa)*, can be understood to tonify Yin and might yield other means of controlling hormone-responsive urinary incontinence. Early experimentation with the use of Alfalfa in my (SM) practice indicates that Alfalfa is effective in at least some cases of hormone-responsive urinary incontinence. A *suggested starting dose* of Alfalfa extract, either in alcohol or in glycerine, is 0.2 ml per 5 lb of body weight, divided into two daily doses.
- Other Yin tonics that are not necessarily estrogenic also seem to serve this function in dogs, including those present in **Sang Piao Xiao San.** Sang Piao Xiao San thus acts to restore the Heart and Kidney connection in two ways: tonifying the Kidney to cool the Heart, and descending the Heart to reconnect with the Kidney. It is a good first choice for animals with nocturia that seem generally deficient, and it has been used successfully in practice. A different clinical presentation calling for Sang Piao Xiao San is the excitable, anxious, incontinent dog with floating, forceful pulses and a pink tongue. In this type of patient, the heavy mineral elements of the formula "drag" consciousness downward to the lower body and the bladder. Acupuncture points useful in such a patient include GV 20, SI 3, and GV 3 or 4. **Restore Integrity**, a modern

formula that is a combination of Sang Piao Xiao San and Suo Quan Wan, has been useful in some practices.

- Points to calm the spirit include GV 20, PC 6, HT 7, and ear Shen Men. Points to tonify Kidney Yin, such as BL 23, BL 20, CV 4, ST 36, and KI 6, can be considered.

Damp Heat Accumulation in the Lower Body

- The third main cause of incontinence is the accumulation of Damp Heat in the lower body, which produces a frequent and sometimes irresistible urge to urinate small amounts. Very strong Heat-clearing formulas such as **Long Dan Xie Gan Tang** (Gentian Purge the Liver Decoction) have been used for enuresis of this type in humans. **Si Miao San** (Four Miracles Powder) is a safer alternative for long-term use because it is not as vigorously cooling and is more supportive of Spleen Qi and digestion. A *suggested starting dose* of granular concentrate for each of these formulas is ¼ tsp per 10 to 15 lb of body weight, or 60 to 75 mg/kg of body weight, divided into two daily doses.
- Formulas used to treat urinary tract infections may also be considered for use in incontinence. This is particularly true for mass lesions in the trigone area, which may respond to Blood-moving formulas, such as **Jia Wei Wu Lin San** (Augmented Five Herbs to Eliminate Painful Urination Powder) and **Shao Fu Zhu Yu Tang** (Drive Out Stasis in the Lower Abdomen Decoction). Adding 15 g of Hua Shi to Shao Fu Zhu Yu Tang enhances its efficacy. A *suggested starting dose* of granular concentrate for both of these formulas is ¼ tsp per 10 to 15 lb of body weight, or 60 to 75 mg/kg of body weight, divided into two daily doses.
- Extreme cases of Damp causing urinary incontinence in humans have responded to use of strong diuretic formulas such as **Zhu Ling Tang** (Polyporus Decoction). Although seemingly contraindicated, diuretic formulas are applied to "disinhibit urination," resulting in thorough voiding and a reduced sense of urinary retention and urgency. A *suggested starting dose* of granular concentrate is ¼ tsp per 10 to 15 lb of body

weight, or 60 to 75 mg/kg of body weight, divided into two daily doses.

- Acupuncture points that may be useful for this disorder include BL 28, BL 22, BL 39, SP 9, SP 6, and CV 3.

Other Acupuncture Methods

- **Scar therapy** (injecting ovariohysterectomy scars) may help some dogs. This is an aquapuncture-like treatment in which Vitamin B_{12}, saline, lidocaine, or a mixture of all or some of these is injected proximal and distal to the scar and into nearby meridians.

Chiropractic

- It is common to find lower lumbar and sacral vertebral fixations in animals with urinary incontinence. Release of fixations alone using chiropractic technique seems to relieve nerve root pressure sufficiently in some animals to restore normal continence without any other intervention. Lumbar vertebral fixations are, however, commonly found in dogs affected with Kidney deficiency and Damp Heat accumulation in the lower body. The fixations can thus serve as an indication that some of the formulas mentioned may be beneficial in restoring and maintaining normal continence. Use of the appropriate herbal formula may reduce further tendencies to vertebral fixation.
- Acupuncture may be used in tandem with chiropractic to address incontinence and relax the low back. The practitioner should consider using BL 25 through BL 28, BL 40, BL 60, and CV 3.

Homeopathy

- **Causticum 30C** sid: for unconscious dribbling when standing up or walking, together with tendencies to hind limb weakness.
- **Sepia 30C** sid as needed: for urinary incontinence during the first few hours of sleep.

Cautions

- The use of diuretic herbs, which is frequently recommended in lay publications, may make continence control more difficult. These herbs include Dandelion, Corn Silk, Parsley, and others.

- Herbs with potential hormonal activity (Vitex, Black Cohosh, soy isoflavones, Red Clover, Licorice) may potentiate the effect of diethylstilbestrol.

AUTHORS' CHOICES:

SM: Sang Piao Xiao San; chiropractic; Si Miao San; find replacements for drugs causing polyuria; Shao Fu Zhu Yu Tang for bladder masses in older animals.

SW: Elimination diet; attention to drugs causing polyuria; Chinese herbs; chiropractic.

OXALATE UROLITHS

Therapeutic Rationale

- Use diuresis.
- Reduce urinary calcium excretion.
- Reduce dietary oxalates.
- Reduce excessive levels of dietary calcium.

Alternative Options with Conventional Bases

Nutritional Therapies

- **Dietary phytate:** increases urinary phytate, a crystallization inhibitor in humans (Grases, 2000). Phytates are contained in grains, so low-meat, high-grain, homemade diets may be recommended.
- **Lemon juice:** in the form of lemonade given qid to humans increases urinary citrate levels (Seltzer, 1996). Compliance could be a problem if given to dogs or cats in this form.

Herbs

- **Fenugreek** *(Trigonella foenum-graecum):* reduced calcium oxalate stone deposition in kidneys of rats in an induced model (Ahsan, 1989).
- **Diuretic herbs:** see the section on Calculi for more information. Caution should be exercised until it is

known if these herbs enhance calcium excretion. Horsetail and Uva-Ursi may be most appropriate for these cases. Dandelion is said to contain substantial amounts of oxalates. I (SW) was unable to find firm support for this common claim; if it is true, Dandelion should be avoided.

- **Cranberry:** has multiple effects that may affect formation of oxalate stones. In one study it was shown to decrease urinary calcium excretion (Light, 1973). Cranberry is often recommended for acidifying urine, which is contraindicated in oxalate urolithiasis. However, urinary acidification caused by Cranberry ingestion occurs inconsistently or not at all according to most studies published to date. Also, Cranberries contain oxalates and have been shown to increase urinary oxalate levels in humans (Terris, 2001). In general, it appears that Cranberry should not be given to patients with calcium oxalate formation tendencies.
- ***Alisma orientele*** (Ze Xie in Chinese, or Takusha in Kampo): a single herb found in many Chinese formulas for urinary tract inflammation, including Choreito (Polyporus Combination). This herb was shown in a rat model of calcium oxalate calculus formation to slow accumulation of stones (Koide, 1995; Yasui, 1999).
- ***Dendrobium styracifolium:*** an extract of this Chinese herb was shown to reduce calcium oxalate stone formation in a rat model (Hirayama, 1993).

Chinese Herbs

- The most common type of urolith in humans is calcium oxalate stones, and they are often treated with **Shi Wei San** (Pyrrosia Leaf Powder). As mentioned in the sections on Calculi and on FLUTD, herbs often added to this formula to enhance its ability to dissolve and expel stones include Jin Qian Cao (Lysimachia), Hai Jin Sha (Lygodium Spores), and Ji Nei Jin (Chicken Gizzard Lining). Despite its widespread use and studies demonstrating its clinical effectiveness, the mechanisms by which this formula dissolves stones or reduces their formation are not known. A *suggested starting dose* of granular concentrate is ¼ tsp per 10 to 15 lb of body

weight, or 60 to 75 mg/kg of body weight, divided into two daily doses.

Cautions

- Herbal diuretics may add to the effect of conventional diuretics, such as hydrochlorothiazide, and should be used cautiously with these drugs.
- Herbal diuretics may have effects on mineral secretion that are undesirable, but as yet uncharacterized.

AUTHORS' CHOICES:

SM: Calcium restriction.
SW: Low-meat, high-grain diet; avoid dry foods; potassium citrate supplementation.

STRUVITE UROLITHS

Therapeutic Rationale

- Control infection that is the predisposing factor in dogs.
- Reduce dietary magnesium.
- Induce urinary acidification.
- Reduce urine concentration by increasing water in the diet.

Alternative Options with Conventional Bases

Nutritional Therapies

- **Ascorbic acid:** may acidify urine, but most studies have shown equivocal results or negative results (Castellow, 1996; Hetey, 1980). Interestingly, one study in horses suggested that Vitamin C is effective in reducing urine pH (Wood, 1990). If persistently alkaline urine is characteristic of the case after negative urine cultures, a trial of Vitamin C given tid will probably be risk free.

Herbs

- **Cranberry:** may be effective in preventing recurrent bacterial infections, an important part of managing struvite stones in dogs. See the Urinary Tract Infection section for more information on Cranberry.

- **Diuretic herbs,** such as Dandelion Leaf, in combination with increasing dietary water may help keep urinary specific gravity low. (See the section on Calculi.)

Chinese Medicine

- Crystals and calculi represent a more severe form of Damp Heat accumulation in the Bladder than that discussed in the Chinese medical section for urinary tract infections. Dampness is present in such abundance that it is congealing into uroliths.
- The Chinese herbal formula typically advocated in Chinese medicine for urolithiasis in humans is **Shi Wei San** (Pyrrosia Leaf Powder). This formula drains Dampness, clears Heat, and expels stones. Its antilithic properties are reportedly enhanced with the addition of Jin Qian Cao (Lysimachia), Hai Hin Sha (Lygodium Spores), and Ji Nei Jin (Chicken Gizzard Lining). Hematuria can be reduced with the addition of Xiao Ji (Small Thistle), Pu Huang (Bulrush Pollen), and Mu Dan Pi (Moutan Bark) to the base formula. A *suggested starting dose* of granular concentrate is ¼ tsp per 10 to 15 lb of body weight, or 60 to 75 mg/kg of body weight, divided into two daily doses.

Western Herbs

- Clinical experience with the combination of Hydrangea, Stone Root, Gravel Root, and Corn Silk discussed in the section on Western herbal treatment of urinary tract infections suggests that this formula is an effective urinary acidifier. Clinical experience in my (SM) practice demonstrates that it has been effective in acidifying urine pH and dissolving uroliths in dogs. This benefit exists even when acidifying diets are not used. However, uroliths in successfully treated cases were not chemically analyzed. Extended use of this formula over several months yielded no toxic effects.
- In Chinese medicine, Dampness is considered a type of unusable body fluid that is manufactured by faulty

digestion. This underscores the recognized link between diet and uroliths. Dietary control of struvite uroliths seems to be more than a matter of including urinary acidifiers and controlling magnesium levels, however. Excess levels of congealed Dampness and Phlegm commonly correlate with food allergies or sensitivities and incomplete digestion. It is noteworthy that one of the Chinese "herbs" used specifically for urinary calculi is Chicken Gizzard Lining. Metabolites of its content of ventriculin are credited with producing a delayed increase in secretion of gastric juices, which in turn increases gastric acidity and completeness of digestion. This increased acid secretion may play an indirect role in urinary tract acidification.

- The herbal formula containing Hydrangea, Stone Root, Corn Silk, and Gravel Root may also help acidify urine by regulating circulation through the bladder wall so that tendencies to hematuria are lessened. Blood and transudates seem to have an alkalinizing effect on urine, and the apparent benefit of herbs that regulate microcirculation suggests that chronic low-grade cystitis is an antecedent event to many cases of urethral obstruction.

Cautions

- Uva-Ursi and Horsetail may alkalinize urine and would not be recommended for patients with struvite uroliths.

AUTHORS' CHOICES:

SM: Hydrangea, Stone Root, Corn Silk, and Gravel Root combination.
SW: Increase water in diet; identify and treat concurrent bacterial infections; correct diet.

URINARY TRACT INFECTION

Therapeutic Rationale

- Identify and treat infection.

Alternative Options with Conventional Bases

- **Cranberry:** human clinical trials have shown that ingestion of cranberry juice reduces frequency of bacteruria (Avorn, 1994). Cranberry appears to irreversibly inhibit the expression of P-fimbriae of *Escherichia coli* (Ahuja, 1998). Cranberry does appear to help with recurrent infections; however, resistant bacteria may also develop when Cranberry is used for the long term, especially in insufficient doses.
- **Uva-Ursi** or **Bearberry:** the leaves contain arbutin, which is converted in alkaline urine to hydroquinone. German and Czech literature apparently indicates that this lends antibacterial and antiinflammatory action, and Commission E monographs list urinary tract infections and urinary inflammation as indications for use of Uva-Ursi. High-quality dog and cat diets may contain enough meat to give these omnivorous and carnivorous pets more acidic urine, except during active bacterial infection when the urine pH does rise. It is possible that Uva-Ursi stops working in these animals as soon as the bacterial population is reduced to the extent that the infection no longer causes alkaline urine.
- **Buchu:** Buchu leaves have diuretic and very mild antimicrobial properties (Lis-Balchin, 2001).
- **Pippsissewa** *(Chimaphila umbellata, C. maculata):* a traditional treatment for urinary inflammation, Pippsissewa also contains hydroquinone constituents.
- **Juniper:** the berries and oil are diuretic and have been used for urinary tract inflammation.

Paradigmatic Options

Homeopathy

- **Cantharis 30C** sid to tid: for hematuria and dysuria. Clinical experience with this remedy shows it to be frequently effective in acute uncomplicated cystitis and in the prevention of recurrences of FLUTD.
- **Staphysagria 30C** sid to tid: for infectious and sterile cystitis. The owners of cats that benefit the most from this remedy often report that their animals appear to be resentful and bear a grudge. The owners may also state

that their cat either is exceptionally gentle or is bullied by other cats. This remedy also appears useful for marking behavior by cats when the urinary tract is not inflamed but when resentment or repression seems to be present.

Chinese Medicine

- Although several pathophysiologic mechanisms in Chinese medicine lead to cystitis in humans, acute urinary tract infections in dogs and cats are caused primarily by accumulations of Damp Heat in the Bladder. Dampness is an unusable type of body fluid that is a by-product of faulty digestion. A potential link is therefore seen between diet, digestion, and the tendency toward urinary tract inflammation. Like fluid in general, Dampness tends to drain downward and accumulate in the lower reaches of the body. Colitis, cystitis, and vaginitis are all examples of Damp Heat, which explains how they may coexist in the same patient from the Chinese medical perspective.
- A prominent symptom of Dampness accumulation in the colon or Bladder is straining. The explanation for this symptom is basically the same in Chinese medicine as in conventional medicine. Accumulations of fluid in the viscus produce a constant sensation of distention attended by an urge to eliminate. Damp Heat also produces a burning sensation.
- Other signs of Damp Heat are blood and crystalluria. Bleeding is produced when Blood is sufficiently "agitated" by the Damp Heat to "leap" from the vessels. When Dampness is especially "turbid," it is manifested as more congealed forms, such as crystals, mucus, or stones.
- The Chinese medical view of the progression of cystitis mirrors conventional understanding of the pathology of the bladder. As Dampness continues to accumulate in the bladder wall in chronic conditions, obstructions to normal circulation occur. Initially, pain might come and go and have a distending quality characteristic of Qi stagnation. Qi is the motive force for Blood circulation, and as obstructions become more

established, the Blood circulation itself becomes involved. Blood stagnation in the Bladder is attended by focal stabbing persistent pain and perhaps the elaboration of bleeding masses. These masses may be manifested as fibrosis, polyps, and tumors.

- Goals of Chinese medical treatment of cystitis in small animals depend on the chronicity of the condition. Priorities for acute conditions are to drain Dampness and clear Heat. Goals in chronic conditions are to transform obstructing Dampness and Phlegm, drain Dampness, clear Heat, and stop bleeding.

Chinese Herbs

- For all of the formulas listed below, a *suggested starting dose* of granular concentrate is ¼ tsp per 10 to 15 lb of body weight, or 60 to 75 mg/kg of body weight, given in divided doses twice daily. Higher doses may be used as needed if the formula is well tolerated.
- **Ba Zheng San** (Eight Rectifiers Powder) is the formula most commonly used for simple acute cystitis in human Chinese medicine. Constituent herbs contain both antiinflammatory and antimicrobial compounds. This formula is not to be used in weak or debilitated patients.
- As cystitis proceeds from simple Damp Heat accumulations to a condition of Blood stasis, formulas with hemostatic and Blood-moving herbs are used. **Wu Lin San** (Five Herbs to Relieve Painful Urination Powder; Gardenia and Hoelen Formula) can be considered for conditions of Damp Heat progressing to Blood stasis. **Jia Wei Wu Lin San** (Augmented Five Herbs to Relieve Painful Urination Powder) may be even more effective.
- When Blood stasis has progressed to the development of bleeding masses, **Shao Fu Zhu Yu Tang** (Drive Out Blood Stasis in the Lower Abdomen Decoction) should be considered. This formula is especially appropriate for the older chilly animal. The practitioner may add 15 g of Hua Shi (Talc; note this is not the scented cosmetic, but a mineral) to 100 g of the base formula to "guide" the formula's Blood-moving effects to the

Bladder. Hua Shi may also help soften masses and address Damp Heat accumulations. Hua Shi should probably be avoided, however, in cases of struvite urolithiasis, since it has a high magnesium content. Shao Fu Zhu Yu Tang may debulk or eliminate bleeding masses, especially when San Leng (Sparganium) and E Zhu (Zedoaria) are added.

- **Xiao Ji Yin Zi** (Decoction of Small Thistle) may be used for cases that are not attended by polyps or tumor, but in which significant hematuria attends chronic cystitis.
- Patients with tendencies to Damp-Heat accumulation in the lower jiao, such as colitis and cystitis, may be given **Si Miao San** (Four Miracles Powder) to prevent recurrences.

Acupuncture

- Acupuncture points to consider for patients with urinary tract infection are CV 3, BL 28, SP 9, SP 6, and SP 10. The first two points are the Alarm and Association points of the Bladder. SP 9 drains Damp and clears Heat from the lower burner and strengthens the Spleen to reduce the production of obstructing Dampness. SP 6 is a major point to move stagnant Qi and Blood in the lower burner. SP 10 also moves and cools Blood.

Western Herbs

- As previously discussed, several Western herbs are credited with antibiotic properties that appear to be useful in cystitis. Some of the most useful herbs, however, seem to have minimal or no antimicrobial activity. These include Gravel Root, Hydrangea, Stone Root, and Corn Silk. A formula advocated by Hoffman that contains these four herbs is a urine-acidifying formula. I (SM) use alcohol extracts of the four herbs in a 2:2:1:1 ratio. A *suggested starting dose* is 0.2 ml per 5 lb of body weight, divided into two daily doses. In addition to acidifying the urine, the formula is effective in both infectious and sterile cystitis, of both an acute and a recurrent nature. Evaluation of the constituent herbs in light of Chinese medicine suggests that Gravel Root drains Damp and clears Heat, Hydrangea moves Qi, Stone Root moves Blood, and Corn Silk acts as a soothing demulcent and a Dampness-draining herb. The actions of this formula are thus fully in accord with Chinese medicine's treatment goals for acute and chronic cystitis.

- For bleeding masses, different Western herbs are used. Alcohol extracts of Horsetail, Cleavers, Gravel Root, and Hydrangea are combined in approximately equal amounts. Horsetail seems to soften or transform obstructions to blood circulation, thereby finding use in chronic hematuria associated with fibrotic and polypoid disorders of the Bladder. Cleavers aids Horsetail in softening fibrotic tissues. Hydrangea is used to relieve Bladder pain by moving Qi, and Gravel Root is used to drain Dampness and clear Heat.
  A *suggested starting dose* is 0.2 ml per 5 lb of body weight, divided into two daily doses.

AUTHORS' CHOICES:

SM: Gravel Root, Hydrangea, Corn Silk, and Stone Root combination; Shao Fu Zhu Yu Tang for masses and chronic hematuria; Cantharis 30C in simple acute cases.

SW: Antibiotics based on culture and sensitivity. For chronic recurrent infections, rotate among Cranberry, Buchu, and Uva-Ursi, or appropriately chosen Chinese herbs.

VAGINITIS, PERSISTENT (ALSO SEE CHAPTER 17)

Therapeutic Rationale

- Identify predisposing cause (anatomic, irritation, neoplasia, infection, etc.).

Paradigmatic Options

- Treatment of vaginitis and vulvitis in small animals involves addressing accumulations of Dampness and Damp Heat in the lower body.

Chinese Herbs

- For all of the formulas listed below, a *suggested starting dose* of granular concentrate is ¼ tsp per 10 to 15 lb of body weight, or 60 to 75 mg/kg of body weight, given in divided doses twice daily. Higher doses may be used as needed if the formula is well tolerated.
- **Long Dan Xie Gan Tang** (Gentian Purge the Liver Decoction) for excess-type patients with a brick-red tongue, forceful pulses, irritability, raw and weeping lesions, suppurative discharges, and pain. Use should be discontinued immediately if loss of appetite or fatigue develops.
- **Si Miao San** (Four Marvels Powder) for more deficient patients in which lesions may appear the same as in patients benefiting from Long Dan Xie Gan Tang, but the pulse is more feeble, the tongue is less dark, or there is an intolerance of Long Dan Xie Gan Tang. Other signs consistent with an underlying Spleen Qi deficiency might be present (see the Case Report in Chapter 17).
- Clear vaginal discharge sometimes appears in Spleen-deficient animals that are being treated for some other disorder. Successful treatment of this disorder will usually rectify the discharge.
- Formulas more specifically developed to treat vaginitis with foul yellow discharges caused by Damp Heat in the lower body include **Yu Dai Wan** (Cure Discharge Pill) and **Zhi Dai Tang** (Stop Leukorrhea Decoction). For milder clear or white discharges in Spleen-deficient animals that possibly have a tendency to prolapse, **Yi Zhi Tang** (Boosting Wisdom Decoction) can be considered.

Western Herbs

- Several Western herbs, either alone or in combination, have been advocated for use in vaginal discharges in women and may have application to canine disorders. All of these herbs are more for use in infectious conditions and are given orally:
  - Blue Cohosh *(Caulophyllum thalictroides)*.
  - Bethroot *(Trillium erectum)*.

- Nettles—especially when extreme itch is present.
- Cranesbill *(Geranium maculatum)*—especially if the discharge is bloody.
- A *suggested starting dose* of the above herbs, whether alone or in combination, is 0.2 ml per 5 lb of body weight, divided into two daily doses.

AUTHORS' CHOICES:

SM: Appropriate Chinese herbal formula.
SW: Probiotics; Chinese herbs.

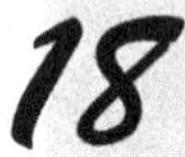

CASE REPORT
Recurrent Urinary Tract Infection in a Dog

HISTORY

Maggie, a 6-year-old, female, spayed Golden Retriever, was referred for alternative medical treatment for recurrent lower urinary tract infections spanning a 3-year period.

Signs of the infection initially included frequent passage of a small amount of occasionally bloody urine, followed by unproductive straining. The odor of the urine was "musty" and offensive. A culture of the urine identified *Proteus mirabilis* as the pathogen. The organism was sensitive to cephalexin, and the drug was administered at a dosage of 1000 mg twice daily.

Maggie's response to the drug was immediate, and was confirmed by negative urine cultures. Within several weeks, however, the *Proteus* infection had returned and was again successfully treated. An ultrasound was performed on Maggie's bladder to identify any persistent nidus of infection, but it showed only a slightly thickened cranial bladder wall. Repeated courses of antibiotics reliably resolved the infection, only for it to recur within a month of stopping the drugs. A biopsy of the bladder wall was suggested, but the owner declined surgery in favor of more antibiotics. These continued to be effective, but the *Proteus* infection continued to recur after their cessation.

The owner consulted a veterinary herbalist who prescribed a formula containing several herbs known for their antimicrobial effect on the urinary tract. The formula may have provided some significant symptomatic relief for Maggie, but her urine culture continued to test positive for *Proteus mirabilis* despite continued use of the herbs. A repeat ultrasound showed the thickening of the bladder wall to be progressing, particularly near the apex. Surgery and contrast cystography were recommended, but the owner again declined in favor of another prolonged course of antibiotic therapy. Five weeks after the cessation of antibiotics, Maggie's bladder was once again infected, this time with *Enterococcus.* At this point, Maggie and her owner were referred to me (SM).

At the time of examination Maggie's urinary tract infection was relatively asymptomatic, with only a slight increase in frequency of urination noted in the evening. Maggie also had slightly increased thirst. Her urine was very yellow, with no unusual odor. She had a tendency to become too hot but was not unduly restless. She had a good appetite and was energetic and affectionate.

PHYSICAL EXAMINATION

Maggie's physical examination was unremarkable, although note was taken of her tongue and pulse characteristics for the purpose of evaluating her condition from a Chinese medical perspective. Her tongue had appeared dark-red and wet in previous examinations by other practitioners, but it was now a normal color, with a light coating.

Maggie's pulses were consistently wiry on one side and slippery on the other. A wiry pulse refers to increased tension in the vessel wall so that it resists compression. In Chinese medicine this pulse suggests impaired circulation.

A slippery pulse refers to a pulse that feels engorged and forceful, yet with very little tone in the vessel wall. The pairing of a slippery pulse with a wiry pulse suggests that the cause of obstructed circulation is some pathologic accumulation.

ASSESSMENT

From a conventional standpoint, Maggie's clinical presentation was consistent with a possible persistent urachal diverticulum, given the thickening of the bladder wall at the apex of the bladder. The change from a *Proteus* to an *Enterococcus* infection may simply reflect a new infection developing after eradication of a previous one.

Although a persistent urachal diverticulum is a condition that requires surgery, reduction of bladder wall inflammation offered some hope in resolving it, simply by decongesting the bladder wall enough to promote a complete emptying of the pouch during voiding. Decongesting the bladder wall also would be expected to allow better access of the immune system to the infected area. Conventional medical goals thus focused on the improvement of bladder wall circulation.

From a Chinese perspective, improving circulation through the bladder wall was likewise the prime objective. Cystitis in Chinese medicine frequently arises from the accumulation of Dampness in the Bladder, promoting the eventual obstruction of Qi and Blood circulation. As this obstruction progresses, Heat is elaborated. This Damp Heat manifests as a red, wet tongue, and the obstructed Qi flow leads to a wiry pulse. Both of these features were present in Maggie.

TREATMENT

In an effort to address both the conventional and Chinese medical assessments of Maggie's condition, a combination of four herbs was prescribed. Alcohol extracts of *Hydrangea arborescens*, *Eupatorium purpureum*, *Collinsonia canadensis*, and *Zea mays* were combined in equal quantities and administered at a dosage of 30 drops three times daily. As discussed in the text, these herbs seem to improve bladder wall circulation from a Chinese medical perspective and may also do so from a conventional perspective. The formula may also hinder microbial growth through its acidifying action, but none of the herbs are specifically antimicrobial.

RESPONSE TO TREATMENT

Maggie responded quickly to the formula. A culture of her urine proved sterile after she was given the herbs for approximately 4 weeks. No antibiotics had been given for 4 months. The owner also noted that Maggie was more energetic than she had been in many months, suggesting that Maggie may have been in some degree of pain that was relieved by the formula. Many months later, Maggie's urine continued to show no microbial growth with intermittent use of the formula whenever an abnormal odor was detected in her urine.

SM

REFERENCES

Ahsan SK, Tariq M, Ageel AM, al-Yahya MA, Shah AH. Effect of *Trigonella foenum-graecum* and *Ammi majus* on calcium oxalate urolithiasis in rats. *J Ethnopharmacol* 26(3):249-254, 1989.

Ahuja S, Kaack B, Roberts J. Loss of fimbrial adhesion with the addition of

Vaccinum macrocarpon to the growth medium of P-fimbriated *Escherichia coli*. *J Urol* 159(2):559-562, 1998.

Avorn J, Monane M, Gurwitz JH, Glynn RJ, Choodnovskiy I, Lipsitz LA. Reduction of bacteriuria and pyuria after ingestion of cranberry juice. *J Am Med Assoc* 271(10):751-754, 1994.

Barsanti JA, Finco DR, Mahaffey MM, Fayrer-Hosken RA, Crowell WA, Thompson FN Jr, Shotts EB. Effects of an extract of *Serenoa repens* on dogs with hyperplasia of the prostate gland. *Am J Vet Res* 61(8):880-885, 2000.

Brown SA, Finco DR, Brown CA. Is there a role for dietary polyunsaturated fatty acid supplementation in canine renal disease? *J Nutr* 128(12 Suppl):2765S-2767S, 1998.

Buffington CA, Blaisdell JL, Komatsu Y, Kawase K. Effects of choreito and takushya consumption on in vitro and in vivo struvite solubility in cat urine. *Am J Vet Res* 58(2):150-152, 1997a.

Buffington CA, Blaisdell JL, Kawase K, Komatsu Y. Effects of choreito consumption on urine variables of healthy cats fed a magnesium-supplemented commercial diet. *Am J Vet Res* 58(2):146-149, 1997b.

Buffington CA, Blaisdell JL, Komatsu Y, Kawase K. Effects of choreito consumption on struvite crystal growth in urine of cats. *Am J Vet Res* 55(7):972-975, 1994.

Castello T, Girona L, Gomez MR, Mena Mur A, Garcia L. The possible value of ascorbic acid as a prophylactic agent for urinary tract infection. *Spinal Cord* 34(10):592-593, 1996.

Cerulli J, Grabe DW, Gauthier I, Malone M, McGoldrick MD. Chromium picolinate toxicity. *Ann Pharmacother* 32:428-431, 1998.

Doan DD, Nguyen NH, Doan HK, Nguyen TL, Phan TS, van Dau N, Grabe M, Johansson R, Lindgren G, Stjernstrom NE. Studies on the individual and combined diuretic effects of four Vietnamese traditional herbal remedies *(Zea mays, Imperata cylindrica, Plantago major,* and *Orthosiphon stamineus). J Ethnopharmacol* 36(3):225-231, 1992.

Ehling D. *The Chinese Herbalist's Handbook,* revised ed. Santa Fe, NM, 1996, Inword Press.

Grases F, Melero G, Costa-Bauza A, Prieto R, March JG. Urolithiasis and phytotherapy. *Int Urol Nephrol* 26(5):507-511, 1994.

Grases F, March JG, Prieto RM, Simonet BM, Costa-Bauza A, Garcia-Raja A, Conte A. Urinary phytate in calcium oxalate stone formers and healthy people—dietary effects on phytate excretion. *Scand J Urol Nephrol* 34(3):162-164, 2000.

Guilford G. Proceedings of the North American Veterinary Conference, Orlando, Fla, 1999.

Habash MB, Van der Mei HC, Busscher HJ, Reid G. The effect of water, ascorbic acid, and cranberry-derived supplementation on human urine and uropathogen adhesion to silicone rubber. *Can J Microbiol* 45(8):691-694, 1999.

Hetey SK, Kleinberg ML, Parker WD, Johnson EW. Effect of ascorbic acid on urine pH in patients with injured spinal cords. *Am J Hosp Pharm* 37(2):235-237, 1980.

Hirayama H, Wang Z, Nishi K, Ogawa A, Ishimatu T, Ueda S, Kubo T, Nohara

T. Effect of *Desmodium styracifolium*–triterpenoid on calcium oxalate renal stones. *Br J Urol* 71(2):143-147, 1993.

Ishani A, MacDonald R, Nelson D, Rutks I, Wilt TJ. *Pygeum africanum* for the treatment of patients with benign prostatic hyperplasia: a systematic review and quantitative meta-analysis. *Am J Med* 109(8):654-664, 2000.

Kinney AB, Blount M. Effect of cranberry juice on urinary pH. *Nurs Res* 28(5):287-290, 1979.

Koide T, Yamaguchi S, Utsunomiya M, Yoshioka T, Sugiyama K. The inhibitory effect of kampou extracts on in vitro calcium oxalate crystallization and in vivo stone formation in an animal model. *Int J Urol* 2(2):81-86, 1995.

Lappin MR, Jensen WA, Chandrashekar R, Kinney SD. Parenteral administration of FVRCP vaccines induces antibodies against feline renal tissues. Proceedings of the ACVIM Forum, Dallas, Tex, 2002.

Leishi L. *Rheum officinale:* a new lead in preventing progression of chronic renal failure. *Chin Med J* 109(1):35-37, 1996.

Li CP. Chinese Herbal Medicine, 1974. (DHEW publication # 75-732) John E. Fogarty International Center for Advanced Study in the Health Sciences, U.S. Department of Health, Education and Welfare, NIH, Rockville, Md, pp 21-22.

Light I, Gursel E, Zinnser HH. Urinary ionized calcium in urolithiasis: effect of cranberry juice. *Urology* 1(1):67-70, 1973.

Lis-Balchin M, Hart S, Simpson E. Buchu *(Agathosma betulina* and *A. crenulata, Rutaceae)* essential oils: their pharmacological action on guinea-pig ileum and antimicrobial activity on microorganisms. *J Pharm Pharmacol* 53(4):579-582, 2001.

Lu GW, Miura K, Yukimura T, Yamamoto K. Effects of extract from *Clerodendron trichotomum* on blood pressure and renal function in rats and dogs. *J Ethnopharmacol* 42(2):77-82, 1994.

Mills S, Bone K. *Principles and Practice of Phytotherapy.* Philadelphia, Pa, 2000, Churchill Livingstone.

Mitsuma T, Yokozawa T, Oura H, Terasawa K, Narita M. [Clinical evaluation of kampo medication, mainly with wen-pi-tang, on the progression of chronic renal failure]. *Nippon Jinzo Gakkai Shi* 41(8):769-777, 1999.

Perez Gutierrez RM, Laguna GY, Walkowski A. Diuretic activity of Mexican *Equisetum. J Ethnopharmacol* 14(2-3):269-272, 1985.

Racz-Kotilla E, Racz G, Solomon A. The action of *Taraxacum officinale* extracts on body weight and diuresis of laboratory animals. *Planta Med* 26:212-217, 1974.

Sanderson SL, Osborne CA, Lulich JP, Bartges JW, Pierpont ME, Ogburn PN, Koehler LA, Swanson LL, Bird KA, Ulrich LK. Evaluation of urinary carnitine and taurine excretion in 5 cystinuric dogs with carnitine and taurine deficiency. *J Vet Intern Med* 15(2):94-100, 2001.

Sebekova K, Dammrich J, Krivosikova Z, Heidland A. The effect of oral protease administration in the rat remnant kidney model. *Res Exp Med* 199(3):177-188, 1999.

Seltzer MA, Low RK, McDonald M, Shami GS, Stoller ML. Dietary manipulation with lemonade to treat hypocitraturic calcium nephrolithiasis. *J Urol* 156(3):907-909, 1996.

Su ZZ, He YY, Chen G. [Clinical and experimental study on effects of man-shen-ling oral liquid in the treatment of 100 cases of chronic nephritis]. *Zhongguo Zhong Xi Yi Jie He Za Zhi* 13(5):259-260, 269-272, 1993.

Terris MK, Issa MM, Tacker JR. Dietary supplementation with cranberry concentrate tablets may increase the risk of nephrolithiasis. *Urology* 57(1):26-29, 2001.

Tsukada K, Tokunaga K, Iwama T, Mishima Y, Tazawa K, Fujimaki M. Cranberry juice and its impact on peristomal skin conditions for urostomy patients. *Ostomy Wound Manage* 40(9):60-62, 64, 66-68, 1994.

Wasser WG, Feldman NS, D'Agati VD. Chronic renal failure after ingestion of over-the-counter chromium picolinate [letter]. *Ann Intern Med* 126:410, 1997.

Wilt T, Ishani A, MacDonald R, Stark G, Mulrow C, Lau J. Beta-sitosterols for benign prostatic hyperplasia. *Cochrane Database Syst Rev* 2:CD001043, 2000.

Wood T, Weckman TJ, Henry PA, Chang SL, Blake JW, Tobin T. Equine urine pH: normal population distributions and methods of acidification. *Equine Vet J* 22(2):118-121, 1990.

Yasui T, Fujita K, Sato M, Sugimoto M, Iguchi M, Nomura S, Kohri K. The effect of takusha, a kampo medicine, on renal stone formation and osteopontin expression in a rat urolithiasis model. *Urol Res* 27(3):194-199, 1999.

Yeung H. *Handbook of Chinese Herbal Formulas.* Los Angeles, 1996, Self-published.

Yeung H. *Handbook of Chinese Herbs.* Los Angeles, 1996, Self-published.

Zhang G, el Nahas AM. The effect of rhubarb extract on experimental renal fibrosis. *Nephrol Dial Transplant* (1):186-190, 1996.

Appendix A

Guidelines for Homemade Diets

Published dog and cat nutritional requirements are based on known minimums and *speculated* optimums. From the holistic point of view, one table of optimum nutrient intakes cannot begin to address an animal's individual genetic nutrient requirements to stay well, much less manage the many illnesses that may develop as an animal ages. Homemade diets provide variety, unprocessed food constituents that may have unrecognized importance in animal health, and the flexibility to change as the animal's health changes. These are just a few of the reasons that holistic practitioners recognize the utility of homemade diets and actively recommend them.

The pet owner who does not have the time or inclination to maintain proper balance in a homemade diet is a danger to the pet. For these owners a variety of commercial diets are available, and they can address many of the concerns of holistic practitioners for ill patients. For a certain number of these clients, *supplementing* commercial diets with fresh food may benefit the animal. For owners who can consistently and properly balance and supplement homemade diets, these foods can be safe and provide another dimension to the health care of these animals provided they are regularly monitored by a sympathetic veterinarian. Veterinarians should not underestimate the number of owners who are willing and enthusiastic animal chefs.

CLASSIC RECOMMENDATIONS

There are a few rules for preparing home-cooked diets for dogs and cats. The following information is derived from the excellent book *Small Animal Clinical Nutrition*, ed. 4 (Hand, 2000).

Remillard describes a Six-Step Formulation Method for designing a homemade pet food (Hand, 2000). These steps are:

1. Calculate nutrient requirements for the patient, especially energy and protein requirements.
2. Provide a fat source.
3. Provide a carbohydrate and fiber source.
4. Accommodate the nutrients of concern, especially if the patient has a condition that can be managed with diet.
5. Add minerals and vitamins.
6. Make a final assessment of the recipe.

This is undoubtedly the method with the best track record and can be used with a substantial investment of time and energy. Alternatively, a veterinary nutritionist can be consulted. If one is not available locally or at a nearby veterinary college, a commercial service such as PetDiets.com (www.petdiets.com) can be a great boon for busy veterinarians.

Diets that have been balanced by computer and that meet the allowances of the American Association of Feed Control Officials have been used successfully for years and may be found in a number of books, such as those by Richard Pitcairn *(Natural Health for Dogs and Cats)*, Monica Segal *(K9 Kitchen: Your Dogs' Diet: The Truth Behind the Hype)*, and Donald Strombeck *(Home Prepared Dog and Cat Diets)*. *Small Animal Clinical Nutrition* contains a number of recipes that can be adapted according to a pet's health characteristics and locally available ingredients. Below are two examples from *Small Animal Clinical Nutrition:*

Balanced Generic Formula for Healthy Adult Dogs (enough for one 18-kg dog daily)

Carbohydrate, cooked	240 g
Meat, cooked	120 g
Fat	10 g
Fiber (high-fiber cereal)	30 g
Bone meal or dicalcium phosphate	4 g
Potassium chloride	1 g
Human multivitamin-mineral tablet	1 tablet

Balanced Homemade Generic Formula for Healthy Adult Cats (enough for one 4.5-kg cat daily)

Carbohydrate, cooked	60 g
Meat, cooked	40 g
Fat	10 g

Bone meal or dicalcium phosphate	1.2 g
Salts (sodium chloride or potassium chloride)	1.0 g
Taurine	0.5 g
Human multivitamin-mineral tablet	0.5 tablet

ALTERNATIVE DIETS

Veterinarians have recommended homemade diets for many years, and some of these are extreme variations on the proportions and amounts listed in the classically balanced recipes just described. In the absence of computer balancing, it would appear that a built-in safety factor in homemade diets is the variety usually provided.

Nutrient sources *must* include the following:

- **Protein source (40% to 80%):** unless allergies preclude them, animal proteins are the preferred source. These can include poultry, fish, and animal meat and organs, eggs, and milk products. If vegetable protein must be used, soybean products, beans, and peas will do.
- **Fat source:** oils or high-fat meat.
- **Carbohydrate and fiber sources (0 to 60%):** grains such as oatmeal, rice, corn, barley, and wheat, and their products such as pasta and bread. Fiber is provided by whole grains, brans, seeds, and vegetables. Cats do not require carbohydrates as an energy source, nor do most dogs, although some will experience a drop in energy without them. Fiber is probably important for most animals and should always be included. Some veterinarians provide fiber and reduce digestible carbohydrates by using mostly vegetables and not using grains.
- **Macromineral sources:** primarily calcium and phosphorus.
- **Trace element and vitamin sources:** from a complete vitamin-mineral supplement.

The two diets below are recommended in the text and used frequently in my practice (SW). They are often recommended for short-term use or for animals with serious diseases. Since they are not balanced when analyzed by computer, we recommend providing variety in the ingredients. Pets eating these diets should be seen regularly by the veterinarian, and any suspected metabolic problems should be investigated with an eye to nutritional as well as nonnutritional diseases.

Paleolithic Diet

Many holistic practitioners have used a paleolithic diet that is similar to the one below. This is the diet that I (SW) recommend for most patients with cancer (for approximately 50 lb of dog, daily):

Meat, cooked with fat	10 oz
Grains	0-1oz
Mixed vegetables	6-7 oz
Menhaden or salmon oil; flax oil only if necessary	6 T
Lite salt	1-1½ tsp
Calcium carbonate (600 mg tablet)	3 tablets
Multivitamin-mineral tablet (a human product)	1 tablet
If feeding a cat, add 250 to 500 mg taurine daily.	

Hypoallergenic Diet

Hypoallergenic homemade diets are indicated for some animals with chronic skin, gastrointestinal, or immune-mediated diseases. Here are some guidelines (for 30 to 40 lb of pet daily):

Cooked millet, amaranth, or potato with skin	8-12 oz
Cooked rabbit, fish, venison, quail, duck, or goat	8-12 oz
Mixed vegetables, *nonstarchy*	2-4 oz
Olive or flaxseed oil	4 tsp
Dicalcium phosphate, bone meal, or other calcium source	1 tsp
Salt or salt substitute	½ tsp
Hypoallergenic multivitamin-mineral supplement	1 tablet
If feeding a cat, add 500 mg taurine daily.	

Raw Diet

Many pet owners are firm believers in feeding their pets according to principles recently espoused in books by authors who advocate feeding raw meaty bones, such as chicken backs, wings, and necks, for consumption whole. Alternatively, some pet owners use commercially prepared raw food diets and provide precut raw bones from large animal sources. As horrified as any well-trained veterinarian will be on hearing this, many dogs and cats do well on raw diets. Two main risks are associated with feeding raw diets: obstruction or perforation by bones, and infection with food-borne pathogens (Box A-1).

The risks are real. Pathogenic organisms are recognized risks in our food supply. Some veterinarians worry that handling raw meat in preparing these diets is a risk to the owner; owners counter that proper handling is safe if they follow instructions for handling their own food. Owners who feed their pets

BOX A-1 Food-Borne Pathogens

Bacterial
Salmonella spp.
Escherichia coli
Campylobacter spp.
Yersinia spp.
Vibrio spp.
Mycobacterium spp.
Brucella spp.
Cyclospora spp.
Listeria monocytogenes

Rickettsial
Neorickettsia spp.

Protozoan
Toxoplasma gondii
Neospora canis
Cryptosporidium spp.

Metazoan
Echinococcus spp.
Trichinella spiralis

Toxicants
Clostridium botulinum
Bacillus cereus
Staphylococcus aureus
Mycotoxins

raw food claim that healthy animals are not susceptible to infection with pathogenic organisms; in fact, a recent report indicated that for 10 dogs eating BARF (biologically appropriate raw food) diets, 80% of the meals submitted contained *Salmonella* serovars, and 30% of the stool samples taken from the dogs eating these meals were positive for *Salmonella*. No illness was reported in these dogs during the study period (Joffe, 2002). Whether or not dogs are at dramatic risk for infection by enteropathogenic bacteria, the potential for zoonotic infection requires that owners who feed raw meat to their dogs be warned about the potential for passing pathogenic bacteria into the environment, a risk especially for small children.

Some manufacturers of commercially prepared raw food diets are taking an initiative to answer the food safety concerns by performing bacteria counts on their products through random cultures as a component of quality control. These manufacturers report no growth of microorganisms, although a reliable third-party reporting system is not in place in the industry. Manufacturers credit the reported sterility of their products to rapid food processing in a refrigerated environment followed immediately by deep freezing. Raw poultry products in grocery stores are not processed in a similar manner and are generally not sold with the intention of being fed raw. Food safety concerns may therefore be more of an imperative for homemade raw food diets than those that have been commercially prepared.

For clients who continue to feed their animals raw diets, two main recommendations can be made to increase safety somewhat. First, blanching or scalding the meat surface will kill surface bacteria (clearly, ground meat cannot be treated this way). Although this method will not eliminate internal cysts, it increases protection from the more common enteropathogenic bacteria. Freezing to −12° C for over 24 hours kills *Toxoplasma* and possibly *Neospora* tissue cysts in meat, but most household freezers do not reliably freeze to this temperature.

Second, the bones can be ground. Some clients use home grinders. Owners who feed their animal a raw diet have had success with the following grinders:

Maverick Grinder or VillaWare Grinder
Pierce Food Service Equipment Co. Inc.
Chef's Mart
9685 West 55th Street
Countryside, Illinois 60525
Toll free: 877-354-1265
Telephone: 708-354-1265
Fax: 708-354-1361
www.pierceequipment.com

Moulinex Grinder
Moulinex
112 Doncaster Avenue
Thornhill, Ontario
Canada L3T 1L3
Telephone: 905-764-1188
Fax: 905-764-1199
http://www.cayneshousewares.com/cgi-bin/shopping.cgi

PARADIGMATIC PERSPECTIVES (see Appendix B for specific recommendations)

Practitioners and pet owners are subjected to a variety of dietary rhetoric. Raw, cooked, vegetarian, and all-meat diets all have their proponents who have convincing arguments for their use. The paradigmatic perspective of Chinese medicine appears to lend support to more paleolithic diets, such as the one previously discussed. These diets have a very low carbohydrate content. Their macronutrients are supplied chiefly by protein and vegetable matter.

Chinese medicine demonstrates that certain dynamics predominate in dogs and cats, based on consistent responses to various Chinese herbal treatment strategies. For the dog the chief problem is Blood deficiency. For the cat the chief issue is Dampness elaborated by Spleen deficiency. Diets and herbal formulas are available to address each of these conditions. Indeed, herbal medicine was initially developed in China as a means to enhance diets used to treat disease.

Blood deficiency in dogs arises from two main mechanisms. Some dogs become Blood deficient in response to decreased Spleen function. Others are "primarily" Blood deficient. Foods that directly tonify Blood include viscera, which has recently been excluded from many commercial dry and canned foods because of public perception that viscera (known generically as "by-products") is a substandard protein source.

Other dogs, like cats, appear to require diets that reinforce Spleen function. Spleen problems also are abundant in humans, and reduced carbohydrate-to-protein ratios in the diet are increasingly recommended. Many cases of carbohydrate intolerance are manifested in humans as Dampness from Spleen deficiency. My (SM) early clinical experience with low-carbohydrate diets in dogs and cats supports the hypothesis that carbohydrates may "overburden" the Spleens of dogs and cats, leading to secondary Blood deficiency and accumulations of Dampness. The bias of feline liver metabolism toward a reliance on protein as the chief carbohydrate source in the body is consistent with the notion that cats, at least, are best adapted to low-carbohydrate diets. While cats and dogs are certainly capable of digesting carbohydrates in their diet, the question arises whether carbohydrate-rich diets are optimal. Most medical systems have acknowledged for centuries that creating optimal living conditions seems to offer the best hope for maximal results in the treatment and prevention of disease.

See Appendix B for a comprehensive listing of food qualities according to traditional Chinese medicine.

REFERENCES

Hand MS, Thatcher C, Remillard RL, Roudebush P. *Small Animal Clinical Nutrition*, ed 4. Topeka, Kan, 2000, Mark Morris Institute.

Joffe DJ, Schlesinger DP. Preliminary assessment of the risk of *Salmonella* infection in dogs fed raw chicken diets. *Can Vet J* 43(6):441-442, 2002.

Pitcairn R, Pitcairn S. *Natural Health for Dogs and Cats*. Emmaus, Penn, 1995, Rodale Press.

Segal M. *K9 Kitchen: Your Dogs' Diet: The Truth Behind the Hype*. Toronto, 2002, Doggie Diner.

Strombeck D. *Home Prepared Dog and Cat Diets*. Ames, Ia, 1998, Iowa State University Press.

Appendix B

Chinese Food Therapy

Foods are recommended in Traditional Chinese medicine to help maintain long-term Yin/Yang balance in the body. Although food therapy does not have dramatic short-term results, it is important for prevention and for maintaining results achieved through herbs and acupuncture. Note that organ meats are often used to treat malfunctioning organs (i.e., organ meats such as heart, stomach, kidney, liver).

Food	Taste	Property	Meridian	Function	Indication	Contraindications
Chicken	Sweet	Warm	SP, ST	Enrich Qi and Blood, tonify KI and Jing	SP Qi deficiency problems, weakness, emaciation, edema, frequent urination	Not for excess conditions
Chicken liver	Sweet	Slightly warm	LIV	Nourish LIV, tonify KI Yang	Improve vision, male impotence	
Eggs	Sweet	Neutral		Nourish Yin and Blood	Prevent abortion	Dampness conditions
Duck	Sweet, salty	Neutral	LU, SP, KI	Nourish Yin, reinforce ST, remove damp	Yin deficiency fever, cough; remove edema	
Turkey	Sweet	Cool	KI, LIV	Yin tonic		
Goose	Sweet	Neutral	SP, LU	Enrich Qi, reinforce deficiency, nourish ST, ease thirst	Emaciation, fatigue, anorexia from weak SP, ST, shortness of breath, diabetes	
Quail	Sweet	Neutral	SP, LIV	Reinforce SP Qi, remove damp	Remove edema, strengthen bones and tendons	
Beef	Sweet	Warm or neutral	SP, ST	Reinforce SP/ST, enrich Qi and Blood	Anorexia, diarrhea, edema, fatigue	
Beef kidney		Neutral				
Beef liver	Sweet	Neutral	LIV	Nourish Blood, reinforce LIV	Improve vision, deficiency of LIV Blood	
Tripe	Sweet	Neutral	SP, ST	Reinforce SP/ST	Anorexia, diarrhea	
Mutton, Lamb, Goat	Sweet	Hot	SP, KI	Warm middle burner; enrich Qi and Blood	Male impotence, cold intolerance, weakness in lower back, profuse clear urine, abdominal pain, cold limbs, fatigue	Exogenous epidemic pathogens or susceptibility to fevers; contraindicated in most heat conditions, including skin disorders

Food	Taste	Property	Meridian	Function	Indication	Contraindications
Lamb liver		Warm				
Lamb kidney		Warm				
Pork	Sweet, salty	Neutral	LU, SP, LIV	Nourish Yin, moisten dryness, enrich Blood	Dry cough, dry mouth, emaciation, fatigue, constipation	
Pork liver		Neutral				
Pork kidney		Neutral				
Rabbit	Sweet	Cool	SP, ST	Reinforce SP, enrich Qi	Anorexia, fatigue, thirst	
Catfish	Sweet	Neutral	SP, ST	Reinforce SP, enrich Qi	Promote production of milk, induce urination, edema	
Cod	Sweet	Cold	SP, KI, LIV	Yin tonic	Use when a nondampening Yin tonic is required	
Salmon	Sweet, salty	Neutral	SP, KI, HT	Qi tonic		
Mackerel	Sweet	Neutral	SP	Tonify SP Qi		
Tuna	Sweet	Neutral	HT, LIV	Blood tonic		
Sardine		Neutral				
Rice, white	Sweet	Warm or Neutral	SP, ST	Nourish SP, harmonize ST, relieve thirst	Vomiting, anorexia, thirst and dry mouth from ST Yin impairment and heat	All carbohydrate sources are quite rich, making them effective Yin tonics, but also a dampening influence
Rice, brown	Sweet	Cool	SP, ST, KI	Regulate SP/ST, clear heat, nourish KI		All carbohydrate sources are quite rich, making them effective Yin tonics, but also a dampening influence

Corn	Sweet	Neutral	SP, ST, LI	Detoxify, regulate ST, improve appetite	Weak ST, diminished urination	All carbohydrate sources are quite rich, making them effective Yin tonics, but also a dampening influence
Millet	Sweet, salty	Slightly cold	SP, ST, KI	Nourish SP and KI; relieve thirst, induce urination	Vomiting, anorexia from weak SP/ST; thirst, difficult urination with fever	All carbohydrate sources are quite rich, making them effective Yin tonics, but also a dampening influence
Barley	Sweet	Cool	SP, ST, BL	Reinforce SP, regulate ST, relieve thirst, induce urination	Weakness of SP/ST with anorexia and diarrhea, thirst, difficult, painful urination	All carbohydrate sources are quite rich, making them effective Yin tonics, but also a dampening influence
Buckwheat	Sweet	Cool	SP, ST, LI	Food stagnation, send down counterflow Qi, reinforce SP, remove damp	Fullness or pain in abdomen, diarrhea, leukorrhea	All carbohydrate sources are quite rich, making them effective Yin tonics, but also a dampening influence

Food	Taste	Property	Meridian	Function	Indication	Contraindications
Oats	Sweet	Warm	SP, KI	Warm KI Yang		All carbohydrate sources are quite rich, making them effective Yin tonics, but also a dampening influence
Wheat	Sweet	Cool	HT, SP, KI	Nourish HT, reinforce SP, relieve thirst, induce urination	Thirst, difficult urination with fever	All carbohydrate sources are quite rich, making them effective Yin tonics, but also a dampening influence
Garlic	Pungent, sweet	Warm	SP, ST, LU	Warm middle burner, reinforce ST	Aid digestion, kill parasites, food stagnation, pain in upper abdomen, food poisoning	Use with caution
Ginger	Pungent	Slightly warm	LU, SP, ST	Warm middle burner, arrest vomiting, warm lungs, arrest cough, arrest invasion at the Wai/Tai Yang level by inducing sweating	Anorexia from SP/ST disharmony or weakness, cough from cold in the LU, Wind-Cold type URI	
Vinegar	Sour, sweet	Warm or neutral	LIV, ST	Food stagnation, anorexia	Hard masses in abdomen, vomiting blood, bloody stools, nosebleed	
Soy Sauce	Salty	Warm	KI	Warms KI, SP		

Salt	Salty	Neutral	SP, KI	Harmonize middle burner, reinforce KI, moisten dryness	KI Yang or Yin deficiency, constipation, Yin deficiency fire
Green beans	Sweet	Neutral or Warm	LIV	Nourish LIV Yin	
Cabbage	Sweet	Neutral	SP, ST	Nourish SP, regulate ST, relieve spasm and pain	SP/ST disharmony; fresh juice is used to address pain in upper abdomen from ulcers
Carrots	Sweet	Neutral	SP, LIV, LU	Reinforce SP, aid digestion, reinforce LIV, enhance vision, send down counterflow Qi, arrest cough, clear heat, detoxify	Indigestion, food stagnation, blurred vision, night blindness, LU heat cough
Spinach	Sweet	Cool	LI, ST, LIV	Moisten dryness, ease bowel motions, promote production of body fluids, quench thirst, nurture LIV, improve vision	Constipation from dryness in geriatric patients, thirst from diabetes or ST heat; LIV heat, LIV Yin deficiency
Broccoli	Sweet	Cool	LIV	Yin tonic, Blood tonic	
Celery	Pungent, sweet	Cool	LIV, ST, BL	Clear heat, calm LIV, reinforce ST, send down central Qi, ease urination	Feverish diseases, agitation from heat, LIV heat, vomiting and anorexia from ST heat, difficult urination from heat, hematuria

Food	Taste	Property	Meridian	Function	Indication	Contraindications
Asparagus	Sweet	Warm	LU, KI	Nourish Yin	Constipation, dry cough, weight loss; Yin deficiency	
Onion	Pungent, bitter	Warm	LU, ST, LI	Activate Yang, dissolve hard masses, send down Qi, aid bowel motions	Chest congestion, chest pain, phlegm coughs, Qi stagnation in the middle burner	Use with extreme caution in small animals
Potato	Sweet	Neutral	SP, ST	Reinforce SP/ST, relieve spasm and pain	Indigestion, weak SP/ST, pain in the upper abdomen from ST/SP disharmony	
Sweet potato	Sweet	Neutral	SP, ST, LI	Reinforce SP and ST, assist bowel motions, promote production of body fluids, quench thirst	Fatigue, constipation, thirst	
Pumpkin	Sweet	Warm	SP, ST	Reinforce middle burner, replenish Qi, dissolve phlegm, promote discharge of pus, expel roundworms	Weak SP, coughing up thick sputum, GI parasites	
Kelp	Salty	Cold	LIV, ST, KI	Dissolve phlegm, soften hard masses, relieve edema	Goiter, edema, hypertension?, heart disease?	

Data from Jilin L, Peck G, eds. *Chinese Dietary Therapy*. New York, 1995, Churchill Livingstone; Schwartz C. *Four Paws, Five Directions*. Berkeley, Calif, 1996, Celestial Arts Publishing; and Xie H, Chi Institute, Reddick, Fla, personal communication.

BL, Bladder; *HT*, Heart; *KI*, Kidney; *LI*, Large Intestine; *LIV*, Liver; *LU*, Lung; *SP*, Spleen; *ST*, Stomach.

Appendix C

Suggested Oral Herb Dosages

This is the first publication of veterinary dosages for herbs in mg/lb form, as far as we know. We are well aware that some dosages may be viewed as arbitrary or incorrect. Practitioners should be aware that this is an initial effort and is based on published human dosages and our experience. These dosages should serve only as a starting point, and the practitioner's judgment should be the final guide in herb form and dosage selection.

We recognize that many pet owners are unable to administer medicines to their animals tid. In some cases, flexibility is possible. Herbs that have short-term effects, such as those with physical effects on the gastrointestinal tract (containing mucilages, tannins, etc.) may require tid-qid doses. On the other hand, some tonics may be given sid if administered over weeks to months.

When herb choices are well suited to the patient from both a paradigmatic and a conventional medical perspective, patients may benefit from smaller doses, but seem tolerant of excessive dosing. Safety during pregnancy is unknown for the majority of herbs in the table; it is best not to give herbs during pregnancy.

HERB FORMS

Dried Forms

Dried bulk herb: the herb is harvested, dried, and sometimes powdered. Dried powdered herb may be supplied as a loose powder or in capsules.

Dried granular extracts: the manufacturer concentrates the herb by simmering it in water, removing the residue, and spraying the concentrated "tea" in a vacuum chamber, resulting in powder or granules of remaining concentrated herbal constituents. These granules may be supplied as a loose powder, in pressed tablets, or in capsules. Tea pills are simply coated balls of granular extracts. One caution in the use of this form is that water extracts may miss active constituents that are only alcohol soluble. A commonly provided form is a 4:1 or 5:1 extract, allowing veterinarians to recommend fewer capsules than if powdered herb is used.

Liquid Extracts

Infusions and decoctions: a hot infusion is made when an herb is steeped in water, like a tea. Cold infusions involve simply placing dried or fresh herb in cold water for a time and might be used with delicately scented herbs, like flowers. Decoctions are like "herb soup"; the herb is boiled in water to a concentrated extract and drunk as a very concentrated tea. Most Chinese herbal formulas are called "decoctions," even when supplied as a granular extract. This is not inaccurate, since the creation of granular extracts, as mentioned above, involves first simmering the herbs to create a decoction.

Liquid concentrated extracts: the herb is extracted in solvent and the residue removed. The infusions and decoctions described above are water extracts. Alcohol extracts are concentrated and potentially absorbed more rapidly from the gastrointestinal tract. Alcohol is also an excellent solvent and is able to dissolve most types of chemicals found in plants, except polysaccharides. Alcohol extracts taste terrible to most dogs and cats, but the small amount required in addition to the ease with which they can be combined make alcohol extracts popular. Glycerin extracts are also available, and glycerin does not taste as bad as alcohol. The sweet taste of glycerin may hide the taste of the herbs, but some herbs may taste bad enough that animals do not accept glycerin extracts readily either. A disadvantage to glycerin extracts is that they are not as concentrated as alcohol extracts, suggesting that they have weaker activity.

The most readily available and easy to use forms in veterinary practice are powdered herb, concentrated granular extract powders (loose or in capsules), tea pills, and alcohol tinctures, for which doses are provided below.

DOSAGE STRATEGY

Dosages should begin at the low end of the recommendations given here. If adverse effects are noted at the recommended dosage, stop administration of the herb for 1 to 2 days, then resume at one third of the dose. If no effects (desired or adverse) are noted at the low end of the recommended range, increase gradually.

Strength and safety rating:
Extremely safe (food-like)
Moderately safe
Powerful herb with side effects likely if overdosed
Toxic; use with extreme caution

Herb	Botanical Name	Dried Herb	Dried Concentrated Extract	Alcohol Tincture*	Contraindications and Side Effects of Large Doses, and Drug Interactions	Principal Uses —Modern and Traditional
Agrimony Herb	*Agrimonia eupatoria, A. pilosa*	35 mg/lb tid		1 drop/lb tid	Possible allergic reactions; may increase photosensitivity	Gargle, mouth wash, tea for GI inflammation, urinary tract astringent
Alfalfa Herb	*Medicago sativa*	35 mg/lb tid or more		2 drops/lb tid	None; however, cats may have increased sensitivity to coumarins contained in alfalfa	Nutritional tonic
Aloe Vera Leaf	*Aloe vera, A. barbadensis*	0.25-1 ml juice/lb tid	1-2.5 mg/lb sid	N/A	May cause diarrhea if taken orally; may cause hypersensitivity topically (rare); may interact with digoxin, diuretics, antiarrhythmics, glyburide, or steroids if taken orally	Wound healing, cathartic, some practitioners use for diarrhea and constipation
Artichoke Leaf	*Cynara scolymus*	50 mg/lb tid	5-8 mg/lb tid	2-3 drops/lb bid	Allergic reactions	Liver disease
Ashwaganda Root	*Withania somnifera*	25 mg/lb tid		2 drops/lb tid	Rarely, nausea, diarrhea, dermatitis, abdominal pain	Tonic, anti-inflammatory, traditionally for chronic debilitating disease
Astragalus Root	*Astragalus membranaceus*	60 mg/lb tid		1-2 drops/lb tid	None reported	Immunostimulant

Baptisia Root	*Baptisia tinctoria*			1 drop/lb bid		Antimicrobial
Barberry Root	*Berberis vulgaris*			1-2 drops/lb bid-tid	Nausea, diarrhea, nephritis, disorientation, hypotension; may interact with doxycycline and tetracycline	Antimicrobial
Bilberry Leaf and Berry	*Vaccinium myrtillus*	25-100 mg/lb tid	5-8 mg/lb tid	2 drops/lb tid	Long-term use of leaf may have gastric and renal effects; possibly interacts with anticoagulants	Retinal disorders, diarrhea, sore throat
Bitter Melon Fruit	*Momordica charantia*			2 drops/lb bid-tid	May enhance effects of other hypoglycemics	Diabetes, cancer, skin disease, and asthma
Black Cohosh Root	*Actea racemosa*	10-25 mg/lb tid	3 mg/lb tid	2 drops/lb bid-tid	Overdose may be associated with disorientation, hypotension, and nausea; a species threatened with extinction	Estrogen replacement, nervine, rheumatism
Blessed Thistle Leaf, Stem, Flower	*Cnicus benedictus*	25-90 mg/lb tid		1 drop/lb tid	Overdose may cause nausea; occasional allergic reactions may occur	Indigestion, liver problems
Bloodroot	*Sanguinaria canadensis*	Powdered root is used topically		Not recommended, but has been given short term at 1 drop/10-20 lb total per day	Oral ingestion of large doses may be associated with diarrhea, hypotension, coma	Dental disease, skin growths, topically only

Herb	Botanical Name	Dried Herb	Dried Concentrated Extract	Alcohol Tincture*	Contraindications and Side Effects of Large Doses, and Drug Interactions	Principal Uses —Modern and Traditional
Blue Cohosh Root	*Caulophyllum thalictroides*	10-15 mg/lb tid		1 drop/lb tid	Has possibly caused congestive heart failure in newborns when used during labor; gastritis, diarrhea, hypertension; signs similar to nicotine overdose	Induce uterine contractions; used to stimulate labor and pass placenta
Boneset Leaf and Flower	*Eupatorium perfoliatum*			1-2 drops/lb tid	Nausea, vomiting, diarrhea, anorexia, hepatotoxicity (contains small amounts of pyrrolizidine alkaloids)	Fever, influenza, bronchitis
Boswellia Tree Resin	*Boswellia serrata*		10 mg/lb tid		Occasional mild gastric upset	Antiinflammatory, expectorant, skin diseases, ulcers, bronchitis
Buchu Leaf Essential Oil	*Agathosma betulina*	25 mg/lb tid		1-2 drops/lb tid	Nausea, vomiting, anorexia, diarrhea, hepatotoxicity, spontaneous abortion (contains pulegone)	Diuretic for genitourinary infections
Bugleweed Leaf and Flower	*Lycopus virginicus*	6-8 mg/lb tid		0.5-1 drop/lb bid-tid	Interacts with thyroid medications	Hyperthyroidism; interacts with sex hormones and may have contraceptive effects

Calendula Flowers	*Calendula officinalis*	Used topically as a wet dressing (from tea) or ointment	N/A	N/A	Be aware of possible cross-reactivity for patients with allergies to the daisy family	Topically for skin irritation, wounds, etc.; traditionally for conjunctivitis and gastric ulcers, and as a lymphatic, diaphoretic, and bitter tonic
Cascara Sagrada Aged Bark	*Rhamnus purshiana*			0.5-1 drop/lb bid	Nausea, vomiting, cramps, diarrhea, dependence	Laxative
Cat's Claw Inner Bark	*Uncaria tomentosa, U. guianensis*	Up to 65 mg/lb divided daily		1 drop/lb tid	Mild GI effects; monitor for bleeding; do not use with antihypertensives	Amazonian remedy for cancer, arthritis, gastroenteritis, skin disorders; used in Europe for cancer and HIV
Cayenne Fruit	*Capsicum annuum*	Up to 15 mg/lb divided daily		1 drop/lb total, divided daily	Burns when applied to skin or swallowed; GI distress	Topically in people for localized pain, neuralgias; also as a nasal spray for chronic allergic rhinitis; traditionally for digestive and cardiovascular weakness

Herb	Botanical Name	Dried Herb	Dried Concentrated Extract	Alcohol Tincture*	Contraindications and Side Effects of Large Doses, and Drug Interactions	Principal Uses —Modern and Traditional
Chamomile Flowers	*Matricaria recutita, Chamaemelum nobilis*	30-50 mg/lb tid		2 drops/lb tid	Allergic cross reactivity with members of the daisy family; may potentiate effects of anticoagulants; cats may be particularly sensitive	Mild gastritis or indigestion; mildly tranquilizing; topically for mucosal irritation or ulcers;
Celandine Leaf and Flower	*Chelidonium majus*	60 mg/lb total daily dose; not recommended		1 drop/lb sid-bid	Hypotension, disorientation, hepatotoxicity, nausea, polyuria and polydipsia, restlessness	GI spastic conditions; not a commonly used herb
Chaste Tree Berry	*Vitex agnus-castus*	25 mg/lb sid	2.5 mg/lb sid	1 drop/lb total daily dose	Nausea, vomiting, urticaria, pruritus	Menstrual problems in women; "anaphrodisiac," galactagogue; apparently does not affect estrogen receptors
Cleavers Herb	*Galium aparine*	Not usually used	Not used	1-2 drops/lb tid	None reported	Diuretic; lymphatic

Clover (Red) Flowers	*Trifolium pretense*	50 mg/lb tid		2 drops/lb bid	Coumarins may interact with anticoagulants; estrogenic effects may be a concern	Topically for skin problems; cough; lymphatic; source of isoflavones that seem useful in human menopause
Coleus Root	*Plectranthus barbatus*		1-1.5 mg bid-tid	1-2 drops/lb tid	Avoid in hypotension and gastric ulcers	Asthma, glaucoma, cardiovascular disease
Coltsfoot Leaf and Flower	*Tussilago farfara*	75 mg/lb tid		1 drop/lb bid	Hypertension, fever, nausea, vomiting, diarrhea; contains pyrrolizidine alkaloids that may cause liver disease; cross-reactive allergens with other members of the daisy family	Asthma, bronchitis
Cranberry Fruit	*Vaccinium macrocarpon*	1-8 ml juice/lb daily	5 mg/lb bid	2 drops/lb bid	Diarrhea; rare hypersensitivity reactions	Urinary tract infections
Cranesbill Root and Herb	*Geranium maculatum*	Usually supplied as a tea		1-2 drops/ lb bid-tid	Indigestion; not for long-term use	Sore throat, stomatitis, diarrhea; astringent

Herb	Botanical Name	Dried Herb	Dried Concentrated Extract	Alcohol Tincture*	Contraindications and Side Effects of Large Doses, and Drug Interactions	Principal Uses —Modern and Traditional
Dandelion Leaf	*Taraxacum officinale*	Fresh young leaves can be eaten as salad addition		2 drops/lb tid	Dermatitis from milky latex (which is why it was used for warts traditionally); use with caution for animals taking antihypertensives; additive effect with other diuretics; may contain oxalates; this is a very safe herb	Potassium-sparing diuretic?, digestive stimulant
Dandelion Root	*Taraxacum officinale*	60 mg/lb tid		3-4 drops/lb bid-tid	Dermatitis from milky latex (which is why it was used for warts traditionally); use with caution for animals taking antihypertensives	Digestive stimulant and cholagogue
Devil's Claw Root	*Harpagophytum procumbens*	10-20 mg/lb bid		0.5-1 drop/lb bid	Contraindicated when GI ulcers are present; may cause mild GI signs; may interact with antiarrhythmics	Arthritis; traditionally for indigestion and skin sores or boils
Dioscorea Root	*Dioscorea villosa*	25-50 mg/lb divided daily		1-2 drops/lb bid-tid	Nausea, vomiting, diarrhea	Traditionally for pain relief of all kinds; inflammatory bowel syndrome

Dong Quai Root	*Angelica sinensis*	50 mg/lb tid	5-7 mg/lb bid	1 drop/lb bid-tid	Diarrhea; possible photosensitization; may cause heavy menses in women	Female reproductive disorders; cardiovascular disorders; hematologic and immune disorders
Echinacea Root or Leaves and Flowers	*Echinacea purpura, E. angustifolia*	12 mg/lb tid	4 mg/lb tid	1-2 drops/lb tid-qid	Vomiting, drooling, lethargy, hyperactivity, allergic hypersensitivity reactions; contraindicated if autoimmune disorder present; aspecies threatened with extinction	Antibacterial; immune stimulant; traditionally for snake bites, toothaches, abscesses
Elderberry Flowers	*Sambucus nigra*			2-4 drops/lb tid	Use only flowers; bark and leaves are poisonous; nausea, vomiting, anorexia; hypersensitivity reactions	Influenza; antioxidant; traditionally for diabetes; upper respiratory astringent
Elecampane Root	*Inula helenium*	35 mg/lb tid		1-2 drops/lb bid-tid	Nausea, vomiting, anorexia, GI spasms; contact dermatitis, hypersensitivity reactions; large overdoses associated with paralysis	Expectorant; antiseptic; cough, bronchitis, asthma

Herb	Botanical Name	Dried Herb	Dried Concentrated Extract	Alcohol Tincture*	Contraindications and Side Effects of Large Doses, and Drug Interactions	Principal Uses —Modern and Traditional
Eleuthero Root	*Eleutherococcus senticosis*	10-15 mg/lb tid	0.03-0.05 mg/lb bid extract standardized on eleutherosides B and E	1 drop/lb tid	Do not use in hypertensive patients	Adaptogenic tonic for improving memory and strength in chronically debilitated patients; immunostimulant
Eyebright Herb	*Euphrasia officinalis*	Used topically in the eye, as a cooled tea; attention to contamination is vital			Nausea, vomiting, anorexia; said to exacerbate seizures; a species threatened with extinction	Topically for conjunctivitis in aqueous form only; traditionally as oral medication for allergic dermatitis, asthma, diarrhea
False Unicorn Root	*Chamaelirium luteum*	15-25 mg/lb tid		1-2 drops/lb bid	Nausea, vomiting; a species threatened with extinction	For female reproductive problems, specifically infertility or cycling problems

Fennel Seed	*Foeniculum vulgare*	20-30 mg/lb tid		1 drop/lb tid	Nausea, vomiting, anorexia; hypersensitivity reactions; seizures; photosensitivity	Carminative for intestinal gas; estrogen-like effects are indicated for human menstrual disorders and to increase milk production
Fenugreek Seed	*Trigonella foecumgraecum*	30-300 mg/lb tid		1 drop/lb tid (not recommended, as seed contains the most activity)	Intestinal gas, diarrhea; may interact with other hypoglycemics	Hypoglycemic agent; galactagogue; topically for boils, ulcers, and inflammatory skin disorders; indigestion (as a tea)
Feverfew Flowering Tops	*Tanacetum parthenium*		1-2 mg/lb bid; standardized to 0.2% parthenolides	0.5 drop/lb bid	Nausea, vomiting, anorexia, hypersensitivity reactions; mouth ulcers if fresh leaves are chewed	Fever, arthritis; migraines in humans

Herb	Botanical Name	Dried Herb	Dried Concentrated Extract	Alcohol Tincture*	Contraindications and Side Effects of Large Doses, and Drug Interactions	Principal Uses —Modern and Traditional
Garlic Bulb	*Allium sativum*	1 clove/40-50 lb	10-30 mg/lb Kyolic	N/A	May cause Heinz body anemia in cats and dogs in high doses; may cause short-term clotting abnormalities and should be used with caution in presence of other anticoagulants; nausea, body and breath odor, flatulence	Antibacterial, antiviral, antihypertensive, hypoglycemic, antihyperlipidemic, antineoplastic
Gentian Root	*Gentiana lutea*	15-20 mg/lb tid		1 drop/lb bid	Nausea, vomiting, anorexia; hypersensitivity reactions	Digestive disorders such as gastritis, inflammatory bowel disease, colitis
Ginger Root	*Zingiber officinale*	25-35 mg/lb bid		1 drop/lb bid-tid	Nausea if taken in large doses on an empty stomach; may enhance bleeding if given with anticoagulants	Antiemetic, antiinflammatory; circulatory stimulant; used in China for acute colds and upper respiratory infections

Ginkgo Leaf	*Ginkgo biloba*		1 mg/lb tid or 3 mg/lb daily of EGb extract	1 drop/lb bid	Enhances bleeding when combined with anticoagulants; seizures have been reported when seeds and fruits (as opposed to leaf) were eaten; allergic reactions	Senile cognitive dysfunction; asthma; antioxidant that may be useful for retinal disorders, cardiovascular, and peripheral vascular disease
Ginseng Root, American	*Panax quinquefolius*	25-35 mg/lb tid	6-8 mg/lb tid	1 drop/lb tid	High blood pressure, nervousness, insomnia	Adaptogenic tonic; hypoglycemic; not as strong as Asian ginseng
Ginseng Root, Asian	*Panax ginseng*	25-35 mg/lb tid	6-8 mg/lb tid	1 drop/lb tid	High blood pressure, nervousness, insomnia; avoid in acute disorders and brittle diabetics	Adaptogenic tonic; hypoglycemic

Herb	Botanical Name	Dried Herb	Dried Concentrated Extract	Alcohol Tincture*	Contraindications and Side Effects of Large Doses, and Drug Interactions	Principal Uses —Modern and Traditional
Goldenseal Root	*Hydrastis canadensis*	15-25 mg/lb tid	4-6 mg/lb tid	1 drop/lb bid-tid	GI signs; various claims that it causes hypotension and hypertension; Berberine displaces bilirubin from albumin; not for use in icteric patients and can cause icterus; nausea, vomiting, abdominal cramping; a species threatened with extinction	Topical antimicrobial agent for stomatitis, vaginitis, conjunctivitis, gastritis; plant is highly endangered in the wild and should not be used unless it is strongly indicated
Gotu Kola Leaf and Root (also known as Brahmi)	*Centella asiatica*	50 mg/lb daily of fresh leaf; can be added as a vegetable to food	1 mg/lb standardized extract sid-bid	5 drops/lb tid	Potentially interacts with anxiolytic medications	Orally: slightly sedative; improves cognition, skin conditions; topically: antiinflammatory; enhances wound healing

Guggul Resin	*Commiphora mukul*		0.5-12.5 mg/lb bid standardized to 2.5%-10% guggulsterones		Minor GI disturbance, nausea; not for use with beta-blockers and calcium channel blockers—may interfere with effectiveness	Reduces cholesterol; antiinflammatory for arthritis
Gymnema Leaf	*Gymnema sylvestre*	50 mg/lb sid	5 mg/lb sid	1 drop/lb bid	May interact with insulin and other hypoglycemics	Diabetes; obesity
Hawthorn Leaves and Flowers, Fruit	*Crataegus oxycantha, C. laevigata*	30 mg/lb bid (fruits)	1-3 mg/lb tid (leaves and flowers)	2 drops/lb bid (fruit)	GI upset if product is high in leaf; may potentiate effect of digitalis, antihypertensives, beta-blockers	Heart disease; digestive disorders
Hops Fruits	*Humulus lupulus*	5-7 mg/lb tid-qid		1 drop/lb tid	Reported to cause malignant hyperthermia–4 of 5 dogs were greyhounds; allergies, contact dermatitis; generally safe as consumed in beer by much of the world's population	Mild sedative; GI spasmolytic
Horehound Herb	*Marrubium vulgare*	25-30 mg/lb bid		1-2 drops/lb tid	Possibly abortifacient; nausea, vomiting, anorexia, diarrhea, hypersensitivity reactions, arrhythmias; hypoglycemic; use with caution with antiarrhythmics, hypoglycemics, ondansetron/granisetron, sumatriptan because it inhibits serotonin action	Dry cough

Herb	Botanical Name	Dried Herb	Dried Concentrated Extract	Alcohol Tincture*	Contraindications and Side Effects of Large Doses, and Drug Interactions	Principal Uses —Modern and Traditional
Horseradish Root	*Cochlearia armoracia*	15-20 mg/lb fresh grated root bid-tid; not easy to do with animals		1 drop/lb bid-tid	Abortifacient; irritant; nausea, vomiting, anorexia, diarrhea, hypersensitivity reactions	Sinusitis, cough, anthelmintic
Horsetail Herb	*Equisetum arvense*	35-40 mg/lb bid		2 drops/lb bid-tid	Thiaminase may be a problem in raw, uncooked herb; hypersensitivity reactions; contains small amounts of nicotine	Diuretic; bone healing, nail and hair growth
Hyssop Leaf and Flower	*Hyssopus officinalis*			1 drop/lb bid	Nausea, vomiting, anorexia, hypersensitivity reactions; abortifacient	Cough; possibly antiviral
Ivy Leaf				1 drop/lb bid	Nausea, vomiting; possibly abortifacient	Cough, asthma, bronchitis
Juniper Berry	*Juniperis communis*	60 mg/lb bid		1-2 drops/lb bid-tid	Nausea, vomiting, anorexia, diarrhea, hypersensitivity reactions; may interact with diuretics; may aggravate glomerulonephritis	Urinary tract infection, GI disorders, diabetes

Kava Kava Root	*Piper methysticum*	20-35 mg/lb divided daily	1-2 mg/lb tid	1-2 drops/lb tid	Not for long-term use; liver failure has been reported with long-term use or as idiosyncratic reaction; occasional GI effects have been observed; scaly dermatitis, low platelet and white blood cell counts noted in humans after long-term use; not for use with other anti-psychotics, tranquilizers, etc.	Sedative; may relieve muscle spasms and have some anticonvulsant activity
Kudzu Root	*Pueraria lobata*	60 mg/lb tid	2 mg/lb bid	1 drop/lb bid	None described	Diarrhea, lower GI disorders, neck pain or stiffness
Linden Flowers	*Tilia vulgaris*			2-3 drops/lb bid	None described	Upper respiratory disorders with mucoid discharges, diarrhea, irritability and anxiety

Herb	Botanical Name	Dried Herb	Dried Concentrated Extract	Alcohol Tincture*	Contraindications and Side Effects of Large Doses, and Drug Interactions	Principal Uses —Modern and Traditional
Licorice Root	*Glycyrrhiza glabra*	20-60 mg/lb tid	10 mg/lb bid	1-2 drops/lb tid	Use with caution in renal, hepatic, or cardiovascular disease (but may be well indicated in some conditions);many documented cases of hyperaldosteronism from prolonged use, causing hypertension, hyperkalemia, sodium and water retention/edema; induces cytochrome P-450–dependent activities; may alter metabolism of many other drugs; not have DGL form does mineralocorticoid effects, but efficacy not as well established	Cough (antitussive and expectorant); mild antiinflammatory; may be antiviral; gastroenteritis and GI ulcers, Addison's disease
Lobelia Leaf	*Lobelia inflata*	As part of combinations only	As part of combinations only	0.5-1 drop/lb bid of vinegar extract only	Acts on nicotine receptors; nausea, dyspnea, hypotension, vomiting, tachycardia; causes respiratory depression	Asthma, COPD, congestive heart failure
Maitake Mushroom Fruiting Body and Mycelium	*Grifola frondosa*	30 mg/lb tid		1-2 drops/lb bid	None described	Antitumor, immunostimulant, antiobesity

Marshmallow Root	*Althea officinalis*	75 mg/lb tid		5 drops/lb tid, but not recommended, since herb mucilage is most active, and may not be present in this form	Nausea, vomiting, anorexia, hypersensitivity reactions,	Gastroenteritis, cough, urinary tract infection
Meadowsweet Flowering Tops	*Filipendula ulmaria*	30-40 mg/lb tid		2 drops/lb bid-tid	Salicylate content makes it potentially dangerous for use in cats	Arthritis, pain from inflammation, digestive disorders
Melissa Herb	*Melissa officinalis*	50 mg/lb tid	2-5 mg/lb tid	2 drops/lb tid	Possibly contraindicated for animals with glaucoma; may interfere with T_4 conversion to T_3	Herpes infections, GI problems; mild sedative
Milk Thistle Seed	*Silybum marianum*	15-20 mg/lb sid	2-5 mg/lb bid-tid (extract standardized to 80% silymarin)	1-2 drops/lb bid	May be associated with mild GI side effects; hypersensitivity reactions	Hepatocellular disease, especially toxic injuries to the liver

Herb	Botanical Name	Dried Herb	Dried Concentrated Extract	Alcohol Tincture*	Contraindications and Side Effects of Large Doses, and Drug Interactions	Principal Uses —Modern and Traditional
Mistletoe Flowering Tops, Leaf	*Viscum album*	35-75 mg/lb bid-tid		0.25 drop/lb bid	Bradycardia, hypotension, gastritis, hepatitis, hypersensitivity reactions; may interact with cardiac glycosides, antihypertensives, CNS depressants, immunosuppressants	Cancer, immunostimulant, hypotensive
Motherwort	*Leonurus cardiaca*	15 mg/lb tid		1 drop/lb bid-tid	None described	Cardiovascular disease—said to suppress arrhythmias generated by stress; mildly sedative; arrhythmias associated with hyperthyroidism; traditionally for menstrual disorders

Mullein Leaf and Flower	*Verbascum thapsis*	50 mg/lb tid		2 drops/lb tid; whole herb may be preferred	Nausea, anorexia, hypersensitivity reactions	Expectorant, antitussive for asthma, bronchitis; topically for ear inflammation
Myrrh Resin	*Commiphora molmol*	Unknown		5-10 drops in 3 oz of water as a "mouth wash" tid	Contact dermatitis	Arthritis, benign prostatic hyperplasia; diuretic
Neem Leaf	*Azadirachta indica*	25 mg/lb bid	1-3 mg/lb tid	0.25 drop/lb sid-bid	Nausea, vomiting, anorexia, hypersensitivity reactions	Most useful topically for external parasites; to a lesser extent orally, since toxicity is possible; may be useful contraceptive; hypoglycemic, immunomodulatory; traditionally used for itching and other skin problems, fevers, especially malaria

Herb	Botanical Name	Dried Herb	Dried Concentrated Extract	Alcohol Tincture*	Contraindications and Side Effects of Large Doses, and Drug Interactions	Principal Uses —Modern and Traditional
Nettles Herb	*Urtica dioica*	20-40 mg/lb tid	3-4 mg/lb tid	1-2 drops/lb tid	Dermatitis on contact with fresh herb; may potentiate action of diuretics	Nutritional tonic; atopic signs; antiinflammatory for arthritis; traditionally as a hemostatic
Nettles Root	*Urtica dioica (root)*		2 mg/lb bid		Nausea, vomiting	Benign prostatic hyperplasia
Noni Fruit	*Morinda citrifolia*		10 drops/lb bid of concentrate juice; 5-7 mg/lb of dried extract		Hyperkalemia is a contraindication, since juice has high potassium content	Arthritis; topically for skin infections, irritations
Oak Tree Bark	*Quercus* spp.	12.5-15 mg/lb tid		1-2 drops/lb bid-tid	Nausea, vomiting, anorexia, hypersensitivity reactions	Most useful for topical astringent effect for inflammatory skin disorders, GI problems, including stomatitis, gingivitis; may have use in prevention of uroliths

Olive Leaf	*Olea europea*		12.5 mg/lb bid	1 drop/lb sid-bid	Gastritis, hypoglycemia	Bacterial and viral infections, hypertension
Oregon Grape Root	*Mahonia aquifolium, Berberis aquifolium*	20 mg/lb bid		1-2 drops/lb bid	Nausea, vomiting, diarrhea, hypersensitivity reactions	Skin disorders, GI disorders, cancer, cardiovascular diseases
Pau d'arco	*Tabebuia avellanedae, T. impestiginosa*	15 mg/lb bid		1 drop/lb sid-bid	High doses of one extract have caused nausea, vomiting, bleeding; no adverse events reported with use of whole herb; use cautiously with anticoagulants	Cancer, viral infections, fungal infections, immune stimulation
Passion Flower Leaf, Stem, and Flower	*Passiflora incarnata*	50 mg/lb tid		2 drops/lb tid	Nausea, vomiting, anorexia, hypersensitivity reactions	Mild sedative; also for "nervous stomach"; muscle relaxant
Peppermint Herb	*Mentha piperita*	25 mg/lb bid	Enteric coated capsules containing oil: 0.005 ml/lb	1-2 drops/lb bid-tid; essential oil: 1 drop bid-tid	Allergic reaction; irritation if oil is placed on mucous membranes	GI antispasmodic; cramping, intestinal gas, borborygmus

Herb	Botanical Name	Dried Herb	Dried Concentrated Extract	Alcohol Tincture*	Contraindications and Side Effects of Large Doses, and Drug Interactions	Principal Uses —Modern and Traditional
Picrorhiza Root	*Picrorhiza kurroa*	5-12.5 mg/lb bid		1 drop/lb bid-tid	Nausea, vomiting, intestinal cramping, skin rashes	Hepatoprotective; asthma; may improve immune function; some reports of autoimmune disease improvement
Prickly Ash Bark	*Zanthoxylum americanum, Z. clava-herculis*			2 drops/lb bid-tid	Hypotension, coagulation problems, nausea, vomiting, anorexia, hypersensitivity reactions, photosensitivity	GI disorders, fever, inflammatory disorders, circulatory disorders
Propolis	A natural product of bees	Best used topically according to product label			hypersensitivity reactions, dermatitis	Wound healing, infection, stomatitis, antiinflammatory
Psyllium Seed	*Plantago ovata*	80 mg/lb tid in moistened food or water/broth because of swelling	Not a useful form	Not a useful form	Intestinal gas; contraindicated when bowel obstruction is a possibility; allergic reactions	Increases fiber in stool; may reduce absorption of glucose and lipids

Pumpkin Seed	*Cucurbita pepo*	60-65 mg/lb bid; much more may be required for treatment of parasites			Nausea, vomiting, anorexia, hypersensitivity reactions; may cause electrolyte loss if used for prolonged periods	Tapeworms, benign prostatic hypertrophy; fiber source
Pygeum Bark	*Pygeum africanum*		1 mg/lb bid of lipophilic extract standardized to 13% total sterols		Nausea, stomach pain	Benign prostatic hypertrophy
Red Raspberry Leaf and Fruit	*Rubus idaeus*	50-100 mg/lb daily		1-2 drops/lb bid-tid	Nausea, diarrhea	Diarrhea, "uterine tonic," astringent for stomatitis and gingivitis
Red Clover Flowers (nonfermented only)	*Trifolium praetense*	50 mg/lb tid		1-2 drops/lb bid-tid	Very safe; may have anticoagulant effects and phytoestrogens may be a concern for some cancers	Isoflavone content makes this a source of phytoestrogens for treatment of gynecologic disorders in women; traditionally for cancer and as a "blood cleanser"; antitussive

Herb	Botanical Name	Dried Herb	Dried Concentrated Extract	Alcohol Tincture*	Contraindications and Side Effects of Large Doses, and Drug Interactions	Principal Uses —Modern and Traditional
Reishi Mushroom Fruiting Body	*Ganoderma lucidum*	40-60 mg/lb bid	10-12 mg/lb tid	1-2 drops/lb tid	Used as food ingredient; rare GI effects, bleeding problems, dizziness have occurred in people using reishi for 3 to 6 months	Said to normalize immune function; used to increase response, as well as for some autoimmune disorders; cancer, cardiovascular disease
Rosemary Herb	*Rosmarinus officinalis*	25-30 mg/lb bid		1 drop/lb tid	Seizure disorders may be a contraindication for use; contact hypersensitivity	GI disorders, especially borborygmus and gas; antioxidant; may improve memory
St. John's Wort Flowering Tops	*Hypericum perforatum*	25 mg/lb bid	2-3 mg/lb bid-tid	1 drop/lb bid-tid	Photosensitivity; serotonin syndrome has been reported when used with SSRIs; nausea, anorexia, vomiting, diarrhea; interferes with the metabolism of numerous other drugs processed through CYP liver system; theoretical potential for increasing agitation if used with $beta_2$ agonists	Antidepressant; antiviral used topically for wounds and neuralgia and nerve pain

Sarsaparilla Root	*Smilax* spp.	40-60 mg/lb bid-tid		1-2 drops/lb bid-tid	Nausea, vomiting; saponins may interfere with absorption of other drugs	Antiinflammatory for arthritis, rheumatoid arthritis, GI disorders, inflammatory bowel disease and "leaky gut"
Saw Palmetto Berry	*Serenoa repens*	15-30 mg/lb bid	2 mg/lb bid	1 drop/lb bid	GI upset, diarrhea; (used as food by Native Americans)	Used to improve urine flow in benign prostatic hypertrophy; also for cystitis and possibly urethrospasm
Schisandra Berry	*Schisandra chinensis*	10-35 mg/lb bid		1-2 drops/lb bid-tid	GI upset, nausea, urticaria; possibly contraindicated in epilepsy	Adaptogen and performance enhancer; hepatoprotective; respiratory disorders
Skullcap Root, Chinese	*Scutellaria baicalensis*	50-75 mg/lb tid		1-2 drops/lb tid	Side effects generally unknown	Rhinitis, asthma; a major herb for clearing "empty heat" in Chinese medicine

Herb	Botanical Name	Dried Herb	Dried Concentrated Extract	Alcohol Tincture*	Contraindications and Side Effects of Large Doses, and Drug Interactions	Principal Uses —Modern and Traditional
Skullcap Herb, American	*Scutellaria laterifolia*	Fresh plant preferred; dried plant has very little activity		2 drops/lb tid	Side effects generally unknown; homeopathic literature suggests disorientation, twitching; reports of hepatotoxicity from products adulterated with germander	Mild sedative and antispasmodic for nervous tremors
Slippery Elm Bark	*Ulmus rubra, U. fulva*	10-20 mg/lb tid		Not recommended; does not contain mucilage that whole herb does	Allergic reactions	For GI inflammatory disorders, ulcers; topically to soothe cough from skin lesions, pharyngitis, and sore throat
Tea Tree Oil	*Melaleuca alternifolia*	Used topically *only;* 5%-15% concentra-tions or less	Not recommended	Not recommended	Fatal reactions in cats; is dangerous in dogs as well; weakness, depression, tremors, paresis; contact dermatitis and irritation are common on skin and oral tissues when animals lick the product	Topically for yeast and dermatophyte infections; possibly too toxic to use in many animals

Thyme Herb	*Thymus vulgaris*	25 mg/lb tid		1-2 drops/lb bid-tid	No problems identified unless using essential oil, which should be administered only highly diluted topically (mouthwash, douche) or via vaporizer	GI upset; expectorant for cough antimicrobial
Turmeric Root	*Cucurma longa*	10-50 mg/lb tid	5 mg/lb bid if standardized extract containing 95% curcumin	1 drop/lb bid	Allergic contact dermatitis; possibly contraindicated when biliary obstruction exists	Hepatoprotective; cancer prevention and possibly treatment; anti-hyperlipidemic
Tylophora Leaf and Root	*Tylophora indica*	2 mg/lb bid		1 drop/lb sid	Nausea, vomiting, mouth soreness	Asthma, bronchitis, possible allergic rhinitis
Usnea lichen	*Usnea barbata*	1-1.5 mg/lb tid		1 drop/lb tid	No problems reported	Upper respiratory infection, cough
Uva-Ursi Leaf	*Arctostaphylos uva-ursi*	35-40 mg/lb tid	4 mg/lb tid	2 drops/lb tid	Contraindicated in kidney disease; may cause GI upset, turn urine greenish; not for use longer than 10 to 14 days; not for use with urinary acidifiers, since effective only in alkaline urine	Urinary antiseptic

Herb	Botanical Name	Dried Herb	Dried Concentrated Extract	Alcohol Tincture*	Contraindications and Side Effects of Large Doses, and Drug Interactions	Principal Uses —Modern and Traditional
Valerian Root	*Valeriana officinalis*	50 mg/lb bid	2-3 mg/lb bid	1-2 drops/lb bid	May produce a stimulating, rather than sedating effect; do not use concurrently with barbiturates or benzodiazepines	Sedative, mild muscle relaxant, mild pain reliever; insomnia; may be more effective for anxiety disorders after 2 to 4 weeks of use
White Willow Bark	*Salix alba*	15 mg/lb tid		1-2 drops/lb tid	Nausea, diarrhea, gastric ulceration; caution is advised with nonsteroidal antiinflammatory drugs	Antiinflammatory pain reliever
Wild Cherry Bark	*Prunus serotina*			1-2 drops/lb tid	Cyanogenic glycosides theoretically pose risk of cyanide toxicity at very high doses	Antitussive
Yarrow Flowering Tops	*Achillea millefolium*	30 mg/lb bid-tid	2 drops/lb tid		Hypersensitivity reactions, contact allergy	GI tract inflammation and bleeding; bleeding disorders such as epistaxis, hemoptysis; topically as a styptic

Yellow Dock Root	*Rumex crispus*		1-2 drops/lb bid	Nausea, vomiting, diarrhea, hypersensitivity reactions	Skin disease; traditionally as a "blood cleanser"; possible iron source
Yucca Root and Stalk	*Yucca schidigera*	¼-½ tsp daily		Possible nausea, gastroenteritis; theoretically can cause hemolysis in vitro, but is safe enough that it is an approved food additive	Arthritis

Data from Brinker F. *Herb Contraindications and Drug Interactions.* Sandy, Ore, 1998, Eclectic Medical Publications; Health Notes Online: http://www.healthwell.com/healthnotes/index/herb_index.cfm; Kuhn M, Winston D. *Herbal Therapy and Supplements: a Scientific and Traditional Approach.* New York, 2001, Lippincott; Mills S, Bone K. *Principles and Practice of Phytotherapy.* New York, 2000, Churchill Livingstone; Wulff-Tilford M, Tilford G. *All You Ever Wanted to Know About Herbs for Pets.* Irvine, Calif, 1999, Bowtie Press; and Wynn SG. *Emerging Therapies: Using Herbs and Nutraceuticals in Small Animals.* Boulder, Colo, 1999, AAHA Press.

CYP, cytochrome P450 enzymes; *GI*, gastrointestinal; *SSRI*, selective serotonin reuptake inhibitor.

*Alcohol tinctures (given in drops) are derived from human doses given in ml. Although droppers are of variable size, we assume in this table that there are 30 drops per ml.

Appendix D

Chinese Herb Cross Reference Table

The reader must keep in mind that the pin yin name is descriptive of the particular plant species (or group of species), as well as the plant part and how it is prepared. See, for instance, the entries Sang Shen, Sang Ye, and Sang Zhi, which represent Mulberry tree fruit, leaf, and twig, respectively. This is why the pin yin name is preferred in this and any other text that discusses Chinese herbs. When a practitioner is learning Chinese herbs, however, it is important to know the pin yin *and* botanical names, the reason for which is well illustrated by the *Aristolochia* disaster.

Aristolochia fangchi is a toxic herb that has led to renal failure and urinary tract cancer when used in a modern weight loss formulations. In pin yin, this herb is known as Guang Fang Ji. A different herb, *Stephania tetrandra,* is more useful and less toxic and is known as Han Fang Ji. Unfortunately, both herbs are sometimes sold as Fang Ji. Yet another herb, *Akebia trifoliata* or *A. quinata,* is known as Mu Tong. In modern times, however, this pin yin name actually denotes *Aristolochia manshuriensis, Clematis armandi,* or *C. montana.* So *Aristolochia* species may sometimes, but not always, be contained in herbs listed as Fang Ji or Mu Tong. Let the buyer beware and be educated when buying Chinese herbs. Fortunately, most Chinese herb granules from North American distributors are currently screened for any content of potentially toxic aristolochic acids.

Pin Yin Name	Botanical Name	Common Name and Medicinal Part
Ai Ye	*Artemisa argyi, A. vulgaris*	Mugwort herb
Ba Dou	*Croton tiglium*	Croton seed
Bai Bu	*Stemona sessilifolia, S. japonica, S. tuberosa*	Stemona root
Bai Dou Kou	*Amomum kravanh*	White cardamon fruit
Bai Fan		Alum
Bai Guo	*Ginkgo biloba*	Ginkgo nut
Bai He	*Lilium brownii, L. colchesteri, L. pumilum, L. longiflorum*	Lily bulb
Bai Hua She	*Agkistrodon acutus, Bungarus ulticinctus*	Multibanded krait (this is an elapid snake or viper, with organs removed)
Bai Hua She She Cao	*Hedyotidis diffusa, Oldenlandia diffusa*	Oldenlandia herb
Bai Ji	*Bletilla striata, B. ochracea*	Bletilla rhizome
Bai Ji Tian	*Morinda officinalis*	Morinda root
Bai Jiang Cao	*Patrinia scabiosaefolia, Sonchus arvensis, S. brachyotus*	Patrinia herb
Bai Jie Zi	*Brassica alba*	White mustard seeds
Bai Mao Gen	*Imperata cylindrica*	Wooly grass rhizome, White grass rhizome, Imperata rhizome
Bai Qian	*Cynanchum stautoni, C. glaucescens*	Cynanchum root and rhizome
Bai Shao; Bai Shao Yao	*Paeonia lactiflora*	White peony root
Bai Tou Weng	*Pulsatilla chinensis, P. dahurica, P. turczaninovii, P. ambigua*	Anemone root
Bai Wei	*Cynanchum atratum, C. versicolor*	Swallowwort root
Bai Xian Pi	*Dictamnus dasycarpus*	Dictamnus root bark, Chinese dittany root bark
Bai Zhi	*Angelica dahurica*	Angelica root
Bai Zhu	*Atractylodes macrocephala*	White atractylodes rhizome
Bai Zi Ren	*Biota orientalis*	Arbor-vitae seed, Biota seed
Ban Bian Lian	*Lobelia chinensis*	Chinese lobelia herb and root
Ban Lan Gen	*Isatis baphicacanthus, I. tinctoria, I. indigotica, Baphicacanthus cusia*	Chinese woad root

Continued

Pin Yin Name	Botanical Name	Common Name and Medicinal Part
Ban Xia	*Pinellia ternata*	Cooked rhizome of Pinellia
Ban Zhi Lian	*Scutellaria barbata*	Barbart scullcap herb
Bi Ba	*Piper longum*	Long pepper fruit
Bi Xie	*Dioscorea hypoglauca, D. septemloba, D. futschauensis*	Yam tuber
Bian Dou	*Dolichos lablab*	Hyacinth bean seed
Bian Xu	*Polygonum avicularis*	Polygonum root, Knotweed root
Bie Jia	*Amydae sinensis*	Tortoise shell
Bing Lang	*Areca catechu*	Betel nut
Bing Pian	*Dryobalanops aromatica, Blumea balsamifera*	Borneol
Bo He	*Mentha haplocalyx, M. arvensis*	Mint herb
Bu Gu Zhi	*Psoralea corylifolia*	Psoralea seed
Can Sha	*Bombyx mori*	Silk worm casting
Cang Er Zi	*Xanthium sibiricum*	Cocklebur fruit, Xanthium fruit
Cang Zhu	*Atractylodes lancea, A. chinensis*	Red atractylodes rhizome
Cao Dou Kou	*Alpinia katsumada*	Galangal seed, Katsumadai seed
Cao Guo	*Amomum tsaoko*	Tsaoko fruit
Cao Wu		Prepared Tsao Wu aconite
Ce Bai Ye	*Biota orientalis*	Biota tops
Chai Hu	*Bupleurum chinensis*	Bupleurum root
Chan Tui	*Periostracum cicadae*	Cicada shed skin
Che Qian Zi	*Plantago asiatica, P. depressa*	Plantain seed
Chen Pi	*Citrus reticulata, C. tangerina*	Aged orange peel
Chen Xiang	*Aquillaria agallocha, A. sinensis*	Aquillaria wood, Aloeswood
Chi Shao	*Paeonia rubra*	Red peony root
Chi Shi Zhi		Red kaolin, Hallyosite
Chou Wu Tong	*Clerondendron trichotomum*	Glorybower leaf
Chuan Bei Mu	*Fritillaria cirrhosa, F. thunbergia, F. unibracteata, F. prezwalskii, F. delavayi*	Fritillary bulb
Chuan Lian Zi	*Melia toosendan*	Sichuan chinaberry
Chuan Niu Xi	*Achyranthes bidentata*	Achyranthes root
Chuan Shan Jia†	*Manis pentadactyla*	Anteater scales
Chuan Xin Lian	*Andrographis paniculata*	Green chiretta herb, Andrographis herb
Chuan Xiong	*Ligusticum chuanxiong*	Szechuan lovage root, Cnidium root
Chun Gen Pi	*Ailanthus altissima*	Ailanthus bark
Ci Ji Li	*Tribulus terrestris*	Tribulus fruit

Pin Yin Name	Botanical Name	Common Name and Medicinal Part
Ci Shi		Magnetite, Loadstone
Cong Bai	*Allium fistulosum*	Spring onion bulb
Da Fu Pi	*Areca catechu*	Areca nut peel
Da Huang	*Rheum palmatum, R. officinale, R. tanguticum*	Rhubarb root and rhizome
Da Ji	*Euphorbia pekinensis, Knoxia valerianoides*	Peking spurge root, Euphorbia root
Da Qing Ye	*Isatis tinctoria, I. indigota, Baphicacanthus cusia, Polygonum tinctorium, Clerodendron cyrtophyllum*	Chinese woad leaf
Da Suan	*Allium sativum*	Garlic bulb
Da Zao	*Ziziphus jujuba*	Chinese date, Jujube fruit
Dai Zhe Shi		Hematite
Dan Dou Chi	*Glycine max*	Prepared soy bean
Dan Shen	*Salvia miltorrhiza*	Salvia root
Dan Zhu Ye	*Lophatherum gracile*	Lopatherum stem and leaf
Dang Gui (Tang kuei) Shen	*Angelica sinensis*	Angelica root
Dang Gui Wei	*Angelica sinensis*	Angelica root tips or tails
Dang Shen	*Codonopsis pilosula*	Codonopsis root
Deng Xin Cao	*Juncus effusa*	Rush pith
Di Fu Zi	*Kochia scoparia*	Kochia fruit, Broom cypress root
Di Gu Pi	*Lycium chinense, L. barbarum*	Lycium root bark, Wolfberry root bark
Di Long	*Pheretima aspergillum, Allolobophora caliginosa*	Earthworm
Di Yu	*Sanguisorba officinalis*	Burnet root
Ding Xiang	*Eugenia caryophyllata*	Cloves
Dong Chong Xia Cao	*Cordyceps sinensis*	Cordyceps caterpillar fungus
Dong Gua Ren	*Benincasa hispida*	Winter melon seed, Wax gourd seed
Dong Kui Zi	*Malva verticillata*	Mallow seed
Du Huo	*Angelica pubescens*	Tu Huo, Angelica root
Du Zhong	*Eucommia ulmoides*	Eucommia bark
E Jiao	*Equus asinus*	Donkey hide gelatin
E Zhu	*Curcuma zedoaria*	Turmeric root
Fan Xie Ye	*Cassia angustifolia, C. acutifolia*	Senna leaf
Fang Feng	*Ledebouriella divaricata, L. sesiloides*	Siler root
Fang Ji: see Guang Fang Ji and Han Fang Ji		

Continued

Pin Yin Name	Botanical Name	Common Name and Medicinal Part
Fu Ling	*Poria cocos*	Poria sclerotium
Fu Pen Zi	*Rubus chingii*	Raspberry fruit
Fu Ping	*Spirodela polyrrhiza*	Duckweed herb
Fu Xiao Mai	*Triticus aestivus*	Light wheat
Fu Zi	*Aconitum carmichaeli*	Prepared aconite root
Gan Cao	*Glycyrrhiza glabra*	Licorice root
Gan Jiang	*Zingiber officinale*	Ginger root
Gan Sui	*Euphorbia kansui*	Gansui root, Kan-sui root
Gao Ben	*Ligusticum sinense, L. jeholense*	Chinese lovage root, Ligusticum root
Gao Liang Jiang	*Alpinia officinarum*	Galanga rhizome, Lesser galangal rhizome
Ge Gen	*Pueraria lobata, P. thunbergiana*	Kudzu root
Ge Jie	*Gecko gecko*	Whole gecko lizard
Gou Ji	*Cibotium barometz*	Chain fern rhizome
Gou Qi Zi	*Lycium chinense*	Wolfberry fruit
Gou Teng	*Uncaria rhyncophylla, U. sinensis*	Gambir stem and thorn
Gu Sui Bu	*Drynaria fortunei, D. baronii*	Drynaria rhizome
Gu Ya	*Oryza sativa*	Germinated rice
Gua Lou	*Tricosanthes kirilowii, T. uniflora, T. rosthornii*	Trichosanthes fruit
Gua Lou Ren	*Trichosanthes kirilowii, T. uniflora, T. rosthornii*	Trichosanthes seed
Guang Fang Ji	*Aristolochia fangchi, Cocculus trilobus*	Aristolochia root, Stephania root
Gui Ban	*Plastrum testudinis*	Turtle shell
Gui Zhi	*Cinnamomum cassia*	Cinnamon twigs
Hai Piao Xiao	*Sepia esculenta, Sepiella maindroni*	Cuttlefish bone
Hai Tong Pi	*Erythrina variegata, E. indica*	Coral bean bark, Erythrina bark
Hai Zao	*Sargassum pallidum, S. fusiforme*	Sargasso seaweed
Han Fang Ji	*Stephania tetrandra, Sinomenium acutum*	Stephania root
Han Lian Cao	*Eclipta prostrata*	Eclipta herb
He Huan Pi	*Albizzia julibrissin*	Mimosa tree bark
He Shou Wu	*Polygonium multiflorum*	Fo-ti root, Polygonum
He Ye	*Nelumbo nucifera*	Lotus leaf
He Zi	*Terminalia chebula*	Terminalia fruit
Hei Zhi Ma	*Sesame indica*	Black sesame seed
Hong Hua	*Carthamus tinctorius*	Safflower
Hou Po	*Magnolia officinalis*	Magnolia bark
Hu Gu*	*Os tigridis*	Tiger bone

Pin Yin Name	Botanical Name	Common Name and Medicinal Part
Hu Huang Lian	*Picrorhiza scrophulariaefolia*	Picrorhiza rhizome
Hu Jiao	*Piper nigrum*	Pepper fruit
Hu Lu Ba	*Trigonella foenum-graecum*	Fenugreek seeds
Hu Po		Amber
Hu Tao Ren	*Juglans regia*	Walnut
Hua Jiao	*Zanthoxylum bungeanum*	Chinese prickly ash fruit, Szechuan pepper
Hua Shi		Talc
Huai Hua Mi	*Sophora japonica*	Sophora flower
(Huai) Niu Xi	*Achyranthes bidentata*	Achyranthes root
Huang Bai	*Phellodendron amurense*	Amur cork-tree bark
Huang Jing	*Polygonum sibiricum, P. cyrtonema, P. kingianum*	Siberian solomon seal rhizome
Huang Lian	*Coptis chinensis, C. deltoidea, C. teetoidess*	Coptis root
Huang Qi	*Astragalus membranaceus*	Astragalus root
Huang Qin	*Scutellaria baicalensis, S. amoena, S. viscidula*	Baical Scullcap root Scullcap root
Huo Ma Ren	*Cannabis sativa*	Cannabis seed, Hemp seed
Huo Xiang	*Agastaches pogostemon, A. rugosa, Pogostemon cablin*	Patchouli herb
Ji Nei Jin	*Endothelium corneum*	Chicken gizzard lining
Ji Xue Teng	*Spatholobus suberectus, Millettia dielsiana, M. reticulata*	Milettia root and vine
Jiang Can	*Bombyx batryticatus*	Silkworm body
Jie Geng	*Platycodon grandiflorum*	Balloon flower root, Platycodon root
Jin Qian Cao	*Lysimachia christinae, Desmodium styracifolium*	Lysimachia herb
Jin Sha Teng	*Lygodium japonica*	Japanese fern leaf, Lygodium leaf
Jin Yin Hua	*Lonicera japonica*	Honeysuckle buds and flowers
Jin Ying Zi	*Rosa laevigata*	Rosehip
Jing Jie	*Schizonepeta tenuifolia*	Schizonepeta herb
Ju Hong	*Citrus erythrocarpus*	Pummelo peel
Ju Hua	*Chrysanthemum morifolium*	Chrysanthemum flowers
Jue Ming Zi	*Cassia obtusifolia, C. tora*	Cassia seed
Ku Shen	*Sophora flavescens*	Sophora root
Kuan Dong Hua	*Tussilago farfara*	Coltsfoot flower
Kun Bu	*Laminaria japonica, Ecklonia kurome*	Laminaria seaweed
Lai Fu Zi	*Raphanus sativus*	Radish seed

Continued

Pin Yin Name	Botanical Name	Common Name and Medicinal Part
Lian Qiao	*Forsythia suspensa*	Forsythia fruit
Lian Zi Xin	*Nelumbo nucifera*	Lotus leaf bud
Lian Zi	*Nelumbo nucifera*	Lotus seed
Ling Yang Jiao	*Cornu antelopes*	Antelope horn
Long Dan Cao	*Gentiana scabra, G. triflom, G. manshurica*	Chinese gentian root
Long Gu		Fossilized bone (usually of mammals)
Long Yan Rou	*Euphoria longan, Arillus euphoria*	Longan fruit
Lu Dou	*Phaseolus radiata, P. mungo*	Mung bean seed
Lu Gen	*Phragmites communis*	Reed rhizome
Lu Hui	*Aloe vera*	Aloe leaf juice concentrate
Lu Rong	*Cervus nippon*	Pilose deer antler
Ma Chi Xian	*Portulaca oleracea*	Purslane herb, Portulaca herb
Ma Dou Ling	*Aristolochia debilis, A. contorta*	Aristolochia fruit, Birthwort fruit
Ma Huang	*Ephedra sinica*	Ephedra stems
Mai Men Dong	*Ophiopogon japonica*	Mondo grass root
Mai Ya	*Hordeum vulgaris*	Malt, germinated barley
Man Jing Zi	*Vitex rotundifolia*	Vitex fruit
Mang Xiao		Sodium sulfate, Glauber's salt, Mirabilite
Mi Meng Hua	*Buddleia officinalis*	Butterfly bush flower bud
Mo Yao	*Commiphora myrrh*	Myrrh resin
Mu Dan Pi	*Paeonia suffruticosa*	Tree peony root bark
Mu Gua	*Chaenomelis lagenaria, C. sinensis, C. speciosa*	Chinese quince fruit
Mu Li	*Ostrea* spp.	Oyster shell
Mu Tong	*Akebia trifoliata, A. quinata* but *Aristolochia manshuriensis, Clematis armandii*, or *Clematis montana* may be substituted for *Akebia* spp.	Akebia vine
Mu Xiang	*Aucklandia lappa*	Costus root, Saussurea
Mu Zei	*Equisetum hiemalis*	Chinese horsetail herb, Scouring rush herb, Shave grass herb
Niu Bang Zi	*Arctium lappa*	Burdock seed, leaf, root
Niu Huang	*Calculus bovis*	Cow gallstone
Nu Zhen Zi	*Ligustrum lucidum*	Privet berry
Pi Pa Ye	*Eriobotrya japonica*	Loquat leaf
Pu Gong Ying	*Taraxacum mongolicum*	Dandelion flowers
Pu Huang	*Typha* spp.	Cat-tail pollen

Pin Yin Name	Botanical Name	Common Name and Medicinal Part
Qian Cao Gen	*Rubus cordifolia*	Madder root
Qian Hu	*Peucedanium praeruptorum, P. decursivum*	Hog fennel root, Peucedanum root
Qian Niu Zi	*Pharbitis nil, P. purpurea*	Morning glory seed
Qian Shi	*Euryales ferocis*	Euryale seed
Qiang Huo	*Notopterygium incisum, N. forbesii*	Notopterygium root, Chiang Huo root
Qin Jiao	*Gentiana macrophylla, G. straminea, G. crassicaulis, G. tibetica*	Large leaf gentian root
Qin Pi	*Fraxinus rhynchophylla*	Korean ash bark
Qing Hao	*Artemisia annua, A. apiacea*	Wormwood herb
Qing Pi	*Citrus reticulata*	Green tangerine peel
Qu Mai	*Dianthus superbus, D. chinensis*	Dianthus flowering tops, Chinese pink flowering tops, Fringed pink flowering tops
Quan Xie	*Buthus martensis*	Whole scorpion
Ren Shen	*Panax ginseng*	Korean ginseng root, Red ginseng root
Rou Cong Rong	*Cistanches deserticola, C. salsa*	Broomrape stem, Cistanche stem
Rou Dou Cou	*Myristica fragrans*	Nutmeg seed
Rou Gui	*Cinnamomum cassia*	Inner bark of cinnamon
Ru Xiang	*Boswellia carterii*	Boswellia carterii resin, Frankincense, Mastic
San Leng	*Sparganium stolonifera*	Sparganium rhizome, Scirpus
San Qi	*Panax pseudoginseng, P. notoginseng*	Pseudoginseng root, Notoginseng root
Sang Bai Pi	*Morus alba*	Mulberry root bark
Sang Ji Sheng	*Viscum coloratum, V. album, Loranthus parasiticus, Taxillus chinensis, T. sutchuensnsis, L. yadoriki*	Mistletoe stems, Loranthus stems
Sang Piao Xiao	*Paratenodera sinensis, P. augustipennis, Statilia maculata, Hierodula patellifera*	Mantis egg case
Sang Shen	*Morus alba*	Mulberry fruit
Sang Ye	*Morus alba*	Mulberry leaf
Sang Zhi	*Morus alba*	Mulberry twig
Sha Ren	*Amomum villosum, A. xanthioides*	Cardamon fruit
(Bei) Sha Shen	*Adenophora glehnia, A. tetraphylla, A. stricta, Glehnia littoralis*	Glehnia root

Continued

Pin Yin Name	Botanical Name	Common Name and Medicinal Part
Shan Dou Gen	*Sophora tonkinensis, S. subprostrata*	Sophora root
Shan Yao	*Dioscorea opposita*	Yam tuber
Shan Zha	*Crataegus pinnatifida, C. cuneata*	Hawthorn fruit
Shan Zhu Yu	*Cornus officinalis*	Cornus fruit
Shang Lu	*Phytolacca acinosa, P. esculenta*	Pokeroot
She Gan	*Belamcanda chinensis*	Belamcanda rhizome
She Xiang	*Moschus*	Musk deer secretion, musk
Shen Qu		Medicated leaven (combination of grains and yeast)
Sheng Di Huang	*Rehmannia glutinosa*	Rehmannia root
Sheng Jiang	*Zingiber officinale*	Fresh ginger root
Sheng Jiang Pi	*Zingiber officinale*	Fresh ginger root peel
Sheng Ma	*Cimicifuga foetida, C. dahurica, C. heracleifolia*	Chinese black cohosh rhizome, Bugbane rhizome
Shi Chang Pu	*Acorus graminei*	Sweetflag rhizome, Acorus rhizome
Shi Gao	*Gypsum fibrosum*	Gypsum
Shi Hu	*Dendrobium nobile, D. fimbriatum, D. loddigesii, D. chrysanthum*	Dendrobium plant
Shi Jue Ming	*Concha haliotidis*	Haliotis shell
Shi Shang Bai	*Selaginella doederleinii*	Selaginella herb
Shi Wei	*Pyrrosia lingua, P. sheareri, P. petiolosa*	Pyrrosia leaf
Shu Di Huang	*Rehmannia glutinosa*	Cooked rehmannia root
Shui Niu Jiao†		Water buffalo horn
Song Jie	*Pinus tabulaeformis, P. massoniana, P. yunnanensis*	Knotty pine wood
Su He Xiang	*Liquidambar orientalis*	Rose maloe resin, Liquidambar, Styrax
Su Zi	*Perilla frutescens*	Perilla fruit and seed
Suan Zao Ren	*Ziziphus spinosa*	Sour jujube seed
Suo Yang	*Cynormorus songaricus*	Cynomorium stem
Tai Zi Shen	*Pseudostellaria heterophylla*	Pseudostellaria root
Tan Xiang	*Santalum album*	Sandal wood heartwood
Tao Ren	*Prunus persica*	Peach kernel
Tian Ma	*Gastrodia elata*	Gastrodia rhizome
Tian Hua Fen	*Trichosanthes kirilowii*	Trichosanthes root
Tian Men Dong	*Asparagus conchinchinensis, A. officinalis*	Asparagus shoot and root

Pin Yin Name	Botanical Name	Common Name and Medicinal Part
Tian Nan Xing	*Arisaema consanguineum, A. amurense, A. heterophyllum*	Jack-in-the-pulpit rhizome, Arisaema rhizome
Ting Li Zi	*Descurainia sophia, Lepidium apetalum*	Lepidium seed
Tu Fu Ling	*Smilax glabra*	Smilax rhizome, Greenbrier rhizome
Tu Si Zi	*Cuscuta chinensis*	Cuscuta seeds
Wang Bu Liu Xing	*Vaccaria segetalis*	Vaccaria seed
Wei Ling Xian	*Clematis chinensis, C. hexapetala, C. uncinata*	Clematis root
Wu Gong	*Scolopendra subspinipes*	Centipede
Wu Jia Pi	*Acanthopanax gracilistylus, A. giraldii, Periploca sepium*	Acanthopanax root bark
Wu Ling Zhi	*Faeces trogopterorum*	Flying squirrel feces, Trogopterus dung
Wu Mei	*Prunus mume*	Black plum fruit
Wu Wei Zi	*Schisandra chinensis*	Schisandra fruit
Wu Yao	*Lindera strychnifolia*	Lindera root
Wu Zhu Yu	*Evodia ruteacarpa, E. officinalis, E. bodinieri*	Evodia fruit
Xi Gua	*Citrullus vulgaris*	Watermelon fruit
Xi Jiao*,†	*Cornu rhinoceri*	Rhinoceros horn
Xi Xian Cao	*Siegesbeckia pubescens, S. orientalis, S. glabrescens*	Siegesbeckia herb
Xi Xin	*Asarum sieboldii, A. heterotropoides, A. mandshuricum*	Chinese wild ginger herb and root
Xi Yang Shen	*Panax quinquefolium*	American ginseng root
Xia Ku Cao	*Prunella vulgaris*	Self-heal herb
Xian He Cao	*Agrimonia pilosia*	Agrimony herb
Xian Mao	*Curculigo orchioides*	Orchid-eye grass rhizome
Xiang Fu	*Cyperus rotundifolia*	Nut grass rhizome, Cyperus rhizome
Xiang Zi	*Celosia argentea*	Celosia seeds
Xiao Hui Xiang	*Foeniculum vulgaris*	Fennel fruit
Xin Yi Hua	*Magnolia liliflora*	Magnolia flower
Xing Ren	*Prunus armeniaca*	Apricot kernel
Xiong Dan	*Vesica fellea*	Bear gall
Xu Duan	*Dipsacus asperus, D. japonicus*	Teasel root, Dipsacus
Xuan Fu Hua	*Inula japonica, I. britannica, I. chinensis*	Inula flower
Xuan Shen	*Scrophularia ningpoensis, S. buergeriana*	Scrophularia root, Ningpo figwort root
Yan Hu Suo	*Corydalis yanhusuo*	Corydalis root

Continued

Pin Yin Name	Botanical Name	Common Name and Medicinal Part
Ye Jiao Teng	*Polygonum multiflorum*	Fleeceflower stem
Yi Mu Cao	*Leonurus heterophylla*	Chinese motherwort herb
Yi Tang	*Saccharum granorum*	Maltose
Yi Yi Ren	*Coix lachryma jobi*	Coix seeds, Job's tears seeds
Yi Zhi Ren	*Alpinia oxyphylla*	Black cardamon
Yin Chai Hu	*Stellaria dichotoma v. lanceolata; Arenaria juncea; Silena jenissensis; Gypsophila oldhamiama*	Stellaria root
Yin Chen Hao	*Artemisia capillaris, A. scoparia*	Capillaris herb, Yinchenhao herb
Yin Yang Huo	*Epimedium grandiflorum*	Epimedium leaf
Yu Jin	*Curcuma longa, C. aromatica, C. kwangsinensis*	Curcuma tuber
Yu Li Ren	*Prunus japonica, P. humulus*	Bush cherry pit
Yu Xing Cao	*Houttuynia cordata*	Houttuynia herb and root
Yu Zhu	*Polygonum odoratum*	Solomon's seal rhizome
Yuan Hua	*Daphne genkwa*	Genkwa flower, Daphne flower
Yuan Zhi	*Polygala tenuifolia*	Polygala root, Chinese senega root
Zao Jiao	*Gleditsia sinensis*	Chinese honeylocust fruit
Ze Lan	*Lycopus lucidum*	Bugleweed herb
Ze Xie	*Alisma orientalis, A. plantago-aquatica v. orientale*	Water plantain rhizome, Alisma rhizome
Zhe Bei Mu	*Fritillaria verticillata*	Fritillaria bulb
Zhen Zhu Mu	*Pteria margaritifera, P. martensii, Hydiopsis cumingii, Cristaria plicata*	Pearl
Zhi Ke	*Citrus aurantium*	Bitter orange fruit
Zhi Mu	*Anemarrhena asphodeloides*	Anemarrhena rhizome
Zhi Shi	*Citrus aurantium*	Immature orange fruit
Zhi Zi	*Gardenia jasminoides*	Gardenia fruit
Zhu Ling	*Polyporus umbellatus*	Polyporus sclerotium
Zhu Ru	*Bambusa brevifolia, Phyllostachys nigra*	Bamboo shavings
Zhu Sha		Cinnabar, a derivative of mercury
Zi Cao Gen	*Lithospermum erythrorhizon, Arnebia euchroma* or *Macrotomia euchroma, Onosma paniculatum*	Lithospermum root, Groomwell root, Arnebia root
Zi He Che	*Placenta hominis*	Human placenta

Pin Yin Name	Botanical Name	Common Name and Medicinal Part
Zi Hua Di Ding	*Viola yedoensitis, V. mandshurica*	Yedeon's violet herb and root
Zi Su Ye	*Perilla frutescens*	Perilla leaf
Zi Wan	*Aster tatarica*	Purple aster root

*These ingredients come from extremely endangered species and should be recognized only with an eye to avoiding and reporting these products.

†These ingredients are probably difficult to obtain in North America because of their animal origins, and are not commonly used in practice despite their historical importance.

Appendix E

Acupuncture Points

The acupuncture points below are described in this way:

IVAS designation	Pin Yin Name, translation	Five Element Command Point

Location:

Special qualities:

Anatomy:

Use:

Comments:

LU 1	**Zhong Fu (central storage)**	
Location:	On the median edge of the brachiocephalicus muscle, medial to the lesser tubercle of the humerus, in the first intercostal space, in the superficial pectoral muscle, 0.5 to 1 cm deep; avoid pneumothorax	
Special qualities:	**Alarm point for the Lung**	
Anatomy:	Pectoralis cranialis; seventh and eighth cervical spinal nerves	
Use:	Diagnostic, respiratory, cough, bronchitis, asthma	
Comments:	Allows Qi to enter the forelimb from the chest; tonifies Lung Qi	
LU 5	**Chi Ze (ulnar marsh)**	**Water**
Location:	On the transverse cubital crease, lateral to the biceps tendon and medial to the extensor carpi radialis, 0.5 to 1 cm deep; the musculocutaneous nerve is deep to this point	
Special qualities:	**He point** **Sedation point**	

Anatomy:	Craniolateral cutaneous antebrachial nerve
Use:	Local point for elbow, cough with phlegm or congestion, asthma, paralysis of distal thoracic limb, afternoon fever, mastitis, hemoptysis
Comments:	CLEARS LUNG HEAT AND PHLEGM-HEAT; useful for that reason in severe bronchopneumonia

LU 6	**Kong Zui (obvious cleft)**
Location:	On the medial aspect of the forelimb, slightly proximal to the midpoint and medial to the extensor carpi radialis muscle (about 5/12 of the distance from the cubital fossa to the carpus)
Special qualities:	**Xi cleft**
Anatomy:	Lateral cutaneous antebrachial nerve
Use:	Pharyngolaryngitis, pain in the elbow and forelimb, cough

LU 7	**Lie Que (missing row)**
Location:	On the medial aspect of the forelimb, proximal to styloid process of radius and medial to the tendon of the extensor carpi radialis, 1.5 cun above the transverse crease of the carpus (slightly less than 1/6 the distance from the carpus to the cubital fossa)
Special qualities:	**Luo point** **Master point for head and neck** **Confluent point for Ren Mai (or CV extra meridian)**
Anatomy:	Craniolateral cutaneous antebrachial nerve, superficial branch of the radial nerve
Use:	EXPELS WIND, WIND COLD; major point for all respiratory disorders, laryngolaryngitis, rhinitis, sinusitis, sneezing, tracheobronchitis, cough, asthma, stiff neck, cervical spondylosis, facial paralysis, local point for carpus; use with KI 6 to regulate the Ren Mai

LU 9	**Tai Yuan (great abyss)**	**Earth**
Location:	On the medial aspect of the carpus, cranial to the tendon of the flexor carpi radialis and immediately distal to the radial styloid process, 0.5 cm deep	
Special qualities:	**Source point** **Tonification point** **Influential point for blood vessels** **Shu Stream point**	
Anatomy:	Craniolateral cutaneous brachial nerve, superficial branch of the radial nerve	
Use:	EXPELS WIND; WIND COLD; PHLEGM; respiratory disorders, vascular disorders, pain in elbow and shoulder, forelimb paralysis	

LU 11 **Shao Shang (minor Shang, weak lung Qi)** **Wood**

Location: On the medial coronary border of the first phalanx of the forefoot, 0.2 cm deep (painful)

Special qualities: **Jing Well point**
Ghost point

Anatomy: Palmar digital nerve of first digit

Use: DISPELS WIND; WIND HEAT; acute emergencies such as respiratory arrest, coma, collapse, epilepsy, high fever

Comments: Like all Jing Well points, has the ability to rapidly and substantially influence the Qi, which flows very superficially here. This gives these points the ability to restore consciousness and act as powerful points to clear Heat.

LI 1 **Shang Yang (Yang of Shang)** **Metal**

Location: On the dorsal forefoot, on the medial coronary border of the second phalanx, 0.2 cm deep (painful)

Special qualities: **Jing Well point**
Horary point

Anatomy: Second palmar common digital nerve

Use: DISPELS WIND; emergencies such as epilepsy, high fever

Comments: Like all Jing Well points, has the ability to rapidly and substantially influence the Qi, which flows very superficially here. This gives these points the ability to restore consciousness and act as powerful points to clear Heat.

LI 4 **He Gu (union valley)**

Location: Between the first and second metacarpal bones at the level of the head of the first metacarpus; when the first metacarpal is missing or removed, the point is at the scar, on the medial side of the second metacarpal, 0.5 cm deep. Some authors believe that to get an equivalent action to what is observed in humans in animals with the first digit removed, the needle must be inserted into the muscle belly ventral to the second metacarpal.

Special qualities: **Source point**
Master point for face and mouth

Anatomy: First dorsal common digital nerve

Use: EXTERNAL WIND, WIND COLD, WIND HEAT; dermatologic disorders, pain in the head and neck, pain in the forelimb and shoulder, acupuncture analgesia, neurodermatitis; an important analgesic point, beneficial for any pain

Comments: An alternate name for this point is Tiger's Mouth, which refers to the ability of this point to directly access the Qi and Yang of the body. This gives the point the ability to tonify Qi and Yang (in combination with

ST 36), move Qi (in tandem with LIV 3), and clear Heat (when used with LU 7).

LI 6 — **Pian Li (sinister course)**

Location: On the cranial surface of the forelimb, at the junction of the extensor carpi radialis and abductor pollicis longus, and lateral to the tendon of the extensor carpi radialis

Special qualities: **Luo point**

Anatomy: Lateral cutaneous antebrachial nerve

Use: Epistaxis, tonsillitis, pain in the forearm

LI 10 — **Shou San Li (hand 3 mile)**

Location: One sixth the distance from the elbow joint to the carpus, between the extensor carpi radialis and the brachioradialis muscles, 1-2 cm deep; the superficial radial nerve is deep to this point

Anatomy: Lateral cutaneous antebrachial nerve

Use: Pain or paralysis of the shoulder and arm, elbow arthritis or arthritis of the elbow joint, diarrhea

Comments: Important tonification point, given its parallel location with ST 36, with which it is paired for this purpose

LI 11 — **Qu Chi (pond in the curve)** — **Earth**

Location: With the elbow flexed, at the lateral end of the cubital crease, halfway between the biceps brachii tendon and the lateral epicondyle of the humerus, 1-2 cm deep

Special qualities: **He point**
Tonification point
Ghost point

Anatomy: Cranial cutaneous antebrachial nerve; the superficial radial nerve is deep to this point

Use: DISPELS WIND, DISPELS HEAT, CLEARS DAMP HEAT, STOPS ITCH, BUILDS WEI QI, COOLS BLOOD; local point for elbow and forelimb, skin disorders, neurodermatitis, endocrine disorders, fever, enhances immune function, good for allergic and infectious diseases

Comments: One of the most important points in the body. The name "pond" is taken from the Chinese character for the point that, literally translated, means "added water." This suggests the point's main role, which is the clearing of Damp Heat. It combines with Spleen 9, another He-Sea point, to create a powerful point combination for the treatment of Damp Heat accumulations. Its cooling properties also allow it to cool the Blood, thus stopping itch. Other Blood-cooling points with which it is often combined are LI 4, BL 40, and SP 10. The placement at the elbow means that the cooling effects of LI 11 are quite powerful, as with the other points at the elbow. It is thus a good point to use in febrile illnesses, especially when combined with GV 14, LI 4, GV 4, and distal extremity points.

LI 14 — **Bi Nao (upper arm)**

Location: At the ventral tip of the deltoideus, cranial to the lateral head of the triceps

Anatomy: Craniolateral cutaneous brachial nerve

Use: Injuries to shoulder joint, pain of the thoracic limb, thoracic acupuncture analgesia

LI 15 — **Jian Yu (shoulder bone)**

Location: At the midpoint between the acromion and the greater tubercle of the humerus, on the cranial margin of the distal part of the deltoideus muscle, 1-2 cm deep. This point may be the same as the traditional point in animals known as Jain Jing (shoulder well).

Anatomy: Branches from the lateral supraclavicular nerve

Use: Shoulder arthritis, Bi syndromes

LI 18 — **Fu Tu (neck)**

Location: At the midpoint of the groove between the sternocephalicus and brachiocephalicus muscles, 0.5-1.5 cm deep

Use: Goiter, cough, bronchial asthma, acupuncture analgesia

LI 20 — **Ying Xiang (welcome aroma)**

Location: Lateral to the wing of the nostril (ala nasi), in the groove between the nasal plane and the hairy skin, 0.5 cm deep

Anatomy: Branches from the infraorbital nerve

Use: DISPELS WIND, DISPELS HEAT; rhinitis, especially cats with upper respiratory infection, nasal obstruction, epistaxis, facial paralysis

ST 1 — **Cheng Qi (receiving tears)**

Location: In the center of the ventral border of the orbit, between the globe of the eye and the orbital rim, 2-4 cm deep

Anatomy: Branches from the maxillary branch of the trigeminal nerve

Use: Local for eyes, chemosis, blepharospasm, conjunctivitis, atrophy of optic nerve, cataract

Comments: This is a traditional point in animals that should be used with extreme caution given its proximity to the eyeball

ST 2 — **Si Bai (4 white)**

Location: At the infraorbital foramen, rostroventral to ST 1, 0.2-0.5 cm deep

Anatomy: Maxillary branch of the trigeminal nerve

Use: Depending on location, local point for eye or facial paralysis, conjunctivitis

ST 4 **Di Cang (earth storage)**

Location: Lateral corner of mouth, 0.5-1 cm deep
Anatomy: Buccal nerve
Use: Toothache, lip fold dermatitis, trigeminal neuralgia, nasal obstruction

ST 6 **Jia Che (cheek wheel)**

Location: At the ventral end of the belly of the masseter muscle, rostral to the angle of the mandible
Special qualities: **Ghost point**
Anatomy: Great auricular nerve
Use: Facial paralysis, toothache, swelling of cheek or face; this is a very important local point for treatment of masticatory myositis

ST 7 **Xia Guan (under the joint)**

Location: In a depression ventral to the zygomatic arch rostral to the condyloid process of the mandible; a traditional canine point
Anatomy: Auriculotemporal nerve
Use: Facial paralysis, mandibular myositis

ST 8 **Tou Wei (head corner)**

Location: This point is not taught in most veterinary acupuncture courses but is an important point in my (SM) opinion; it is located in the center of a domed area of muscle, just dorsal to the midpoint of a line connecting the lateral canthus to the medial insertion of the pinna with the scalp
Special qualities: **Intersection point of the Stomach and Gall Bladder channels**
Use: The symbol for corner is derived from the symbol for a silk net used to catch birds in China. The implication is that this point has an important function in unbinding the head. In humans, it is thus used for headache, and it may be used in animals when there is a suggestion of headache. Its most important use, however, is in treating ocular disease and clearing redness and inflammation from the eye.

ST 9 **Ren Ying (man's reception)**

Location: Level with and just lateral to the larynx; avoid puncturing carotid
Special qualities: **Intersection point of the Gall Bladder and Stomach channels**
Use: Hyperthyroidism in cats, asthma, dysphagia

Comments:	One possible translation of Ying refers literally to allowing entry or passage on presentation of credentials. This suggests this point's crucial role in allowing the entry of ingested food or water into the rest of the body. If entry is refused, food and water is detained here or regurgitated.
ST 25	**Tian Shu (celestial center)**
Location:	Lateral to the umbilicus, midway between the umbilicus and the abdominal milk line (nipples), 0.2-0.5 cm deep. The rectus abdominis muscle is beneath the point; a traditional canine point
Special qualities:	**Alarm point of Large Intestine**
Anatomy:	Tenth and eleventh intercostal nerves
Use:	FOOD ACCUMULATION; diagnostic point for large intestine disorders, gastroenteritis, diarrhea, constipation, vomiting
ST 35	**Du Bi (calf's nose)**
Location:	On the lateral side of the patella, at the junction between the patella and the patellar ligament, 1 cm deep. A traditional animal acupoint includes the medial point (known as Xi Yan) and both together are called Xi Xia (under the kneecap); use caution because of proximity of joint capsule
Anatomy:	Lateral cutaneous femoral and saphenous nerves
Use:	Local point for stifle disorders or pain due to cranial cruciate ligament rupture, patellar luxation, arthritis
ST 36	**Hou San Li (hindleg 3 miles)** **Earth**
Location:	Three-sixteenths the distance from the point ST 35 to cranial tarsus or 3 cun below ST 35, about one digit breadth lateral to the tibial crest, in the lateral portion of the cranial tibial muscle, 1-2 cm deep; a traditional veterinary acupoint
Special qualities:	**He point** **Master point for Abdomen, GI function** **Tonification point** **Horary point**
Anatomy:	Branches from the saphenous nerve; peroneal nerve is deep to the point
Use:	BUILDS QI AND BLOOD, TONIFICATION OF DEFICIENT PATIENTS; most important distal point for GI problems; pelvic limb paralysis, acupuncture analgesia, homeostatic effects in endocrine disorders such as degenerative myelopathy, metabolic disorders
Comments:	The Yang Ming channels represent the areas in the body where Yang Qi consolidates. As a major point on this channel, ST 36 is used to generate Yang Qi when it is lacking. From this Qi and Blood can be manufactured.

Points to use in combination with ST 36 in the generation of Qi and Blood are LI 4 and LI 10. ST 36 also has an important consolidating effect on the Yang Qi, allowing it to help promote the downbearing of Qi and a resultant reduction of hypertension.

ST 37	**Shang Ju Xu (upper great hollow)**
Location:	In the cranial tibialis, the same distance below ST 36 as ST 36 is below the eye of the knee (ST 35)
Special qualities:	**Lower he sea point for Large Intestine**
Use:	FOOD ACCUMULATION; colitis, constipation, abdominal pain, and distention
Comments:	An underused and underappreciated point called for in any large intestine condition, an important point to move Blood, either alone or in combination with ST 39 and BL 11
ST 39	**Xia Ju Xu (lower great hollow)**
Location:	6 cun below ST 36
Special qualities:	**Lower he sea point for Small Intestine**
Use:	Small intestinal diarrhea, lower abdominal pain, an important point to move Blood, either alone or in tandem with ST 37
ST 40	**Feng Long (robust, flourishing, bountiful bulge)**
Location:	At the midpoint of the line between the point ST 35 and the lateral malleolus of the fibula. The point is between the muscles of the cranial tibial and the long digital extensor; 1 cm deep
Special qualities:	**Luo point** **Influential point for Phlegm**
Anatomy:	Superficial peroneal nerve
Use:	TRANSFORMS AND DISPERSES PHLEGM; hind limb paralysis, bronchitis, asthma, phlegm, gastrointestinal disorders, vestibular syndrome, epilepsy, any condition in which there is abundant mucus and thick, ropy saliva
ST 41	**Jie Xi (dispersing brook, relax cramp, ravine divide)** **Fire**
Location:	On the dorsum of the tarsal joint, in a depression between the tendons of the long digital extensor and the tibialis cranialis muscles, approximately at the level of the tip of the malleolus, 0.2-0.5 cm deep
Special qualities:	**Jing River point** **Tonification point**
Anatomy:	Superficial peroneal nerve; the cranial tibial artery and vein and the deep peroneal nerves are deep to the point
Use:	DISPERSES DAMP, DISPELS WIND; local point for hock, pelvic limb paralysis, abdominal disorders

Comments: This is an important point for draining pathogenic Qi out of the Stomach channel. One of the major clinical applications is thus Wei Syndrome, manifesting as hind limb paralysis or degenerative myelopathy, when excess Damp Heat has entered the Stomach channel and desiccated its content of Blood. Once this occurs, Blood is not available in the Stomach channel to nourish the tendons and support movement. Atrophy and spasm occur as a result. When pathogenic Qi has moved from the Stomach channel into the abdomen, producing abdominal disorders, ST 41 can likewise be used to drain the Qi.

ST 42 **Chong Yang (surging Yang)**

Location: On the dorsal aspect of the tarsal joint, at the junction of the second and third tarsal bones and the bases of the second and third metatarsal bones, 0.3 cm deep

Special qualities: **Source point**

Anatomy: Superficial peroneal nerve

Use: Tarsal pain, behavioral disorders, facial disorders

ST 44 **Nei Ting (inner court)** **Water**

Location: On the dorsum of the hindfoot, in the depression between the second and the third proximal phalanges, and proximal to the margin of the digital web

Special qualities: **Ying Spring point**

Anatomy: Superficial peroneal nerve

Use: CLEARS HEAT FROM STOMACH; gingivitis, stomatitis, (especially compulsive eaters that vomit afterward [Stomach Fire]), use in combination with ST 45

ST 45 **Li Dui (severe mouth)** **Metal**

Location: On the lateral coronary border of the second phalanx, at the base of the nail of the hind foot, 0.2 cm deep, painful to needle

Special qualities: **Jing Well point**
Sedation point

Anatomy: Second abaxial dorsal digital nerve

Use: Emergencies, behavioral problems

Comments: Like all Jing Well points, has the ability to rapidly and substantially influence the Qi, which flows very superficially here. This gives these points the ability to restore consciousness and act as powerful points to clear Heat.

SP 1 **Yin Bai (hidden white)**

Location: Medial to the base of the first phalanx of the hind foot

Special qualities: **Jing Well point**
Ghost point

Use: Emergencies, shock, abdominal pain, uterine bleeding

Comments: Like all Jing Well points, has the ability to rapidly and substantially influence the Qi, which flows very superficially here. This gives these points the ability to restore consciousness and act as powerful points to clear Heat. SP 1, even more than SP 4 (below), is noted for its ability to stop hemorrhage caused by Spleen deficiency. Traditionally, the point is warmed with moxibustion to stop hemorrhage.

SP 2 **Da Du (great city)**

Location: Medial to the base of the first phalanx of the hind foot and proximal to SP 1

Special qualities: **Tonification point**

Use: Digestive disorders

SP 3 **Tai Bai (great white)** **Earth**

Location: Medial to the head of the first metatarsal bone in humans, and if dewclaw is present. In dogs, the point location is considered uncertain, but is generally said to be on the midpoint of the medial side of the second metatarsal bone, 0.3 cm deep

Special qualities: **Source point**
Horary point

Anatomy: Second abaxial plantar digital nerve (if on second metatarsal bone)

Use: Abdominal pain, diarrhea, constipation

SP 4 **Gong Sun (grandparent and grandchild; yellow emperor)**

Location: In the depression in the medial aspect of the base of the first metatarsal bone (or dewclaw), or the medial aspect of the base of the second metatarsal bone, if the first is not present, 0.5-1 cm deep

Special qualities: **Luo point**

Anatomy: Second abaxial plantar digital nerve

Use: REGULATES CHONG MAI, REGULATES BLOOD, TONIFIES SPLEEN'S ABILITY TO HOLD BLOOD; for bleeding, especially uterine, gastritis, diarrhea, constipation; to influence the Chong Mai combine with PC 6. See also SP 1 to stop bleeding,

SP 5 **Shang Qiu (shang's hill)** **Metal**

Location: In the depression between the medial malleolus and the head of the talus bone, medial to the tendon of the tibialis cranialis muscle, 0.5-1 cm deep

Special qualities: **Sedation point**

Anatomy: Saphenous nerve

Use: Local point for tarsus, gastrointestinal disorders

SP 6 **San Yin Jiao (3 Yin conjoined, meeting of the three Yin)**

Location: On the medial aspect of the hind limb, caudal to the tibial bone, 3/16 distance from the medial malleolus of the tibia to the stifle joint or 3 cun proximal to the medial malleolus, on the posterior border of the tibia, 0.8-1.5 cm deep

Special qualities: **Master point for caudal abdomen and pelvic organs**

Anatomy: Saphenous nerve; the tibial nerve is deep and slightly caudal

Use: DISPERSES DAMP, DAMP HEAT, TONIFIES QI, BLOOD, AND YIN, TONIFIES SPLEEN; FOR POOR SHEN; urogenital disorders, gastrointestinal disorders, acupuncture analgesia for abdominal surgery and dystocia, general tonification, especially for geriatric patients, fatigue, weakness; allergic and immune disorders, endocrine disorders such as degenerative myelopathy when combined with ST 36, dermatologic disorders; liver, kidney, and pancreatic disorders; pelvic limb disorders

Comments: This point is of great importance when Liver Blood deficiency is perceived to be present, causing Liver Qi stagnation. It is a point *par excellence* for Qi and Blood stagnation in the lower jiao, both within the abdomen and over the lower back and legs. Most of its clinical applications stem from this action, although it is a point to be considered when both Liver and Kidney Yin tonification is required.

SP 9 **Yin Ling Quan (spring of the Yin grave hill) Water**

Location: On the medial aspect of the leg, in the depression ventral to the medial condyle of the tibia, between the caudal border of the tibia and the gastrocnemius muscle, 1-2 cm deep

Special qualities: **He point**

Anatomy: Saphenous nerve; tibial nerve is deep to this point

Use: DISPELS DAMP HEAT; local point for stifle, urogenital disorders, cystitis, balanoposthitis, vaginitis, inguinal dermatitis, ascites, diarrhea

Comments: This point is called for when Spleen deficiency is leading to an accumulation of Damp Heat in the lower jiao, especially the bladder and urogenital tract. It combines well with LI 11 for this purpose.

SP 10 **Xue Hai (sea of blood)**

Location: On the medial aspect of the thigh, proximal to the medial epicondyle along the cranial border of the femur on top of the vastus medialis muscle, 0.5-1.5 cm deep

Anatomy: Cutaneous branches of the lateral cutaneous femoral and genitofemoral nerves

Use: COOLS BLOOD, BUILDS BLOOD (almost as well as SP 6); BLOOD DEFICIENCIES, BLOOD HEAT; fevers, bloody pustules, itch, female reproductive disorders, dermatitis, allergies, infections, urogenital disorders, immune enhancement

SP 21 — **Da Bao (great embracement)**

Location: On the lateral aspect of the chest, in the sixth intercostal space, along the line from the shoulder to the hip joint, 1 cm deep; caution to prevent pneumothorax

Anatomy: Intercostal nerve

Use: "Luo of all luos"—great connecting point; chest pain, lung disorders, dyspnea, digestive disorders, generalized pain, forelimb and hind limb paralysis

HT 1 — **Ji Quan (deep spring)**

Location: In the center of the axilla, medial to the axillary nerve, 0.5-1 cm deep

Anatomy: Intercostobrachial nerve

Use: Cardiac pain, pain in the limb

HT 3 — **Shao Hai (minor sea)** — **Water**

Location: On the medial side of the cubital fossa (of the elbow), at the midpoint between the medial epicondyle of the humerus and the tendon of the biceps brachii, near the origin of the pronator teres muscle, 0.5-1.5 cm deep

Special qualities: **He point**

Anatomy: Medial cutaneous antebrachial nerve

Use: CLEARS HEAT; local point for elbow

HT 5 — **Tong Li (internal connection)**

Location: On the caudal aspect of the antebrachium, in the muscle groove between the flexor carpi ulnaris and the superficial digital flexor muscles, about 1/12 the distance from the carpus to the elbow cubital fossa, 0.5-1 cm deep

Special qualities: **Connecting point to the SI meridian (to SI 4)**
Luo point

Anatomy: Caudal cutaneous antebrachial nerve

Use: Pharyngolaryngitis, carpal pain, behavioral problems

HT 7 — **Shen Men (spirit gate)** — **Earth**

Location: On the caudal aspect of the antebrachium, immediately proximal to the accessory carpal bone, between the tendons of the flexor carpi ulnaris and the superficial digital flexor, 0.5 cm deep

Special qualities: **Source point**
Sedation point

Anatomy: Caudal cutaneous antebrachial nerve; the ulnar nerve is deep to this point

Use: SHEN DISTURBANCES; agitation, anxiety, neurosis, other behavioral problems

HT 8	**Shao Fu (lesser mansion, minor hall)**	**Fire**
Location:	On the palmar surface of the forefoot, at the lateral edge of the metacarpal pad. The point is between the fourth and the fifth metacarpal bones, proximal to the fifth metacarpophalangeal joint.	
Special qualities:	**Horary point**	
Anatomy:	Axial palmar digital nerve of the fifth digit	
Use:	Heat in feet, pruritus of external genitalia	
HT 9	**Shao Chong (minor channel)**	**Wood**
Location:	On the medial aspect of the coronary border (nail bed) of the fifth digit of the front forepaw, 0.2 cm deep (painful)	
Special qualities:	**Tonification point** **Jing Well point**	
Anatomy:	Abaxial palmar digital nerve of the fifth digit	
Use:	CLEARS HEAT; cardiovascular emergency	
Comments:	Like all Jing Well points, has the ability to rapidly and substantially influence the Qi, which flows very superficially here. This gives these points the ability to restore consciousness and act as powerful points to clear Heat.	
SI 1	**Shao Ze (minor marsh)**	**Metal**
Location:	On the dorsum of the forepaw, on the lateral coronary border of the fifth digit, 0.2 cm deep	
Special qualities:	**Jing Well point**	
Anatomy:	Fifth abaxial palmar digital nerve	
Use:	Hypogalactia, mastitis, acute emergencies, mammary disorders	
Comments:	Like all Jing Well points, has the ability to rapidly and substantially influence the Qi, which flows very superficially here. This gives these points the ability to restore consciousness and act as powerful points to clear Heat.	
SI 3	**Hou Xi (caudal brook)**	**Wood**
Location:	On the lateral side of the fifth metacarpophalangeal joint, proximal to the head of the fifth metacarpal bone, 0.5-1 cm deep	
Special qualities:	**Tonification point** **Confluent point to the GV (Du Mai) meridian**	
Anatomy:	Fifth abaxial dorsal digital nerve	
Use:	Cervical vertebral problems, cervical vertebral instability, cervical pain, shoulder pain, seizures, meningitis	
Comments:	This is a major point to influence the Tai Yang meridians and the region that envelops the posterior neck and shoulder region. It also regulates the Du Mai to descend Yang energy when used in tandem with BL	

62. It is an important point for any condition in which the upper jiao has too much "energy" or has become disconnected from the lower jiao. Examples of disorders treated with SI 3 and BL 62 include epilepsy, extreme anxiety and hyperexcitability, and even hormone-responsive urinary incontinence. It is also useful for seizures of feline hyperesthesia syndrome.

SI 6 — **Yang Lao (nursing elders)**

Location: Medial to the styloid process of the ulna and the ulnaris lateralis muscle, 0.5-1.5 cm deep

Special qualities: **Xi cleft point**

Use: Stiff neck, pain in the neck, shoulder, carpus, and forelimb

SI 7 — **Zhi Zheng (branching correctly)**

Location: On the lateral aspect of the forelimb about 5/12 the distance from the carpus to the cubital fossa, on the cranial edge of the ulnaris lateralis muscle, 0.5-1.5 cm deep

Special qualities: **Luo point**

Anatomy: Lateral cutaneous antebrachial nerve

Use: Pain in the elbow, forelimb, and shoulder, behavioral problems

SI 8 — **Xiao Hai (small sea)**

Location: In a depression between the medial epicondyle of the humerus and the olecranon; the ulnar nerve is deep to this point, 0.5 cm deep

Special qualities: **Sedation point**
He point

Anatomy: Medial cutaneous antebrachial nerve

Use: REMOVES OBSTRUCTIONS IN THE CHANNEL; local point for elbow, pain in the elbow, forelimb, and shoulder

SI 9 — **Jian Zhen (steadfast shoulder)**
(may correspond to the traditional point Qiang Feng—robbing the wind)

Location: In a depression between the long head and lateral head of the triceps and the caudal border of the deltoideus muscle, 1-3 cm deep

Anatomy: The cranial lateral cutaneous brachial nerve (branch of the axillary nerve) emerges from this area

Use: Injuries or arthritis of the shoulder and thoracic limb; acupuncture analgesia

SI 18 — **Quan Liao (cleft of the zygomatic bone, cheek bone hole)**
(may correspond to traditional point Kai Guan—open and close)

Location: Ventral to the zygomatic arch at the level of the lateral canthus, 1-3 cm deep depending on angle of insertion

Anatomy: Communicating branch of the buccal nerve is deep to this point

Use: Facial paralysis, acupuncture analgesia for the head

SI 19 **Ting Gong (hearing palace)**

Location: In the depression rostral to the tragus of the ear, 0.5-1.5 cm deep

Anatomy: A branch of the auriculotemporal nerve

Use: Deafness, otitis, facial palsies

BL 1 **Jing Ming (bright eyes)**

Location: Slightly dorsomedial to the medial canthus; a traditional veterinary acupoint, 0.2-0.5 cm deep

Anatomy: Supratrochlear nerve

Use: ELIMINATES WIND, DISPELS HEAT; local point for eyes, conjunctivitis, epiphora, keratitis

BL 2 **Zan Zhu (base of bamboo, bamboo leaf)** (traditional point)

Location: At the medial extremity of the eyebrow, in the supraorbital notch, 0.2 cm deep

Anatomy: Supraorbital nerve

Use: Conjunctivitis, sinusitis, keratitis, diminishes pain

BL 10 **Tian Zhu (celestial pillar)**

Location: On the dorsal aspect of the neck, in the depression at the atlantoaxial junction, medial to the wing of the atlas, at the location of the transverse foramen where the C1 spinal nerve emerges, 0.5 cm deep

Anatomy: Greater occipital nerve

Use: DISPELS WIND; cervical spondylosis, cervical disk disease, improves vision, especially in old dogs

BL 11 **Da Shu (big shuttle)**

Location: In a depression 1.5 cun lateral to the caudal border of the spinous process of the first thoracic vertebra, midpoint between the spinous process and the medial border of the scapula, 0.5-1 cm deep

Special qualities: **Influential point for bone**

Anatomy: Cutaneous branch of the dorsal ramus of the first thoracic nerve

Use: AN IMPORTANT POINT TO MOVE BLOOD; bone and joint disorders, rheumatoid arthritis, cervical spondylosis, cervical disk disease, forelimb pain, Bony Bi. Used with ST 37 and 39 to move Blood,

BL 12 **Fen Men (wind door)**

Location:	1.5 cun lateral to the caudal border of the spinous process of the second thoracic vertebra, midway from spinous process to the medial border of the scapula, 1-3 cm deep
Special qualities:	**Influential point for Trachea, Wind**
Use:	DISPELS WIND, WIND COLD, BUILDS WEI QI; acute attacks of sneezing, asthma
BL 13	**Fei Shu (lung association point)**
Location:	Lateral to the caudal border of the spinous process of the third thoracic vertebra, along the longitudinal line of the costal tubercula. The point is approximately midway between the midsagittal plane and the medial border of the scapula, 0.5-1 cm deep; caution necessary to prevent pneumothorax
Anatomy:	Lateral branch of the dorsal ramus of the third thoracic nerve
Use:	DISPELS WIND, WIND COLD; lung disorders (pneumonia, bronchitis, asthma), dry skin. Moxa for chronic disorders.
BL 14	**Jue Yin Shu (pericardium association point)**
Location:	Lateral to the caudal border of the spinous process of the fourth thoracic vertebra, along the longitudinal line of the costal tubercula, approximately midway between the midsagittal plane and the medial border of the scapula, 0.5-1 cm deep
Anatomy:	Lateral branch of the dorsal ramus of the fourth thoracic nerve
Use:	Cardiovascular disorders
BL 15	**Xin Shu (heart association point)**
Location:	Lateral to the caudal border of the spinous process of the fifth thoracic vertebra, along the longitudinal line of the costal tubercula, 0.5-1 cm deep
Anatomy:	Lateral branch of the dorsal ramus of the fifth thoracic nerve
Use:	Heart and consciousness disorders, such as syncope and epilepsy
BL 16	**Du Shu (governing vessel association point)**
Location:	Lateral to the caudal border of the spinous process of the sixth thoracic vertebra, along the longitudinal line of the costal tubercula, 0.5-1 cm deep
Anatomy:	Lateral branch of the dorsal ramus of the sixth thoracic nerve
Use:	Heart problems, abdominal pain
BL 17	**Ge Shu (diaphragm association)**
Location:	Lateral to the caudal border of the spinous process of

	the seventh thoracic vertebra, along the longitudinal line of the costal tubercula, 0.5-1 cm deep
Special qualities:	**Influential point for Blood**
Anatomy:	Lateral branch of the dorsal ramus of the seventh thoracic nerve
Use:	TONIFIES QI, BUILDS BLOOD, OPENS CHEST, PACIFIES STOMACH; FOR BLOOD STASIS AND BLOOD DEFICIENCY; chronic hemorrhage, spasm of diaphragm, blood dyscrasias, bronchial asthma
Comments:	This point is a major point in canine acupuncture, given the importance of Blood deficiency in so many canine disorders. Use this point when Blood needs to be tonified directly rather than through support of the Spleen.
BL 18	**Gan Shu (liver association point)**
Location:	Lateral to the caudal border of the spinous process of the tenth thoracic vertebra, along the longitudinal line of the costal tubercula, 0.5-1 cm deep
Anatomy:	Lateral branch of the dorsal ramus of the tenth thoracic nerve
Use:	LIVER QI STAGNATION; liver and gall bladder problems, eye problems
BL 19	**Dan Shu (gall bladder association point)**
Location:	Lateral to the caudal border of the spinous process of the eleventh thoracic vertebra, along the longitudinal line of the costal tubercula, 0.5-1 cm deep
Anatomy:	Lateral branch of the dorsal ramus of the eleventh thoracic nerve
Use:	DISPELS DAMP HEAT FROM THE LIVER AND GALL BLADDER, REBELLIOUS QI; local point for intervertebral disk, cholecystitis
Comments:	Most Shu points have an amphoteric action, serving to both tonify deficiencies and remove excesses. Consider this point not only in situations of Liver excess, but also Liver Blood or Yin deficiency.
BL 20	**Pi Shu (spleen association point)**
Location:	Lateral to the caudal border of the spinous process of the twelfth thoracic vertebra, along the longitudinal line of the costal tubercula, 0.5-1 cm deep
Anatomy:	Dorsal cutaneous branch of the twelfth thoracic nerve
Use:	DRAINS DAMP, TONIFIES QI AND BLOOD; local point for intervertebral disk, digestive disorders, pancreatic disorders, diabetes, pancreatitis, vomiting, anemia
BL 21	**Wei Shu (stomach association point)**
Location:	Lateral to the caudal border of the spinous process of the thirteenth thoracic vertebra, along the longitudinal

line of the costal tubercula, 0.5-1 cm deep (landmark—after the last rib)

Anatomy: Dorsal cutaneous branch of the thirteenth thoracic nerve

Use: DRAINS DAMP; local point for intervertebral disk, gastric disorders, vomiting, gastritis, gastric ulcers, Qi and Blood deficiency. It combines well with CV 12 to produce a nice "front and back" treatment for gastric complaints.

BL 22 **San Jiao Shu (triple heater association point)**

Location: Lateral to the caudal border of the spinous process of the first lumbar vertebra, along the longitudinal line of the thoracic costal tubercula, 1 cm deep

Anatomy: Dorsal cutaneous branch of the first lumbar spinal nerve

Use: DRAINS DAMP; endocrine disorders, bloating, diarrhea, stranguria (opens water passage), vomiting

Comments: This is a major point to influence the Triple Heater, which is a corridor connecting the three burners or levels of the body. Qi rises and Moisture descends down the Triple Heater. Because of its content of moisture, the passageway usually accumulates pathologic versions of moisture known as Dampness and Phlegm. This point thus finds use in many Dampness conditions, such as cystitis, edema, ascites, and in conditions in which the descent of Qi and Fluids is disrupted, such as dysphagia. Some sources also locate this point on the Dai Mai as it crosses the spine. The role of Dampness accumulation in the Dai Mai and the lower body in degenerative myelopathy conditions makes BL 22 a major point in the treatment of that disorder.

BL 23 **Shen Shu (kidney association point)**

Location: Lateral to the caudal border of the spinous process of the second lumbar vertebra, along the longitudinal line of the thoracic costal tubercula, 1-3 cm deep

Anatomy: Dorsal cutaneous branch of the second lumbar spinal nerve

Use: TONIFIES KIDNEY YANG AND YIN; renal disorders, urogenital disorders, back pain, spondylosis, hip dysplasia, intervertebral disk, ear disorders, senile deafness, keratoconjunctivitis sicca

Comments: Since Kidney Qi is the fire that warms the Spleen and allows digestion to occur, BL 23 can be used for advanced or long-standing Spleen Qi or Yang deficiency. It combines with CV 4 to tonify the Kidneys.

BL 24 **Qi Hai Shu (sea of Qi association point)**

Location: Lateral to the caudal border of the spinous process of the third lumbar vertebra, along the longitudinal line of the thoracic costal tubercula, 1-2 cm deep

Anatomy: Dorsal cutaneous branch of the third lumbar spinal nerve

Use: Constipation, back pain

Comments: An important point for Spleen and Kidney Qi deficiency

BL 25 **Da Chang Shu (large intestine association point)**

Location: Lateral to the caudal border of the spinous process of the fifth lumbar vertebra, along the longitudinal line of the thoracic costal tubercula, 1-2 cm deep

Anatomy: Dorsal cutaneous branch of the fifth lumbar spinal nerve

Use: Local point for intervertebral disk, gastrointestinal disorders, constipation, chronic colitis

Comments: BL 25 is used in sciatica in humans and seems very important in animals as a point to influence the sciatic nerve to deliver power to the hind limbs; use this point in any case of hind limb weakness. It also seems to be called for in Damp Heat conditions without Large Intestine symptoms, possibly serving to help prevent Damp Heat accumulation that later leads to colitis and other pathologic conditions.

BL 26 **Guan Yuan Shu (enclosed original energy [Qi] association point)**

Location: Lateral to the caudal border of the spinous process of the sixth lumbar vertebra, along the longitudinal line of the thoracic costal tubercula, 0.5-1 cm deep

Anatomy: Dorsal cutaneous branch of the fifth lumbar spinal nerve

Use: Intestinal disorders; constipation, diarrhea, indigestion

Comments: An important point to tonify Qi, Yin, and Yang of the Kidney

BL 27 **Xiao Chang Shu (small intestine association point)**

Location: Lateral to the caudal border of the spinous process of the seventh lumbar vertebra, along the longitudinal line of the thoracic costal tubercula, 1-2 cm deep

Anatomy: Dorsal cutaneous branch of the seventh lumbar spinal nerve

Use: Indigestion, sciatica, cauda equina, bladder disorders, combine with GB 30 to help relieve obstructions to the descent of Qi down the Bladder channel to the leg

BL 28 **Pang Guang Shu (bladder association point)**

Location: Lateral to the second dorsal sacral foramen, in the depression between the sacrum and the medial border of the dorsal iliac spine, 1-2 cm deep

Anatomy:	Dorsal cutaneous branch of the first and second sacral nerves
Use:	Bladder and prostate problems, sciatica, cauda equina
BL 32	**Ci Liao (second sacral foramen)** (the two points below together were the traditional Er Yan)
Location:	Dorsal to the first (BL 31) and second (BL 32) dorsal sacral foramina, deep to the points are the gluteal muscles
Anatomy:	Dorsal branches of the first and second sacral spinal nerves
Use:	Paralysis of the pelvic limb, sciatica, uterine diseases, cauda equina
BL 35	**Hui Yang (meeting of the Yang)**
Location:	In the depression of the ischiorectal fossa lateral to the base of the tail. This point is easily located by lifting the tail. The pudendal nerve is deep to the point; a traditional veterinary acupoint; 1 cm deep.
Anatomy:	Coccygeal nerve
Use:	Flea allergy dermatitis, anal itching, local skin irritation, sacral coccygeal hyperpathia, paresis or paralysis
BL 36	**Cheng Fu (support, bearing and supporting)**
Location:	Ventral to the ischial tuberosity, at the proximal end of the muscle groove between the biceps femoris and the semitendinosus, 1-2.5 cm deep
Anatomy:	Caudal femoral cutaneous nerve
Use:	Back pain, pain in gluteal region, constipation, muscle atrophy, hind limb paresis
BL 39	**Wei Yang (Yang in the bend)**
Location:	On the lateral end of the popliteal fossa, medial to the tendon of the biceps femoris muscle, lateral to BL 40, 0.5-1 cm deep
Anatomy:	Caudal cutaneous sural nerve
Use:	DAMP HEAT IN THE BLADDER; hematuria, cystitis, edema accumulations, incontinence, thoracolumbar disease
BL 40	**Wei Zhong (center of the bend)** **Earth**
Location:	In the center of the popliteal fossa, 0.5-1.5 cm deep; the femoral artery and vein and the tibial nerve are deep to the point
Special qualities:	**Master point for the low back and hips** **He point**
Anatomy:	Caudal cutaneous sural nerve
Use:	COOLS BLOOD; lesions on the hind limb, acute pain, thoracolumbar disk disease, spondylosis, caudal

	paresis or paralysis, enuresis, high fevers (combine with LI 11, LI 4, GV 4, and GV 14)
BL 43	**Gao Huang Shu (between the heart and diaphragm; residence of the noble organs)** (traditional point Bi Lan [shoulder post] in large animals)
Location:	At the caudal angle of the scapula
Anatomy:	Lateral branch of the dorsal ramus of the third thoracic spinal nerve
Use:	Injury or pain of the shoulder area
BL 52	**Zhi Shi (will chamber, room of will)**
Location:	Lateral to BL 23, on the second line of the Bladder meridian, at the level between the second and third lumbar vertebrae, 0.5-1 cm deep
Anatomy:	Dorsal cutaneous branch of the first lumbar nerve
Use:	Chronic renal disease, polyuria, pain in back
BL 54	**Zhi Bian (sequential limit, reaching the margin)**
Location:	Dorsal to the greater trochanter
Use:	Hip dysplasia
BL 57	**Cheng Shan (mountain foothill)**
Location:	At the transaction of the following two lines: the transverse line from the greater trochanter of the femur to the caudal sacrum, and the line of the sacrotuberous ligament. The point is between the two gluteal muscles—gluteus medius and gluteus superficialis, 2-3 cm deep
Anatomy:	Lateral and caudal cutaneous sural nerve
Use:	Sciatica, pain in the pelvic limb
BL 60	**Kun Lun (mountain)** **Fire**
Location:	In the depression between the lateral malleolus of the fibulus and the attachment of the common calcanean tendon to the calcaneal tuber, 0.5 cm deep
Special qualities:	**Jing river point**
Anatomy:	Caudal cutaneous sural nerve
Use:	FOR DEFICIENCY PAIN; chronic pain, such as of the neck or shoulder, lumbar
Comments:	This point regulates the entire Bladder channel and is able to both draw pathogenic Qi out and infuse healthful Qi into the Bladder meridian; some human acupuncturists refer to this point as the "aspirin point," given its strong analgesic properties
BL 62	**Shen Mai (extending vessel)**
Location:	In the depression directly distal to the lateral malleolus of the fibula, 0.2-0.5 cm deep

Special qualities:	**Confluent point for Yang Qiao Mai** **Ghost point**
Use:	Good for lateral tendons; use with KI 6 for keratoconjunctivitis sicca, leg pain; use with SI 3 to regulate the Yang Qiao Mai and Du Mai to stop seizures, descend Yang, and calm the Shen

BL 67 **Zhi Yin (terminal Yin)** **Metal**

Location:	On the lateral coronary border of the fifth digit of the rear foot, 0.3 cm deep (painful)
Special qualities:	**Jing Well point** **Tonification point**
Anatomy:	Fifth abaxial dorsal digital nerve
Use:	DISPELS WIND; pain on bladder channel, dystocia, incontinence, paralysis or paresis, ocular disorders

KI 1 **Yong Quan (fluorish spring, bubbling spring)** **Wood**

Location:	In the center of the plantar surface of the hind foot, at the caudal margin of the metatarsal footpad, 0.5-1 cm deep, (painful)
Special qualities:	**Jing Well point** **Sedation point**
Anatomy:	Plantar metatarsal nerve
Use:	TONIFIES YIN, REDUCES HEAT AND WIND; resuscitation point especially for lightening anesthesia, pododermatitis, epilepsy, shock
Comments:	When Yang Qi is vigorously rising upward, use this point to descend it, such as in hypertension and retinal detachment. When Yang Qi is collapsing, use KI 1 to raise it, such as in patient resuscitation efforts. GV 20 can be paired with KI 1 to treat both problems

KI 2 **Ran Gu (blazing valley)** **Fire**

Location:	This point is not standardly recognized in veterinary acupuncture but is an extremely important point in my (SM) experience. It is immediately ventral to the navicular bone
Use:	Advanced Yin deficiency with Empty Fire that may manifest as a severe upward disturbance of Yang, such as in nocturnal restlessness and pacing, Wei syndrome, and vestibular disorders; it may also manifest as hemorrhage, such as in some cases of ITP or in advanced renal failure with bleeding ulcers
Comments:	In patients with severe Yin deficiency with Empty Fire, the entire region between KI 6 and KI 2 often seems to coalesce into one large acupuncture point. In such a case, apply acupuncture transversely from KI 2 to KI 6.

KI 3	**Tai Xi (great brook)**	**Earth**
Location:	In the depression ventral to the medial malleolus of the tibia, between the malleolus and the talus, 0.5 cm	
Special qualities:	**Source point** **Shu stream point**	
Anatomy:	Saphenous nerve	
Use:	TONIFY KIDNEY; local point for tarsus, urogenital disorders, cystitis, enuresis, chronic renal disease, back pain	
Comments:	This point tonifies both Kidney Qi and Yin	
KI 6	**Zhao Hai (shining sea)**	
Location:	In the depression immediately ventral to the medial malleolus of the tibia, between the malleolus and the talus	
Special qualities:	**Master point of the Yin Qiao Mai**	
Anatomy:	Saphenous nerve	
Use:	KIDNEY YIN DEFICIENCY; constipation, frequent micturition, vulvar pruritus, Wei syndrome, chronic renal failure, cognitive disorders and dementia in aging animals, asthma; see KI 2 above; use with LU 7 to regulate the Yin Qiao Mai	
KI 7	**Fu Liu (flow again, recover flow)**	**Metal**
Location:	On the cranial border of the calcanean tendon and about one cun caudoventral to the point SP 6, approximately 2/16 the distance from the medial malleolus to the stifle joint, 0.5-1 cm deep	
Special qualities:	**Tonification point** **Jing river point**	
Anatomy:	Saphenous nerve	
Use:	KIDNEY YANG DEFICIENCY, DISPELS DAMP; diarrhea, cystitis, nephritis, back pain; may be useful in cooling the upper body and clearing Heart Fire	
PC 3	**Qu Ze (elbow marsh)**	**Water**
Location:	In a depression at the cubital fossa, medial to the tendon of the biceps brachii and lateral to the pronator teres, 0.5-1.5 cm deep; deep insertion can injure the brachial artery	
Special qualities:	**He point**	
Anatomy:	Medial cutaneous antebrachial nerve; median nerve is deep to this point	
Use:	COOLS BLOOD; HEAT SEDATION POINT; local point for elbow; axillary dermatitis	
PC 4	**Xi Men (cleft gate)**	
Location:	In the same groove as PC 6, slightly distal to the midpoint of the forelimb	
Special qualities:	**Xi cleft point**	

Use:	Cardiovascular disorders, neurosis
PC 6	**Nei Guan (inner pass, inner gate)**
Location:	In the muscle groove caudal to the flexor carpi radialis and cranial to the superficial digital flexor muscles, approximately 1/6 the distance from the carpus to the cubital fossa, OR 2 cun above the transverse crease of the wrist, between the tendons of the flexor digitorum superficialis and the flexor carpi radialis, 0.5-1 cm deep; the median nerve and artery are deep to the point
Special qualities:	**Luo point** **Master point for the chest and heart** **Regulates the Yin Wei Mai**
Anatomy:	Medial and lateral cutaneous antebrachial nerves
Use:	CALMS SHEN; asthma, nausea, arrhythmia, "stage fright point," "motion sickness point," cardiovascular disorders, neurosis, epilepsy, cranial abdominal problems, gastric ulcers, gastritis, vomiting
Comments:	This point opens the chest, calms and cools the Heart, and restores the normal downward movement of Qi. Most of its reported clinical uses are derived from one of these three functions. It is one of the most important points in both human and small animal acupuncture. With ST 40 and CV 12, PC 6 stops the formation and accumulation of Phlegm in the Stomach. PC 6 also helps open the Orifices of the Heart when they have been blocked by Phlegm.
PC 7	**Da Ling (large mount)** **Earth**
Location:	Caudal to the tendon of the flexor carpi radialis and immediately proximal to the carpal bone, 0.2-0.5 cm deep
Special qualities:	**Source point** **Sedation point** **Ghost point** **Shu stream point**
Anatomy:	Medial cutaneous antebrachial nerve
Use:	Carpal injuries, behavioral problems
PC 8	**Lao Gong (palace of manual labor)** **Fire**
Location:	On the palmar surface of the forepaw, on the medial side of the metacarpus proximal to the third metacarpophalangeal joint, 0.5-1 cm deep
Special qualities:	**Horary point** **Ying Spring point** **Ghost point**
Anatomy:	Third palmar common digital nerve

Use: CLEARS HEAT, CLEARS HEART FIRE; gastritis, vomiting, nausea, tongue ulceration, foul breath, fungal infections of the foot, sister point to KI 1

PC 9 **Zhong Chong (middle channel)** **Wood**

Location: On the ventrolateral coronary border of the third phalanx, 0.2 cm deep, painful to needle

Special qualities: **Jing Well point**
Tonification point

Anatomy: Third palmar common digital nerve

Use: YIN COLLAPSE, COOLS BLOOD; cardiovascular emergency, shock, coma

Comments: Like all Jing Well points, has the ability to rapidly and substantially influence the Qi, which flows very superficially here. This gives these points the ability to restore consciousness and act as powerful points to clear Heat.

TH 1 **Guan Chong (gate channel)** **Metal**

Location: On the lateral coronary border of the fourth phalanx

Special qualities: **Jing Well point**

Anatomy: Fourth palmar common digital nerve

Use: Pharyngolaryngitis, fever

Comments: Like all Jing Well points, has the ability to rapidly and substantially influence the Qi, which flows very superficially here. This gives these points the ability to restore consciousness and act as powerful points to clear Heat.

TH 3 **Zhong Zhu (central island, middle island)** **Wood**

Location: On the dorsum of the forefoot, between the fourth and fifth metacarpals, in the depression proximal to the metacarpophalangeal joint, medial to SI 3, 0.5 cm deep

Special qualities: **Tonification point**
Shu stream point

Anatomy: Dorsal branch of the ulnar nerve

Use: CLEARS HEAT, USE IN BI SYNDROMES, LIVER STAGNATION; inflammation of the face, thoracic limb problems, carpal problems, eye problems, moodiness

TH 4 **Yang Chi (Yang pond)**

Location: On the dorsum of the forepaw, at the junction of the forelimb and the radial and ulnar carpal bones, caudal to the tendon of the common digital extensor, 0.5-1 cm deep

Special qualities: **Source point**

Anatomy: Dorsal branch of the ulnar nerve and cranial cutaneous antebrachial nerve

Use: Carpal injuries

TH 5	**Wai Guan (lateral pass, outer pass, outer frontier gate)**
Location:	At the most distal 1/6 the distance of the craniolateral antebrachium from the carpus to the cubital fossa (or 2 cun above the carpus), caudal to the tendon of the common digital extensor; at the distal end of the interosseous space between the radius and ulna, 1-2 cm deep
Special qualities:	**Luo point** **Confluent point for Yang Wei Mai**
Anatomy:	Cranial cutaneous antebrachial nerve
Use:	CLEARS WIND HEAT, OPENS YANG WEI MAI, BI SYNDROMES; carpal problems, arthritis, deafness, ear problems, fever, stiff neck, thoracic limb problems, constipation; may increase efficacy of GB 41 in opening the Dai Mai in hind limb paralysis; any neck pain
TH 10	**Tian Jing (celestial well, Heaven's well) Earth**
Location:	1 cun proximal to the olecranon, on the caudal border of the antebrachium in a depression proximal to the olecranon process
Special qualities:	**He point** **Sedation point**
Anatomy:	Superficial branch of the radial nerve
Use:	Local point for elbow, neck stiffness; may be useful in hyperthyroidism, although TH 13 is more classically indicated for this purpose. TH 13 is not an official veterinary acupuncture point, but is located on the posterior margin of the deltoideus, where a line drawn from TH 10 to TH 14 intersects.
TH 14	**Jian Liao (shoulder seam)**
Location:	Caudal and distal to the acromion, on the posterior margin of the deltoideus muscle
Use:	Local point for shoulder
TH 17	**Yi Feng (covered wind)**
Location:	In a depression caudal to the mandible, ventral to the ear base, and cranial to the mastoid process, where the ear canal goes horizontal, 1-2 cm deep; the parotid gland and facial nerve are deep to the point; a traditional veterinary acupoint
Anatomy:	Great auricular nerve
Use:	DISPELS AND EXTINGUISHES WIND; deafness, facial paralysis, otitis

TH 21	**Er Men (ear gate)**
Location:	Rostral to the supratragic notch, directly dorsal to SI 19, at the posterior border of the mandible, dorsal to the condyloid process, with the mouth open
Use:	Local point for ear, deafness, otitis, tinnitus, hematomas, toothache, temporomandibular joint
TH 23	**Si Zhu Kong (silken bamboo hollow)**
Location:	In the depression at the lateral end of the eyebrow, lateral to the supraorbital process, where it connects with the orbital ligament
Use:	DISPELS WIND; local point for eyes, conjunctivitis, keratoconjunctivitis sicca, facial paralysis
GB 1	**Tong Zi Liao (pupillary cleft, pupil seam)**
Location:	Lateral to the lateral canthus, in the depression on the lateral side of the orbit, 0.5 cm deep
Anatomy:	Zygomaticofacial nerve
Use:	ELIMINATES WIND HEAT, DISPELS FIRE; local point for eye conjunctivitis, optic nerve, atrophy, keratitis, retinitis, trigeminal nerve
GB 2	**Ting Hui (confluence of hearing)**
Location:	Rostral to the intertragic notch, directly below SI 19, at the posterior border of the condyloid process of the mandible, with the mouth open
Use:	DISPELS WIND; local point for ears, deafness, otitis, masseter problems, seizures, pyorrhea, toothaches
GB 3	**Shang Guan (upper joint)**
Location:	In the depression caudal to the masseter muscle and dorsal to the zygomatic arch, with the mouth open
Anatomy:	Zygomaticofacial nerve
Use:	Facial paralysis, deafness
GB 14	**Yang Bai (Yang white)**
Location:	1 cun above the midpoint of the eyebrow
Use:	DISPELS WIND, SUBDUES LIVER RISING; epilepsy, facial paralysis, temporomandibular joint, night blindness, glaucoma, biliary disorders
GB 20	**Feng Chi (pond of the wind, wind pool)**
Location:	In the dorsal aspect of the neck, caudal to the occipital bone, in the depression between the upper portion of the sternocleidomastoideus and trapezius muscles
Anatomy:	Greater occipital nerve
Use:	DISPELS WIND, CLEARS HEAT FROM ROSTRAL PART OF BODY, DIMINISHES LIVER STAGNATION; EXTINGUISHES INTERNAL WINDS; clears brain,

cervical problems, headache, hemiplegia, epilepsy, eye disorders

GB 21	**Jian Jing (shoulder well)**
Location:	Midway between GV 14 and the acromion
Special qualities:	**Additional alarm point for Gall Bladder**
Anatomy:	Fifth cervical spinal nerve, supraclavicular nerve
Use:	Local point for shoulder and neck problems, shoulder arthritis, relaxes sinews, promotes lactation, retained placenta
GB 24	**Ri Yue (sun and moon)**
Location:	At the tenth or ninth intercostal space, slightly ventral to the costochondral junction
Special qualities:	**Alarm point for the Gall Bladder**
Anatomy:	Ninth or tenth intercostal nerve
Use:	Liver and gall bladder disorders; upper abdominal pain and "disharmony"
GB 25	**Jing Men (capital gate, capital's door)**
Location:	On the lateral side of the abdomen on the tip of the free end of the thirteenth rib, 0.5 cm deep
Special qualities:	**Alarm point of the Kidney**
Anatomy:	Twelfth intercostal nerve
Use:	Kidney disorders, pain in the renal region, water metabolism disorders, liver and gall bladder disorders; part of the kidney belt with GV 4, BL 23, and BL 52
GB 29	**Ju Liao (stationary seam)** (known as Huan Tiao in traditional point system)
Location:	In the depression cranial to the greater trochanter
Use:	Hip formula point, lumbar pain, removes obstructions from the gall bladder channel
GB 30	**Huan Tiao (ring jumping, circular jump)** (traditional point is known as Huan Hou)
Location:	Midway between the bony protrusion of the cranial ventral iliac spine (caudolateral end of the tuber coxae) and the greater trochanter of the femur, in the shallow depression between the gluteus medius and the tensor fasciae latae muscles
Anatomy:	Gluteus cranialis nerve, lateral cutaneous femoral nerve, and cutaneous branches of the sacral nerves; the sciatic nerve trunk is deep to the point
Use:	Regulates Qi of the hind leg; hip formula point, hindquarter paralysis, hip dysplasia; hind limb weakness and lameness
Comments:	Some authors place this point dorsal to the greater trochanter in the depression in the gluteal muscles, making it akin to BL 54.

GB 31 — **Feng Shi (wind market, windy city)**

Location: On the lateral aspect of the thigh, 7 cun above the transverse popliteal crease (7/18 the distance from the lateral condyle of the femur to the greater trochanter of the femur)

Use: DISPERSES WIND; generalized pruritus, pain in thigh and lumbar spine

GB 33 — **Xi Yang Guan (knee Yang gate, knee Yang point)**

Location: When the knee is flexed, the point is 3 cun above GB 34; on the lateral aspect of the stifle joint, in the depression at the level of the patella's dorsal margin, dorsal to the lateral epicondyle of the femur, between the tendon of the biceps femoris and the bone, 0.5 cm deep

Anatomy: Lateral to the cutaneous femoral nerve

Use: Local point for knee or leg pain. It is the Xi-Cleft point of the Gall Bladder meridian.

GB 34 — **Yang Ling Quan (spring of Yang grave, Yang mound spring)**

Location: In the depression anterior and distal to the head of the fibula, in the interosseous space, proximal to the bifurcation of the deep and peroneal nerves, 1-2 cm deep

Special qualities: **He point**
Influential point for muscles and tendons

Use: QI STASIS; local point for knee; disorders of pelvic limb, disorders of liver and gall bladder, muscle and tendon disorders, myopathies, intervertebral disk

Comments: As a Shao Yang organ, the Gall Bladder accesses the Yang Qi that allows the movement of the limbs, just as the Triple Heater accesses the Yang Qi used by the internal organs. Yang Ling Quan refers to the ability of GB 34 to profoundly affect movement by serving as the locale through which Yang Qi bubbles up to the surface for use by the limbs. As such, it can be used to treat all limb movement disorders. It may be especially called for when Blood deficiency is leading to an increased tendency to spasm and Qi stagnation. It has a special ability to move Qi that is stagnating along the costal arch and producing flank pain.

GB 39 — **Xuan Zhong (hanging bell)**

Location: 3 cun above the tip of the lateral malleolus, or 3/16 the distance from the tarsus joint to the stifle joint, in the depression between the posterior border of the fibula and the tendons of the peroneus longus and brevis muscles, directly across from SP 6, 0.5 cm deep

Special qualities:	**Influential point for marrow** **Lower uniting point of the three leg channels**
Use:	Myelopathy, anemia, blood dyscrasias, pelvic limb disorders, indigestion; allows simultaneous treatment of all three leg channels at once, such as in musculoskeletal disorders
GB 40	**Qiu Xu (hill ruins, abandoned hill)**
Location:	Ventrocranial to the lateral malleolus of the fibula
Special qualities:	**Source point**
Anatomy:	Fourth dorsal common digital nerve
Use:	Tarsal injury, chest pain
GB 41	**Zu Lin Qi (foot overlooking tears, near weeping)** **Wood**
Location:	On the dorsum of the foot, in the depression distal to the base of the fourth and fifth metatarsal bones, on the lateral side of the tendon of the extensor digitorum longus muscle
Special qualities:	**Horary point** **Shu stream point** **Master point of the Dai Mai**
Use:	DAMP HEAT IN THE GENITAL AREA, BI SYNDROME, LIVER STAGNATION; arthritic pain in hips, epiphora, cranial abdominal pain
Comments:	The name of this point is said to be reflective of its importance in treating eye disorders. I (SM) would offer a different interpretation, however. The Chinese character for Lin also means to arrive and depicts a minister for the emperor traveling from city to city over a large territory. Qi is a character that depicts someone weeping while standing. Combination of the two characters, especially when combined with Zu or "foot," might therefore suggest the notion of endurance, of continuing to move despite pain or discomfort. This is certainly in keeping with the main use of GB 41 in small animal acupuncture, which is in the treatment of lower limb weakness and paralysis. This point in tandem with TH 5 also regulates the Dai Mai, which provides a foundation for being able to stand and move. Finally, as a distal point, GB 41 has a profound effect over the proximal reaches of the channel, allowing it to drain pathogenic Qi from the entire channel all the way up to the head.
GB 44	**Zu Qiao Yin (Yin portals of the foot)** **Metal**
Location:	On the lateral coronary border of the fourth phalanx
Special qualities:	**Jing Well point**
Anatomy:	Fourth abaxial dorsal proper digital nerve
Use:	Emergency, shock, problems in the head area

Comments:	Like all Jing Well points, has the ability to rapidly and substantially influence the Qi, which flows very superficially here. This gives these points the ability to restore consciousness and act as powerful points to clear Heat.
LIV 1	**Da Dun (large hump)** **Wood**
Location:	Lateral to the coronary border of the first phalanx, rear foot
Special qualities:	**Jing Well point** **Horary point**
Use:	Emergencies, epilepsy, orchitis, acute metabolic disturbances
Comments:	Like all Jing Well points, has the ability to rapidly and substantially influence the Qi, which flows very superficially here. This gives these points the ability to restore consciousness and act as powerful points to clear Heat.
LIV 2	**Xing Jian (between the two columns, going into the space)** **Fire**
Location:	On the medial aspect of the second toe, distal to the metatarsal phalangeal joint, midway between the dorsal and medial aspect of the bone
Special qualities:	**Sedative point** **Ying spring point**
Use:	LIVER FIRE, DISPELS WIND; aggression, seizures, urogenital disorders; historically, an important point for low back pain and hind limb weakness arising from Qi stagnation, especially when combined with GB 25; calms the Heart
LIV 3	**Tai Chong (great surge, grand impact)** **Earth**
Location:	On the medial aspect of the second toe, proximal to the metatarsal phalangeal joint, midway between the dorsal and medial aspects of the bone, 0.5-1 cm deep
Special qualities:	**Source point** **Shu stream**
Anatomy:	Deep peroneal nerve
Use:	LIVER STAGNATION, DISPELS WIND; epilepsy, liver and gall bladder problems, gastrointestinal, urogenital, endocrine, and metabolic disorders
Comments:	This point is a powerful Qi mover, as suggested by its name. Its Qi-moving properties are enhanced when it is combined it with LI 4. It is also the Source point for the Liver, and can be used to directly nourish Liver Blood and Yin. Finally, this point is a less powerful but still useful point to clear Liver Heat. Some authors feel that to get the same effects as LIV 3 in humans, the muscle belly inferior to the second metatarsal bone must be needled, rather than the skin over the bone.

LIV 5 | **Li Gou (wormwood canal)**

Location: On the medial side of the leg, caudal to the tibia and cranial to the gastrocnemius muscle, 5/16 the distance from the medial malleolus of the tibia to the stifle joint, 0.5-1 cm deep

Special qualities: **Luo point**

Anatomy: Saphenous nerve

Use: Hepatitis, reproductive problems in females, inguinal lesions or pain, pain along the liver channel

LIV 8 | **Qu Quan (curve spring, spring in the curve) Water**

Location: On the medial side of the stifle; when the knee is flexed, the point is in the depression between the medial condyle of the femur and the insertion of the semimembranosus muscle, opposite GB 33, 1-1.5 cm deep

Special qualities: **He point**
Tonification point

Anatomy: Saphenous nerve

Use: DAMP HEAT IN THE LOWER JIAO; local point for stifle, scrotal swelling, vaginitis, inguinal dermatitis, urinary tract infection, diarrhea, uterine prolapse

LIV 13 | **Zhang Men (completion gate)**

Location: On the ventrolateral side of the abdomen, at the costal cartilage of the twelfth rib, 0.5-1 cm deep (very deep insertion could puncture the liver)

Special qualities: **Alarm point of the Spleen**
Influential point for Yin organs

Anatomy: Eleventh intercostal nerve

Use: FOOD ACCUMULATION, DISPELS DAMP; hepatitis, enteritis, indigestion, liver and gall bladder disorders

Comments: The most important use of this point is to harmonize the Liver and Spleen when it appears Wood is overcontrolling Earth.

LIV 14 | **Qi Men (gate of hope, last gate, cycle gate)**

Location: On the mammary line in the sixth intercostal space, 0.5 cm; be careful of pneumothorax

Special qualities: **Alarm point of Liver**

Anatomy: Sixth intercostal nerve

Use: QI STASIS, FOOD ACCUMULATION; liver and gall bladder disorders, lactation disorders, mastitis, gastritis

Comments: This point harmonizes the Liver and the Stomach when it appears Wood is overcontrolling Earth

CV 1 | **Hui Yin (Yin meeting, united Yin)**

Location: In the depression between the anus and the scrotum or vulva, on the midline of the perineum, 0.5-1 cm deep

Special qualities: **Ghost point**
Anatomy: Ventral perineal nerve
Use: Vaginitis, urogenital disorders, uterine prolapse, genital diseases, urethrospasm, feline lower urinary tract disease, anuria, constipation, incontinence

CV 3 **Zhong Ji (middle peak, central pole)**

Location: 4 cun caudal to the umbilicus, on the midline (2/3 the distance from the umbilicus to the pubic tubercle), 0.5-1.5 cm deep, evacuate bladder before needling
Special qualities: **Alarm point of the Bladder**
Anatomy: Lateral cutaneous branches of iliohypogastric nerve
Use: Cystitis, urogenital disorders, incontinence, urine retention, any Damp Heat in the lower jiao; may be beneficial as a point on the front of the body to treat hind limb and low back weakness or pain

CV 4 **Guan Yuan (enclosed original energy)**

Location: On the ventral midline of the abdomen, 3 cun caudal to the umbilicus, on the midline (at the middle of the distance between the umbilicus and the pubic tubercle), 0.5-1 cm deep
Special qualities: **Alarm point for the Small Intestine**
Use: TONIFIES BLOOD; YANG COLLAPSE, YIN DEFICIENCY, JING DEFICIENCY; urogenital disorders, urine retention, incontinence, enuresis

CV 5 **Shi Men (stone gate)**

Location: On the ventral midline of the abdomen, 1/3 the distance from the umbilicus to the pubic tubercle, 0.5-1 cm deep
Special qualities: **Alarm point of the Triple Heater**
Anatomy: Lateral cutaneous branch of the first lumbar spinal nerve
Use: Abdominal pain, dysentery, edema, urinary tract infection

CV 6 **Qi Hai (sea of Qi, sea of vital energy)**

Location: On the ventral midline, 1/4 the distance from the umbilicus to the pubic tubercle (1.5 cun caudal to the umbilicus)
Anatomy: Lateral cutaneous branches of the thirteenth thoracic nerve
Use: TONIFIES QI AND BLOOD, BUILDS QI IN THE LOWER JIAO; YANG COLLAPSE, JING DEFICIENCY; CONSOLIDATES QI WHEN IT REBELS IN DEFICIENT PATIENTS; SPLEEN QI DEFICIENCY

CV 8 **Shen Que (spirit gate)**

Location: Umbilicus; acupuncture here is prohibited in humans but has been performed on animals with safety; moxibustion may be used here in place of needling

Use: YANG COLLAPSE, DISPELS DAMP, SPLEEN QI TONIFICATION; abdominal pain, borborygmus, rectal prolapse

CV 12 **Zhong Wan (central outlet, middle stomach)**

Location: Halfway between the umbilicus and the xiphoid process on the midline, 0.5-1 cm

Special qualities: **Alarm point for the Stomach**
Influential point for Yang organs

Anatomy: Ninth intercostal nerves

Use: TONIFIES SPLEEN; DISPELS DAMP; FOOD ACCUMULATION; gastrointestinal disorders, vomiting, diarrhea, gastroenteritis, liver disorders, epilepsy, vestibular disorders, degenerative myelopathy

Comments: This point may be more important than ST 36 in regulating the middle jiao in animals. It may be combined with PC 6 and ST 40 to stop Phlegm formation. Some sources show the Dai Mai crossing the conception vessel at this point, making CV 12 useful in cases of Dai Mai obstruction such as degenerative myelopathy.

CV 14 **Ju Que (large void, large palace gate)**

Location: Halfway between CV 12 and the xiphoid process, on the midline, 0.5 cm deep

Special qualities: **Alarm point for the Heart**

Anatomy: Eighth intercostal nerve

Use: REBELLIOUS STOMACH QI; cardiac or gastric responses to stressful conditions, behavioral problems; a major point for epilepsy

CV 17 **Shan Zhong (chest center, center of the sternum)**

Location: On the ventral midline, at the level of the fourth intercostal space, approximately 2/3 the distance from the tip of the manubrium to the xiphoid process of the sternum

Special qualities: **Alarm point for the Pericardium**
Influential point for Qi

Use: REGULATES THE QI OF THE CHEST; SOME AUTHORS RECOMMEND IT FOR DEFICIENCY CONDITIONS

Comments: This point overlies where the Lung gathers Qi before dispersing it into the channels and meridians and descending it to the Kidneys. Traditionally, its main use was in cases in which Qi and Blood were stagnating in the chest and not dispersing.

CV 20 **Hua Gai (florid canopy, pretty cover)**

Location: On the ventral midline, at the first intercostal space, 0.5 cm

Anatomy: First intercostal nerve

Use: Asthma, bronchitis

CV 22	**Tian Tu (celestial chimney, protrude to heaven)**
Location:	At the cranial tip of the manubrium, on the midline
Use:	DESCENDS LUNG QI, CLEARS HEAT; cough, swallowing problems, throat problems
GV 1	**Hou Hai (caudal sea)** Transposed from the human point, **Chang Qiang** (lasting and strong, lasting strength)
Location:	In the depression between the anus and base of the tail, 1-3 cm deep
Anatomy:	Ventral branches of the sacral and coccygeal nerves
Use:	RELIEVES DAMP HEAT IN THE ANAL AREA; diarrhea, rectal or anal paralysis, rectal prolapse, back pain
GV 2	**Wei Gen (tail base)** (Transpositional point from the human point known as **Yao Shu** [Lumbar Point])
Location:	On the dorsal midline between the second and third sacral vertebrae
Special qualities:	**Association point for the loin, lumbar Shu**
Anatomy:	Cutaneous branches of the dorsal sacral nerves
Use:	Paralysis of the pelvic limb or tail, rectal prolapse, constipation, diarrhea
Lumbosacral point	**Yao Bai Hui (also taught as GV 20 [lumbar hundred meetings])**
Location:	On the dorsal midline in the depression at the lumbosacral junction, 1-2 cm deep
Anatomy:	Medial branch of the seventh lumbar nerve
Use:	Sciatica, pelvic limb paralysis, rectal prolapse, any lumbar or pelvic limb disorder
Comments:	Nomenclature for this point is confusing. Some sources use the term Bai Hui for this point, and GV 20 for the point at the vertex of the head. Other authors believe Bai Hui should be applied to the vertex of the head, and the point described here listed as an extra point. The latter authors contend there must be a convergence of Yang to balance the convergence of Yin at Yin Hui (CV 1) and that convergence must be at the opposite pole of the body to CV 1. They argue that a meeting of the Yang at the top of an animal's head is an essential dictate of basic body energetics. In practice, GV 3 is more commonly palpably active in animals with low back and hind limb complaints.
GV 3	**Yao Yang Guan (lumbar Yang gate)**
Location:	Variable—the largest depression between the dorsal spinous processes of L4-5, L5-6, or L6-7
Anatomy:	Medial branch of the fourth lumbar nerve

Use: STRENGTHENS YANG; strengthens lower back, reproductive problems, endometritis, lumbar spondylosis, arthritis, hind limb weakness

GV 4 **Ming Men (life gate)**

Location: On the dorsal midline between the dorsal spinous processes of L2-3, 1-2 cm deep

Anatomy: Medial branch of the second lumbar nerve

Use: DISPELS COLD, TONIFIES MING MEN (KIDNEY YANG); YANG DEFICIENCY; CLEARS SEVERE HEAT; disk disease, pelvic limb disorders, acupuncture analgesia, urogenital disorders, chronic gastrointestinal disorders, extreme pruritus, fever

GV 5 **Xuan Shu (suspended center)**

Location: On the dorsal midline between the spinous processes of T13-L1, 1-2 cm

Anatomy: Medial branch of the thirteenth thoracic spinal nerve

Use: Thoracolumbar disorders, gastrointestinal disorders, diarrhea

GV 6 **Ji Zhong (center of the spine)**

Location: On the midline between the dorsal spinous processes of T11-12, 0.5-1 cm

Anatomy: Medial branch of the eleventh thoracic nerve

Use: Loss of appetite, gastrointestinal disorders, diarrhea, hepatitis, hind limb paresis or paralysis

GV 7 **Zhong Shu (central point)**

Location: On the dorsal midline between the spinous processes of the tenth and eleventh thoracic vertebrae, 1-2 cm deep

Anatomy: Medial branch of the tenth thoracic spinal nerve

Use: Loss of appetite, gastritis, thoracolumbar hyperpathia, epilepsy, Spleen deficiency

GV 10 **Ling Tai (spiritual platform)**

Location: On the dorsal midline between the spinous process of the sixth and seventh thoracic vertebrae, 1-3 cm deep

Anatomy: Medial branch of the sixth thoracic spinal nerve

Use: Stomach upset, infection of the liver or lung

GV 12 **Shen Zhu (column of body, support of personality)**

Location: On the dorsal midline between the spinous processes of the second and third thoracic vertebrae, 2-4 cm deep

Anatomy: Medial branch of the third thoracic nerve

Use: Pneumonia, bronchitis, shoulder pain

GV 13 **Tao Dao (way of content)**

Location: On the median plane between the spinous processes of the first and second thoracic vertebrae

Anatomy: Medial branch of the first thoracic spinal nerve
Use: Pain in the neck or shoulder area, cervical spondylosis, epilepsy, fever

GV 14 **Da Zhui (large spinous process)**

Location: On the midline between the dorsal spinous processes of the last cervical and the first thoracic vertebrae
Anatomy: Medial branch of the eighth cervical spinal nerve
Use: DISPELS WIND, DISPELS HEAT, TONIFIES WEI QI, OPENS ALL YANG MERIDIANS, TONIFIES OR DRAINS YANG; allergies, asthma, "stiff back," fever, cervical spondylosis, epilepsy, immunodeficiencies, neck pain, forelimb lameness

GV 16 **Feng Fu (storage of wind)**

Location: Base of occiput on the dorsal midline, 0.5-1 cm deep (do not puncture the epidural space)
Use: DISPELS WIND; epilepsy, cervical hyperpathia

GV 20 **Bai Hui (hundred meetings)**

Location: On the dorsal midline of the skull, on a line between the cranial edge of the base of the ears, in the notch between the sagittal crest and the frontal crest
Anatomy: Branches from the greater occipital, auriculotemporal, and supraorbital nerves
Use: CLEARS MIND, STRENGTHENS SPLEEN, GOOD FOR LIVER FIRE, LIVER YANG RISING, LIVER STAGNATION (SOME AUTHORS BELIEVE IT IS THE ENDING POINT OF INTERNAL LIVER MERIDIAN), YANG DEFICIENCY AND COLLAPSE, BLOOD EXHAUSTION, DISPELS WIND; good for prolapses

GV 25 **Shan Gen (hill foot)**

Transposed as human point Su Liao (simple bone cleft)

Location: On the median plane of the dorsal surface of the nose, just rostral to the hairline—peck for hemoacupuncture
Anatomy: Nasal branch of the infraorbital nerve
Use: Acute emergency, rhinitis, sinusitis, cold or initial state of canine distemper

GV 26 **Ren Zhong (center of the upper lip)**

Location: In the intersection of the T formed below the nose, in the philtrum; needle deep with aggressive pecking (on the median plane of the upper lip, at the junction of its dorsal and middle third)
Special qualities: **Ghost point**
Use: DISPELS HEAT; YIN COLLAPSE; RESUSCITATION

REFERENCES

Cheng X, editor. *Chinese Acupuncture and Moxibustion.* Beijing, China, 1987, Foreign Languages Press.

Ellis A, Wiseman N, Boss K. *Grasping the Wind: An Exploration into the Meaning of Acupuncture Point Names.* Brookline, Mass, 1989, Paradigm Publications

Schoen A, editor. *Veterinary Acupuncture: Ancient Art to Modern Medicine.* St. Louis, 2001, Mosby.

Lee-Kin. *A Handbook of Acupuncture Treatment for Dogs and Cats.* Hong Kong, 1994, Medicine and Health Publishing.

International Veterinary Acupuncture Society, class notes, 1996-1997, Albuquerque, NM.

Appendix F

Suppliers

PRIMARILY VETERINARY

Animal Health Options
500 Corporate Cir., #A
Golden, CO 80401
Phone: 303-271-0491
Toll free: 800-845-8849
Fax: 303-271-0512
www.animalhealthoptions.com

Animals' Apawthecary
P.O. Box 212
Conner, MT 59827
Phone: 406-821-4090

Genesis/Resources LTD
4093 Oceanside Blvd., Suite B
Oceanside, CA 92056
Phone: 760-631-6225
Toll free: 877-P-E-T-S-4-L-I-F-E
Fax: 760-631-6227 FAX
www.genesispets.com

Healing Herbs for Pets
4292-99 Fourth Ave.
Ottawa, Ontario
Canada K1S 5B3
Phone: 613-230-9966
Fax: 613-230-0750
email: wwilmot@petherbs.com

Hilton Herbs, Ltd.
Downclose Farm
North Perott, Crewkerne
Somerset TA18 7SH
England
(In the U.S.:
Chamisa Ridge
3212–A Richards Ln.
Santa Fe, NM 87507
Toll free: 800-743-3188
www.chamisaridge.com)

Jing Tang Herbal Company
9791 NW 160th St.
Reddick, FL 32686
Phone: 352-591-3165
Fax: 352-591-0988

Rx Vitamins for Pets
200 Myrtle Blvd.
Larchmont, NY 10538
Phone: 914-834-1804
Toll free: 800-792-2222
www.rxvitamins.com

Thorne Research, Inc.
25820 Hwy. 2 West
P.O. Box 25
Dover, ID 83825
Toll free: 800-228-1966
www.thorne.com

Vetri-Science Laboratories
20 New England Dr., C 1504
Essex Junction, VT 05453-1504
Toll free: 800-882-9993
www.vetri-science.com/

Wysong
1880 North Eastman Rd.
Midland, MI 48640
Toll free: 800-748-0188
www.wysong.net

HUMAN SUPPLY COMPANIES

Western Herbs

Agapi Sales
#132–1135 Stevens Rd.
Kelowna, British Columbia
Canada V1Z 2S8

Eclectic Institute, Inc.
14385 S.E. Lusted Rd.
Sandy, OR 97055
Toll free: 800-332-4372

Frontier Herbs
3021 78th St.
P.O. Box 299
Norway, IA 52318
Toll free: 800-669-3275

Gaia Herbs
108 Island Ford Rd.
Brevard, NC 28712
Toll free: 800-831-7780

Herb Pharm
P.O. Box 116
Williams, OR 97544
Toll free: 800-348-4372
Fax: 541-846-6112

Herbalist and Alchemist
P.O. Box 553
Broadway, NJ 08808-0553
Phone: 908-689-9020
Toll free: 800-611-8235
Fax: 908-689-9071

Mediherb
Standard Process, Inc.
1200 West Royal Lee Dr.
PO Box 904
Palmyra, WI 53156-0904
Phone: 262-495-2122
Toll free: 800-848-5061 (USA)
Fax: 262-495-2512
www.standardprocess.com/mh_catalog_search.asp

Murdock Pharmaceuticals, Inc.
1400 Mountain Springs Park
Springville, UT 84663
Toll free: 800-962-8873

Northeast School of Botanical Medicine
P.O. Box 6626
Ithaca, NY 14851
Phone: 607-564-1023

Wise Woman Herbals
P.O. Box 279
Creswell, OR 97426
Phone: 541-895-5152
Fax: 541-895-5174

Chinese Herbs

Brion Corporation
9200 Jeronimo Rd.
Irvine, CA 92718
Toll free: 800-333-4372

Crane Enterprises—Jade Pharmacy
45 Samoset Ave., RFD #1
Plymouth, MA 02360
Toll free: 800-227-4118

East Coast Herbs Distributor
2525 South Mount Juliet Rd.
Mt. Juliet, TN 37122
Toll free: 800-283-5191

Eastern Currents Distributing Ltd.
#200A-3540 West 41st Ave.
Vancouver, British Columbia
Canada V6N 3E6

Golden Flower Chinese Herbs
P.O. Box 781
Placitas, NM 87043
Toll free: 800-729-8509

Health Concerns
8001 Capwell Dr.
Oakland, CA 94621
Toll free: 800-233-9355

Institute of Traditional Medicine
2017 SE Hawthorne
Portland, OR 97214
Phone: 503-233-4907

K'an Herb Company
6001 Butler Ln.
Scotts Valley, CA 95066
Toll free: 800-543-5233

KPCanada
492 Main St.
Winnipeg, Manitoba
Canada R3B 1B7
Toll free: 877-942-0950
Fax: 204-942-0405

Lotus Herbs
1124 N. Hacienda Blvd.
La Puente, CA 91744
Phone: 626-916-1070
Fax: 626-917-7763

MayWay Trading Company
1338 Cypress St.
Oakland, CA 94607
Phone: 510-208-3113

McZand Herbal, Inc.
P.O. Box 5312
Santa Monica, CA 90409
Toll free: 800-800-0405

Nuherbs Co.
3820 Penniman Ave.
Oakland, CA 94519
Toll free: 800-233-4307

Qualiherb
13340 E. Firestone Blvd., Suite N
Santa Fe Springs, CA 90670
Toll free: 800-533-9067

Spring Wind Herbs
2325 4th St., #6
Berkeley, CA 94710
Toll free: 800-588-4883

Ayurvedic

Ayush Herbs, Inc.
2115 112th NE
Bellevue, WA 98006
Phone: 206-637-1400
Fax: 206-451-2670
email: ayurveda@ayush.com

Index

C

H

I

Q

S

T

W